RENAL STONE DISEASE

RENAL STONE DISEASE

1st Annual International Urolithiasis Research Symposium

Indianapolis, Indiana 2 – 3 November 2006

EDITORS

Andrew P. Evan
Indiana University School of Medicine
Indianapolis, Indiana

James E. Lingeman
Methodist Hospital Institute for Kidney Stone Disease
Indianapolis, Indiana

James C. Williams, Jr.
Indiana University School of Medicine
Indianapolis, Indiana

All papers have been peer-reviewed

SPONSORING ORGANIZATION
International Kidney Stone Institute

AMERICAN INSTITUTE OF PHYSICS

Melville, New York, 2007

AIP CONFERENCE PROCEEDINGS ■ VOLUME 900

Editors:

Andrew P. Evan, Ph.D.
Department of Anatomy and Cell Biology
Indiana University School of Medicine
635 Barnhill Drive, MS 5035
Indianapolis, IN 46202-5120
United States

E-mail: evan@anatomy.iupui.edu

James E. Lingeman, M.D.
Methodist Hospital Institute for Kidney Stone Disease
1801 North Senate Boulevard
Suite 220
Indianapolis, IN 46207-7168

E-mail: jlingeman@clarian.org

James C. Williams, Jr., Ph.D.
Department of Anatomy and Cell Biology
Indiana University School of Medicine
635 Barnhill Drive, MS 5035
Indianapolis, IN 46202-5120
United States

E-mail: williams@anatomy.iupui.edu

L.C. Catalog Card No. 2007923523
ISBN 978-0-7354-0406-9
ISSN 0094-243X
Printed in the United States of America

Contents

III. INSIGHTS INTO HYPERCALCIURIA AND STONE DISEASE

IV. UPDATE OF CRYSTAL-CELL ATTACHMENT, PROTEIN INHIBITORS, AND URINARY DETERMINATES OF CRYSTALLIZATION

V. NEW TECHNOLOGIES FOR TREATING STONE DISEASE

VI. URETERAL PHYSIOLOGY AND STENTS

VII. SHOCK WAVE LITHOTRIPSY: MECHANISMS OF SHOCK WAVE ACTION AND STRATEGIES FOR IMPROVED SWL

VIII. OTHER TOPICS IN UROLITHIASIS RESEARCH

PREFACE

This is an exciting time in stone research. We are entering a new paradigm in which urolithiasis is seen not as a single entity but, rather, as a spectrum of stone diseases. Progress in recent years has opened our eyes to the possibility of multiple mechanisms for stone formation, and exciting findings now push us toward the inevitability that urinary calculi are the consequence of systemic disease. Indeed, at this point we do not know how many primary etiologies may exist for the retention and growth of stones in the urinary tract, but there is clearly more than one. As we face the prospect of multiple and complex etiologies, we need to prepare for the challenge that this brings.

It is into this unique time that the International Kidney Stone Institute has been born. The Institute, based here in Indianapolis, has as its mission the support of clinical and basic science research and education for the detection, management and prevention of kidney stone disease. The Institute was established in 2004, to guide research in stone disease and to channel resources toward projects that deliver positive results in stone disease treatment and prevention.

Recognizing recent advances that impact basic research and the clinical treatment of stone disease, the Institute was convinced that the time was right for a meeting to bring these two areas together. The First Annual Urolithiasis Research Symposium, held in Indianapolis in November of 2006, was a smashing success. We are pleased to bring the information presented at the Symposium together in this volume, which we believe will stand as a valuable reference for time to come.

We would like to express our appreciation to the researchers who joined us in Indianapolis to share their latest work and best thinking. We are also appreciative to the many attendees who contributed importantly to the meeting, participating in the stirring discussions that were stimulated by the presentations. Of course, a meeting of this quality could not occur without the substantial and dedicated efforts of the International Kidney Stone Institute staff, Katy Cantor, Katie Marlow, and Hillary McCarley, as well as the tireless efforts of Cathy Sprunger. We are also deeply appreciative for the support of the Methodist Health Foundation, of which the International Kidney Stone Institute is a component, and Clarian Health Partners for their support. Finally, this proceedings would not exist were it not for the tireless efforts of Dr. James Williams, who undertook the task to organize and execute this substantial body of work.

James E. Lingeman, M.D.
Andrew P. Evan, Ph.D.

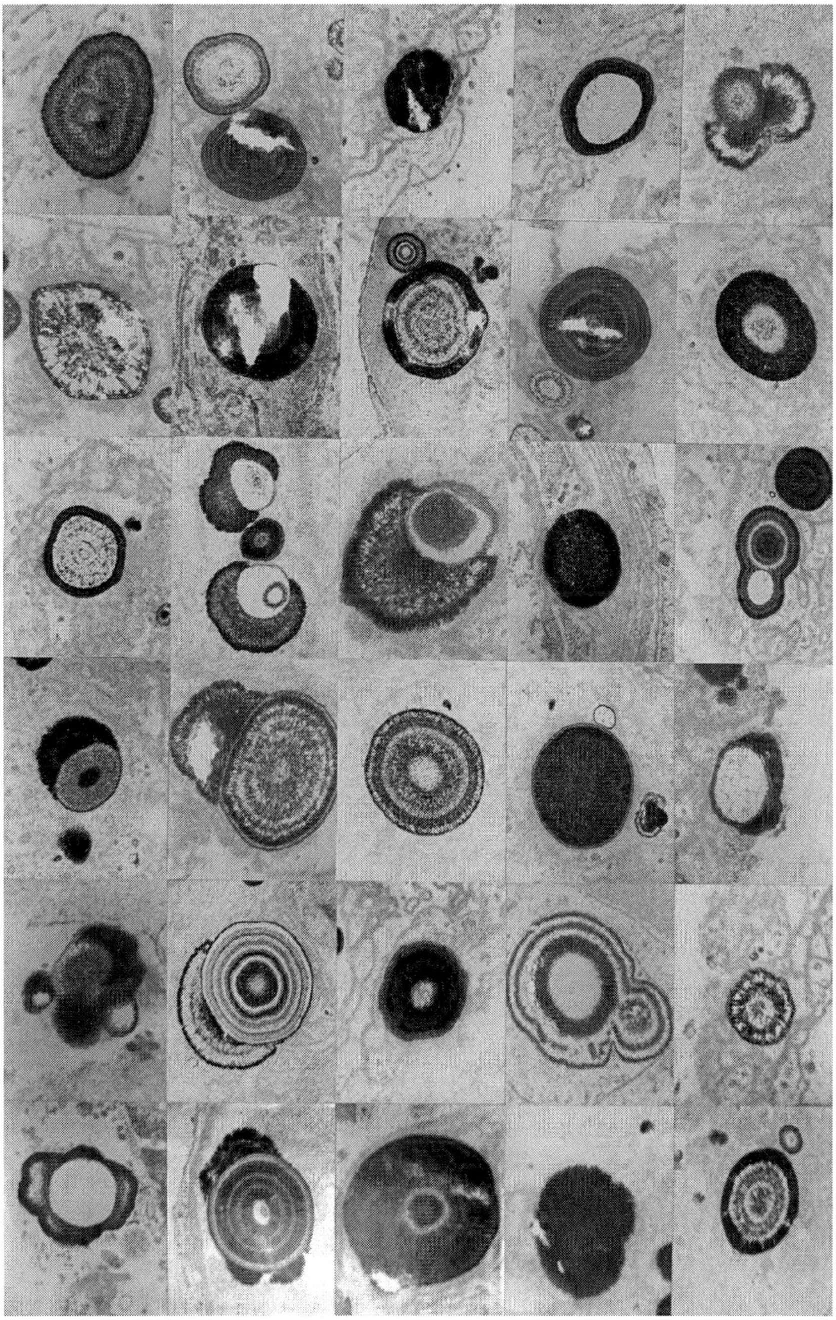

Cover image. Electron micrographs of particles of Randall's plaque, found in biopsies of kidneys from calcium oxalate stone formers. These are the earliest sites of mineralization found in the kidneys of idiopathic calcium oxalate stone formers, most commonly in the basement membranes of the thin limbs of Henle's loop. Sizes of the particles shown range from 0.05-0.4 μm in diameter. Image courtesy of A.P. Evan and Y. Shao.

THE INTERNATIONAL KIDNEY STONE INSTITUTE

The International Kidney Stone Institute (IKSI) is a charitable organization dedicated to supporting clinical and basic science research and education for the detection, management and prevention of kidney stone disease.

The Institute was established in 2004 by urologist James E. Lingeman, M.D. and kidney researcher Andrew P. Evan, Ph.D., to guide research in stone disease and to channel resources toward projects that deliver positive results in stone disease treatment and prevention. The International Kidney Stone Institute recognizes the accomplishments of kidney researchers and physicians who have:

- pioneered advances in minimally invasive treatments to clear stones from the body;
- dramatically refined the medical management of stone patients; and
- localized the site of stone formation in the kidney, a critical step toward developing strategies to prevent stones from forming.

Research initiatives of the International Kidney Stone Institute include:

- shock wave lithotripsy improvement
- studies in percutaneous kidney stone removal
- Randall's plaque and the prevention of stone disease
- dietary studies
- study of kidney stones in the bariatric population
- stone treatment and hypertension/bone disease

Education initiatives of the International Kidney Stone Institute include:

- Programs and conferences

  The International Kidney Stone Institute will host its 2nd International Urolithiasis Research Symposium on March 27-29, 2008, in Indianapolis.

  In addition, the Institute is developing educational programs and materials that will provide patients, medical care providers, school-age children and the general public with helpful information regarding kidney stone disease.

- Online atlas

  A Web-based reference and resource of images and clinical scenarios from representative stone patients is now in development and will enable researchers and physicians worldwide to explore diagnoses, clinical decision-making, treatment options and outcomes.

- Fellowships

  A two-year fellowship in stone disease and minimally invasive urology has been offered since 1990 by Methodist Hospital in affiliation with the Indiana University School of Medicine. The fellowship provides urologists who have completed their residency with an extensive clinical and basic science experience in all aspects of kidney stone disease. The fellowship is organized and approved by the Endourology Society.

INTERNATIONAL KIDNEY STONE INSTITUTE

Co-Directors

James Lingeman, M.D.
Andrew Evan, Ph.D.

Advisory Board Members

Drew Carey
Fredric Coe, M.D.
James Davis, D.D.
Daniel Evans, Jr.
Richard Hamilton, D.D.
Stephan Jay, M.D.
Bruce Kidd
Julia Lacy
L. Ben Lytle, *Ex Officio* Member
David Mann
Ron Meeusen
Daniel Newman, M.D.
Gary Schahet
Mark Sherman
Betty Stilwell
Morris Thomas, Jr.
Scott Willis
Gordon Wishard
Stephen Zinkan

IKSI Staff

Katy Cantor, Associate Vice President
Hillary McCarley, Development Officer

www.iksi.org

Mission Statement

The International Kidney Stone Institute (IKSI) is a charitable organization established to raise funds for clinical and basic science research, and education for the prevention, detection, and management of kidney stone disease. Further, it is the goal of the International Kidney Stone Institute to promote the highest standards of Urological clinical care.

SPONSORS FOR THE
1st ANNUAL INTERNATIONAL UROLITHIASIS
RESEARCH SYMPOSIUM

Platinum

Boston Scientific Corporation

Gold

Clarian Health Partners
Cook Urological, Inc.
Gyrus ACMI
Laser Peripherals/Clarus Medical
Methodist Health Foundation
National Institutes of Health (NIH)

Silver

Direx
Dornier MedTech
Litholink
Lumenis, Inc.
Richard Wolf Medical Instruments Corp.
Mission Pharmacal and Quest Diagnostics
Olympus Surgical America

Crystal

American Urological Association
HealthTronics, Inc.
Indiana University School of Medicine
Smith Barney

Corporate Donors

American Urological Association, Inc.
Clarian Health Partners, Inc.
CyberSonics, Inc.
Indiana University School of Medicine,
Department of Anatomy & Cell Biology
Methodist Health Foundation
Methodist Urology, LLC

Funding for this conference was made possible (in part) by grant R13 DK078503 from the National Institute of Diabetes and Digestive and Kidney Diseases (NIDDK). The views expressed in written conference materials or publications and by speakers and moderators do not necessarily reflect the official policies of the Department of Health and Human Services; nor does mention of trade names, commercial practices, or organizations imply endorsement by the U.S. Government.

1st Annual International Urolithiasis Research Symposium

Organizing Committee

Andrew P. Evan, PhD.
James E. Lingeman, M.D.
Fredric L. Coe, M.D.
John R. Asplin, M.D.
Elaine M. Worcester, M.D.
James A. McAteer, Ph.D.
James C. Williams, Jr., Ph.D.
Philip M. Blomgren

With special thanks to:
Katy Cantor
Katie Marlow
Hillary McCarley
and
Cathy Sprunger

Sponsoring organization:
The International Kidney Stone Institute
P.O. Box 7168
Indianapolis, IN 46207-7168
(317) 962-9043
www.iksi.org

1st Annual International Urolithiasis Research Symposium

The Westin Hotel, Indianapolis, Indiana

Thursday, November 2, 2006

7:30-7:45 a.m.	Stone disease: a prelude	Fredric L. Coe, M.D. *Chicago, Illinois*
Session 1	**Specific links of stone disease to other systemic disorders** Moderators: Fredric L. Coe, M.D., *Chicago, Illinois* Dawn S. Milliner, M.D., *Rochester, Minnesota*	
7:45-8:00 a.m.	Changes in renal function and blood pressure	Elaine M. Worcester, M.D. *Chicago, Illinois*
8:10-8:25 a.m.	Urinary pH as a risk factor for stone type	Khashayar Sakhaee, M.D. *Dallas, Texas*
8:35-8:50 a.m.	Stone disease as consequence of bariatric surgery	John R. Asplin, M.D. *Chicago, Illinois*
9:00-9:15 a.m.	Disorders of PTH	Philippe Jaeger, M.D. *Nice, France*
9:25-9:40 p.m.	What insights can epidemiology offer to understanding systemic disorders and stone disease?	Gary C. Curhan, M.D. *Boston, Massachusetts*
9:50-10:05 a.m.	Links between stone disease and bone disease	David A. Bushinsky, M.D. *Rochester, New York*
Session 2	**New technologies in stone disease** Moderators: James E. Lingeman, M.D., *Indianapolis, Indiana* Gerhard J. Fuchs, M.D., *Los Angeles, California*	
10:35-10:50 a.m.	Improvements in intracorporeal lithotriptors: the Cyberwand	Ramsay L. Kuo, M.D. *Indianapolis, Indiana*
11:00-11:15 a.m.	Lasers – Erbium laser	Joel M.H. Teichman, M.D. *Vancouver, British Columbia*
11:25-11:40 a.m.	Lasers – Holmium pulse width	Demetrius H. Bagley, M.D. *Philadelphia, Pennsylvania*
11:50-12:05 p.m.	Perc access: renal structural and functional changes in a porcine model	Rajash K. Handa, Ph.D. *Indianapolis, Indiana*
Session 3	**Insights into hypercalciuria and stone disease** Moderators: Andrew P. Evan, Ph.D., *Indianapolis, Indiana* Michael E. Moran, M.D., *Albany, New York*	
1:30-1:45 p.m.	Mechanisms for hypercalciuria: human studies	Fredric L. Coe, M.D. *Chicago, Illinois*
1:55-2:10 p.m.	Adenylyl cyclase in hypercalciuria: link to stone disease	Orson W. Moe, M.D. *Dallas, Texas*
2:20-2:35 p.m.	Improving future knockout models for hypercalciuric stone disease: what new clinical data are needed?	Rene Bindels, Ph.D. *Nijmegen, Netherlands*
2:45-3:00 p.m.	Hypercalciuria: the role of genes	Giovanni Gambaro, M.D. *Verona, Italy*

Session 4 — **Ureteral physiology and stents**

Moderators: Stephen Y. Nakada, M.D., *Madison, Wisconsin*
John D.A. Honey, M.D., *Toronto, Ontario*

3:30-3:45 p.m.	The role of ureteral peristalsis in stone passage	Francis X. Keeley, M.D. *Bristol, United Kingdom*
3:55-4:10 p.m.	The role of adrenergic receptor blockade in medical expulsive stone therapy: a molecular analysis	Erdal Erturk, M.D. *Rochester, New York*
4:20-4:35 p.m.	Role of pharmacology in ureteral physiology and expulsive therapy	Travis J. Jerde, Ph.D. *Madison, Wisconsin*
4:45-5:00 p.m.	Novel stent designs	John D. Denstedt, M.D. *London, Ontario*
5:10-5:25 p.m.	Everting ureteral access sheath	Marshall L. Stoller, M.D. *San Francisco, California*

6:30-8:30 p.m. Reception/Poster Session

Friday, November 3, 2006

Session 5 — **Randall's plaque as a mechanism of stone formation**

Moderators: Glenn M. Preminger, M.D., *Durham, North Carolina*
Filiberto Zattoni, M.D., *Verona, Italy*

7:30-7:45 a.m.	Histopathology predicts the mechanism of stone formation	Andrew P. Evan, Ph.D. *Indianapolis, Indiana*
7:55-8:10 a.m.	Stone morphology suggestive of Randall's plaque	Michel Daudon, Ph.D. *Paris, France*
8:20-8:35 a.m.	CaOx stones in IH patients are fixed to plaque	Brian R. Matlaga, M.D. *Baltimore, Maryland*
8:45-9:00 a.m.	Molecular biology of the renal interstitium in stone formation	Matthew D. Breyer, Ph.D. *Nashville, Tennessee*
9:10-9:25 a.m.	Interstitial hyaluronan and stone formation	Carl F. Verkoelen, Ph.D. *Rotterdam, Netherlands*
9:35-9:50 a.m.	The role of the papillary epithelium in stone growth	Kristen Bergsland, Ph.D. *Chicago, Illinois*

Session 6 — **Update of crystal-cell attachment, protein inhibitors, and urinary determinates of crystallization**

Moderators: Dean G. Assimos, M.D., *Winston-Salem, North Carolina*
Marguerite Hatch, Ph.D., *Gainesville, Florida*

10:20-10:35 a.m.	Macromolecules relevant to stone formation	Rosemary Ryall, Ph.D. *Adelaide, Australia*
10:45-11:00 a.m.	Pathogenesis of hyperoxaluria in mutant mice lacking the anion transporter Slc26a6	Peter Aronson, M.D. *New Haven, Connecticut*
11:10-11:25 a.m.	Oxalate transporters in the kidney and gut	David Mount, Ph.D. *Boston, Massachusetts*
11:35-11:50 a.m.	Lessons in stone formation and growth from an *in vitro* stone farm	John Kavanagh, Ph.D. *Manchester, England*
12:00-12:15 p.m..	The phosphatonins in disorders of mineral homeostasis	Rajiv Kumar, M.D. *Rochester, Minnesota*
12:25-12:40 p.m.	Urinary oxalate: where does it come from?	Ross P. Holmes, Ph.D. *Winston-Salem, North Carolina*
12:50-1:05 p.m.	JESS: What can it teach us about stone disease?	Allen L. Rodgers , Ph.D. *Cape Town, South Africa*

Session 7 **Shock wave lithotripsy: mechanisms of shock wave action and strategies for improved SWL**

Moderators: Christian G. Chaussy, M.D., *Munich, Germany*
Michael R. Bailey, Ph.D., *Seattle, Washington*

2:00-2:15 p.m.	Shock wave trauma to the kidney: an overview of acute and chronic effects	James A. McAteer, Ph.D. *Indianapolis, Indiana*
2:25-2:40 p.m.	Is diabetes a consequence of SWL?	Amy E. Krambeck, M.D. *Rochester, Minnesota*
2:50-3:00 p.m.	LESS — Long-term effects of shockwaves study	Thomas Knoll, M.D. *Mannheim, Germany*
3:10-3:25 p.m.	The acoustics of lithotripsy	Robin O. Cleveland, Ph.D. *Boston, Massachusetts*
3:35-3:50 p.m.	Innovations in lithotripsy technology	Pei Zhong, M.D. *Durham, North Carolina*
4:20-4:35 p.m.	Improving outcomes with the equipment at hand: the advantage of slower SW rate	Kenneth T. Pace, M.D. *Toronto, Ontario*
4:45-5:00 p.m.	Using helical CT to assess stone fragility at diagnosis	James C. Williams, Ph.D. *Indianapolis, Indiana*
5:10-5:25 p.m.	The future of shock wave lithotripsy: a global perspective	Uwe Köhrmann, M.D. *Mannheim, Germany*
5:35-5:55 p.m.	Stone disease: a postlude	Fredric L. Coe, M.D. *Chicago, Illinois*
5:55-6:15 p.m.	Discussion	
6:15 p.m.	Adjourn	

PROLOGUE

Introduction: Kidney Stone Research, Lessons From Human Studies

Fredric L. Coe

Department of Medicine, Nephrology Section, University of Chicago, Renal Section MC 5100
5841 S. Maryland Ave.Chicago, IL, 60637, USA

Abstract. About 5% of American women and 12% of men will develop a kidney stone at some time in their life, the prevalence has been rising in both sexes. Approximately 80% of stones are composed of calcium oxalate, and calcium phosphate; 10% of struvite; 9% of uric acid; and the remaining 1% are composed of cystine or ammonium acid urate or are diagnosed as drug-related stone. Stones ultimately arise because of an unwanted phase change of these substances from liquid to solid state. In this introduction, I have outlined our current thinking of the possible mechanisms involved in stone formation based on our biopsy data collected from a series of human kidney stone formers. In addition, I have presented a set of questions as a means of focusing future research in this field.

Keywords: kidney biopsy, kidney anatomy, renal injury, histopathology, kidney stones
PACS: 01.30.Ce; 87-19.Xx

SITES OF RANDALL'S PLAQUE IN IDIOPATHIC CALCIUM STONE FORMERS (ICSF)

We have had the good fortune, and privilege, to inspect human tissues obtained at stone surgery, and it seems to me an obligation to go further and point out open questions raised by what the tissues show. In particular I will focus on questions raised by interstitial—so called Randall's—plaque, apatite deposits that plug inner medullary collecting ducts (IMCD) in certain kinds of stone formers (SF), and the high urine pH of patients with calcium phosphate stones. All three human phenomena would benefit greatly from basic science studies to determine mechanisms, and consequences of what, in humans, we can mainly observe.

Everyone has seen these pictures. Interstitial plaque begins in the basement membranes of thin loops of Henle, where it appears as black dots with Yasue stain under light microscopy (Fig. 1a) and as laminated micro-spherules of crystal, white in this TEM (Fig. 1b), alternating with organic matrix (black) that contains osteopontin [1, 2]. From there it appears to spread into the interstitial compartment (Fig. 1c), where particles fuse into a syncytium in which islands of white crystal float in a black organic sea. Eventually the plaque makes its way into the deep papillum (Fig. 1d) and appears, to the surgeon, as white material (Fig. 1e) just under the papillary epithelium.

CP900, *Renal Stone Disease, 1st Annual International Urolithiasis Research Symposium,*
edited by A. P. Evan, J. E. Lingeman, and J. C. Williams, Jr.

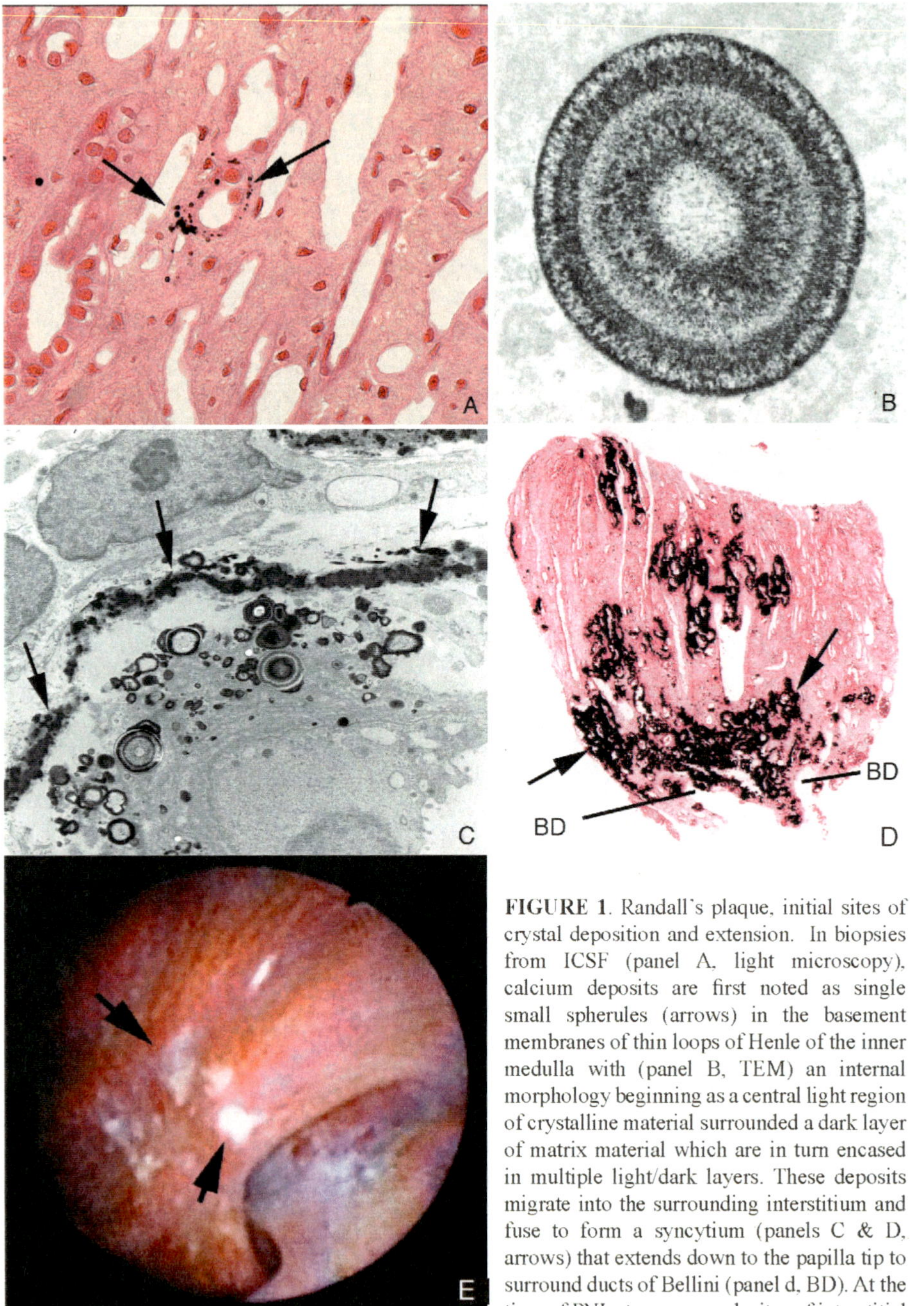

FIGURE 1. Randall's plaque, initial sites of crystal deposition and extension. In biopsies from ICSF (panel A, light microscopy), calcium deposits are first noted as single small spherules (arrows) in the basement membranes of thin loops of Henle of the inner medulla with (panel B, TEM) an internal morphology beginning as a central light region of crystalline material surrounded a dark layer of matrix material which are in turn encased in multiple light/dark layers. These deposits migrate into the surrounding interstitium and fuse to form a syncytium (panels C & D, arrows) that extends down to the papilla tip to surround ducts of Bellini (panel d, BD). At the time of PNL stone removal, sites of interstitial plaque are visualized through an endoscope as whitish, irregular regions (arrows) usually at the papilla tip (panel E). Panels A, D & E from [1] and panel B from [2]; used with permission.

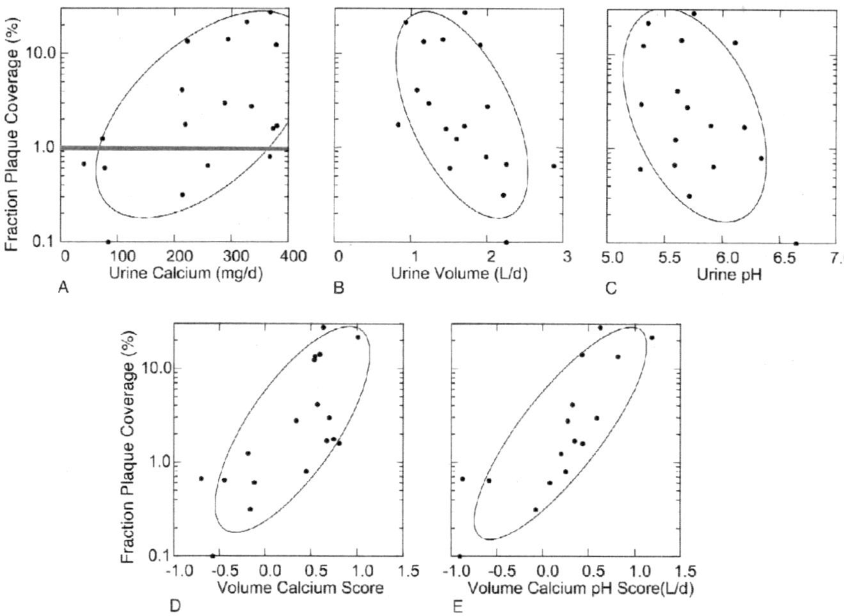

FIGURE 2: Urine correlates of Randall's plaque. Fractional plaque coverage per papillum varies inversely with urine volume (panel a) among stone formers (closed circle, above red line) and non-stone forming control subjects (open circles, below red line). Plaque coverage varies with urine calcium excretion (panel b) and in inverse to urine pH (panel c). A composite multivariate regression score using volume and calcium excretion (panel d) and one that includes urine pH as well (panel e) strongly correlates with plaque coverage. Figure from [3]; used with permission

Although plaque is present in normal people, it covers less than 1% of the renal papillum (Fig. 2a), points below the red line) [3]. Idiopathic calcium oxalate stone formers (ICSF), range up to 10 and even 20% coverage (Fig. 2a, points above red line). The percent of coverage rises with urine calcium, and falls with urine volume and pH (Fig. 2b-e). So plaque, like hypercalciuria itself, is present in normals but exaggerated greatly in ICSF.

Pertinent Research Questions Concerning Plaque

I have taken the liberty of listing some research issues related to plaque.

1. How does it form in thin limb basement membranes?
2. What is its matrix composed of, and where is it made?
3. Will plaque particles form in cultured cell systems?
4. Does plaque affect renal interstitial cells?
   Are there markers in human tissue to show such an effect?
   Is maximum urine osmolality affected?
   Can we look for interactions between coated apatite and interstitial cells in culture?

5. Is plaque an example of bone formation in the kidney?
6. Is plaque related to the documented higher blood pressure of stone formers?
7. Is plaque related to the increased loss of renal function in stone formers with age?
8. How can urine calcium, volume and pH affect plaque abundance?
9. Can one produce an animal model of human renal apatite plaque?
   -That model would have to have interstitial apatite plaque.
   -No crystals would be found in the epithelial cell compartment.
   -Has to be related to hypercalciuria, and inverse to urine pH and volume.
10. Can we quantitate plaque radiographically?
   These are by no means all of the questions that one could ask but are the ones that have occurred to me.

STONES IN ICSF ARE ATTACHED TO PAPILLUM

If you look at a calcium oxalate stone attached to a human papillum, you can see white plaque peeking around its edges (Fig. 3a). Remove the stone and the white plaque underpinning is clear (Fig. 3b). The mass of stones (Fig. 3c) resides on white

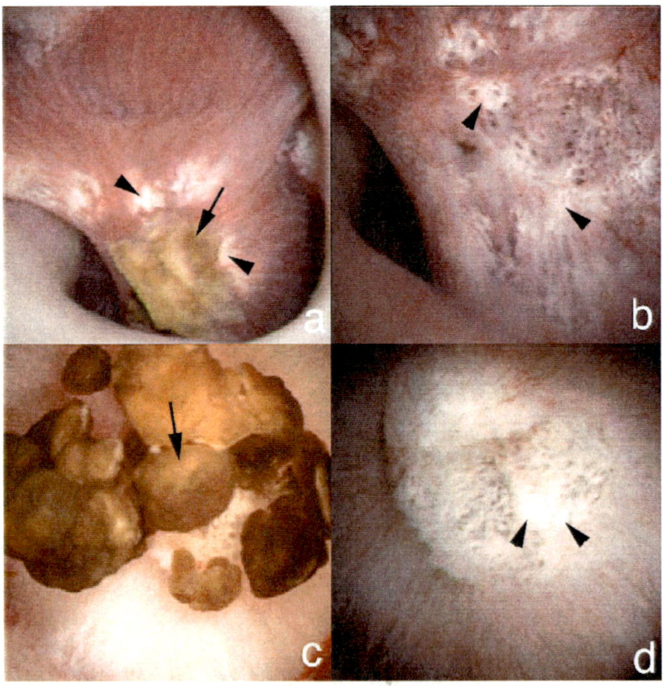

FIGURE 3: Two examples of attached stones to sites of Randall's plaque. In panel **a** a single stone (arrow) and in panel **c** multiple stones are seen attached to the tip of a renal papilla. Note the areas of white plaque (arrowheads) at the margins of these attached stones. After the stones were detached, plaque (arrowheads) was clearly seen at sites beneath and at the sides of the stones.

plaque you can see under them and especially well when they are removed (Fig. 3d). These pictures show that CaOx stones can grow on plaque [4]. Others at this meeting will present statistical data showing that attachment to plaque is the usual occurrence.

Pertinent Research Questions Concerning Stone-Plaque Junction

There are many research issues related to the stone-plaque junction.

1. How is the epithelial barrier breached?
   -Do urine ions pass through intact papillary epithelium and crystallize on plaque?
   -Does plaque affect the papillary epithelium so that there is apoptosis with erosion?
   -Does it signal cells to separate?
2. Can overgrowth from urine on coated crystals be modeled in the laboratory so that one can look at effects of different coating proteins that are interstitially derived?
   -Look at the urine from stone formers vs. normals.
   -Look at effects of individual urine macromolecules.
   -Determine whether inhibition measurements reflect effects on overgrowth such as crystal growth inhibition, upper limit of metastability or aggregation.
3. What is the matrix on stones at the attachment site?
4. Can animal models of attached stones (on apatite plaque) be produced?

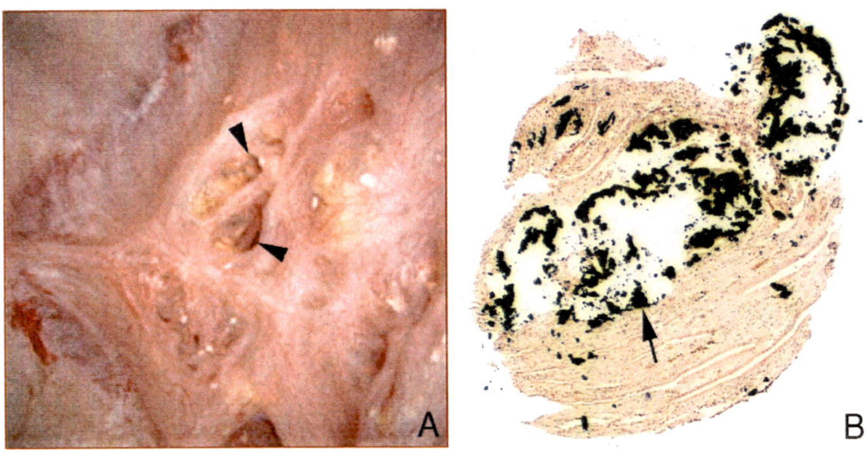

FIGURE 4: Endoscopic and histological images from brushite SF. Panel A shows an endoscopic view of a malformed papilla characterized by flattened appearance and numerous depressions (arrowheads) that represent dilated openings of ducts of Bellini lined by varying amount of yellowish crystal deposits. Few sites of Randall's plaque are noted. Histological examination of such a papilla (panel B) reveals greatly dilated ducts of Bellini and inner medullary collecting ducts (arrow) filled with hydroxyapatite crystals. Figure from [5]; used with permission.

STONE FORMERS WITH APATITE PLUGGING OF IMCD

Patients who form brushite stones [5], or who form apatite stones because of distal renal tubular acidosis [6], or patients with calcium oxalate stones due to obesity bypass procedures [1] plug IMCD with apatite deposits that can reach immense proportions, and lead to total destruction of the epithelial cells. Whereas in over 3000 serial sections from 32 ICSF we have never found a single crystal in the epithelial cell compartment, in these aforementioned specialized populations we find prominent deposits, always of biological apatite. In this patient, the effects have led to gross papillary deformity, a not uncommon outcome. The large mouth of a malformed papillum (Fig. 4a) shows crystals blocking it. In Fig. 4b one sees a duct of Bellini enlarged twenty-fold, filled with crystals and there are no viable epithelial cells.

Phosphate stones have been increasing during the past three decades in women (Fig. 5, closed symbols) and men; these data are from my own clinic [7]; Mandel [8] has published similarly from his extensive VA experience. So the histopathology I just showed you must be becoming more common.

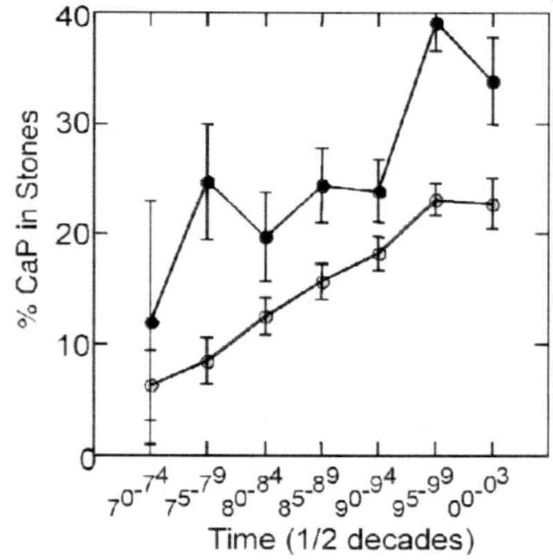

FIGURE 5: Change in stone calcium phosphate (CaP) over three decades. Mean values for stone CaP% are plotted against the time period (half decade) of the stone analysis. For stones from females (closed circles) and males (open circles) alike. CaP% in stones rose between 1970 and 2003. Females were higher throughout. The increases for both sexes over time were significant using analysis of variance with post-hoc contrasts as was the higher female CaP%. Figure from [7]; used with permission.

Urine supersaturation with respect to brushite faithfully mirrors stone composition in rising progressively (Fig. 6a, y axis) with the percent of calcium phosphate in stones (x axis). This increase is driven mostly by increasing urine pH (Fig. 6b). See how the urine pH rises from 5.9 in a group of patients with hardly any CaP in their stones to reach astronomical levels of 6.2 to 6.3 in patients with increasing amounts of CaP in their stones. Partly, the CaP stone is worse in hypercalciuria (Fig. 6c). This is particularly true in women and men up to the 50-70% CaP in stones point. Thereafter, urine calcium in men remains high and in women is actually going down. So this is an irregular relationship. Urine volume (Fig. 6d), phosphate excretion (Fig. 6e), and citrate

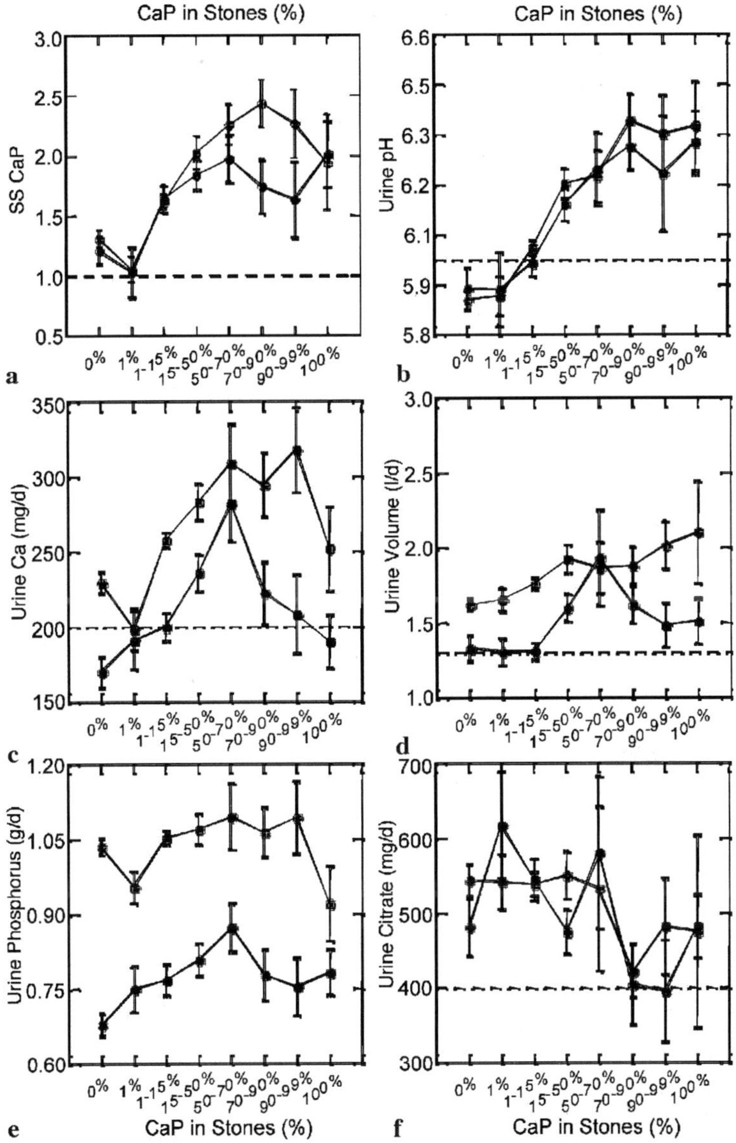

FIGURE 6: Urine stone risk factors with increasing stone CaP%. As expected, CaP supersaturation (SS) rose with stone CaP% (panel **b**, y and x axis respectively) among men (gray circles) and women (black circles, values are mean ± SEM)). Urine pH rose progressively (panel **b**), which would increase CaP SS. Urine calcium excretion (panel **c**) rose to a plateau in men., but rose and fell in women. Urine volumes were higher at high CaP% values in both sexes (panel **d**). Urine phosphorous excretion was variable with no specific pattern (panel **e**). Urine citrate excretion was lowest when CaP% was highest (panel **f**), but SEM values were very wide and generally overlapping and no significant trend could be proven. Figure from [7]; used with permission.

excretion (Fig. 6f) are poorly correlated at best. Unlike the mysteries of apatite plaque and overgrowth on plaque, formation of apatite deposits in IMCD and formation of CaP stones themselves seems reasonably straightforward: Urine pH is too high, and tubule fluid pH is too high in IMCD, calcium phosphate supersaturation is increased, and crystals form. The unsolved problems concern why the pH is high, and the details of apatite effects on IMCD cells.

Some Research Issues Related To IMCD Plugging

IMCD plugging like phosphate stone formation really leads to a group of related questions

1. Do apatite crystals affect proton secretion by IMCD cells?
2. Do apatite crystals affect ammonia transporters in IMCD cells?
3. Do apatite crystals affect paracellular proton movement in IMCD cells?
4. Is urine pH high in some CaOx SF who later convert to CaP stones?
5. Is there a familial tendency to high urine pH (not the rare dRTA)?
6. What are the pathways to IMCD cell injury by biological apatite?
   -Can we study it with plain (uncoated) apatite in cultured cells, with coated crystals (probably with urine proteins)?
   -Can we study the mechanisms of attachment?
7. Can one find urine markers of IMCD cell injury early detection?
8. Why is CaP stone prevalence increasing?
   -Is it shock wave lithotripsy treatment?
   -Is it related to a greater use of potassium citrate salts?
9. Can IMCD and BD plugging be distinguished from plaque radiographically?
10. Can we obtain an animal model of IMCD and BD apatite plugging?

TABLE 1. Summary of stone phenotypes thus far

Phenotype	Stones	Interstitium	IMCD BD
ICSF	CaOx	Heavy Plaque	Nothing
Obesity Bypass	CaOx	No Plaque	Apatite Plugs
CaP SF	Brushite	Plaque	Apatite Plugs
	Apatite	Plaque	Apatite Plugs
dRTA	Apatite	Normal Plaque	Apatite Plugs
Cystinuria	Cystine	Normal Plaque	Apatite & Cystine Plugs

SUMMARY

I would like to summarize the findings from the human biopsies in a more compact form showing the phenotype, the type of stones, what is forming in IMCD and ducts of Bellini (Table 1). ICSF have CaOx stones, of course, heavy plaque and nothing in the epithelial compartment. Obesity bypass patients form CaOx stones; they have no plaque (i.e. below what one finds in normal people) and apatite plugging in IMCD. Calcium phosphate stone formers with brushite stones have plaque above normal and apatite plugging of IMCD and ducts of Bellini Apatite stone formers have plaque in modest abundance above normal and apatite plugging. Distal renal tubular acidosis (dRTA) patients form apatite stones; they have no more plaque than that of normal people and have apatite plugging. Patients with cystinuria form cystine stones; they have normal amounts of plaque (i.e. as in normals) and they have apatite and cystine plugs in their IMCD and ducts of Bellini.

This is what we have found and we offer it as a kind of contribution to world research in stone disease. It is not that we have been the least bit original here, we have simply made biopsies and observed what nature has done and we offer these findings for your interest and consideration.

ACKNOWLEDGMENTS

This study was supported by a grant from the NIH (PO1 DK 56788).

REFERENCES

1. A.P. Evan, J.E. Lingeman, F.L. Coe, J.H. Parks, S.B. Bledsoe, Y. Shao, A.J. Sommer, R.F. Paterson, R.L. Kuo and M. Grynpas *JCI* **111**, 607-616 (2003).
2. A.P. Evan, F.L. Coe, S.R. Ritting, S.M. Bledsoe, Y. Shao, J.E. Lingeman and E.M. Worcester *Kidney Intl* **68**, 145-154 (2005).
3. R.L. Kuo, J.E. Lingeman, A.P. Evan, R.F. Paterson, J.H. Parks, S.B. Bledsoe,L.C. Munch and F.L. Coe *Kidney Intl* **64**, 2150-2154 (2003).
4. B.r. Matlaga, J.C. Williams, Jr., S.C. Kim, R.L. Kuo, A.P. Evan, S.B.Bledsoe, F.L. Coe, E.M. Worcesster, L.C. Munch and J.E. Lingeman *J Urol* **175,** 1720-1724 (2006).
5. A.P. Evan, J.E. Lingeman, F.L. Coe, Y. Shao, J.H. Parks, S.B. Bledsoe, C.L. Phillips, S. Bonsib, E.M.Worcester, A.J. Sommer, S.C. Kim, W.W. Tinmouth and M. Grynpas *Kidney Intl* **67,** 576-591 (2005).
6. A.P. Evan, J.E. Lingeman, F.L. Coe, Y. Shao, N. Miller, B. Matlaga, C. Phillips, A. Sommer and E. Worcester *Kidney Intl* (In Press).
7. J.H. Parks, E.M. Worcester, F.L. Coe, A.P. Evan and J.E. Lingeman *Kidney Intl* **66,** 777-785 (2004).
8. N.S. Mandel and G.S. Mandel *J Urol* **142,** 1516-1521 (1989).

I. RANDALL'S PLAQUE AS A MECHANISM OF STONE FORMATION

Histopathology Predicts the Mechanism of Stone Formation

Andrew P. Evan

Department of Anatomy and Cell Biology, Indiana University School of Medicine, Indianapolis, IN 46202-5120, USA

Abstract. About 5% of American women and 12% of men will develop a kidney stone at some time in their life and these numbers appear to be on the rise. Despite years of scientific research into the mechanisms of stone formation and growth, limited advances have been made until recently. Randall's original observations and thoughts on the mechanisms for kidney stone formation have been validated for idiopathic calcium oxalate stone formers (ICSF) but not for most other stone forming groups. Our current studies on selected groups of human stone formers using intraoperative papillary biopsies has shown overwhelming evidence for the presence of Randall's plaque in ICSF and that stone formation and growth are exclusively linked to its availability to urinary ions and proteins. Intense investigation of the plaque-stone junction is needed if we are to understand the factors leading to the overgrowth process on exposed regions of plaque. Such information should allow the development of treatment strategies to block stone formation in ICSF patients. Patients who form brushite stones, or who form apatite stones because of distal renal tubular acidosis (dRTA), or patients with calcium oxalate stones due to obesity bypass procedures, or patients with cystinuria, get plugged inner medullary collecting ducts (IMCD) which leads to total destruction of the lining cells and focal sites of interstitial fibrosis. These stone formers have plaque but at levels equal to or below non-stone formers, which would suggest that they form stones by a different mechanism than do ICSF patients.

Keywords: kidney stones, Randall's plaque, papilla biopsies
PACS: 01.30.Cc; 87-19.Xx

INTRODUCTION

There may be many types of stone disease, each requiring a specific plan of medical management. The idea that different types of stones are formed in different ways, and that the complications that develop in one group of patients may be different from those of others, is a new concept. Little attention has been paid to how stones are formed in each of the different groups of stone formers, whether stone formation involves pathological changes in the kidney, and if there are specific systemic effects associated with the development of stones of a given type. If "stone disease" is really many separate, distinct stone diseases, then the best medical management for a given patient needs to be tailored to his specific disease, and to treat not just the kidney, but solve the systemic complications as well. Our goal is to characterize the various types of stone disease in order to understand their specific renal abnormalities and systemic complications, so that treatment can be targeted specifically and effectively.

CP900, *Renal Stone Disease, 1st Annual International Urolithiasis Research Symposium,*
edited by A. P. Evan, J. E. Lingeman, and J. C. Williams, Jr.

THEORIES OF STONE FORMATION AND GROWTH

Fixed and Free Particle Theories

Three theories of stone formation and growth are currently being investigated. The "Free Particle" concept suggests that crystal nuclei form by homogenous nucleation in the lumen of the nephron under conditions of a phase change (due to increasing supersaturation) in the dissolved salts present in the ultrafiltrate. The theory then states that these nuclei would have to grow to sufficient size to eventually lodge in the lumen of the distal nephron resulting in tubular obstruction. The second theory is termed the "Fixed Particle" model. Like the "Free Particle" model, crystal nuclei also form in the lumen of the nephron, but these crystals then adhere to the apical surface of the tubular epithelium. While a number of mechanisms have been proposed to model this crystal-cell attachment step, the most commonly cited model requires renal cell injury, probably as a result of high tubular oxalate levels. Once the crystal-cell attachment step has occurred, the crystal nuclei would be fixed in position and exposed to the potentially supersaturated ultrafiltrate that would facilitate further growth of these crystals. Clearly both of these theories could result in plugging of the nephron and lead to intratubular calcification, termed tubular nephrocalcinosis. Randall in his historic paper in 1940 described such findings of intraluminal calcification (papillary lesion type II) or nephrocalcinosis in only 23 cases and compared it to the more common finding (204 cases) of interstitial plaque (papillary lesion type I) and placed the type II lesion in a different category than type I [1]. We have shown that patients who form brushite stones [2], or who form apatite stones because of distal renal tubular acidosis (dRTA) [3] or patients with calcium oxalate stones due to obesity bypass procedures [4] or patients with cystinuria [5], plug (tubular nephrocalcinosis) their inner medullary collecting ducts (IMCD) which leads to total destruction of the lining cells and focal sites of interstitial fibrosis. However, it is unclear how the "Free or Fixed Particle" theories could lead to clinical stone formation (i.e. a stone in the renal pelvis large enough to obstruct the ureter) in such stone forming patients, except that either the "Free or Fixed Particle" process or both are occurring in the renal pelvis independent of events in the tubular lumen.

Randall's Plaque Theory

The third theory suggests that crystals in the urine can become attached to a site of exposed crystalline deposits of interstitial calcium phosphate (termed Randall's plaque) following loss of the normal epithelial covering of the renal papilla. An anchored nidus of urinary crystals could form as an overgrowth on the interstitial plaque, permitting a fixed stone to form and potentially grow over many years. This theory is explicit in stating that sites of interstitial plaque are the initiating lesion. Alexander Randall presented his data and theory over six decades ago after examining 1,154 pairs of cadaveric kidneys [1]. After carefully opening the renal pelvis of a kidney, he examined each papilla visually and with a hand lens. His first twenty-seven kidneys were normal in appearance. However, the next kidney revealed an "innocent" appearing lesion that was a cream-colored area near the papillary tip and appeared to be subsurface or subepithelial in location. This lesion was seen in 20.5% of all the kidneys he studied. By light microscopy, the lesion was found to be a plaque of calcium salts deposited in the interstitial tissue and definitely not intraluminal in location. Evidence of inflammation was rarely found. The deposits were localized initially to interstitial collagen material and tubular basement membranes. Subsequently the deposits appeared to fill much of the intertubular space. Chemical analysis of the regions of plaque showed calcium, nitrogen, carbon dioxide and phosphorus. His next major observation was finding a small stone (2 mm) that projected into the lumen of the renal pelvis. It was firmly attached to an area of visible calcium plaque and found to be composed of calcium phosphate. Such stones were found attached to papillae in 65 kidneys. Randall was able to study several stones still attached to the papillary wall and concluded from these studies that 1) attached stones are growing from and are supported by interstitial calcium plaque, 2) the sites of interstitial plaque can lose their epithelial cell covering allowing the plaque to be exposed to the calyceal urine, and 3) that some detached stones have a concave surface with patches of phosphate material (possibly representing the attachment site to the interstitial plaque). Fig. 1 shows an attached stone we have observed in our human studies. This attached stone is probably very similar to what Randall observed. Note that the stone has a concave surface that faced the papilla with a projection of mineral (probably calcium phosphate) and a convex smooth surface that faced the urinary space just like Randall's description. More recent studies of Cifuentes-Delatte [6] and Daudon and colleagues (7, a paper in this proceedings) have also observed a "footprint" of the papilla as a depressed zone ("umbilication") on the concave surface of the stone which corresponds to the shape of the tip of the papilla and this concave surface contains mineral detached from interstitial plaque. These findings give support to Randall's observations and ideas. The observations Randall made from 1,154 pairs of post-mortem kidneys were earth-shattering in their importance and originality. However, what Randall was not able to determine, because of the techniques available to him in the 1930's, was the composition of the mineral in the plaque, the type of crystalline material that formed right at the site of overgrowth, and the transition of mineral type (i.e. calcium oxalate, uric acid, calcium phosphate) from the site of attachment into the body of the stone.

RANDALL'S PLAQUE IS UNIQUE TO IDIOPATHIC CALCIUM OXALATE STONE FORMERS (ICSF)

Our group set out to test the hypothesis that regions of Randall's plaque develop in unique anatomical sites of the kidney, and that their formation is conditioned by specific stone-forming pathophysiologies. To test this hypothesis, we employed state-of-the-art digital endoscopic equipment during percutaneous nephrolithotomy (PNL) for stone removal. We chose to study ICSF patients as our primary group of stone formers in that they represent about 75% of all stone formers [4]. This protocol allowed us to

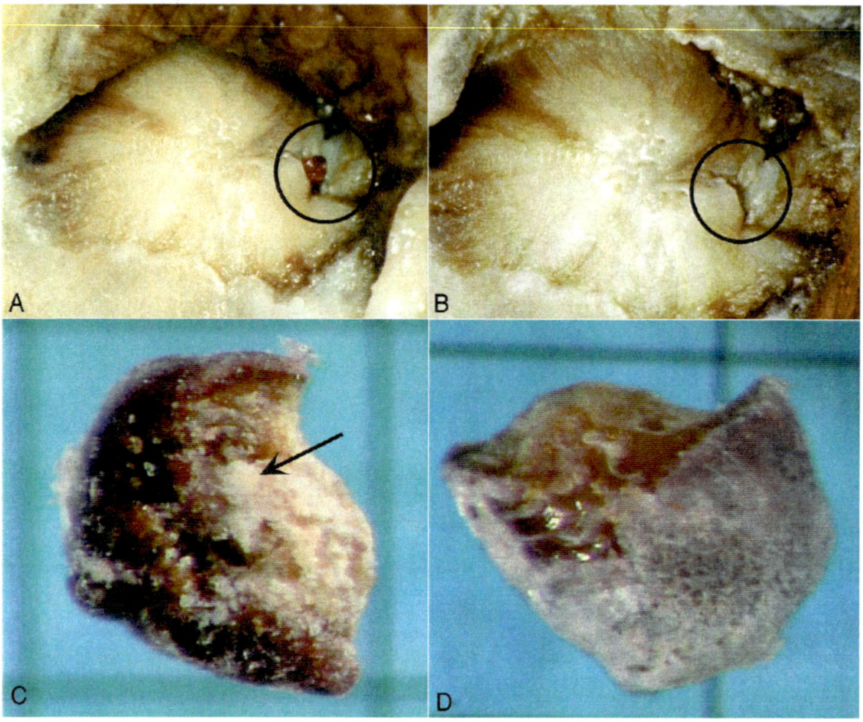

FIGURE 1. Light microscopy photomicrographs of a papilla from a ICSF patient. In panel **A**, a single stone (within circle) is seen fixed to the side of this papilla. After the stone has been detached (panel **B**), an area of plaque (within circle) is visible at the site of stone attachment. This stone has an irregular concave surface (panel **C**) that faced the papilla and a stock or umbilicus (arrow). The opposite side of the stone was convex and smooth (panel **D**).

obtain digital images of all papillae for plaque surface determinations and permitted us to obtain papillary biopsies of regions with and without plaque. During intraoperative endoscopy, we identified irregularly shaped regions of whitish material generally located on the papillary tip and usually surrounding the openings of the ducts of Bellini (Figs. 2**A** & **B**), the same plaque material described by Randall. The plaque is located deep to the epithelium (subepithelial) with a smooth outer surface, except where it is pitted due to the removal of an attached stone (Fig. 2**B**). Light microscopic examination of Yasue stained papillary biopsies revealed minute deposits of mineral first laid down in the basement membrane beneath cells of a specific portion of the urinary tubule, the thin limbs of Henle as they pass near the tip of renal papilla—close to where urine drips into the renal pelvis (Figs. 2**C** & **D**). Initially, these mineral deposits are seen as electron dense, spherically shaped objects of about 50 nm, but larger deposits are seen as multilayered spheres with alternating light (mineral layer) and dark (matrix layer) rings or bands (Fig. 2**C**, insert). The individual deposits appear to then coalesce on the collagen bundles in the interstitial space and become embedded in an electron dense matrix material generating islands of plaque. These islands extend down to the basal

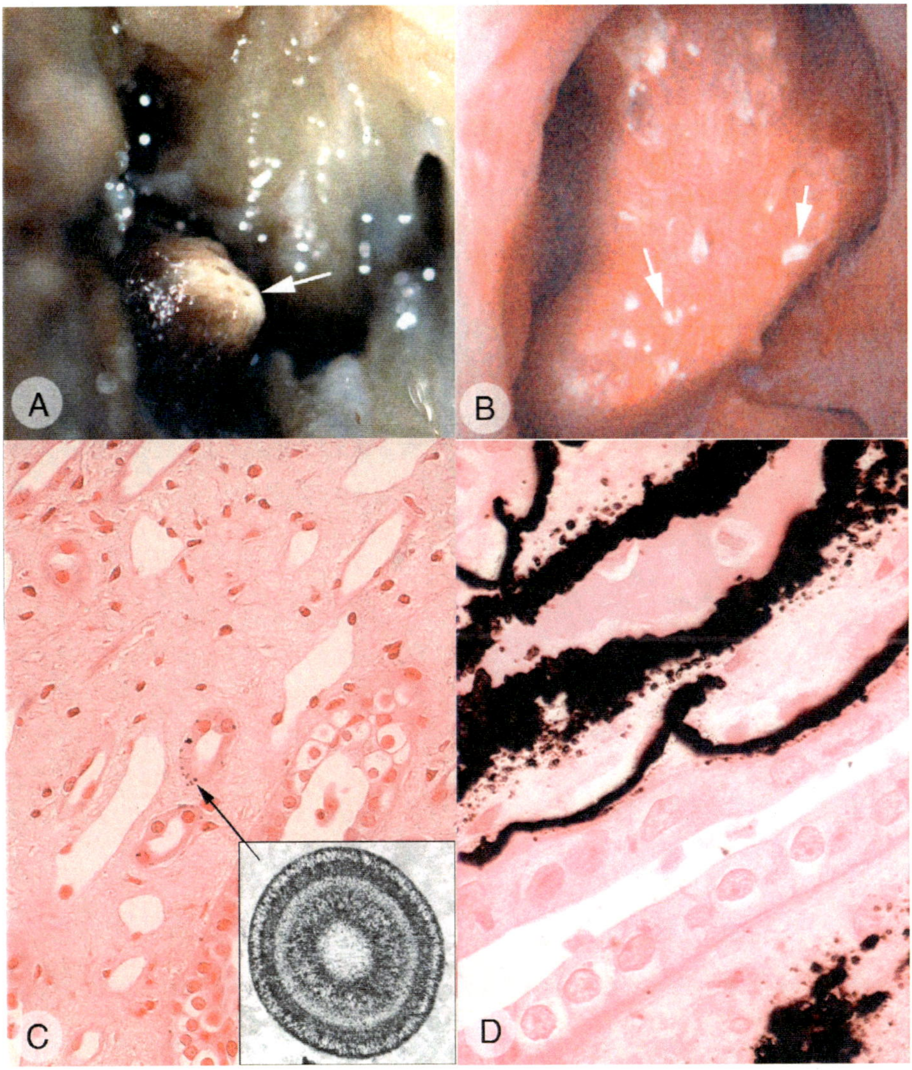

FIGURE 2. Endoscopic and histologic images of Randall's plaque in a ICSF patient. Panel **A** is a light microscopy photomicrograph showing a papilla from an ICSF patient that possesses a large cream-colored area (arrow) at the tip of papilla. This is the interstitial plaque material Randall discovered. Panel **B** shows a papilla from another ICSF patient imaged by endoscopic digital equipment at the time of a PNL procedure for stone removal. Note numerous irregular whitish areas (arrows) of Randall's plaque scattered around the papilla. Histologic examination of a light microscopic Yasue stained section of a papillary biopsy with minimal plaque shows spherically shaped, brown-black deposits only in the basement membranes of the thin loops of Henle (panel **C**, arrow). The insert at the lower right side of panel **C** shows such a deposit by transmission electron microscopy. Note the multilayered appearance with alternating light and dark rings. Panel **D** shows a denser region of plaque where the individual deposits are embedded in a continuous layer of calcified matrix material.

side of the epithelium and encase the ducts of Bellini. In order to determine the mineral composition of the interstitial plaque, we developed a protocol to analyze these small sites of crystalline material using μ-Fourier transform infrared microspectroscopy (μ-FTIR) (Fig. 3). The mineral in the plaque was determined to always be biological apatite (calcium phosphate). In addition, we have identified osteopontin as one of the proteins forming the matrix layers [8]. Other potential matrix proteins are bikunin, prothrombin fragment 1, and fetuin-A. Ryall and colleagues have reviewed the macromolecules relevant to stone formation in a paper in this proceedings [9]. No evidence of cell injury, inflammation, interstitial fibrosis or intratubular crystalline material was detected in any of the ICSF papillary biopsies.

Our biopsy and mapping studies have now included not only ICSF patients but patients with brushite stones [2], those who form apatite stones because of distal renal tubular acidosis (dRTA) [3], patients with calcium oxalate stone due to obesity bypass

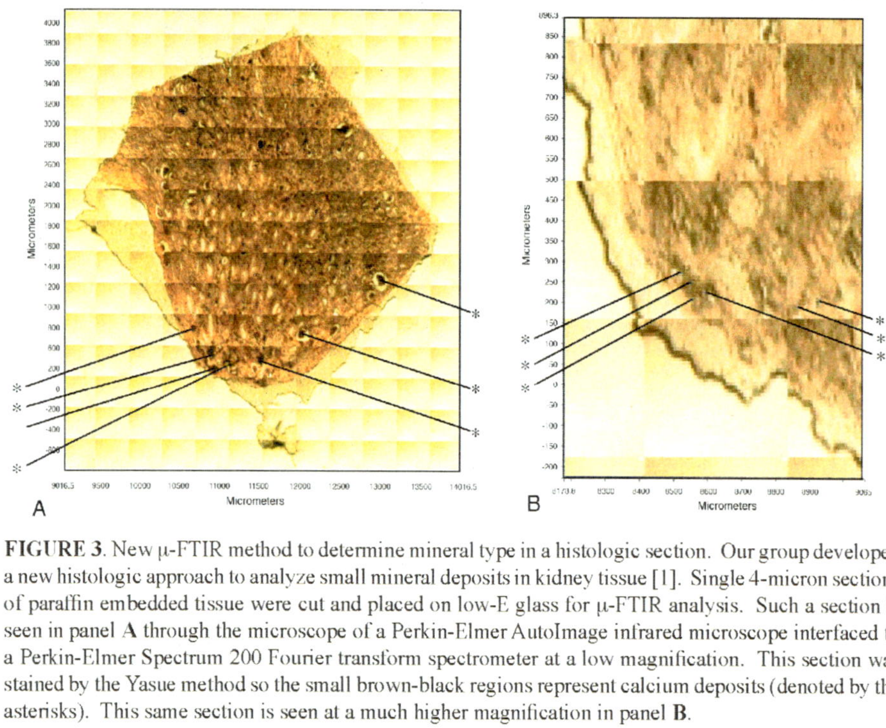

FIGURE 3. New μ-FTIR method to determine mineral type in a histologic section. Our group developed a new histologic approach to analyze small mineral deposits in kidney tissue [1]. Single 4-micron sections of paraffin embedded tissue were cut and placed on low-E glass for μ-FTIR analysis. Such a section is seen in panel **A** through the microscope of a Perkin-Elmer AutoImage infrared microscope interfaced to a Perkin-Elmer Spectrum 200 Fourier transform spectrometer at a low magnification. This section was stained by the Yasue method so the small brown-black regions represent calcium deposits (denoted by the asterisks). This same section is seen at a much higher magnification in panel **B**.

procedures [4], and patients with cystinuria [5]. A table in Coe's paper in this proceedings summarizes the different histopathologic changes for each these stone formers [10]. Randall's plaque is unique to ICSF while the other stone forming groups show varying degrees of plugging of their inner medullary collecting ducts (IMCD), which leads to total destruction of the lining cells and focal sites of interstitial fibrosis. The non-ICSF stone forming groups that we have studied so far have regions of Randall's plaque equal to or below the levels of non-stone forners.

STONES IN ICSF ARE ATTACHED TO THE PAPILLUM

Counting Attached Stones

Randall was convinced that interstitial plaque was a prequisite for stone formation and growth. Unfortunately, he was not able to collect kidneys from carefully selected groups of stone formers, so his theory was stated in very general terms. That is to say, he was not able to determine if all stone formers made plaque or if only a selected group presented such a histopathologic characteristic. Our research program has allowed us that selectivity. So we began collecting data at the time of PNL to determine if all stones in ICSF patients were attached to a papillum, and if so, were they attached at regions of

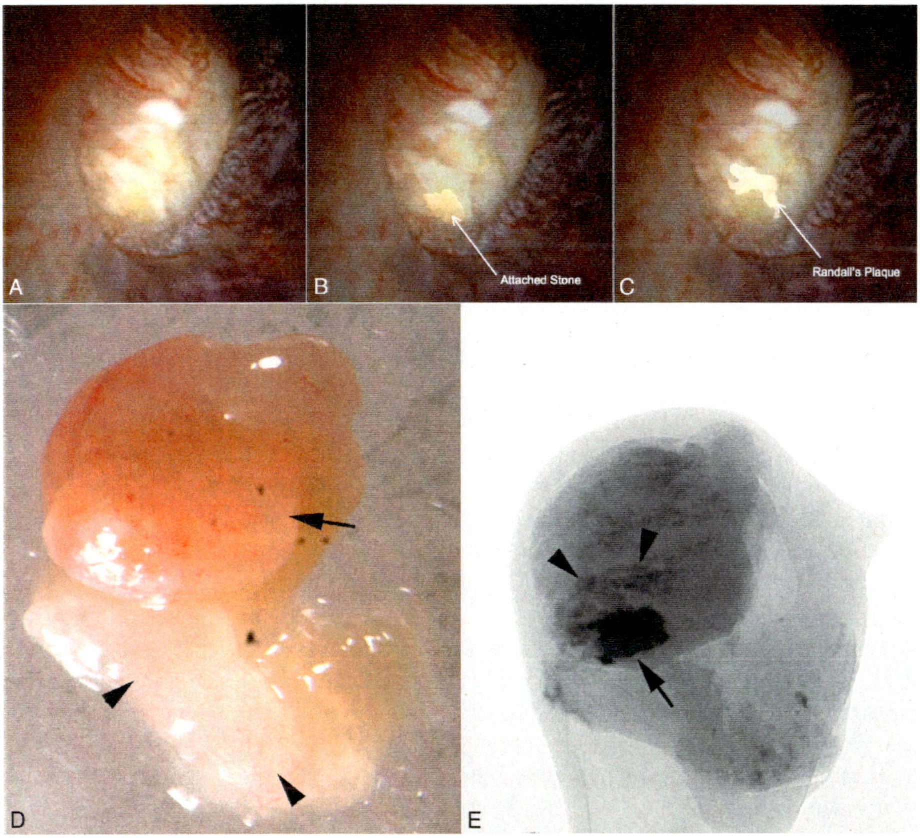

FIGURE 4. Endoscopic and μ-CT profile images of a small stone attached to a papilla tip. Panel **A** shows the endoscopic view of a 0.5 mm attached stone surrounded by white plaque. This stone is highlighted in panel **B** while the plaque is enhanced in panel **C**. The entire stone-tissue sample is seen in panel **D** immediately after biopsy retrieval of this sample. The arrow indicates the stone while the arrowheads point out a large region of white plaque that was associated with this stone. The plaque-stone interface is clearly seen in the μ-CT profile image of this sample (**E**). Again the stone is indicated by the arrow and the regions of plaque by several arrowheads.

Randall's plaque. Figs. **4A-C** show such a stone fixed to the papillum at a site of plaque. Matlaga and colleagues show similar images of attached stones in their paper in this proceeding [11]. The hypothesis of this study stated that if Randall's plaque were a prequisite to future stone formation in ICSF patients, all or most observed stones would be seen attached to the papilla at sites of plaque. Matlaga presented evidence at this symposium in support of this hypothesis in that 11 of 23 patients studied retrospectively had attached stones, with 91% of these stones at sites of plaque [11,12]. These numbers are much higher than those reported by Randall. We are conducting a new prospective study to determine if all stones are indeed attached and, if so, are they attached by means of plaque. Such a study requires the surgeon to inspect and video record all papillae prior to stone removal. This same study would need to be repeated in other types of stone formers to determine the validity of the hypothesis. Those stone forming groups that do not make interstitial plaque should form stones by a process very different than ICSF patients. Those with intraluminal plugging of the ducts of Bellini (like cystine and brushite stone formers) may have pelvic stones attached to the distal ends of such plugs and thereby mimic the Randall's type II papillary lesion [1]. Other types of stone formers may simply form free-floating stones in the renal pelvis.

Stone-Plaque Junction

As stated earlier in this paper, those attached stones that have been plucked off from the papilla, generally have been found to have an irregular concave surface that fit against the papilla and a smooth convex surface that faced the urinary space (Fig. 1). Often the concave surface was found to have a stock or umbilicus (Fig. **1A**, arrow) thought to be made up of plaque and that this plaque was in continuity with the interstitial plaque before the stone was detached from the papilla. Daudon and colleagues have reported at this symposium an analysis of 5,401 stones with an umbilication [7]. They found the main mineral component of this plaque material to be carbapatite (91%) with lesser amounts of amorphous carbonated calcium phosphate, sodium hydrogen urate or uric acid. Matlaga and colleagues using μ-CT have also examined the mineral content of three stones that were observed during PNL to be attached to sites of Randall's plaque [11]. Their proceedings report shows each of these stones to have a small region of apatite in an otherwise large volume of calcium oxalate. These observations again support the ideas laid out by Randall [1]. Thus, calcium oxalate stones in ICSF patients appear to grow like stalactites adherent to the tips of kidney papillae and, typically, are made of layers of calcium oxalate surrounding a core of apatite.

All of these findings lead us to the next critical question: What is the mineral that forms the overgrowth on the interstitial plaque? By answering this question, we will have insight into the initiating event for stone growth on interstitial plaque, which can then be possibly used to determine ways to block this process from occurring. Randall desperately attempted to address this question but failed. We presently have the techniques necessary to carry out such an analysis. The first step requires the selection of a documented ICSF patient and one that requires PNL to remove a stone burden.

At the time of surgery, the smallest (< 0.5 mm), visible attached stone should be selected and biopsied with its underlying papillary tissue so that the entire stone-plaque interface can be sectioned (Fig. 4). If the stone is small, one should be able to cut the sample without demineralizing the stone to allow for μ-FTIR analysis and still keep the plaque/stone junction intact and minimize tissue/stone shredding. A set of serial sections should be prepared for sequential analysis by light microscopic histochemistry and μ-FTIR. Similar samples will need to be demineralized and studied by transmission electron microscopy. Such experiments are currently on their way in our laboratory.

DISRUPTION OF THE UROTHELIAL BARRIER

Randall's theory of stone formation also requires erosion of the epithelium over sites of plaque as a means of exposing the interstitial plaque to the urine in the renal pelvis. Such an event would allow minerals and proteins from the urine to attach to the regions of exposed plaque, and initiate stone formation. To date no one has actively worked on this problem. Bergsland has a paper in this proceedings detailing the known properties of the papillary epithelium, which again is sparse [13,14]. She presents several pathophysiological factors that might cause the epithelial barrier to become leakier and thereby induce a loss of epithlelial integrity. Additional mechanisms of epithelial cell injury and loss are presented in Fig. 5. In panel **A**, the interstitial plaque positioned at the basolateral cell surface of the urothelial cells induces alterations in the integrity of the apical surface of these cells allowing attachment of crystals to the cell surface. In this model, the epithelial layer is not lost but becomes incorporated into the stone-plaque

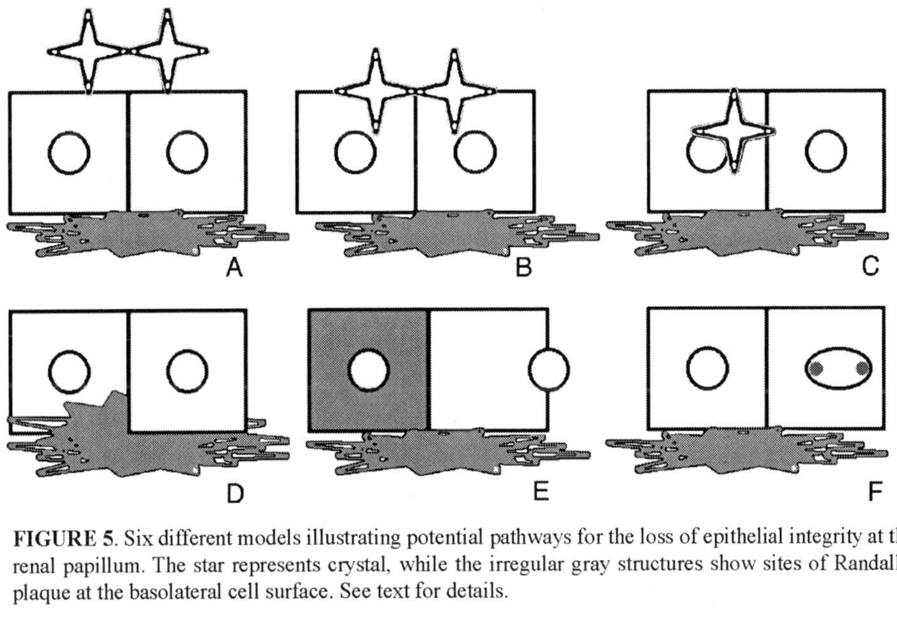

FIGURE 5. Six different models illustrating potential pathways for the loss of epithelial integrity at the renal papillum. The star represents crystal, while the irregular gray structures show sites of Randall's plaque at the basolateral cell surface. See text for details.

complex. In panel **B**, urinary crystals attach to and damage the epithelial cells allowing these crystals to merge with the interstitial plaque. The third model (panel **C**) suggests that calcium and oxalate ions enter the epithelial cells, form intracellular crystals which then injure these cells and allow the crystals to merge with the interstitial plaque. In panel **D**, the interstitial plaque grows through or between the epithelial cells and into the urinary space allowing overgrowth to occur. The fifth model (panel **E**) suggests that the interstitial plaque triggers apoptosis or necrosis of the overlying epithelial cells allowing the plaque to be exposed to the urine and subsequent overgrowth. In panel **F**, a random apoptotic event occurs in epithelial cells overlying a site of interstitial plaque, resulting in a loss of those epithelial cells and exposing the plaque to the urine. It may be that none of these models are useable; however, the issue of how a compromise in epithelial cell integrity might occur during the process of kidney stone formation needs serious investigation.

SUMMARY

In summary, Randall's original thoughts on the mechanisms for kidney stone formation appear valid for idiopathic calcium oxalate stone formers (ICSF) but not for most other stone forming groups. Our current studies on selected groups of human stone formers using intraoperative papillary biopsies have shown overwhelming evidence for the presence of Randall's plaque in ICSF patients and that stone formation and growth are exclusively linked to its availability to urinary ions and proteins. Intense investigation of the plaque-stone junction is needed if we are to understand the factors leading to the overgrowth process on exposed regions of plaque. Such information should allow the development of treatment strategies to block stone formation in ICSF patients. Stone formation in brushite, dRTA, cystine and intestinal bypass stone formers appears to occur by other mechanisms, which are not yet well understood.

ACKNOWLEDGMENTS

This work was supported by NIH grant P01 DK56788.

REFERENCES

1. A. Randall *J Urol* **44**, 580-589 (1940).
2. A.P. Evan, J.E. Lingeman, F.L. Coe, Y. Shao, J.H. Parks, S.B. Bledsoe, C.L. Phillips, S. Bonsib, E.M. Worcester, A.J. Sommer, S.C. Kim, W.W. Tinmouth and M. Grynpas *Kidney Intl* **67**, 576-591 (2005).
3. A.P. Evan, J.E. Lingeman, F.L. Coe, Y. Shao, N. Miller, B. Matlaga, C. Phillips, A. Sommer and E. Worcester *Kidney Intl* (In Press).
4. R.L. Kuo, J.E. Lingeman, A.P. Evan, R.F. Paterson, J.H. Parks, S.B. Bledsoe, L.C. Munch and F.L. Coe *Kidney Intl* **64**, 2150-2154 (2003).
5. A.P. Evan, J.E. Lingeman, Y. Shao, B.R. Matlage, S.C. Kim, S.B. Bledsoe, A.J. Sommer, M. Grynpas, C.L. Phillips and E.M. Worcester *Kidney Intl* **69**, 2227-2235 (2006).
6. L. Cifuentes-Delatte, J. Minon-Cifuentes and J.A. Medina *J Urol* **137**, 1024-1029 (1987).
7. M. Daudon, O. Traxer, P. Jungers and D. Bazin. A paper in this proceedings, pp. 26-34.
8. A.P. Evan, F.L. Coe, S.R. Rittling, S.M. Bledsoe, Y. Shao, J.E. Lingeman and E.M. Worcester *Kidney Intl* **68**, 145-154 (2005).
9. R.L. Ryall, A.F. Cook, L.A. Thurgood and P.K. Grover. In this proceedings, pp. 129-140.
10. F.L. Coe. A paper in this proceedings, pp. 3-11.
11. B.R. Matlaga, J.C. Williams, Jr., A.P. Evan, and J.E. Lingeman. In this proceedings, pp. 35-41.
12. B.R. Matlaga, J.C. Williams, Jr., S.C. Kim, R.L. Kuo, A.P. Evan, S.B. Bledsoe, F.L. Coe, E.M. Worcester, L.C. Munch and J.E. Lingeman *J Urol* **175**, 1720-1724 (2006).
13. K.J. Bergsland. A paper in this proceedings, pp. 42-48.
14. A. Gerard *Traffic* **5**, 117-128 (2004).

Stone Morphology Suggestive of Randall's Plaque

Michel Daudon[*], Olivier Traxer[†], Paul Jungers[‡], Dominique Bazin[§]

[*]*Service de Biochimie A, Hôpital Necker, 149 Rue de Sèvres, 75015 Paris, France*
[†]*Service d'Urologie, Hôpital Tenon, 4 Rue de la Chine, 75020 Paris, France*
[‡]*Service de Néphrologie, Hôpital Necker, 149, Rue de Sèvres, 75015 Paris, France*
[§]*Laboratoire de Physique des Solides, Bat. 510, Université Paris-Sud, 91405 Orsay, France*

Abstract. Randall's plaques are found in a number of calcium oxalate stone formers. Stones developed on a Randall's plaque typically present a small depressed zone ("umbilication") corresponding to the tip of the papilla and containing material detached from the plaque. By examining the morphology and infrared composition of 45,774 calculi referred to our laboratory over the past three decades, we identified 8,916 umbilicated calculi (19.5%). We have selected three periods of time corresponding to the first years of each decade. Over these periods, we analyzed 26,182 consecutive calculi. Among them, we identified 5,401 umbilicated calculi, of which 91.5% had an identifiable plaque. We analyzed the relative prevalence of umbilicated stones over time and the respective composition of Randall's plaque and stones. The proportion of umbilicated stones rose significantly from 10% in period 1 (1978-1984) to 21% in period 2 (1990-1993) and 22.2% in period 3 (2000-2006), with a parallel rise in the prevalence of stones with identifiable Randall's plaque. The main component of plaques was carbapatite in 90.8% of cases, whereas other components such as amorphous carbonated calcium phosphate, sodium hydrogen urate or uric acid were found in other cases. The morphology of plaques made of carbapatite was diverse, as was their carbonate content, thus suggesting variable pathophysiological mechanisms. Stones were made of whewellite as the main component in 51.4% of cases, or admixed with weddellite in 26.8%, predominant weddellite in 12.5% and other components (mainly uric acid) in 7.5% of cases. Our findings confirm that Randall's plaques are made of carbapatite in the great majority of cases, but with the stones more frequently composed of calcium oxalate monohydrate (which is associated with hyperoxaluria) than of calcium oxalate dihydrate (associated with hypercalciuria). In conclusion, in our country, stones developed on a carbapatite Randall's plaque are as frequently made of monohydrate than dihydrate calcium oxalate, thus suggesting a role for a high urine concentration in both oxalate and calcium ions in the lithogenic process.

Keywords: Randall's plaque, stone morphology, calcium oxalate, whewellite, weddellite.
PACS: 81.10.Dn; 87.19.Xx

INTRODUCTION

Based on a large study of autopsy material, Randall first described whitish, calcified, "plaque" deposits beneath the epithelium near the tip of renal papillae, in 20.5% of kidneys from 1154 subjects [1]. He suggested that such plaques, made of calcium phosphate and calcium carbonate crystals, could act as an anchored nidus for calcium oxalate (CaOx) overgrowth, leading to stones. As a matter of fact, Randall

CP900, *Renal Stone Disease, 1st Annual International Urolithiasis Research Symposium*, edited by A. P. Evan, J. E. Lingeman, and J. C. Williams, Jr.

reported examples of stones exhibiting a concave region, suggesting they had developed while attached on a renal papilla, inasmuch as patches of the same phosphate material were found at the bottom of the hollow [2]. Such a 'footprint' of a papilla was found in 12% of 500 spontaneously passed stones analyzed by Cifuentes-Delatte et al. [3]. More recently, endoscopic techniques have shown Randall's plaques to be common on papillae of CaOx stone formers and also—although much less frequently—in subjects without a history of stones [4]. Evan et al. [5], taking advantage of percutaneous nephrolithotomy procedures in 15 recurrent CaOx stone formers, nicely showed that interstitial apatite plaque particles first appear in the basement membranes of the thin loops of Henle. In addition, they showed that stone formation activity was proportional to the surface of papillae covered by Randall's plaques [6], and that the mean fractional plaque coverage was higher in CaOx stone formers with the highest urinary calcium concentration [7].

For years, we have observed that a number of CaOx stones (especially those preponderantly made of whewellite) had at their surface a small depression which we term an "umbilication," containing a material similar to that of Randall's plaques. In the present epidemiologic study, we evaluated the proportion of umbilicated stones among the large series of calculi examined at our laboratory over the past 3 decades (and the evolution of their relative prevalence over time), and the nature of the deposits found in the umbilications.

MATERIALS AND METHODS

All calculi referred to our laboratory were first examined by stereomicroscopy to identify the morphological type of their surface according to our morpho-constitutional classification of urinary stones [8]. Whenever an umbilication was seen, we selectively analyzed the Randall's plaque, which was isolated using a needle under the stereomicroscope. Then the stone was cut, its inner structure was observed and its characteristics were summarized by morphological type. Finally, we used morphological data to guide the selection of appropriate, representative samples of the stone material for compositional analysis. The Randall's plaque and the other samples of the stone were analyzed by infrared spectroscopy as previously described [9]. Spectra were recorded with a Fourier transform infrared spectrometer (Vector 22; Bruker Optics, Wissembourg, France), with a resolution of 4 cm^{-1}. For each sample, 32 scans were recorded against air as reference.

We determined the proportion of stones developed on Randall's plaque among the whole series of 45,774 calculi referred to our laboratory from various parts of France. Then, in order to assess possible changes with time in the occurrence of Randall's plaque, we reviewed records of consecutive stones referred over three periods of time, namely the beginning of the eighties (n=2,814 stones), the beginning of the nineties (n=5,234 stones) and the beginning of the twenty-first century (n=18,142 stones). We also examined the distribution of the stones with Randall's plaque according to patients' age and gender. The results were expressed as polynomial tendency curves to best reflect possible changes in the distribution of the stones.

RESULTS

Epidemiological Data

The overall proportion of stones with an umbilication was 19.5%, and 91% of those stones had identifiable Randall's plaque. Umbilicated stones were more frequent in males (21.5%) than in females (14.7%, $p<0.0001$). The proportion of umbilicated stones strikingly increased from 10% in the first period to 22.2% in recent years, with a parallel increase in the proportion of stones with Randall's plaque, which increased from 8.9% in the early eighties to 20.6% between 2000 to 2006 (Fig. 1). Significant differences were observed according to the patient age. The patients who appear more prone to develop stones from a Randall's plaque were aged 30-50 years. Of note, the proportion of such stones in young patients increased with time. In the age class 20-29 years, stones from Randall's plaque were found in 5.7% of patients in the first period, 17.9% in the second period and 23.3% in the recent years. As illustrated in Fig. 1, nearly 30% of male stone formers aged 35-40 years developed their stone from a Randall's plaque during the most recent period.

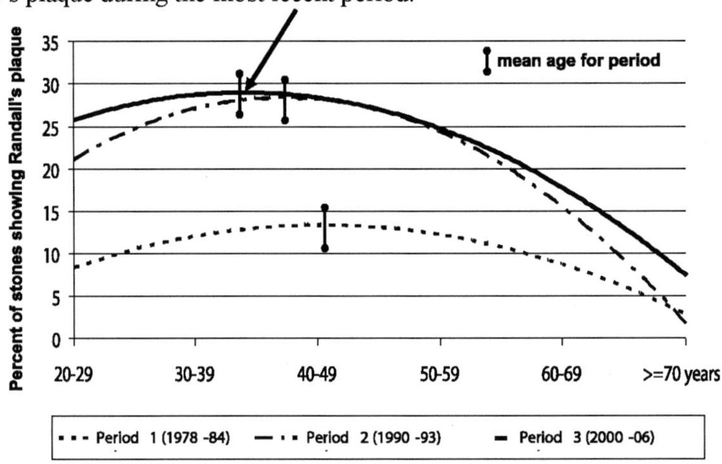

FIGURE 1 Prevalence of Randall's plaques in stones from male patients according to the period and patient age. About 30% of male stone formers had stones developed on a Randall's plaque in the age class 35-40 years in the most recent years (arrow).

As shown in Table 1, significant differences were observed according to gender. Men were especially at risk to form stones from a Randall's plaque, the proportion of such stones increasing with time.

Stone Morphology

The umbilication area corresponds to a small cavity of variable depth and width at the surface of the stone, containing a Randall's plaque and/or a proteinaceous attachment point to the tissue (Fig. 2). Because the anatomy of the papilla may be diverse, we observed different appearances for the umbilication, which may be large and shallow, deep and narrow, very irregular or, more rarely, displaying the aspect of a prominent area rather than of a cavity.

TABLE 1. Occurrence of Randall's plaque according to patient gender.

	Men	Women	Total
	Period 1 (1978-1984)		
Number of stones	1,866	948	2,814
Umbilicated stones (%)	213 (11.4)	68 (7.2)	281 (10.0)
Occurrence of Randall's plaque (%)	189 (10.1)$^{\circ}$	60 (6.3)	249 (8.9)
	Period 2 (1990-1993)		
Number of stones	3,720	1,506	5,226
Umbilicated stones (%)	857 (23.0)$^{*,\circ}$	240 (15.6)*	1,097 (21.0)*
Occurrence of Randall's plaque (%)	746 (20.0)$^{*,\circ}$	218 (14.5)*	964 (18.4)*
	Period 3 (2000-2006)		
Number of stones	12,607	5,535	18,142
Umbilicated stones (%)	3,132 (24.8)$^{*,x,\circ}$	891 (16.1)	4,023 (22.2)
Occurrence of Randall's plaque (%)	2,884 (22.9)$^{*,xx,\circ}$	848 (15.3)	3,732 (20.6)^{xx}

*$p<0.0001$ vs period 1 - $^{x}p<0.05$; $^{xx}p<0.01$ vs period 2 – $^{\circ}p<0.001$ vs women

Most stones with Randall's plaque are predominantly made of CaOx monohydrate (Fig. 2a) and/or dihydrate (Fig. 3a), corresponding to the Ia and IIa types of our morphological classification [8]. Several types may coexist in the same stone (Fig. 2d). We assessed the distribution of these types among 7,260 calculi presenting with an umbilication. The results are summarized in Table 2, which illustrates the high proportion of the Ia type.

TABLE 2. Prevalence of the various types of umbilicated calculi

Morphological type	Number	Prevalence (%)	Stone composition
Type Ia	3,730	51.4	Whewellite
Type Ia > IIa	2,074	28.6	Whewellite>weddellite
Type IIa > Ia	907	12.5	Weddellite>whewellite
Other types	549	7.5	Various components

The cross-section of type Ia stones usually presents a compact crystalline structure made of concentric layers, each of them with a radial organization of the crystals, which converge to the Randall's plaque located in the umbilication (Fig. 2b).

The color of the stone is important to consider. In the case of type Ia stones, the color is usually brownish; this aspect corresponds to a dormant stone (Fig. 2a and 2e). In contrast, a surface partly covered by a grayish thin deposit of new crystals of whewellite is indicative of an active stage of the lithogenic process (Fig. 2c and 2f).

Although CaOx stones are by far the most frequent calculi developed from a Randall's plaque, CaOx is not always the main component of such calculi. Indeed, in 7.5% of cases, umbilicated stones were composed of brushite, carbapatite, uric acid or cystine or an admixture of CaOx and calcium phosphate.

Plaque Morphology

The morphological characteristics of the Randall's plaque found within the umbilication are diverse, thus suggesting differences in composition and origin. For example, Randall's plaque may be laminated as in Figs. 2a and 2f, or bulky as in Fig. 2e.

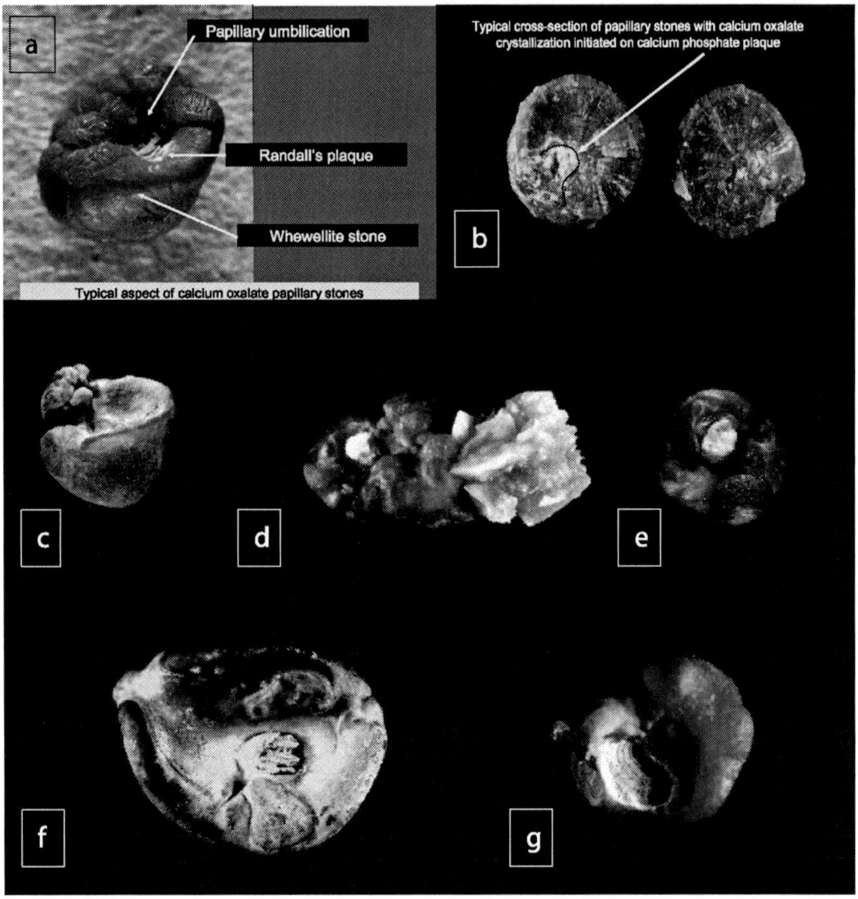

FIGURE 2. Morphological aspects of some papillary stones and Randall's plaques

When a bulky plaque remains anchored to the papilla, the umbilicated stone shows only the impression of the plaque (Fig. 2g). A cylindrical "plaque" is likely to correspond to a tubular cast rather than a papillary calcification (Fig. 3c). A wide plaque may show visible holes corresponding to calcified tubules (Fig. 3b); in contrast, the plaque may appear as a small point (Fig. 3a).

Not exceptionally, no plaque is visible on the surface of the umbilication and only the anchorage point may be seen (Fig.2c). In such a case, this point is shown by infrared spectroscopy to be composed of proteins and carbapatite, thus corresponding to a part of a wider plaque which apparently remained attached to the tissue.

Two other situations may be observed. First, some papillary stones arise from a plaque made of needle-shaped crystals with a radiating organization. Second, some presumed papillary stones have no umbilication but present with a tunnel through the stone (Fig. 3d). This tunnel seems to act as a core, surrounded by carbapatite, subsequently covered by CaOx monohydrate (Fig. 3e).

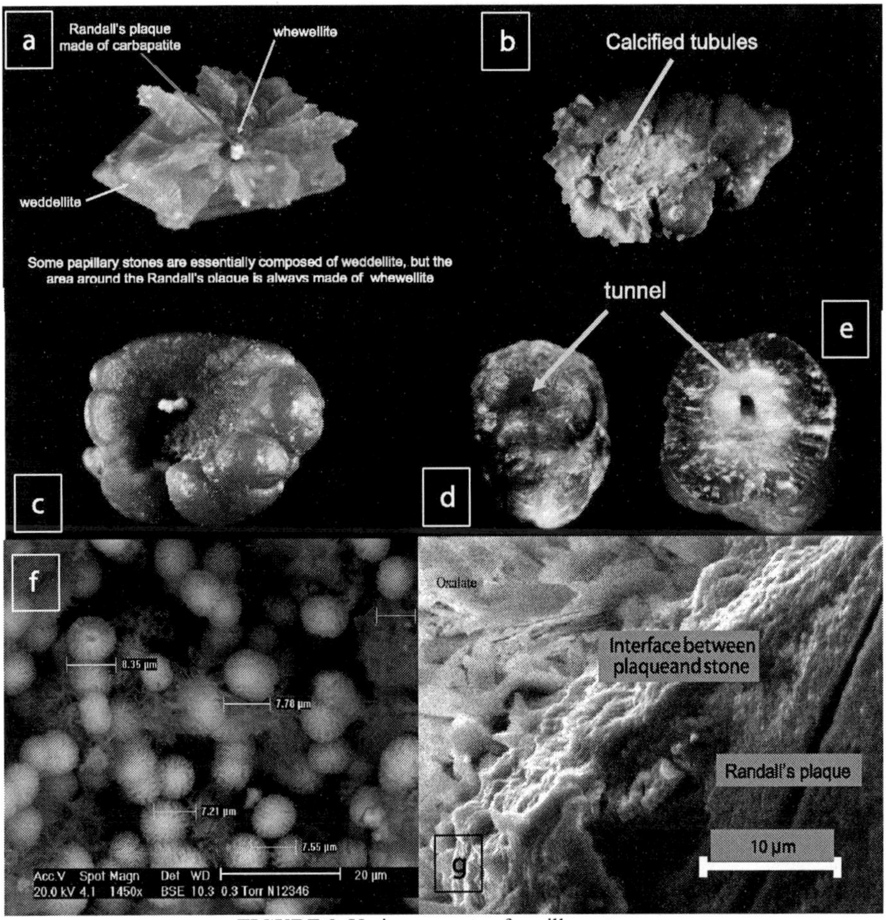

FIGURE 3. Various aspects of papillary stones

As observed by scanning electron microscopy, crystals in carbapatite stones (Fig.3f) form needles aggregated as spherulites. In contrast, the interface between CaOx and Randall's plaque does not show such crystals (Fig. 3g), suggesting that amorphous material (ACCP and proteins) could be prevalent in such an area.

Of note, the size of crystallites assessed by neutron diffraction was revealed to be markedly smaller for carbapatite (5-12 nanometers) than for other components (70-120 nanometers for calcium oxalate monohydrate).

Infrared Analysis

Main Component of the Stones

Most umbilicated stones formed on a renal papilla contain CaOx as the main component (Table 2). However, some of these stones also contain high proportions of carbapatite, especially in patients with medullary sponge kidney. Among CaOx crystalline species, whewellite is always present and is the only form of CaOx in 51.4% of the stones. In other cases, it coexists with various proportions of weddellite. In rare cases, weddellite may be the predominant form of CaOx (Fig. 3a). Not rarely, in patients beyond 50 years, a CaOx stone attached to the papilla by a calcium phosphate Randall's plaque may be covered by uric acid as the main component of the stone. Exceptionally, cystine stones may develop on a Randall's plaque in cystinuric patients. The same is observed for other components such as uric acid, sodium hydrogen urate or brushite stones, but all these cases represent a small proportion of the stones formed on a Randall's plaque [9].

Composition of the Randall's Plaque Attached to the Stone

The infrared spectra of umbilicated stones reveal that the Randall's plaque accounts for 0.5% up to 25% of the stone mass (median proportion 2%). The Randall's plaques are composed of carbapatite in 90.8% of cases, this crystalline phase being admixed with proteins and various proportions of whewellite. In a number of cases, glycosaminoglycans and a small proportion of lipids are also found. The Randall's plaque is not always made of a unique crystalline species, but it also may contain amorphous carbonated calcium phosphate (ACCP) or sodium hydrogen urate and, less frequently, whitlockite, uric acid or brushite (Table 3). The carbonate content of the calcium phosphate found in Randall's plaque ranges from 2% to 25%.

TABLE 3. Relative prevalence of the main components of Randall's plaques

Component	Prevalence (%)	Component	Prevalence (%)
Carbapatite	90.8	Other phosphates	0.4
ACCP	4.6	Other urates	0.1
Sodium hydrogen urate	3.5	Other compounds	<0.1
Uric acid	0.5	Total	100.0

DISCUSSION

The increasing prevalence of CaOx stones formed on a papillary Randall's plaque over the past three decades cannot be explained by genetic changes during such a short period of time. Rather, it reflects a true epidemiological change due to modifications in dietary habits of the population and, possibly, to iatrogenic factors. Because 1) the plaque is the consequence of a long process of calcium phosphate deposition in the interstitium of the inner medulla, 2) it precedes the stone grown on the papilla, and 3) stone formers with a carbapatite plaque are younger and younger, we may hypothesize that changes in dietary habits or excessive supplementations with calcium and/or vitamin D in teenagers or in infants may contribute to hypercalciuria and Randall's plaques formation.

Are all Randall's Plaques of the Same Origin?

The answer is not so clear. As for calcium phosphate plaques, at least two parameters have to be considered. The first one is the composition of the plaque, i.e., the presence of carbapatite alone, or combined with another calcium phosphate species such as ACCP, brushite, octacalcium phosphate or whitlockite, or with other components, such as sodium urate or uric acid. Most of these associations suggest that part of the plaque was formed through urine supersaturation after it has emerged at the surface of the papilla. The second parameter is the carbonate content of the calcium phosphates (carbapatite and ACCP).

Convincing arguments have shown that the plaque is initiated in the inner medulla and progressively expands to the papillary epithelium [5]. Among umbilicated stones, we found a high carbonate content of carbapatite in 42% of cases, a finding in agreement with the physico-chemical conditions in the medulla where the bicarbonate concentration is high. However, in 30% of cases, the very low carbonate content of the carbapatite, i.e., less than 7%, can hardly be compatible with the composition of the interstitial medulla. Thus, such so-called Randall's plaques might result from an accumulation on the surface of the papilla of calcium phosphate deposits coming, at least in part, from the lumen of the collecting ducts where the bicarbonate content is very low. Among papillary stones that are likely to develop from carbapatite of tubular origin are those presenting a tunnel (Figs. 3d and 3e), which were observed in 1.2% of CaOx monohydrate stones. Such calculi presumably come from carbapatite crystals formed on the surface of proteinaceous bridges linking two neighboring papillae. In these cases, calcium phosphate likely does not originate from the interstitium but from tubules as suggested by its low carbonate content (<10%).

Plaques made of sodium hydrogen urate are likely to originate from urines with a high concentration of both sodium and urate ions. Indeed, most of these patients also had documented hyperuricemia. Of interest, two thirds of the plaques containing sodium urate also contained carbapatite crystals.

Covering plaques with the presence of calcified collecting ducts may correspond to an extensive Randall's plaque process, as such plaques were mainly observed in patients with a long history of stone disease. Cylindrical deposits probably are tubular casts and therefore do not correspond to true Randall's plaques, even if composed of carbapatite. Interestingly, their carbonation rate is low and a number of such casts contain both carbapatite and sodium urate (Fig. 3c).

Metabolic Factors Involved in Stone Growth

Evan et al hypothesized that apatite particles which constitute the initial step of Randall's plaques form because fluid in the thin limbs of Henle is supersaturated with respect to calcium phosphate salts. They proposed that hypercalciuria could be the driving force [10], because the extent of renal papilla coverage by Randall's plaque was proportional to urine calcium concentration [7] and the number of stones formed in their patients was proportional to papillary surface covered by Randall's plaques [6].

Our data are in general accordance with this hypothesis, but also suggest that other factors may be operative. Indeed, of our 6311 calculi developed on a Randall's plaque, nearly half (47.2%) were mainly made of weddellite with a type II morphology, characteristic of a lithogenic process related to high urinary calcium concentration [11]. However, nearly as many umbilicated stones were mainly composed of whewellite, a crystalline phase dependent on a high urinary oxalate concentration, rather than hypercalciuria. These findings can be explained if we consider that both calcium and oxalate ions are in high concentration in the papillary area [12]. Thus, crystals of whewellite or weddellite can easily be deposited on the plaque. Bushinsky et al. [10] hypothesized a role for peaks of urinary calcium concentration following meals. Post-prandial peaks of urine oxalate content similarly occur following consumption of oxalate-rich foods and may be an alternative explanation.

Further studies, examining 24 hour-urine parameters and composition of CaOx stones with and without umbilication are needed to clarify factors associated with the presence of Randall's plaques and development of whewellite or weddellite CaOx calculi.

REFERENCES

1. Randall, *Ann Surg* **105**, 1009-1027 (1937).
2. Randall, *J Urol* **44**, 580-589 (1940).
3. L. Cifuentes-Delatte, J. Minon-Cifuentes J. and J.A. Medina, *J Urol* **137**, 1024-1029 (1987).
4. R.K. Low and M.L. Stoller, *J Urol* **158**, 2062-2064 (1997).
5. A.P. Evan, J.E. Lingeman, F.L. Coe, J.H. Parks, S.B. Bledsoe, Y. Shao, A.J. Sommer, R.F. Paterson, R.L. Kuo and M. Grynpas, *J Clin Invest* **111**, 607-616 (2003).
6. S.C. Kim, F.L. Coe, W.W. Tinmouth, R.L. Kuo, R.F. Paterson, J.H. Parks, L.C. Munch, A.P. Evan and J.E. Lingeman, *J Urol* **173**, 117-119 (2005).
7. R.L. Kuo, J.E. Lingeman, A.P. Evan, R.F. Paterson, J.H. Parks, S.B. Bledsoe, L.C. Munch and F.L. Coe, *Kidney Int* **64**, 2150-2154 (2003).
8. M. Daudon, C.A. Bader and P. Jungers, *Scanning Microsc* **7**, 1081-1106 (1993).
9. L. Estepa and M. Daudon, *Biospectroscopy* **3**, 347-369 (1997).
10. D.A. Bushinsky, *J Clin Invest* **111**, 602-605 (2003).
11. M. Daudon and P. Jungers, *Nephron Physiol* **98**, 31-36 (2004).
12. R. Hautmann, A. Lehmann and S. Komor, *J Urol* **123**, 317-319 (1980).

Calcium Oxalate Stones Are Frequently Found Attached to Randall's Plaque

Brian R. Matlaga*, James C. Williams, Jr.†, Andrew P. Evan†, and James E. Lingeman‡

** James Buchanan Brady Urological Institute, The Johns Hopkins University School of Medicine, 4940 Eastern Ave / Room A 345, Baltimore, Maryland 21224, USA*
† Departments of Anatomy & Cell Biology, Indiana University School of Medicine, 635 Barnhill Dr / MS 5035, Indianapolis, Indiana, 46202, USA
‡ Methodist Hospital Institute for Kidney Stone Disease, 1801 N. Senate Blvd, Suite 220, Indianapolis, Indiana, 46202, USA

Abstract. The exact mechanisms of the crystallization processes that occur during the formation of calcium oxalate calculi are controversial. Over six decades ago, Alexander Randall reported on a series of cadaveric renal units in which he observed calcium salt deposits on the tips of the renal papilla. Randall hypothesized that these deposits, eponymously termed Randall's plaque, would be the ideal site for stone formation, and indeed in a number of specimens he noted small stones attached to the papillae. With the recent advent of digital endoscopic imaging and micro computerized tomography (CT) technology, it is now possible to inspect the renal papilla of living, human stone formers and to study the attached stone with greater scrutiny.

Keywords: Kidney, Calculi.
PACS: 01.30.Cc

INTRODUCTION

Our knowledge of the inciting lesion in the pathogenesis of kidney stones is rudimentary. One of the critical elements of this process, though, is certain to be particle retention, which enables the forming stone to develop into a clinically significant calculus [1]. Particle retention is required, because in normal physiologic settings the flow rate of urine through the intra-renal collecting system is such that clusters of crystals will pass before they can grow to a sufficient size to be retained. Over six decades ago, Alexander Randall addressed the subject of stone pathogenesis when he conducted a detailed examination of the papillae of more than 1,000 non-selected cadaveric renal units [2]. He observed calcium salt deposits in the tip of the renal papillum in 19.6% of individuals studied. These deposits, which he termed plaque, were interstitial in location, composed of calcium, and not observed in the tubular lumen. Randall noted that these areas of plaque would be an ideal site for an overgrowth of calcium oxalate to develop into a calculus.

In fact, Randall reported that in a number of kidneys there were small stones were fixed to the surface of the renal papillae, anchored at the location of plaque. Building

CP900, *Renal Stone Disease, 1st Annual International Urolithiasis Research Symposium,* edited by A. P. Evan, J. E. Lingeman, and J. C. Williams, Jr.

on Randall's findings, a critical issue in the pathogenesis of stone disease arises: Does every calcium oxalate stone begins as a papilla-attached stone, or do only a minority of stones form in this way? This question has remained irresolvable, as data have been lacking on the true incidence of attached stones in a population of stone forming patients. Randall's studies were confined to a population of non-selected cadavers, and until our present work there have been no other studies directly addressing the attached renal calculus.

To more completely define the attached stone phenomenon, we performed a study to assess the prevalence of attached renal calculi in a well characterized population of common calcium oxalate stone-formers. We also sought to investigate the structure of attached stones using new technology that allows the study of stone morphology and composition. Specifically, we captured the images of attached stones with high resolution, digital endoscopic equipment. The stones were subsequently removed from the renal papillae, and investigated with micro computed tomography (CT), a technology that is capable of distinguishing different minerals common in urinary stones, and displaying the structural relationship of these components.

PREVALENCE OF ATTACHED RENAL CALCULI

We have anecdotally noted that when endoscopically examining the renal papillae of patients, oftentimes stones attached to the papillae are encountered. Low and Stoller have also reported this phenomenon [3]. However, Randall observed attached stones in only 5.6% of the renal units in his series. It is important to recognize, though, that Randall studied a non-selected cohort of subjects. We hypothesized that the prevalence of attached renal calculi in an exclusively stone-forming population would be greater than the 5.6% prevalence Randall observed.

We endeavored to address this issue when we performed an Institutional Review Board-approved study of patients undergoing percutaneous nephrolithotomy. All patients fulfilled the criteria for common, idiopathic calcium oxalate stone-formers [4]; in all patients, at least one stone was analyzed and shown to be composed of calcium oxalate and no stones contained uric acid, struvite, cystine, or over 50% calcium phosphate. None of the patients had systemic disorders such as primary hyperparathyroidism, sarcoidosis, vitamin D excess, hyperthyroidism, or renal tubular acidosis.

Following percutaneous nephrolithotomy, all accessible papillae were sequentially visualized with either flexible or rigid digital endoscopes. A total of 172 renal papillae were endoscopically identified and inspected in 24 kidneys of 23 patients. One hundred fifty-six papillae (91%) had plaque, and all renal units in the study had plaque on at least one papillum. Forty-nine papillae (28.5%) had attached calculi, and all of these papillae possessed plaque. Further, all attached stones were attached to regions that visually appeared to be plaque. Conversely, no papillae lacking plaque had attached stones.

The quality of digital imaging provides incontrovertible evidence of stone attachment to plaque. Figure 1 demonstrates a typical single calcium oxalate stone attached at the papillary tip (Fig. 1A). After stone removal plaque is clearly evident at the site of stone attachment (Fig. 1B).

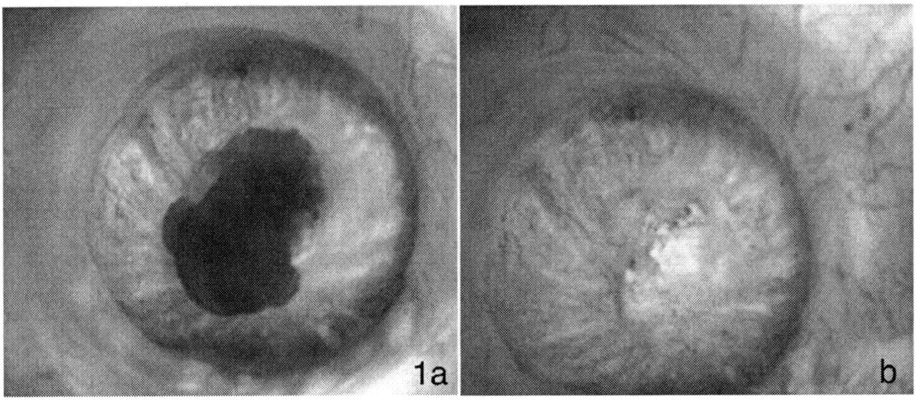

FIGURE 1. A. Digital photograph of a calcium oxalate monohydrate stone attached to the tip of a renal papillum. **B.** The papillum from panel A following stone removal demonstrates extensive plaque at the site of stone attachment. From [5], used with permission.

Figure 2 demonstrates another example of a single calcium oxalate stone attached to a region of plaque on a renal papillum (Fig. 2A). Exposed openings of inner medullary collecting ducts are evident following stone detachment (Fig. 2B).

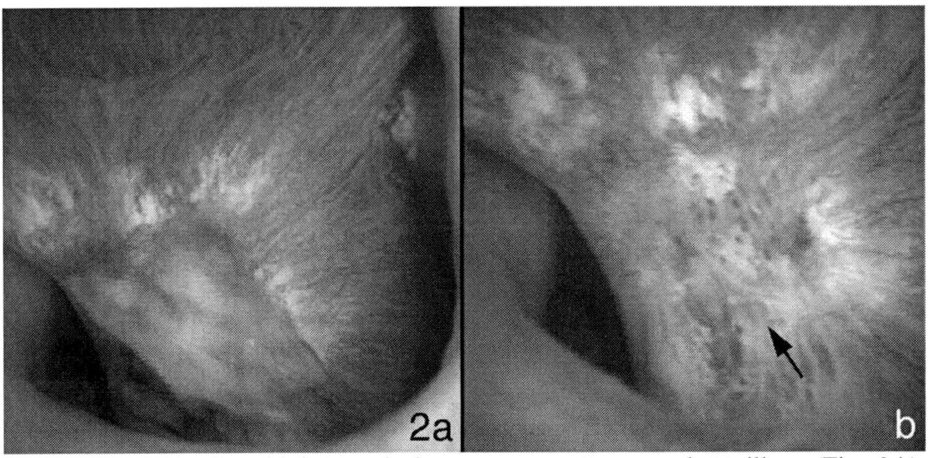

Removal of multiple attached stones on a compound papillum (Fig. 3A) reveals (Fig. 3B) underlying plaque with residual stone material.

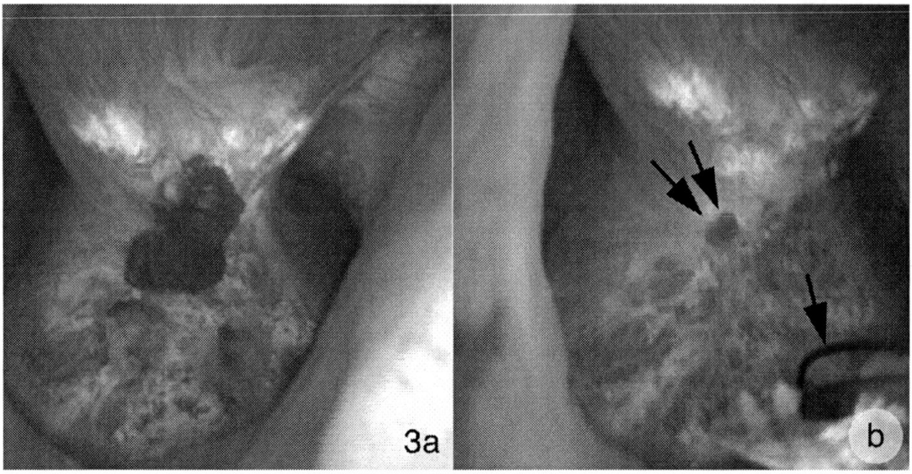

FIGURE 3. A. A compound papillum demonstrating multiple attached calcium oxalate stones. **B.** A stone is being removed from the papillum in Fig. 2A (arrow). A small calcium oxalate stone remains attaché at the site of plaque (double arrow). From [5], used with permission.

Attached calculi were observed in 11 of 23 patients (48%), which far exceeds the prevalence found by Randall (Table 1) in an unselected cadaveric population, confirming our hypothesis that the prevalence of attached renal calculi in an exclusively stone forming population would be greater than that encountered by Randall in an unselected population. Additionally, as only one kidney was examined for 22 of the 23 patients in the series and because in this study multiple stones on a single papillum were recorded as a single stone occurrence, the prevalence of attached stones in stone-forming patients is almost certain to be even higher. Furthermore, all of the stone-forming patients in the present study were seen to have Randall's plaque; indeed plaque was present in 91% of the papillae examined. The prevalence of plaque and attached stones in this population is consistent with the model of stone formation proposed by Randall [2]. Further supporting the hypothesis of a relationship between plaque and stone formation, Kim and associates have demonstrated in a cohort of calcium oxalate stone-formers that the amount of papillary plaque coverage of a renal papillum directly correlates with the number of stone events [6].

TABLE 1. Prevalence of papillary plaque and attached renal calculi ([5], used with permission)

	Matlaga et al.	**Randall et al.**
No. in Total Cohort	23	1,154
No. Individuals with Plaque (%) *	23 (100)	226 (19.6)
No. Individuals with Attached Stones (%) *	11 (48)	65 (5.6)
Mean Stones per Kidney (range)	2.1 (0-9)	Not Recorded

* Chi-square test $p<0.0001$.

Detailed analyses of spontaneously passed calculi also support a link between the development of an attached renal calculus and Randall's plaque. With the aid of scanning electron microscopy and x-ray dispersive elemental analysis, Cifuentes found that 63 of 87 passed calcium oxalate stones had evidence of plaque [7]. Observation of uncalcified tubular lumens found in conjunction with these plaques was presented as being consistent with an interstitial papillary tip origin of this material. These investigations suggest that the spontaneously passed calculi studied were likely to have been, at one time, attached to the renal papillum. Our observation of dilated duct openings at the base of a removed stone (Fig. 2B) is fully consistent with Cifuentes' finding of tubule remnants attached to the site of plaque on stones.

Based on the aforementioned evidence from Randall and Cifuentes, it may be reasonably hypothesized that attached renal calculi are calcium oxalate overgrowths on subepithelial interstitial papillary apatite plaque [2,7]. Since all plaque deposits we have studied to date reveal that apatite crystals are fully coated by organic matrix, it seems most likely that the interface between calcium oxalate and plaque will be the organic matrix and not a direct crystal to crystal attachment [8.9].

THE COMPOSITION OF ATTACHED RENAL CALCULI

The attached calcium oxalate stone is frequently encountered, as we observed this finding in almost half of our idiopathic stone forming patients. As best we can determine by visual endoscopy, the attachment site is Randall's plaque. The prevalence of the attached stone suggests that it may be a common early stage in the formation of calcium oxalate stones. The attached stone is intriguing, as it represents a moment in time when the forming calcium oxalate stone is still fixed to its hypothesized site of origin. As such, data that permit the further characterization of the attached stone are both unique and exceedingly valuable.

The introduction of Micro Computerized Tomography (CT) technology, a high resolution laboratory instrument that is capable of non-destructively distinguishing hydroxyapatite and calcium oxalate, has significantly advanced our efforts to define the structural and compositional make-up of renal calculi. Our first efforts to characterize the structural details of the attached renal calculus have centered on the investigation of papilla-attached stones with such a micro CT. Initially, we obtained these papilla-attached stones as surgical discards, the stones having been observed as attached to the renal papilla when removed during routine endourologic procedures. As before, all patients were idiopathic calcium oxalate stone formers, with cohort stones confirmed to be composed of calcium oxalate. In total, three stones were examined; two of which were removed during ureteroscopy, and one of which was removed during percutaneous nephrolithotomy. Stones were imaged in a Scanco Micro CT20 scanner, and mineral compositions were inferred from x-ray attenuation values. Mineral compositions were subsequently confirmed by infrared microspectrometry.

Micro CT of the stone in Fig. 4a demonstrated that the vast majority of the stone was of calcium oxalate composition, with the exception of the very tip of the stone, where the higher attenuation values correspond to that of apatite. The stone in Fig. 4b exhibits two distinct constituencies: calcium oxalate and apatite. The third stone examined, presented as Figure 4c, exhibited a different architectural appearance, but again, contained calcium oxalate and apatite interposed within the stone.

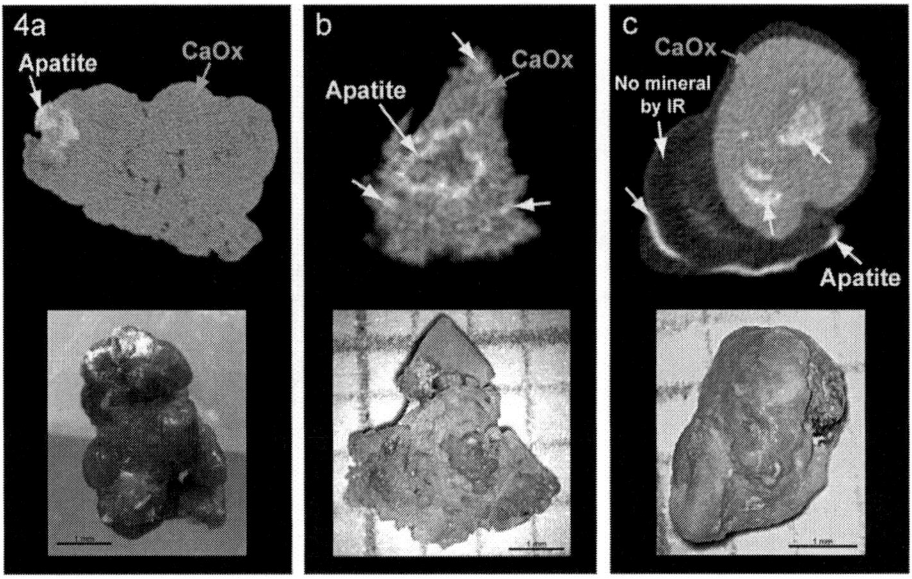

FIGURE 4. Papilla-attached renal stones. Photograph of stones (below), and micro CT image (above). Note regions of apatite intermingled with calcium oxalate, both within and at surface of stones.

It would be very tempting to ascribe the point of apatite as the definitive point by which the stones were attached to the renal papilla. However, critically, the orientation of the stones on the renal papilla before removal was not known with any certainty. Furthermore, the presence or absence of Randall's plaque on the renal papillae could also not be confirmed. Nonetheless, although it is not possible to infer any unassailable conclusions on the pathogenesis of these particular stones, and hypotheses concerning how the stones came to be attached to the papilla remain conjectures, the compositional arrangement of the stones are consistent with Randall's hypothesis.

CONCLUSIONS

Attached calcium oxalate stones are frequent and the attachment site appears to be Randall's plaque, as best we can determine by visual endoscopic evaluation. In our present work with idiopathic calcium oxalate stone-formers, the prevalence of attached renal calculi is significantly greater than that noted by Randall in his study of non-selected cadavers. Our finding that half of these calcium oxalate stone-formers harbored attached renal calculi supports the hypothesis that the attached stone is a common early stage in the formation of calcium oxalate stones. The compositional heterogeneity of the attached calcium oxalate stone can be complex, as evidenced by micro CT imaging. Nonetheless, the ultrastructure of these stones can be reconciled with Randall's hypothesis of kidney stone pathogenesis. Further work will be required to better define the nature of these earliest stages of calcium oxalate stone formation.

ACKNOWLEDGMENTS

This work was funded by United States National Institutes of Health grants P01DK56788 and R01DK59933.

REFERENCES

1. Hess, B., Kok, D.J.: Nucleation, growth, and aggregation of stone-forming crystals. In: *Kidney Stones: Medical and Surgical Management.* Edited by F. L. Coe, Favus, M.J., Pak, C.Y.C., Parks, J.H., Preminger, G.M. Philadelphia, Lippincott-Raven Publishers, 1996, pp. 3-32.
2. Randall, A.: Papillary pathology as a precursor of primary renal calculus. *J Urol*, 44, 580 (1940).
3. Low, R. K., Stoller, M. L.: Endoscopic mapping of renal papillae for Randall's plaques in patients with urinary stone disease. *J Urol*, 158, 2062 (1997).
4. Coe, F. L., Parks, J. H., Asplin, J. R.: The pathogenesis and treatment of kidney stones. *N Engl J Med*, 327, 1141, (1992).
5. Matlaga, B.R., Williams, J.C., Kim, S.C., Kuo, R.L., Evan, A.P., Bledsoe, S.B., *et al.* Endoscopic evidence of calculus attachment to Randall's plaque, *J Urol* 175, 1720 (2006).
6. Kim, S. C., Coe, F. L., Tinmouth, W. W., Kuo, R. L., Paterson, R. F., Parks, J. H. *et al.*: Stone formation is proportional to papillary surface coverage by Randall's plaque. *J Urol* 173, 117, (2005).
7. Cifuentes Delatte, L., Minon-Cifuentes, J. L., Medina, J. A.: Papillary stones: calcified renal tubules in Randall's plaques. *J Urol*, 133, 490, (1985).
8. Evan, A. P., Lingeman, J. E., Coe, F. L., Parks, J. H., Bledsoe, S. B., Shao, Y. *et al.*: Randall's plaque of patients with nephrolithiasis begins in basement membranes of thin loops of Henle. *J Clin Invest*, 111, 607, (2003).
9. Evan, A. P., Coe, F. L., Rittling, S. R., Bledsoe, S. M., Shao, Y., Lingeman, J. E. *et al.*: Apatite plaque particles in inner medulla of kidneys of calcium oxalate stone formers: osteopontin localization. *Kidney Int*, 68, 145, (2005).

The Role of the Papillary Epithelium in Stone Growth

Kristin J. Bergsland

Litholink Corporation, 2250 W. Campbell Park Drive, Chicago, IL 60612, USA

Abstract. The papillary surface epithelium (PSE) covers the renal papilla in mammalian kidneys and serves as a diffusion barrier between the urine on the apical surface and the interstitium on the basolateral surface. The PSE also plays a physiological role in transport of solutes between the urine and interstitium both by active transport and paracellular pathways. Permeability of the PSE may be affected by alterations in specific transporters, components of intercellular tight junctions, cell surface glycosaminoglycans and urine composition. In idiopathic calcium oxalate (CaOx) stone formers, apatite deposits known as Randall's plaque form in the papillary interstitium and lodge beneath the PSE. The presence of plaque may perturb the normal function of the PSE, possibly by provoking the up-regulation of pro-inflammatory cytokines such as TNFα in the interstitium. Disruption of the epithelial barrier may lead to increased permeability and exposure of the plaque matrix to urine constituents, followed by loss of the PSE and growth of CaOx stone over the plaque. To investigate the role of the PSE in stone development, new experimental systems are needed, including animal models of plaque formation as well as cell culture systems for papillary epithelial cells.

Keywords: renal papilla, epithelium, calcium, oxalate, calculi, plaque, permeability, barrier.
PACS: 87.19.Xx

INTRODUCTION

The role of the papillary epithelium in stone growth is neither well studied nor well understood. Hence, the purpose of this paper is threefold: 1) to summarize what is known about the papillary surface epithelium, 2) to suggest possible ways the PSE may be involved in stone formation, and 3) to point out directions for future research that may advance our understanding of how stones form.

STRUCTURE OF THE PAPILLARY SURFACE EPITHELIUM

In mammalian kidneys, the surface of the renal papilla is covered by simple cuboidal epithelium [1]. This single cell layer covers the papilla and lines the pelvic recesses [2]. It is distinct from the transitional epithelium (urothelium) that covers the outer surface of the pelvic space and the rest of the urinary tract, including the bladder, which has a more complex, stratified structure with three cell layers [3]. The simple papillary surface epithelium is a single layer of cells that is continuous with the lining of the collecting tubules, but has distinct morphology. Papillary collecting duct cells

CP900, *Renal Stone Disease, 1st Annual International Urolithiasis Research Symposium*, edited by A. P. Evan, J. E. Lingeman, and J. C. Williams, Jr.

are tall and columnar, transitioning to the more cuboidal PSE cells near the duct of Bellini openings at the papillary tip [4]. Microvilli are present on the apical surface of the PSE as is typical of many types of epithelial cells [3].

There is evidence that stone disease, especially the formation of idiopathic CaOx stones, involves the PSE. In CaOx stone formers, many stones are found attached to the renal papilla over regions of intra-papillary apatite crystal deposit known as Randall's plaque [5]. Evan and colleagues have investigated the origins of Randall's plaque in the papillary interstitium of CaOx stone patients [6]. Initially, apatite deposits form in the basement membranes of the loops of Henle; then, as extensive crystal deposits accumulate around the loops of Henle, they begin to spread into the nearby interstitial space, and eventually lodge under the PSE. Plaque under the papillary surface without stones is almost always covered by an intact epithelial layer without obvious cell damage [7]. It is thought that, ultimately, by some as yet unknown mechanism, the PSE proceeds to erode and exposes plaque matrix to urine, and this exposed plaque serves as a nucleation site for CaOx crystallization and stone formation [8]. Thus, an important question essential to understanding how stones form over plaque is how does the breach of the PSE occur, thereby breaking the barrier between the urine and the interstitial plaque matrix?

FUNCTIONS OF THE PAPILLARY SURFACE EPITHELIUM

Permeability Barrier

In order to address this question, it is useful to consider the structure and functions of the papillary epithelium. In general, the primary function of epithelia is to serve as a diffusion barrier between compartments of very different fluid and solute compositions [9]. Specifically, the PSE is exposed to pelvic urine on the apical surface and papillary interstitium on the basolateral surface. There are several elements to this barrier function. First, the epithelial cells themselves, with plasma membranes and highly specific membrane transport systems, form an obstacle to passage of molecules into the interstitium. Second, there is intercellular space between cells in the papillary surface epithelial layer that must be sealed to form an intact barrier. Tight junction (TJ) protein complexes sit like a bottleneck at the apical end of these spaces. The degree of dilation of the TJ pore can enhance or detract from the impermeability of the epithelium [10]. Third, on top of the apical membrane surface is a thin mucus or glycosaminoglycan layer that is thought to shield the cell surface from urinary solutes, proteins, bacteria and crystals [7,11]. These glycosaminoglycans (or GAGs), mainly heparan sulfate and chondroitin sulfate [12], are highly negatively charged, and have a high affinity to bind water. The bound layer of trapped water molecules acts to prevent adherence to the underlying cells [11]. All of these elements (transporters, TJs and GAGs) contain molecular targets that if altered could change the permeability state of the PSE.

Active Transport

In addition to its barrier function, the PSE also has a physiological role in transport of solutes between the urine and interstitium. This may involve both active, or transcellular, transport pathways and passive permeability, or paracellular, pathways through intercellular tight junctions. Several active transport pathways have been shown to function in the PSE. Potassium and proton transport occurs via H-K-ATPase at the apical surface, resulting in a net acid excretion that may play a role in inhibiting crystallization at the cell surface [13]. A Na-K-Cl co-transporter also located in the apical membrane, along with Na-K-ATPase in the basolateral membrane, could be important for stabilization of intracellular composition against rapid changes in apical osmolality [1,4]. Urea transport via urea transporter B (UT-B) is detected mainly in the basolateral membrane [14]. Urea permeability of the PSE is relatively low, and transport of urea across the PSE is unlikely to be a major source of urea to the interstitium. However, UT-B may be involved in regulation of cell volume during changes in interstitial urea concentration. Oxalate transport is also known to occur across both the apical and basolateral membranes [15]. The PSE shows a net uptake of oxalate which may be important in modulating local renal forniceal oxalate concentration or as a potential source of interstitial oxalate. The exact mechanism of PSE oxalate transport is not clear, but is likely to be anion exchange driven, probably by a sulfate/oxalate transporter similar to those described in proximal tubule and intestine [15,16]. Peter Aronson and others have studied a mouse knockout model of such an oxalate transporter, CFEX (SLC26A6), and found these mice to have a high frequency of CaOx urolithiasis due to severe hyperoxaluria [16,17].

Paracellular Transport

In contrast to active transport, paracellular transport is exclusively passive and is driven by electro-osmotic gradients [18]. It is mediated by TJs which form a selective barrier in the paracellular space that limits the movement of ions, solutes and water. TJs are formed by interweaving protein strands including occludin and members of the claudin family, a group of approximately 24 homologous proteins, each of which shows a unique tissue expression pattern [10,19]. Different epithelial types have different claudins, and different numbers of rows and levels of cross-bridging. This leads to variations in solute permeabilities, ion charge selectivity, and size discrimination differences between different epithelia. The TJ is a continuation of the cytoskeleton, and the TJ proteins are connected to actin filaments and other associated molecules. Changes in structural components of the TJ might be expected to alter the epithelial barrier properties. Claudins are key components of the TJ pore, and, in fact, mutations in some claudins are known to result in specific defects in electrolyte homeostasis. For example, in the kidney, claudin-16 (also called paracellin-1) is exclusively expressed in epithelial cells of the thick ascending limb of the loop of Henle, which is also the location of renal reabsorption of Mg^{2+} by paracellular flux. Mutations in claudin-16 have been identified in individuals with a familial syndrome of hypomagnesemia with hypercalciuria and nephrocalcinosis [20]. Symptoms include severe Mg^{2+} wasting, as well as kidney stones. At least eight other claudins are expressed in various locations in the kidney [19], and although their expression in the papillary epithelium is unclear, their potential role in regulating paracellular permeability and electrolyte homeostasis makes them interesting targets for study.

Physiological Regulation of Tight Junction Permeability

A number of signaling molecules have been implicated in regulating permeability of TJ structures. For example, the protein kinase C family and myosin light chain kinase, when activated, lead to opening of tight junctions [10]. TJ permeability can also be affected by pathological stimuli such as bacterial toxins, cytotoxic compounds, hypoxia, and certain cytokines, and generally the effect is to make the epithelial barrier leakier. The pro-inflammatory cytokine tumor necrosis factor alpha (TNFα) has been shown to cause barrier disruption in a number of epithelia through activation of myosin light chain kinase [21]. TNFα has been shown to induce apoptosis in intestinal epithelial cells, but also exerts apoptosis-independent direct effects on TJs of non-apoptotic cells [10]. The process by which TNFα perturbs a barrier can occur with just transient and mild disruptions to the barrier, and surprisingly little impairment. This is interesting to note, since the PSE layer covering Randall's plaque generally appears intact, without notable damage. Alternatively, apoptosis can occur, and even single cell apoptosis has been shown to cause a significant transepithelial leak in intestinal epithelial layers.

TNFα Signaling

TNFα is produced by a wide variety of cells including monocytes and macrophages, but is also produced by tubular epithelial cells in the renal medulla, where it plays an established role in the initiation or progression of tubulointerstitial damage [22,23]. Although monocytes and macrophages are not typically seen in the interstitium in regions with plaque, TNFα is expressed at a basal level in normal medullary tissue itself, and can be up-regulated in response to pro-inflammatory stimuli [23,24]. There is also evidence to suggest that hyperglycemia can induce TNFα production in the kidney, which is of interest given what is known about elevated blood glucose in people with hypercalciuria, and diabetes as a risk factor for stone formation [25,26]. In addition, basic calcium phosphate crystals in arthritic joints, which are similar in composition to the apatite in Randall's plaque, induce TNFα synthesis, and inhibition of this process with monoclonal antibodies to TNFα is currently used to treat rheumatoid arthritis [27,28]. Taken together, these data suggest that inhibition of TNFα signaling can restore normal epithelial barrier function [21], and that further research on the role of TNFα in the etiology of stone disease or as a possible therapeutic target might be worthwhile.

Protective Glycosaminoglycan Layer

Another important contributor to maintaining the integrity of the PSE is the cell surface glycosaminoglycan layer. Loss or reduced function of these molecules can lead to loss of the anti-adherence and impermeability properties of the papillary epithelium [12]. In experiments with bladder epithelium, treatment with dilute acid or detergent to remove the GAG layer resulted in increased permeability and microcrystal adherence to the cell surface. However, addition of exogenous GAGs such as heparin and pentosan polysulfate restored anti-adherence activity [29]. In fact, such molecules are given as "GAG replacement therapy" to patients with interstitial cystitis, a disease of the bladder urothelium in which the GAG layer is lost or damaged, resulting in epithelial leakage [30]. Possible causes for GAG deficiency in the PSE include: reduced synthesis of GAGs, reduced sulfation of the polysaccharides, chronic neutralization of the anionic surface charge due to cationic urine protein or crystal binding, presence of a GAG-inactivating substance in urine such as quaternary amines, or dysfunction of other urine macromolecules such as Tamm-Horsfall protein that would normally bind to and sequester toxic cations or crystals [11,31].

A MODEL FOR THE ROLE OF THE PSE IN STONE GROWTH

All together, this information suggests that the role of the papillary epithelium in stone growth is likely to be related to disturbance of its function as a diffusion barrier between the urine and the interstitium. One possible model is similar to a model of intestinal permeability in inflammatory bowel disease [21]. Pathophysiological factors described above may perturb the normal pathways that regulate epithelial permeability, resulting in barrier dysfunction of the PSE that may trigger a breach in the epithelium. This would allow urinary solutes to migrate into the interstitium and to contact underlying Randall's plaque matrix. Overgrowth of CaOx on the plaque may then occur. Barrier disruption and increased permeability may create a vicious cycle in which continued leakage stimulates a pro-inflammatory response that can in turn promote further leakiness and, ultimately, loss of epithelial cells and progression of stone growth.

SUMMARY

In summary, the effect of disease processes on epithelial barriers is almost always to make them leakier, and this is true in a diverse range of disease states including chronic inflammatory diseases, diabetes, microbial infections, cancer and interstitial cystitis [10]. The renal papillary epithelium is perhaps unusual among epithelia in that it is potentially subject to disturbance from both the apical and basolateral sides. From above, increased PSE permeability could result from changes in the form or function of specific transporters, TJs, the GAG layer, or in urine composition (concentrations of toxins, proteins, crystals and inhibitors). Alternatively, from beneath, the presence of Randall's plaque could provoke the up-regulation of pro-inflammatory cytokines. In any case, disruption of the epithelial barrier may lead to exposure of the plaque matrix to urine, loss of the PSE and growth of CaOx stone over the plaque. The exact role of these elements in modulating permeability of the PSE, and the contribution of the PSE to the development of stone disease are unclear, but merit further investigation.

FUTURE RESEARCH

The proposed model is highly speculative, and there is a great need for experimental systems for studying the PSE, both *in vivo* and *in vitro*. Animal models of plaque formation are needed, as well as cell culture systems for papillary epithelial cells. In this regard, the laboratory of Hari Koul at the University of Colorado has made some progress in culturing human papillary epithelial cells which they reported at the meeting of the R.O.C.K. (Research On Calculus Kinetics) Society in June 2006. There are many questions to be asked and few answers at this point, but clearly this is a ripe area for future research.

ACKNOWLEDGMENTS

The author thanks Fred Coe for helpful discussions.

REFERENCES

1. R.K. Packer, J.M. Sands and M.A. Knepper, *Am. J. Physiol. Renal Physiol.* **257**, F218-F224 (1989).
2. P.S. Chandhoke, R.K. Packer and M.A. Knepper, *Am. J. Physiol. Renal Physiol.* **258**, F893-F899 (1990).
3. R. Romih, P. Korošec, W. de Mello Jr. and K. Jezernik, *Cell Tissue Res.* **320**, 259-268 (2005).
4. J.M. Sands, M.A. Knepper and K.R. Spring, *Am. J. Physiol. Renal Physiol.* **251**, F475-F484 (1986).
5. B.R. Matlaga, J.C. Williams Jr., S.C. Kim, R.L. Kuo, A.P. Evan, S.B. Bledsoe, F.L. Coe, E.M. Worcester, L.C. Munch and J.E. Lingeman, *J. Urol.*. **175**, 1720-1724 (2006).
6. A.P. Evan, J.E. Lingeman, F.L. Coe, J.H. Parks, S.B. Bledsoe, Y. Shao, A.J. Sommer, R.F. Paterson, R.L. Kuo and M. Grynpas, *J. Clin. Invest.* **111**, 607-616 (2003).
7. A.P. Evan, J.E. Lingeman, F.L. Coe and E.M. Worcester, *Kidney Int.* **69**, 1313-1318 (2006).
8. F.L. Coe, "Stone Disease: a Prelude" in First Annual International Urolithiasis Research Symposium, Conference Proceedings, 2007, pp. 3-11.
9. E.E. Schneeberger and R.D. Lynch, *Am. J. Physiol. Cell Physiol.* **286**, C1213-C1228 (2004).
10. J.M. Mullin, N. Agostino, E. Rendon-Huerta and J.J. Thornton, *Drug Discov. Today* **10**, 395-408 (2005).
11. C.L. Parsons, *World J. Urol.* **12**, 38-42 (1994).
12. R.E. Hurst, *World J. Urol.* **12**, 3-10 (1994).
13. J.W. Verlander, R.M. Moudy, W.G. Campbell, B.D. Cain and C.S. Wingo, *Am. J. Physiol. Renal Physiol.* **281**, F357-F365 (2001).
14. J.-Y. Jung, K.M. Madsen, K.-H. Han, C.-W. Yang, M.A. Knepper, J.M. Sands and J. Kim, *Am. J. Physiol. Renal Physiol.* **285**, F1210-F1224 (2003).
15. P.S. Chandhoke and J. Fan, *J. Urol.* **164**, 1724-1728 (2000).
16. Z. Jiang, J.R. Asplin, A.P. Evan, V.M. Rajendran, H. Velazquez, T.P. Nottoli, H.J. Binder and P.S. Aronson, *Nat. Genet.* **38**, 474-478 (2006).

17. P.S. Aronson, "Pathogenesis of Hyperoxaluria in Mutant Mice Lacking the Anion Transporter SLC26A6" in First Annual International Urolithiasis Research Symposium, Conference Proceedings, 2007, pp. 141-148.
18. C.M. Van Itallie and J.M. Anderson, *Physiology* **19**, 331-338 (2004).
19. M. Furuse and S. Tsukita, *Trends Cell Biol.* **16**, 181-188 (2006).
20. D.B. Simon, Y. Lu, K.A. Choate, H. Velazquez, E. Al-Sabban, M. Praga, G. Casari, A. Bettinelli, G. Colussi, J. Rodriguez-Soriano, D. McCredie, D. Milford, S. Sanjad and R.P. Lifton, *Science.* **285**, 103-106 (1999).
21. D.R. Clayburgh, L. Shen and J.R. Turner, *Lab Invest.* **84**, 282-291 (2004).
22. M. Ruiz-Ortega, M. Ruperez, O. Lorenzo, V. Esteban, J. Blanco, S. Mezzano and J. Egido, *Kidney Int. Suppl.* **82**, 12-22 (2002).
23. S.B. Khan, H.T. Cook, G. Bhangal, J. Smith, F.W.K. Tam and C.D. Pusey, *Kidney Int.* **67**, 1812-1820 (2005).
24. C. von Schnakenburg, J. Strehlau, J.H.H. Ehrich and A. Melk, *Nephrol. Dial. Transplant.* **17**, 573-579 (2002).
25. K. Kalantarinia, A.S. Awad and H.M. Siragy, *Kidney Int.* **64**, 1208-1213 (2003).
26. F.L. Coe, personal communication.
27. E.S. Molloy and G.M. McCarthy, *Curr. Opin. Rheumatol.* **18**, 187-192 (2006).
28. M. Feldmann, *Nat. Rev. Immunol.* **2**, 364-371 (2002).
29. C.L. Parsons, C. Stauffer and J.D. Schmidt, *Science* **208**, 605-607 (1980).
30. V.R. Anderson and C.M. Perry, *Drugs* **66**, 821-835 (2006).
31. V. Kumar, L. Peña de la Vega, G. Farell and J.C. Lieske, *Kidney Int.* **68**, 1784-1792 (2005).

Renal Medullary Interstitial Cells

Reena Rao, Chuan-Ming Hao, and Matthew D. Breyer

Division of Nephrology, Department of Medicine, Vanderbilt University Medical School, S-3223 Medical Center North, Nashville, TN 37232-2372, USA

Abstract. Renal medullary interstitial cells (RMICs) are specialized fibroblast-like cells that reside in the renal medulla among the vasa recta, the thin limbs of Henle's loop, and medullary collecting ducts. These cells are characterized by abundant lipid droplets in the cytoplasm. The lipid droplets are composed of triglycerides, cholesterol esters and free long-chain fatty acids, including arachidonic acid. RMICs are also a major site of cyclooxygenase2 (COX-2) expression, and thus a major site of COX-2 derived prostanoid biosynthesis. RMICs are also a potential target of hormones such as angiotensin II and endothelin. The RMIC COX-2 expression and the abundance of lipid droplets change with salt and water intake. These properties of RMICs are consistent with an important role of these cells in modulating physiologic and pathologic processes of the kidney.

Keywords: arachidonic acid, cyclooxygenase, blood pressure regulation
PACS: 87.17.–d

INTRODUCTION

The medullary interstitium of the kidney contains a very unique and relatively poorly studied cell type, designated the renal medullary interstitial cell (RMIC). These cells are present throughout the inner medulla and the inner stripe of the outer medulla. They have been described as the prominent lipid-laden type-1 medullary interstitial cells. by several investigators in humans [1], mouse [2], rat [3], and rabbit [4,5]. RMICs have long cytoplasmic projections, which give them a stellate appearance, and a single cell may be in contact with several vessels and collecting ducts by virtue of these long cytoplasmic processes [6]. They are often found arranged in rows between loops of Henle and the vasa recta, with their long axis perpendicular to that of adjacent tubules and vessels, resembling the rungs of a ladder [6].

MORPHOLOGY OF RENAL MEDULLARY INTERSTITIAL CELLS

The cells contain large amounts of rough endoplasmic reticulum (ER) that is often continuous with elements of the smooth cytoplasmic membranes. Mitochondria are sparse and scattered randomly in the cytoplasm. A small number of lysosomes are present, but endocytic vacuoles are sparse, although interstitial cells are capable of endocytosis of particulate material. An unusual type of cylindrical body, measuring

CP900, *Renal Stone Disease, 1st Annual International Urolithiasis Research Symposium*, edited by A. P. Evan, J. E. Lingeman, and J. C. Williams, Jr.

0.1-0.2 μm in diameter, believed to be derived from the ER, has been described in the RMICs [7,8]. These structures were observed originally in dehydrated rats and believed to represent a response to severe dehydration [7], though subsequent studies have shown their presence under normal conditions [8]. The walls of the cylinders consist of triple layered membranes and these have been observed to be connected to the ER. Their functional significance remains unknown.

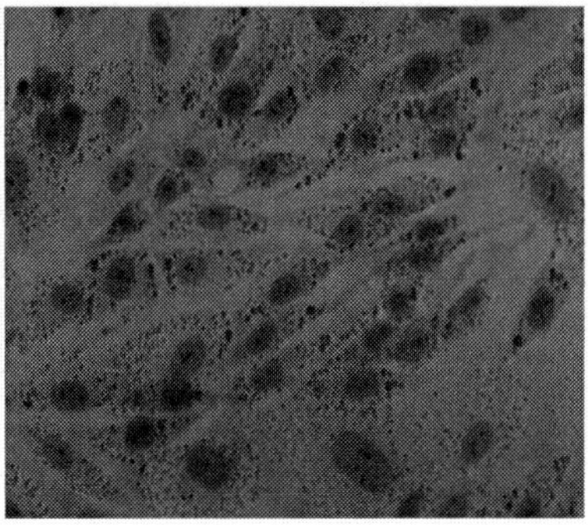

FIGURE 1. Renal medullary interstitial cells, showing intracellular lipid droplets (oil red O stain).

Lipid Droplets

RMICs are characterized by numerous lipid inclusions or droplets in the cytoplasm (Fig. 1), that have long puzzled investigators. The droplets were reported to have a homogeneous content of triglycerides, cholesterol esters and free long-chain fatty acids [9] and surrounded by whorls of cyto-membrane, rather than a limiting membrane [3,6,10]. The droplet/nucleus ratio in RMICs demonstrates a considerable variation in relation to change in water and salt balance and they seem to readily empty under certain conditions like diuresis [11]. Hence, the cells were considered to be secretory in nature and the lipid droplets were expected to contain substances that might play a physiological role in the functioning of the kidney. Similarly, the number and size of the lipid inclusions in RMICs vary considerably, depending on the physiological state of the animal [11,12] and the species [13]. In the rat, lipid droplets constitute 2% to 4% of the interstitial cell volume and the volume depends largely on the physiologic state of the animals [14], The lipid droplets were originally reported to increase in number following a brief period of salt repletion in salt depleted rats [12] and decrease in both size and number after 24 h of dehydration [11].

FUNCTION OF RENAL MEDULLARY INTERSTITIAL CELLS

The function of the RMICs is remains unclear. Accumulating evidence suggest that RMICs could be actively involved in many processes including organogenesis, tumorigenesis, fibrosis, pathological sclerosis and maintenance of normal homeostasis [15-19]. The close proximity of these cells with the tubules and capillaries also suggests a possible interaction between these structures.

RMICs As Secretory Cells

The presence of a well developed ER and lipid droplets suggest a secretory nature for these cells. Muehrcke *et al.* suggested that the interstitial cells might possess a secretory function, and it was emphasized that both erythropoietin and an antihypertensive factor seemed to originate in the renal medulla. It was also suggested that the differences found in the number of lipid droplets in the interstitial cells of the renal papilla during salt depletion and salt repletion could be the result of the lipid droplets containing physiologically active substances, which were accumulated during salt depletion and were released during salt repletion [20]. Nissin showed that the prostaglandin precursor, arachidonic acid, constitutes a significant fraction of the triglyceride long-chain fatty acids in the lipid droplets found in the RMICs [21]. Later investigators established RMICs in cell culture, reproducing the natural characteristics of these cells *in vitro*. This enabled investigators to narrow down the metabolites produced by the RMICs to prostaglandins, including PGE2, PGI2, PGF2 and thromboxane A2 (TxA2).

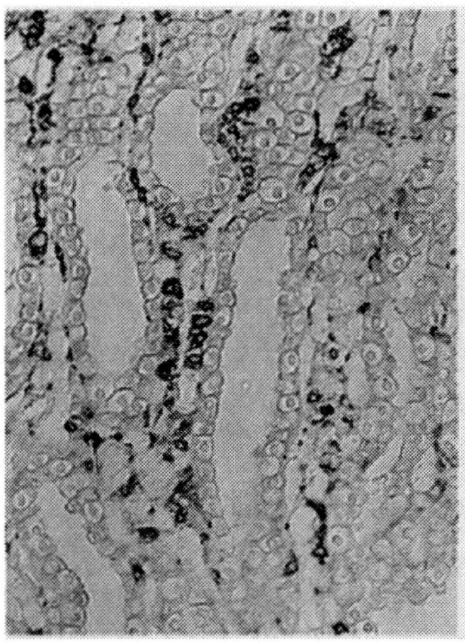

FIGURE 2. COX-2 immunostaining of renal medullary interstitial cells.

The renal medulla is a major site of prostaglandin synthesis and abundant COX-1 and COX-2 expression [22,23]. The enzymatic activity of COX mediates the initial step in the metabolism of arachidonic acid to the prostanoids. Arachidonate is converted to PGH2, which is subsequently metabolized to more stable biologically active prostanoids, including PGE2, PGI2, PGF2a, PGD2 and TxA2, by distinct synthases. The two COX isoforms exhibit differential compartmentalization within the medulla, with COX-1 predominating in the medullary collecting ducts and COX-2 in the renal medullary interstitial cells (Fig. 2) [24-27]. Dynamic regulation of medullary COX-2 expression is an important component of the renal response to physiological stress, including water deprivation and lipopolysaccharides [25]. After dehydration, renal medullary COX-2 mRNA and protein expression are significantly induced primarily in renal medullary interstitial cells [25]. In contrast, COX-1 expression in the mouse kidney is unaffected by water deprivation. Although hormonal factors may also contribute to COX-2 induction, shifting RMICs to hypertonic media (by the addition of NaCl or mannitol) is sufficient to directly induce COX-2 expression.

Regulation of Renal Blood Pressure

RMICs might have an endocrine antihypertensive function [28]. Muirhead and co-workers demonstrated that transplantation of renal papillary tissue [29,30] and cultured RMICs [28] into hypertensive animals was followed by a reduction in blood pressure [31,32] and subsequently reported the source of these antihypertensive lipid substances as RMICs [33]. Muirhead described a feedback blood-pressure control system operating from the renal medulla called the medullipin system. In contrast to the renin-angiotensin system, which upregulates pressure, the medullipin system downregulates blood pressure. His studies indicated that a rise in arterial pressure stimulates secretion of medullipin I, which circulates to the liver, where it is converted to the active hormone, medullipin II, by a P-450 cytochrome oxidase pathway. This results in reduction of arterial pressure with an increase in the urinary excretion of sodium and water coupled with systemic arterial vasodilation by medullipin II [34-38]. A deficiency of medullipin could lead to hypertensive states similar to that observed following loss of renomedullary interstitial cells by bilateral nephrectomy, renal surgical papillectomy, chemical papillectomy, papillary atrophy or necrosis, or a decrease in number and/or damage to renomedullary interstitial cells in accelerated experimental hypertension and malignant hypertension of humans and dysfunction of renomedullary interstitial cells, as mediated by angiotensin II [39].

Other studies suggest that angiotensin II may regulate prostaglandin production in the renal medulla. Investigators have demonstrated angiotensin receptors in cultured RMICs [40] and prostaglandin biosynthesis is stimulated by angiotensin. The presence of an angiotensinase that is capable of degrading angiotensin in the type-1 renomedullary interstitial cells was also reported in rodents [41], which could be yet another mechanism of regulation of the prostaglandin production by angiotensin in the renal medulla.

Regulation of Renal Blood Flow and Salt Absorption

Medullary interstitial cells, being a major source of renal prostaglandin synthesis, also play an important role in modulating renal medullary blood flow and salt absorption. The RMICs, which are interposed between the vasa recta, loops of Henle and collecting ducts, appear to play an important role in regulating salt absorption and renal medullary blood flow.

The precise identity of the substances elaborated by RMICs which are involved in regulation of salt absorption and renal medullary blood flow remain incompletely characterized; however, PGE2 was identified as an important component of this activity [42]. In the context of the current knowledge, COX-2 would appear to be a critical source for PGE2 and possibly other vasodepressors derived from RMICs as well. A high-salt diet markedly increases medullary COX-2 expression, both *in vivo*

[43] and *in vitro*, where increased extracellular salt potently augments RMIC COX-2 expression [44]. Yang *et al.* reported that a high salt diet increases renal medullary COX-2 expression. Selective renal medullary COX-2 inhibition via an intramedullary catheter is associated with increase in systemic blood pressure following a high salt diet, consistent with a critical role of renal medullary COX-2 in modulating blood pressure [43]. Our unpublished data also indicate that intramedullary infusion of PGE2 increases urine volume and urine sodium output. When considered with studies showing that COX-2 inhibition reduces urine salt excretion and the findings of the hypertensive effects of intramedullary COX-2 inhibition, a physiological feedback system can be constructed whereby increased salt intake augments RMIC COX-2 expression and prostaglandin production, thereby promoting increased renal salt excretion. Whether this system also includes elaboration of a renal medullary COX-2 dependent systemic vasodepressor activity remains to be clarified. The identity of these antihypertensive products and the receptors controlling the tone of vascular tissue and promoting renal salt excretion remains to be established.

Several mechanisms contribute to enhanced salt retention with non-steroidal anti-inflammatory drug (NSAID) use, including effects on glomerular hemodynamics, renal epithelial salt absorption, and medullary blood flow. Maintenance of adequate renal medullary blood flow and interstitial pressure is critical. Renal medullary interstitial pressure is positively correlated with medullary blood flow (MBF), and is a potent regulator of sodium and water reabsorption [45]. Selectively increasing renal medullary blood flow by local infusion of the vasodilator, bradykinin, into the renal medulla significantly decreased sodium excretion [46]; conversely, decreasing renal medullary blood flow markedly increased sodium excretion [45,47]. Chronic infusion of captopril into the renal medullary interstitial space increased medullary blood flow in the spontaneously hypertensive rat by 40%, reduced mean arterial pressure by 20 mmHg, and produced net sodium loss [48]. These data support a critical role for the renal medulla in maintaining blood pressure and, by implication, an important role for interstitial cells in the renal medulla.

Survival of RMICS in the Renal Medullary Environment

The ability of the kidney to generate a medullary interstitial tonicity exceeding 1000-3000 mOsm/kg is critical for the generation of concentrated urine. Cells residing in this harsh environment must not only survive rapid changes in sodium chloride and urea concentration associated with changing states of hydration, but also function normally. This, of course, applies to renal medullary interstitial cells, which must not only survive but also function normally in the hypertonic environment that is normally present and critical to the production of concentrated urine. Hyperosmotic stress produces profound cellular responses, including activation of signaling cascades critical for both cell death and the promotion of cell survival. Several mechanisms have been proposed as to how RMICs adapt to the hypertonic stress, including accumulation of organic osmolytes [2,49,50], and induction of heat shock proteins [51,52]. Our recent studies suggest that COX-2 is also involved in the adaptation mechanism of renal medullary interstitial cells exposed to hypertonic stress *in vitro* or following water deprivation *in vivo* [4,22]. COX-2-selective inhibitors cause RMICs to die when exposed to otherwise non-lethal hypertonic stress [18,53]. These results may also account for the finding that RMICs are an early site of papillary injury caused by COX-inhibiting analgesics and NSAIDs [19]. Studies also show that damage of renal interstitial cells, as happens after the use of NSAIDs or other papillotoxins, may lead to degenerative changes in the other structures in the kidney including capillaries, loops of Henle, and collecting ducts [54]. Since chronic ingestion of large amounts of cyclooxygenase-inhibiting NSAIDs has been implicated in renal disease, an important role for renal prostaglandins in the maintenance of interstitial survival has been suggested [22,44].

Role in Maintaining Normal Structure

The RMICs also probably provide structural support in the medulla because of their special ladder-like arrangement that is perpendicular to the tubules and vessels. By virtue of their anatomic location and arrangement, RMICs may hinder axial dissipation of the concentration gradient, thereby aiding urinary concentration. A more active role in urinary concentration has been postulated on the basis of speculations about RMIC contractile potential. Vasopressin and endothelin can reduce RMIC surface area and increase F-actin microfilament staining, demonstrating that RMICs in culture are contractile. The possibility has been raised that contraction of RMICs plays a role in modifying urinary concentration as well as regulation of other renal medullary functions [55].

SUMMARY

Accumulating evidence suggests that renal medullary interstitial cells play an important role in maintaining functional and structural integrity of the normal kidney. Substantial evidence indicates that RMICs are involved in regulation of systemic blood pressure, renal medullary blood flow, and renal sodium excretion. However, the potential role of these cells in kidney stone formation and other physiological aspects remains to be further elucidated, partially due to the limited research approach to these cells. Further research on these cells should provide valuable information in the understanding the physiology and pathophysiology of the kidney.

ACKNOWLEDGMENTS

The authors acknowledge a beginning grant-in-aid from the American Heart Association to R. Rao and DK071876 to C.-M. Hao.

REFERENCES

1. Bulger RE, Tisher CC, Myers CH, et al.: Human renal ultrastructure. II. The thin limb of Henle's loop and the interstitium in healthy individuals. *Lab Invest* 16:124-141, 1967

2. Moeckel GW, Zhang L, Fogo AB, et al.: COX-2 activity promotes organic osmolyte accumulation and adaptation of renal medullary interstitial cells to hypertonic stress. *J Biol Chem* 278:19352-19357, 2003
3. Bulger RE, Trump BF: Fine structure of the rat renal papilla. *Am J Anat* 118:685-721, 1966
4. Hao CM, Komhoff M, Guan Y, et al.: Selective targeting of cyclooxygenase-2 reveals its role in renal medullary interstitial cell survival. *Am J Physiol* 277:F352-359., 1999
5. Rao R, Hao CM, Breyer MD: Hypertonic stress activates glycogen synthase kinase 3beta-mediated apoptosis of renal medullary interstitial cells, suppressing an NFkappaB-driven cyclooxygenase-2-dependent survival pathway. *J Biol Chem* 279:3949-3955, 2004
6. Bohman SO: The ultrastructure of the rat renal medulla as observed after improved fixation methods. *J Ultrastruct Res* 47:329-360, 1974
7. Bulger RE, Griffith LD, Trump BF: Endoplasmic reticulum in rat renal interstitial cells: molecular rearrangement after water deprivation. *Science* 151:83-86, 1966
8. Ledingham JM, Simpson FO: Bundles of intracellular tubules in renal medullary interstitial cells. *J Cell Biol* 57:594-598, 1973
9. Nissen HM: On lipid droplets in renal interstitial cells. I. A histochemical study. *Z Zellforsch Mikrosk Anat* 83:76-81, 1967
10. Osvaldo L, Latta H: Interstitial cells of the renal medulla. *J Ultrastruct Res* 15:589-613, 1966
11. Nissen HM: On lipid droplets in renal interstitial cells. 3. A histological study on the number of droplets during hydration and dehydration. *Z Zellforsch Mikrosk Anat* 92:52-61, 1968
12. Nissen HM: On lipid droplets in renal interstitial cells. II. A histological study on the number of droplets in salt depletion and acute salt repletion. *Z Zellforsch Mikrosk Anat* 85:483-491, 1968
13. Bohman SO, Jensen PK: The interstitial cells in the renal medulla of rat, rabbit, and gerbil in different states of diuresis. *Cell Tissue Res* 189:1-18, 1978
14. Bohman SO, Jensen PK: Morphometric studies on the lipid droplets of the interstitial cells of the renal medulla in different states of diuresis. *J Ultrastruct Res* 55:182-192, 1976
15. Hayward SW: Approaches to modeling stromal-epithelial interactions. *J Urol* 168:1165-1172, 2002
16. Liotta LA, Kohn EC: The microenvironment of the tumour-host interface. *Nature* 411:375-379, 2001
17. Nishikawa M, Tahara T, Hinohara A, et al.: Role of the microenvironment of the embryonic aorta-gonad-mesonephros region in hematopoiesis. *Ann N Y Acad Sci* 938:109-116, 2001
18. Pupa SM, Menard S, Forti S, et al.: New insights into the role of extracellular matrix during tumor onset and progression. *J Cell Physiol* 192:259-267, 2002
19. Silberstein GB: Tumour-stromal interactions. Role of the stroma in mammary development. *Breast Cancer Res* 3:218-223, 2001
20. Muehrcke RC, Mandal AK, Epstein M, et al.: Cytoplasmic granularity of the renal medullary interstitial cells in experimental hypertension. *J Lab Clin Med* 73:299-308, 1969
21. Nissen HM, Bojesen I: On lipid droplets in renal interstitial cells. IV. Isolation and identification. *Z Zellforsch Mikrosk Anat* 97:274-284, 1969
22. Hao CM, Redha R, Morrow J, et al.: Peroxisome proliferator-activated receptor delta activation promotes cell survival following hypertonic stress. *J Biol Chem* 277:21341-21345., 2002
23. Komhoff M, Wang JL, Cheng HF, et al.: Cyclooxygenase-2-selective inhibitors impair glomerulogenesis and renal cortical development. *Kidney Int* 57:414-422, 2000
24. Guan Y, Breyer MD: Peroxisome proliferator-activated receptors (PPARs): novel therapeutic targets in renal disease. *Kidney Int* 60:14-30, 2001
25. O'Banion MK, Winn VD, Young DA: cDNA cloning and functional activity of a glucocorticoid-regulated inflammatory cyclooxygenase. *Proc Natl Acad Sci U S A* 89:4888-4892, 1992
26. Qi Z, Hao CM, Langenbach RI, et al.: Opposite effects of cyclooxygenase-1 and -2 activity on the pressor response to angiotensin II. *J Clin Invest* 110:61-69, 2002
27. Smith WL, Langenbach R: Why there are two cyclooxygenase isozymes. *J Clin Invest* 107:1491-1495, 2001
28. Muirhead EE, Germain GS, Armstrong FB, et al.: Endocrine-type antihypertensive function of renomedullary interstitial cells. *Kidney Int* Suppl:S271-282, 1975

29. Muirhead EE, Brooks B, Pitcock JA, et al.: Renomedullary antihypertensive function in accelerated (malignant) hypertension. Observations on renomedullary interstitial cells. *J Clin Invest* 51:181-190, 1972
30. Muirhead EE, Brooks B, Pitcock JA, et al.: Role of the renal medulla in the sodium-sensitive component of renoprival hypertension. *Lab Invest* 27:192-198, 1972
31. Cowley AW, Jr.: Franz Volhard Lecture. Evolution of the medullipin concept of blood pressure control: a tribute to Eric Muirhead. *J Hypertens* Suppl 12:S25-34, 1994
32. Muirhead EE, Pitcock JA: The renal antihypertensive hormone. *J Hypertens* 3:1-8, 1985
33. Muirhead EE, Rightsel WA, Leach BE, et al.: Reversal of hypertension by transplants and lipid extracts of cultured renomedullary interstitial cells. *Lab Invest* 36:162-172, 1977
34. Muirhead EE: The renomedullary system of blood pressure control. *Am J Med Sci* 295:231-233, 1988
35. Muirhead EE: The medullipin system of blood pressure control. *Am J Hypertens* 4:556S-568S, 1991
36. Muirhead EE, Brooks B, Byers LW, et al.: Medullipin system. Generation of medullipin II by isolated kidney-liver perfusion. *Hypertension* 18:III158-163, 1991
37. Muirhead EE, Brooks B, Byers LW, et al.: Secretion of medullipin I by isolated kidneys perfused under elevated pressure. *Clin Exp Pharmacol Physiol* 18:409-417, 1991
38. Muirhead EE, Brooks B, Byers LW, et al.: Antihypertensive action of medullipin I given by mouth. *Hypertension* 17:1092-1096, 1991
39. Muirhead EE: Renal vasodepressor mechanisms: the medullipin system. *J Hypertens* Suppl 11:S53-58, 1993
40. Brown CA, Zusman RM, Haber E: Identification of an angiotensin receptor in rabbit renomedullary interstitial cells in tissue culture. Correlation with prostaglandin biosynthesis. *Circ Res* 46:802-807, 1980
41. Kugler P: Angiotensinase A in the renomedullary interstitial cells. *Histochemistry* 77:105-115, 1983
42. Daniels EG, Hinman JW, Leach BE, et al.: Identification of prostaglandin E2 as the principal vasodepressor lipid of rabbit renal medulla. *Nature* 215:1298-1299, 1967
43. Yang T, Singh I, Pham H, et al.: Regulation of cyclooxygenase expression in the kidney by dietary salt intake. *Am J Physiol* 274:F481-489, 1998
44. Hao CM, Yull F, Blackwell T, et al.: Dehydration activates an NF-kappaB-driven, COX-2-dependent survival mechanism in renal medullary interstitial cells. *J Clin Invest* 106:973-982, 2000
45. Cowley AW, Jr., Mattson DL, Lu S, et al.: The renal medulla and hypertension. *Hypertension* 25:663-673, 1995
46. Mattson DL, Cowley AW, Jr.: Kinin actions on renal papillary blood flow and sodium excretion. *Hypertension* 21:961-965, 1993
47. Cowley AW, Jr.: Control of the renal medullary circulation by vasopressin V1 and V2 receptors in the rat. *Exp Physiol* 85 Spec No:223S-231S, 2000
48. Lu S, Mattson DL, Cowley AW, Jr.: Renal medullary captopril delivery lowers blood pressure in spontaneously hypertensive rats. *Hypertension* 23:337-345, 1994
49. Burg MB: Renal osmoregulatory transport of compatible organic osmolytes. *Curr Opin Nephrol Hypertens* 6:430-433., 1997
50. Garcia-Perez A, Burg MB: Renal medullary organic osmolytes. Physiol Rev 71:1081-1115., 1991
51. Cohen DM, Wasserman JC, Gullans SR: Immediate early gene and HSP70 expression in hyperosmotic stress in MDCK cells. *Am J Physiol* 261:C594-601., 1991
52. Neuhofer W, Muller E, Burger-Kentischer A, et al.: Hypertonicity affects heat shock protein 27 and F-actin localization in Madin-Darby canine kidney cells. *Kidney Int* Suppl 67:S165-167., 1998
53. Nishimura G, Yanoma S, Mizuno H, et al.: A selective cyclooxygenase-2 inhibitor suppresses tumor growth in nude mouse xenografted with human head and neck squamous carcinoma cells. *Jpn J Cancer Res* 90:1152-1162., 1999
54. Bach PH, Nguyen TK: Renal papillary necrosis--40 years on. *Toxicol Pathol* 26:73-91, 1998
55. Hughes AK, Barry WH, Kohan DE: Identification of a contractile function for renal medullary interstitial cells. *J Clin Invest* 96:411-416, 1995

Hyaluronan in Tubular and Interstitial Nephrocalcinosis

Carl F. Verkoelen

Department of Urology, Erasmus Medical Center, Rotterdam, The Netherlands

Abstract. Hyaluronan (HA) is the major glycosaminoglycan (GAG) component of the renal medullary interstitium. HA is extremely large (up to 104 kDa) and composed of thousands repeating disaccharides of glucuronic acid (GlcUA) and N-acetylglucosamine (GlcNAc). HA is synthesized by hyaluronan synthases (HASs) and degraded by hyaluronidases (Hyals). The production of HA by renomedullary interstitial cells is mediated by local osmolality. When excess water needs to be excreted, increased interstitial HA seems to antagonize water reabsorption, while the opposite occurs during water conservation. Hence, papillary interstitial HA is low and Hyal high during anti-diuresis, whereas during diuresis HA is high and Hyal low. The polyanion HA plays a role in the reabsorption of hypotonic fluid by immobilizing cations (Na^+) via the carboxylate (COO^-) groups of GlcUA. The binding of Ca^{2+} to anionic HA is probably also responsible for the fact that the papilla does not become a stone despite the extremely high interstitial phosphate and oxalate. HA is also an excellent crystal binding molecule. The expression of HA at the luminal surface of renal tubular cells leads to tubular nephrocalcinosis (tubular NC). Calcium staining methods (Von Kossa, Yasue) demonstrated that crystallization inhibitors cannot avoid the occasional precipitation of calcium phosphate in the papillary interstitium (interstitial NC). These crystals are probably immediately immobilized by the gel-like HA matrix. After ulcerating through the pelvic wall the calcified matrix becomes a Randall's plaque. The attachment of calcium oxalate crystals from the primary urine to plaque may ultimately lead to the development of clinical stones in the renal calyces (nephrolithiasis).

Keywords: Hyaluronan, tubular nephrocalcinosis, interstitial, nephrocalcinosis, renal calcification mechanisms.
PACS: 82.39.-k

Calcification Processes in the Kidney

There are three major forms of renal calcification, tubular nephrocalcinosis (the retention of crystals in the renal tubules)[1], interstitial nephrocalcinosis (calcium phosphate precipitations in the renal medullary interstitium that may give rise to Randall's plaques)[2] and nephrolithiasis (stones in the renal calyces and pelvis) [3] (Fig.1).

Urodynamic Events in the Renal Pelvis

The wall of the renal pelvis is equipped with a pacemaker that is responsible for urine transport in the upper urinary tract. Rhythmic contractions of the renal pelvis empty the limbs of Henle and collecting ducts during diuresis [4]. As the peristaltic

CP900, *Renal Stone Disease, 1st Annual International Urolithiasis Research Symposium,* edited by A. P. Evan, J. E. Lingeman, and J. C. Williams, Jr.

wave moves down over the renal papilla, tubular fluid is pushed through the ducts of Bellini in boluses and subsequently propelled toward the bladder [5]. Anyone who has passed a kidney stone knows that the peristaltic contractions continue into the ureter.

Hyaluronan in the Renal Medulla

The renal medullary interstitium is rich in hyaluronan (HA), a glycosaminoglycan (GAG) that is almost undetectable in other areas of the healthy kidney (Fig. 2). HA is a uniformly repetitive linear molecule composed of multiple disaccharides of glucuronic acid and N-acetylglucosamine ([GlcUA-GlcNAc]n). It is extremely large, with a molecular mass in the range of 1,000-10,000 kDa. HA differs from other GAGs in that it is not generally covalently linked to proteins to form proteoglycans, it does not contain sulphate groups and in contrast to other GAGs it is not synthesized in the Golgi apparatus but by hyaluronan synthases (HAS) located just beneath the plasma membrane [6].

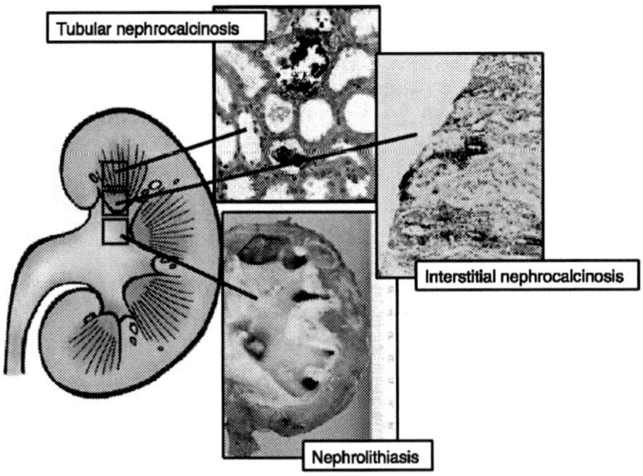

FIGURE 1. The three major forms of renal calcification processes.

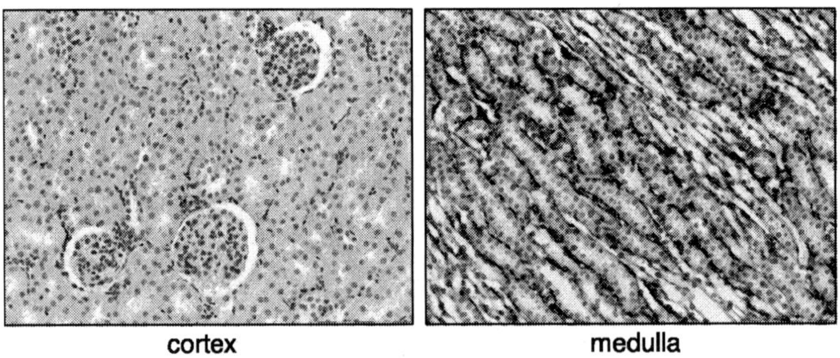

FIGURE 2. In the healthy kidney hyaluronan is expressed in the medullary interstitium but not in the cortical interstitium. Hyaluronan is normally not expressed in the renal tubules.

Peristaltic Contractions and Water Reabsorption in the Medulla

The force of the peristaltic contraction not only pushes tubular fluid down the collecting ducts, but also into the cells lining the duct via water-selective channels in the apical membrane. During rebound the negative interstitial hydrostatic pressure moves water from the basolateral membrane of the epithelial cells into the interstitium and the ascending vasa recta. Due to the carboxylate (COO-) groups of glucuronic acid, HA should be considered a polyanion. HA is strongly hydrophilic and adopts highly expanded, stiffened random-coil conformations that occupy a huge volume relative to its mass. When HA is compressed during the peristaltic contraction of the pelvic wall, the repulsive force of neighboring COO- groups is partly overcome by immobilization of cations (i.e. Na+, K+, Mg2+, Ca2+). In fact, HA serves as a soluble cation exchanger in the interstitium which during compression allows the slightly hypotonic fluid to escape the inner medulla via the ascending vasa recta [7].

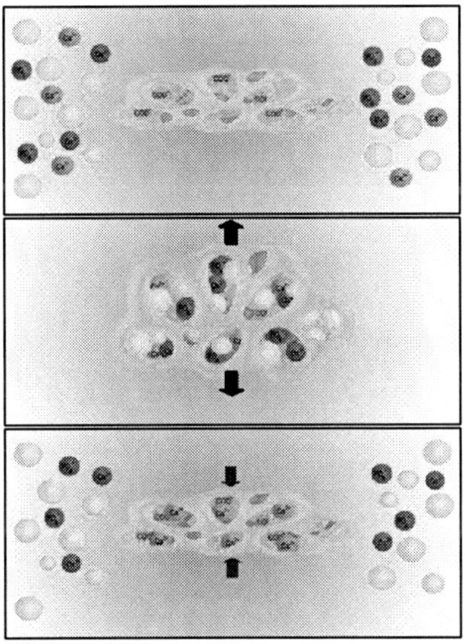

FIGURE 3. Top panel: Components relevant for the development of nephrocalcinosis in the inner medullary interstitium: green matrix=HA, yellow=calcium, brown= phosphate, purple=oxalate, blue=water. **Middle panel**: During rebound, solutes and water are taken up in the inner medullary interstitial HA matrix when the interstitial hydrostatic pressure is negative. **Lower panel**: The inner medullary interstitial matrix is compressed by the force of the pelvocalyceal contractions. Free cations including calcium are sequestered during compression. Slightly hypotonic fluid is squeezed out of the matrix and moves into the ascending vasa recta during the next rebound.

Medullary Hyaluronan and Water Homeostasis

When excess water needs to be excreted, water reabsorption is antagonized by increased papillary interstitial HA, while the opposite occurs during water conservation [8]. In the medullary interstitium HA is produced by renomedullary interstitial cells [9]. Cell culture studies demonstrated that the HA content in the supernatant of renomedullary interstitial cells decreases under hyperosmotic, hypoxic conditions. This may explain why renal papillary HA is decreased during anti-diuresis and increased during water diuresis [10, 11].

Medullary Hyaluronan as Crystallization Inhibitor

The binding of interstitial Ca2+ to COO- may prevent its binding to phosphate (PO43-) to form poorly soluble calcium phosphate. This may explain why the papilla usually is not entirely calcified despite the high concentrations of Ca2+, oxalate (Ox2-) and PO42-. The presence of calcium phosphate deposits in the renal medullary interstitium in recurrent calcium stone formers suggests that interstitial HA was no longer capable to prevent precipitation. At this point in time we can only speculate about the underlying mechanisms leading to calcium phosphate deposition. It is possible that the renal medullary interstitium of recurrent calcium stone formers contains more Ca2+ and PO43-, or less HA. Another possibility is that the frequency of the renal papillary peristaltic contractions is higher in stone formers generating an increased corticomedullary concentration gradient with elevated levels of calcium phosphate supersaturation. The pH must be relatively high in the medullary interstitium since the calcium precipitates invariably consist of phosphate and not of oxalate.

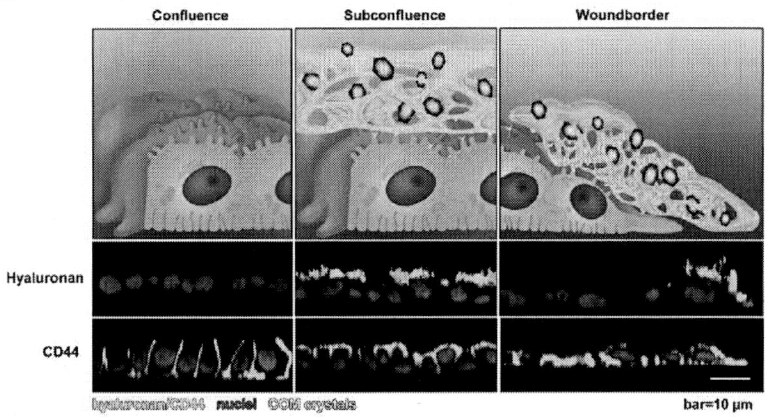

FIGURE 4. Hyaluronan as a crystal binding molecule in the etiology of tubular nephrocalcinosis [1].

Hyaluronan as Crystal Binding Molecule

Previously, we demonstrated that HA plays an important role in the etiology of tubular nephrocalcinosis [1, 12]. The general picture is that calcium crystals preferentially bind to non-differentiated/regenerating epithelial cells in the renal tubules. Various disorders are associated with tubular nephrocalcinosis and each disorder seems to have its specific reasons for the expression of the crystal binding phenotype. Preterm infants, for example, express non-differentiated renal tubular cells because their kidneys are not fully developed yet, while renal transplant patients express a comparable phenotype as a result of injury-repair due to various forms of post-transplantation renal damage (e.g. ischemia/reperfusion, calcineurin inhibitors, periods of acute rejection) (Fig.4).

Due to its polyanionic nature and glue-like properties, high molecular mass HA indeed is an excellent calcium crystal binding molecule (Fig.5).

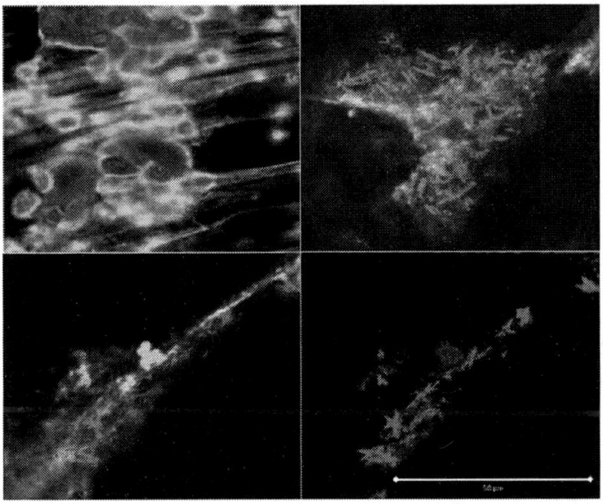

FIGURE 5. Hyaluronan has a high affinity for calcium crystals. **Top left**; HA visualized with biotinylated hyaluronan binding protein (HABP) expressed at the surface of mobile MDCK strain I cells in culture. Cell nuclei are stained in red using propidiumiodide. **Top right**; HA at the surface of MDCK-I cells with many calcium oxalate monohydrate (COM) crystals attached. **Bottom left**; cables of HA at the surface of MDCK-I cells with COM crystals (red reflecting particles). **Bottom right**; the same image as bottom left, but without visualizing bHABP, showing only COM crystals reflecting in laser light.

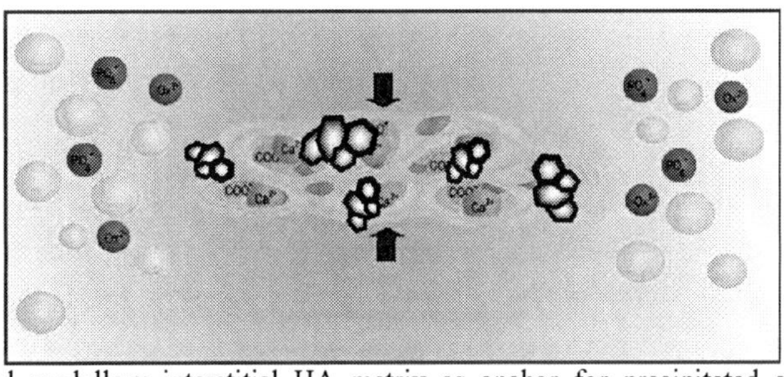

FIGURE 6. Renal medullary interstitial HA matrix as anchor for precipitated calcium phosphate crystals.

When calcium phosphate precipitates in the papillary interstitium during periods of dehydration because the calcium and phosphate concentrations are too high or the amount of HA is too low, it is likely that the same HA that initially served as a crystallization inhibitor, now becomes an anchor for calcium phosphate crystals (Fig.6).

Preliminary studies performed with kidneys removed on oncological indication demonstrated the co-localization of HA and Yasue-positive material in the renal medullary interstitium (Fig.7). It is conceivable that the HA-filled interstitium in principle has a large storage capacity for precipitated calcium phosphate. Randall's plaques may form only when the interstitium is overloaded with calcium phosphate.

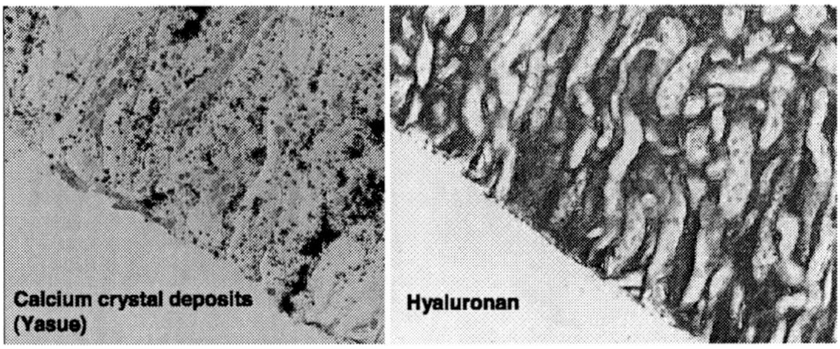

FIGURE 7. Calcium deposits (left) and hyaluronan expression (right) in the renal medullary interstitium. Both the calcium deposits and hyaluronan are located exclusively in the renal papillary interstitium.

Hyaluronan in the Organic Stone Matrix

Calcium oxalate stones were dissolved in EDTA, after which the remaining organic matrix was stained with biotinylated hyaluronan binding protein to detect the localization of HA in the stone matrix. The expression of HA was limited to a small band at the edge of the matrix. This band may be the interface between the stone and a fixation point in the kidney (Fig 8).

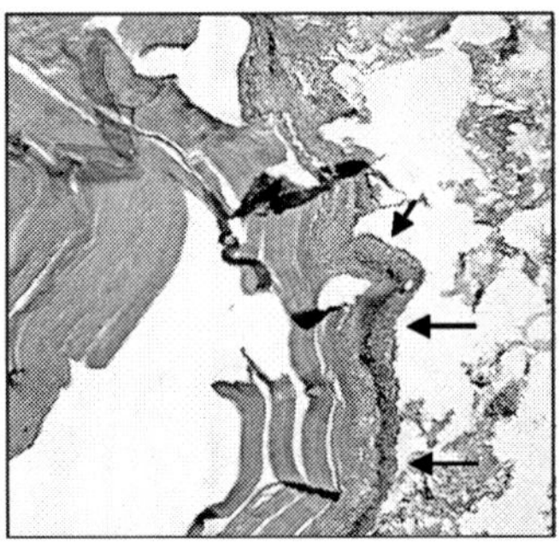

FIGURE 8. Organic calcium oxalate stone (100% COM) matrix stained for HA (arrows).

Conclusions

HA plays an important role in renal tubular nephrocalcinosis. The co-localization of HA with calcium phosphate in the renal papillary interstitium suggests that HA also plays a role in interstitial nephrocalcinosis. Once the interstitial plaque penetrates the wall of the renal pelvis it is not unlikely that HA is also responsible for the binding of circulating calcium oxalate crystals to plaque and their growth into clinical stones.

ACKNOWLEDGMENTS

I would like to thank my collaborators, Marc De Broe, Anja Verhulst, Benjamin Vervaet and Patrick d'Haese from the Laboratory of Pathophysiology, University of Antwerp, Belgium. This work was supported by The Foundation Scientific Urological Research (SUWO), and the Oxalosis and Hyperoxaluria Foundation (OHF).

REFERENCES

1. Verkoelen CF: Crystal retention in renal stone disease: a crucial role for the glycosaminoglycan hyaluronan? *J Am Soc Nephrol* 17:1673-1687, 2006
2. Evan A, Lingeman J, Coe FL, Worcester E: Randall's plaque: Pathogenesis and role in calcium oxalate nephrolithiasis. *Kidney Int* 69:1313-1318, 2006
3. Coe FL, Evan A, Worcester E: Kidney stone disease. *J Clin Invest* 115:2598-2608, 2005
4. Constantinou CE: Renal pelvic pacemaker control of ureteral peristaltic rate. *Am J Physiol* 226:1413-1419, 1974
5. Dwyer TM, Schmidt-Nielsen B: The renal pelvis: machinery that concentrates urine in the papilla. *News Physiol Sci* 18:1-6, 2003
6. Toole BP: Hyaluronan is not just a goo! *J Clin Invest* 106:335-336, 2000
7. Knepper MA, Saidel GM, Hascall VC, Dwyer T: Concentration of solutes in the renal inner medulla: interstitial hyaluronan as a mechano-osmotic transducer. *Am J Physiol Renal Physiol* 284:F433-446, 2003
8. Hansell P, Goransson V, Odlind C, Gerdin B, Hallgren R: Hyaluronan content in the kidney in different states of body hydration. *Kidney Int* 58:2061-2068, 2000
9. Goransson V, Hansell P, Moss S, Alcorn D, Johnsson C, Hallgren R, Maric C: Renomedullary interstitial cells in culture; the osmolality and oxygen tension influence the extracellular amounts of hyaluronan and cellular expression of CD44. *Matrix Biol* 20:129-136, 2001
10. Goransson V, Johnsson C, Nylander O, Hansell P: Renomedullary and intestinal hyaluronan content during body water excess: a study in rats and gerbils. *J Physiol* 542:315-322, 2002
11. Ginetzinsky AG: Relationship between urinary hyaluronidase and diuresis. *Nature* 189:235-237, 1961
12. Verhulst A, Asselman M, De Naeyer S, Vervaet BA, Mengel M, Gwinner W, D'Haese PC, Verkoelen CF, De Broe ME: Preconditioning of the distal tubular epithelium of the human kidney precedes nephrocalcinosis. *Kidney Int* 68:1643-1647, 2005

II. LINKS OF STONE DISEASES TO OTHER SYSTEMIC DISEASES

Changes in Renal Function and Blood Pressure in Patients with Stone Disease

Elaine M. Worcester

Department of Medicine, Nephrology Section, MC 5100, University of Chicago, 5841 South Maryland Avenue, Chicago, Illinois, 60637, USA

Abstract. Stone disease is a rare cause of renal failure, but a history of kidney stones is associated with an increased risk for chronic kidney disease, particularly in overweight patients. Loss of renal function seems especially notable for patients with stones associated with cystinuria, hyperoxaluria, and renal tubular acidosis, in whom the renal pathology shows deposits of mineral obstructing inner medullary collecting ducts, often diffusely. However, even idiopathic calcium oxalate stone formers have a mild but significant decrease in renal function, compared to age, sex and weight-matched normals, and appear to lose renal function with age at a slightly faster rate than non-stone formers. There is also an increased incidence of hypertension among stone formers, although women are more likely to be affected than men.

Keywords: Kidney stones, chronic kidney disease, hypertension, calcium oxalate, glomerular filtration rate
PACS: 01.30.Cc

STONES AND RENAL DISEASE

Stone disease is, fortunately, a rare cause of end-stage renal disease (ESRD). In the United States, the Renal Data System categories "Nephrolithiasis, obstruction, gouty nephropathy" and "Nephrocalcinosis" accounted for 1.2% and 0.1%, respectively, of cases of ESRD, a total of 6453 patients, from 2000-2004 [1]. This is somewhat lower than the frequency of nephrolithiasis-associated ESRD of 3.2% reported in patients starting dialysis at Necker Hospital (Paris, France) between 1989 and 2000; however, the rate dropped from 4.7% in 89-91 to 2.2% in 98-2000, suggesting that this entity is becoming less common [2].

Urolithiasis may result in loss of function by two general mechanisms: 1) episodic events, such as ureteral obstruction during stone passage, or because of procedures needed for stone removal, and their attendant complications, or 2) continuous events, as a result of a disordered physiology that underlies stone formation [3]. Nephrectomy, at one time a relatively common outcome of stone disease, especially in patients with staghorn calculi – such as from struvite or cystine stones – is uncommon in the era of modern endourologic approaches. However, renal dysfunction may still occur in patients with stone disease, via one or both of these mechanisms. As even moderate renal dysfunction is associated with increased long-term cardiovascular morbidity [4], the issue deserves the attention of those who treat patients with stones.

CP900, *Renal Stone Disease, 1st Annual International Urolithiasis Research Symposium,*
edited by A. P. Evan, J. E. Lingeman, and J. C. Williams, Jr.

Nephrolithiasis Is Associated with an Increased Risk of Chronic Kidney Disease

A history of kidney stones may be a risk factor for chronic kidney disease (CKD). In a case control study comparing 548 patients with newly diagnosed CKD from diverse causes to 514 age, sex, and race matched controls, a history of kidney stones was reported significantly more often by the subjects with CKD than by controls (16.8 vs. 6.4% respectively, $p<0.001$) [5]. Stone formers (SF) had an increased risk of CKD (odds ratio 1.9, 95% CI 1.1-3.4) after adjustment for multiple confounders. Among subjects with hypertension, CKD was 3 times more common among those with stones than those without.

This association between stones and CKD was borne out by data from the Third National Health and Nutrition Examination Survey (NHANES III) [6]. This survey, conducted between 1988 and 1994, was designed to provide estimates of health status in the non-institutionalized U.S. population. Participants were asked if they had ever had a kidney stone. Renal function was estimated using the Modification of Diet in Renal Disease (MDRD) equation, and individuals who reported having ever had a stone were compared to those with no such history. The median body mass index (BMI) among SF in this sample was 27 kg/m^2, and initial analysis of the relationship between stone history and glomerular filtration rate (GFR) revealed a significant interaction between stones and BMI. In subjects with BMI<27, history of stones did not increase the relative risk for decreased GFR. However, among subjects with BMI≥27, SF had a significantly increased risk of having Stage 2 or Stage 3 CKD (using the Kidney Disease Outcomes Quality Initiative definitions for reduced renal function [7]), after adjustment for age, gender, race, systolic blood pressure (BP), diabetes, smoking, cardiovascular disease and health insurance. The odds of having Stage 2 CKD (GFR 60-90 ml/min/1.73 m^2) was 1.66-fold higher in SF compared to non-SF, while the odds for stage 3 CKD (GFR 30-60 ml/min/1.73 m^2) was 1.87-fold higher, relative to having a GFR greater than 90 ml/min/1.73 m^2. Among SF in this survey, 19% had had surgery for stone removal, and 7% had ESWL; neither was associated with increased risk for loss of renal function in this analysis. As well, 40% of patients reported taking medication for stones; use of such medication was also not associated with loss of GFR. Thus, among overweight persons, a history of kidney stones significantly increased the risk of having decreased GFR compared to comparably overweight non-stone formers, after adjustment for multiple confounders.

Association of Specific Stone Types with Reduced GFR

These studies cannot give any detail about association of stone type with loss of function. We have used data from SF investigated at the University of Chicago Kidney Stone Program between 1969 and 2005 to look into such associations [8]. All patients had 3 24-hour urines collected prior to starting therapy, and creatinine clearances were calculated for each of the 1856 patients (581 females) in our program with at least one stone analysis; 153 normal subjects (63 female) were used as a comparison (Fig. 1).

Clinical phenotypes were also determined, including the presence of bowel disease, jejunoileal bypass for obesity, renal tubular acidosis, and hyperparathyroidism. Compared with the controls, virtually all the SF groups had some decrease in renal function, but certain types of patients stand out as being at special risk.

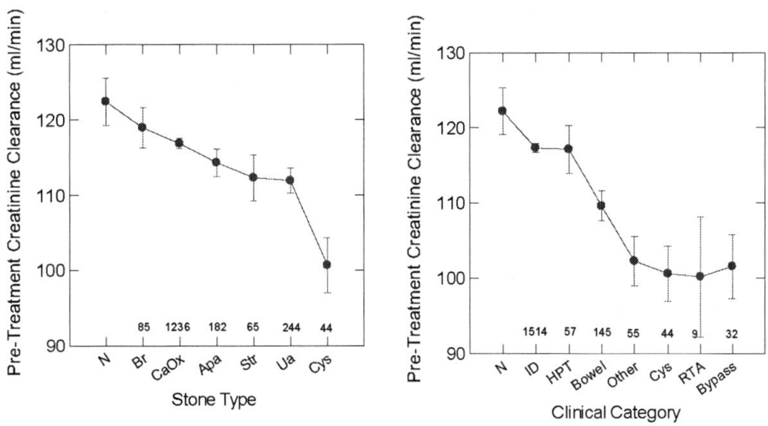

FIGURE 1. Pretreatment creatinine clearances by stone type or clinical category, adjusted for age, weight, and gender, shown as means ± SEM. Patients are from the University of Chicago Kidney Stone Program. Numbers represent patients in each category; overall, 1856 stone formers, 153 normal subjects. N, normal; Br, brushite; CaOx, calcium oxalate; Apa, apatite; Str, struvite; Ua, uric acid; Cys, cystine; ID, idiopathic; HPT, hyperparathyroid; Bowel, bowel disease with or without surgery; Other, rare diseases such as sarcoidosis, drug stones, eating disorders; RTA, renal tubular acidosis; Bypass, obesity bypass. [reprinted from [8], used by permission from American Urological Association].

One example would be inherited diseases with life-long renal excretion of large amounts of insoluble materials, such as patients with cystinuria. Patients with cystine stones are well known to be at risk for renal insufficiency [9]. The fact that these stones may become quite large, are frequently recurrent, and that cystine SF often require many procedures for stone removal, could explain the virtually universal decrease in renal function among cystine SF. However, loss of renal function appears early in the course of cystine stone formation, and creatinine clearance remains below that of idiopathic SF at all ages. Fortunately, ESRD is a rare occurrence, at least among treated patients, in whom procedure rates diminish, although they continue to be higher than among other groups of SF.

The renal pathology of cystinurics suggests another reason that they may experience decreased renal function [10]. During percutaneous nephrolithotomy (PCNL) it is common to find abnormalities of most or all papillae in these patients, with dilated Bellini ducts containing masses of crystal, although some patients, early in their course, have little damage. Histopathologic analysis of papillary biopsies reveals deposition of cystine crystals, and often apatite crystals, that fill inner medullary collecting duct (IMCD) lumens and result in obstruction of these tubules, with damage to the lining cells. Fibrosis surrounds dilated crystal-filled tubules, and is associated with glomerular obsolescence. This diffuse tubule plugging seems likely to contribute to decreased renal function, although there is not yet data correlating the extent of plugging with level of GFR.

Patients with renal tubular acidosis (RTA) also exhibit marked decreases in renal function. These patients, like cystinurics, have a systemic disease, and usually have diffuse involvement of all papillae with deposits of apatite, which is seen on X-ray as nephrocalcinosis, and on papillary biopsy as deposits of apatite filling tubule lumens in most papillae [11]. The diffuse involvement of almost all papillae is a striking feature of patients with either cystinuria or RTA.

Excretion of large amounts of oxalate is also associated with a risk for renal insufficiency. Renal failure is seen in many patients with primary hyperoxaluria type I, because of deposition of calcium oxalate in renal tissue, and may occur before the diagnosis of their underlying disease has been made [12]. Acquired hyperoxaluria may also lead to loss of renal function, as in patients with ileal resection or bypass, in whom intra-tubular crystal deposits are also seen [13]. Recent reports suggest that newer bariatric surgery may also carry a risk for hyperoxaluria, and consequently the potential for renal damage because of increased oxalate transport through the kidney [14].

Overall, the worst kidney dysfunction is seen among patients with stone types associated with crystal plugging, seen most often in the IMCD and Bellini ducts, which is often associated with interstitial fibrosis. That these diseases are also associated with formation of large stones, requiring multiple procedures, is also likely to result in renal injury.

Whether surgical treatment for stones may result in injury to the kidney, with resultant loss of GFR, is unclear. There have been rare reports of acute renal failure after extra-corporeal lithotripsy (ESWL) [15], and studies in animals that have undergone lithotripsy document renal damage accompanied by reduction in GFR [16, 17]. In humans, data about the effects on renal function of repeated episodes of lithotripsy is lacking.

Uric acid stones are associated with risk for CKD as well. Recent work has linked this type of stone to the presence of insulin resistance, obesity, and often frank diabetes [18, 19].

Routine Calcium Oxalate Stone Formers May Not Have Normal Renal Function

The groups noted in Fig. 1 to have the greatest decrease in renal function are those in which diffuse tubular obstruction with crystals could lead to a drop in kidney function. However, these diseases are relatively rare, and unlikely to account for the increased risk of CKD in stone formers noted in the large groups described by Gillen [6] or Vupputuri [5]. Therefore, it is of interest that among the University of Chicago cohort, even routine calcium stone formers—those with calcium oxalate (CaOx) stones and without systemic disorders—also had renal function that was slightly, but significantly, below that of normals, adjusted for sex, age and weight (115±1 vs.

122±2, p=0.02, SF vs. normal) [8]. The reason is not obvious; we do not have data on procedures or stone numbers, which might have an effect on renal function. Since these patients make up the majority of SF, this abnormality, although in general mild, may still be significant.

Tubule obstruction with crystals is not likely to account for decreased renal function in these patients. Routine CaOx SF have not been found to have intra-tubular deposits of mineral. Instead, subepithelial apatite deposits, Randall's plaque, have been found in all those studied to date [13]. These deposits appear to originate in the basement membrane of the thin limb of Henle, and spread into the interstitium. Tubule epithelium is intact, and interstitial fibrosis is not noted. The impact of these deposits on renal function has not been determined; glomerular anatomy appears normal.

Our cross-sectional data suggests some alterations in the renal function of SF; we wished to know also if SF lose renal function with age at the same rate as non-stone formers. When the rate of loss of GFR with age among the SF in the University of Chicago program was compared with data from studies of normal subjects in the literature, renal function among SF began to decline at a later age than among normals, but after the age of 45 male SF lost renal function more rapidly, compared to normals [20]. The pattern for women was similar, but did not reach statistical significance. Whether loss of GFR with age is truly accelerated among stone formers will need to be confirmed by further study, and the associations with underlying stone type and metabolic abnormalities clarified.

STONE DISEASE AND HYPERTENSION

One condition that may impact renal function in this group of patients is the reported association between stone formation and hypertension (HTN). A number of epidemiologic studies have suggested that the incidence of hypertension is increased among patients who make kidney stones. Madore et al. have found an association between stone history and development of hypertension in large cohort studies of women aged 34 to 59 years [21], and men aged 40 to 75 [22]; the relationship was not explained by dietary intake of calcium, sodium or potassium, but was stronger in women. We have found a similar association using data from NHANES III [23]. In this cross-sectional survey, SF's were significantly more likely to report a history of HTN (32.7% vs. 24.6%, SF and non-SF, respectively, p=0.001). We found that the relationship between stone formation and blood pressure was dependent on sex and BMI; among women in the upper 2 quintiles of BMI, systolic BP among SF was 7.62 mm Hg (95% CI 1.04-14.2, p=0.024) and 4.36 mm Hg (95% CI 0.30 to 8.42, p=0.036) greater in SF compared with non-SF; diastolic BP was also increased modestly. A similar trend among males did not reach statistical significance.

The association between nephrolithiasis and HTN does not imply a causal relationship. It is possible that renal damage related to stone formation could lead to increased blood pressure; in animals, tubulo-interstitial injury can lead to a salt-sensitive form of hypertension [24]. As we have seen, many stone formers have some degree of tubulo-interstitial injury; whether these SF are particularly prone to HTN has not been settled. Among cystine SF studied in our program, we did not find higher BP than among routine SF; however, the numbers studied are relatively small, and we cannot know the degree of tubulo-interstitial injury in any given patient, at present. Alternatively, there may be genetic mechanisms that are linked to increased risk for both stones and hypertension. Hypercalciuria may be a link between the two diseases [25].

IS KIDNEY DONATION SAFE FOR STONE FORMERS?

One of the questions that physicians who care for SF are sometimes faced with is whether such individuals can safely donate a kidney. Because calcium stones are quite common, and onset is usually in early to mid-adulthood in otherwise healthy people, SF may present for evaluation as potential donors for a family member with renal failure. Does stone formation pose an unacceptable risk to these potential donors? Are they at risk for more rapid loss of renal function with age?

There have been no systematic studies looking at SF who have donated a kidney. In order to see if the loss of a kidney would lead to significant risk for CKD among SF, we have studied a group of 115 SF (58 male) who lost a kidney for reasons including obstruction and infection [16]. In a cross-sectional analysis, loss of renal function with age in the single kidney SF was not accelerated, compared to two-kidney SF, among the women, nor among men over the age of 45; loss of GFR may be increased among younger male stone formers who have lost a kidney. Stone recurrence was not increased among the single-kidney patients, who were all being treated for their stone disorder. Overall, from this study one would conclude that donation would not automatically be ruled out for SF, but in view of the accumulating data linking stone formation to some risk for renal impairment, careful screening would be important, and treatment to prevent stone recurrence with careful follow-up should be advised to any such donors.

ACKNOWLEDGMENTS

This work was supported by NIH NIDDK P01 56788.

REFERENCES

1. U.S. Renal Data System, USRDS 2006 Annual Data Report: Atlas of End-Stage Renal Disease in the United States, National Institutes of Health, National Institute of Diabetes and Digestive and Kidney Diseases, Bethesda, MD, 2006.
2. P. Jungers, D. Joly, F. Barbey, G. Choukroun and M. Daudon, *Am J Kidney Dis* **44**, 799-805 (2004).
3. G. Gambaro, S. Favaro and A. D'Angelo, *Am J Kidney Dis* **37**, 233-243 (2001).
4. D. E. Weiner, H. Tighiouart, M. G. Amin, P. C. Stark, B. Maclead, J. L. Griffith, D. N. Salem, A.S. Levey and M. J. Sarnak, *J Am Soc Nephrol* **15**, 1307-1315 (2004).
5. S. Vupputuri, J. M. Soucie, W. McClellan and D. P. Sandler, *Ann Epidemiol* **14**, 222-228 (2004).
6. D. L. Gillen, E. M. Worcester and F. L. Coe, *Kidney Int* **67**, 685-690 (2005).

7. National Kidney Foundation, *Am J Kidney Dis* **39**, suppl 2, S1-S266 (2002).
8. E. M. Worcester, J. H. Parks, A. P. Evan and F. L. Coe, *J Urol* **176**, 600-603 (2006).
9. E. M. Worcester, F. L. Coe, A. P. Evan and J. H. Parks, *BJU International* **97**, 1285-1290 (2006).
10. A. P. Evan, F. L. Coe, J. E. Lingeman, Y. Shao, B. R. Matlaga, S. C. Kim, S. B. Bledsoe, A. J. Sommer, M. Grynpas, C. L. Phillips and E. M. Worcester, *Kidney Int* **69**, 2227-2235 (2006).
11. A. P. Evan, S. Bledsoe, J. Lingeman, A. Sommers, F. L. Coe, N. Miller and E. M. Worcester, *Kidney Int* in press (2007).
12. D. S. Milliner, *Am J Nephrol* **25**, 154-160 (2005).
13. A. P. Evan, J. E. Lingeman, F. L. Coe, J. H. Parks, S. B. Bledsoe, Y. Shao, A. J. Sommer, R. F. Paterson, R. L. Kuo and M. Grynpas, *J Clin Invest* **111**, 607-616 (2003).
14. W. K. Nelson, S. G. Houghton, D. S. Milliner, J. C. Lieske and M. G. Sarr, *Surg Obes Relat Dis* **1**, 481-485 (2005).
15. W. S. McDougal, *J Urol*, **174**, 1024 (2005).
16. L. R. Willis, A. P. Evan, B. A. Connors, Y. Shao, P. M. Blomgren, J. H. Pratt, N. S. Fineberg and J. E. Lingeman, *J Endourol* **19**, 90-101 (2005).
17. L. R. Willis, A. P. Evan, B. A. Connors, R. K. Handa, P. M. Blomgren and J. E. Lingeman, *J Am Soc Nephrol* **17**, 663-673 (2006).
18. M. Daudon, O. Traxer, P. Conort, B. Lacour and P. Jungers, *J Am Soc Nephrol* **17**, 2026-2033 (2006).
19. N. Abate, M. Chandalia, A. V. Cab0-Chan, Jr., O. W. Moe and K. Sakhaee, *Kidney Int* **65**, 386-392 (2004).
20. E. Worcester, J. H. Parks, M.A. Josephson, R. A. Thisted and F. L. Coe, *Kidney Int* **64**, 2204-2213 (2003).
21. F. Madore, M. J. Stampfer, W. C. Willett, F. E. Speizer and G. C. Curhan, *Am J Kidney Dis* **32**, 802-807 (1998).
22. F. Madore, M. J. Stampfer, E. B. Rimm and G. C. Curhan, *Am J Hypertens* **11**, 46-53 (1998).
23. D. L. Gillen, F. L. Coe and E. M. Worcester, *Am J Kidney Dis* **46**, 263-269 (2005).
24. R. J. Johnson, J. Herrera-Acosta, G. F. Schreiner and B. Rodriguez-Iturbe, *N Engl J Med* **346**, 913-923 (2002).
25. A. Mente, R. J. D'A. Honey, J. M. McLaughlin, S. B. Bull and A. G. Logan, *J Am Soc Nephrol* **17**, 2567-2575 (2006).

Urinary pH as a Risk Factor for Stone Type

Khashayar Sakhaee

Department of Internal Medicine,
Charles and Jane Pak Center for Mineral Metabolism and Clinical Research,
University of Texas Southwestern Medical Center,
5323 Harry Hines Boulevard, Dallas, Texas, 75390-8885, USA

Abstract: A high urinary pH is main risk factor for the calcium phosphate stone formation; however, its pathophysiologic mechanism has not been fully understood. The introduction of Topiramate in the treatment of various neurological disorders has been complicated by metabolic acidosis, significant hypocitraturia, elevated urinary pH, and calcium phosphate stone formation. This model provides a probe to investigate the pathophysiologic mechanism of calcium phosphate stone formation and perhaps to develop appropriate countermeasures in the future. On the other hand an unduly acidic urine predisposes one to uric acid nephrolithiasis. Our recent investigation linking low urinary pH, and defective renal ammoniagenesis to insulin resistance provides new knowledge to unfold the pathophysiology of uric acid nephrolithiasis. The metabolic profile leading to uric acid stone may emerge as one of the components of metabolic syndrome.

Keywords: urinary pH, Topiramate, nephrolithiasis, calcium phosphate stones, uric acid stones, metabolic syndrome
PACS: 81.10.Dn; 87.19.Xx

URINARY pH AS A RISK FACTOR FOR STONE TYPE

Physicochemical and Pathophysiologic Bases of Elevated Urine pH

Urinary pH is a major determinant for kidney stone formation. However, the importance of urinary pH as a major risk factor for kidney stone formation has not been well recognized by practicing urologists and nephrologists. Kamel *et al.* [1] suggested that urine pH approximately near 6.0 reduces the risk of kidney stone formation. However the risk of uric acid and calcium stone formation increases progressively at urinary pH<5.5 and >6.5, respectively [1]. Until recently the prevalence of calcium phosphate stone formation was reported to be low and mainly associated with distal renal tubular acidosis. However, prevalence of calcium phosphate stones has risen for three decades [2]. One potential association for this change is suspected to be overzealous treatment with alkali, and aggressive extracorporeal shock wave lithotripsy (ESWL) treatment [2]. Moreover, recently the widespread and escalating use of Topiramate (TPM) underscores the importance of considering a possible long-term effect of this drug on kidney stone formation [3].

CP900, *Renal Stone Disease, 1st Annual International Urolithiasis Research Symposium,*
edited by A. P. Evan, J. E. Lingeman, and J. C. Williams, Jr.

TPM is a novel neuromodulatory agent which is now prescribed for many neurological disorders including migraine headache prophylaxis and treatment of seizure disorders [4-12]. TPM is known to inhibit isoenzymes of carbonic anhydrase (CA) II and IV which are localized in proximal and distal renal tubular cells [4-11]. We recently reported the largest series of biochemical stone risk profile in 32 TPM treated subjects [3]. TPM resulted in mild metabolic acidosis, marked hypocitraturia and increased urinary pH, which increases the propensity to form calcium phosphate stone. These biochemical features are shared with patients with distal renal tubular acidosis (dRTA) [13].

Despite the lack of kidney stone surveillance with this agent, the reported incidence is estimated to be 1.5% with TPM treatment, which is 2-4 times greater than the stone incidence in a similar, untreated population [14]. Thus the treatment with TPM may be used as a probe to investigate the physicochemical and pathophysiologic bases of calcium stone formation. Potassium citrate is a widely-used and effective treatment against calcium stone formation via multiple actions. Potassium citrate raises urinary citrate excretion, increases soluble complexation of calcium and reduces ionized calcium concentration, thereby reducing calcium oxalate and calcium phosphate supersaturation [13,15,16]. In addition, urinary citrate also antagonizes crystallization of calcium salts directly through inhibition of spontaneous nucleation, crystal growth, and crystal agglomeration of calcium phosphate crystals and preformed calcium oxalate [17-21]. However there may be a concern that potassium citrate may raise urine pH further in TPM-treated subjects, which will convert phosphate to its divalent form, promote calcium-phosphate complexation and thereby attenuate the beneficial effects of the rise in urinary citrate (Fig. 1) [22].

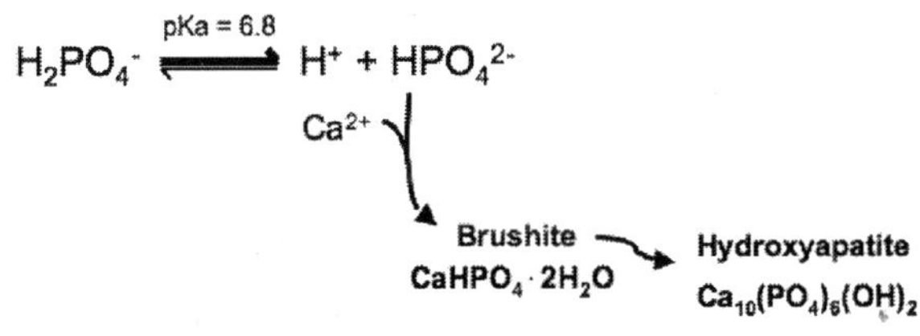

FIGURE 1. Crystallization of calcium phosphate.

Physicochemical Basis of Uric Acid Stone Formation

Urinary pH is the principal determinant of uric acid crystallization. Uric acid is weak organic acid with a pK_a of 5.5 [23]. At this unduly low urinary pH, sparingly soluble uric acid precipitates to form uric acid stones (Fig. 2). Moreover, urate solubility is influenced by urinary cations [24,25]. It has been shown that monopotassium urate has higher solubility than monosodium urate [24,25]. The latter physicochemical characteristic is responsible for formation of calcium oxalate stones through heterogeneous nucleation or by binding of inhibitors of calcium oxalate crystallization [26].

Pathophysiology of Uric Acid Nephrolithiasis

The three important factors responsible for development of uric acid nephrolithiasis are low urine volume, hyperuricosuria, and unduly acidic urine pH [27]. The most invariable factor in development of uric acid nephrolithiasis is unduly acidic urinary pH (≤5.5). Low urinary volume may occur from excessive sweating and chronic diarrheal conditions. The low urinary pH that usually accompanies these clinical states further accelerates the formation of uric acid stones. Hyperuricosuria may occur due to genetic and environmental influences. The genetic disorders include hereditary enzymatic disorders of uric acid metabolism and a recently described mutation in urate transporters [28-32]. Urate overproduction has been proposed as one of the mechanisms for uric acid stone formation in patients with idiopathic primary gout, although it has not been found in the recent studies in uric stone formers [33,34].

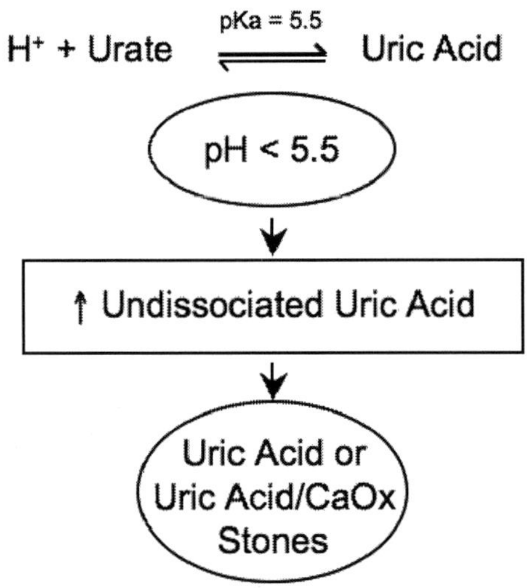

FIGURE 2. Crystallization of uric acid stones.

Pathophysiology of Low Urinary pH

The pathophysiologic mechanisms for low urinary pH in patients with idiopathic uric acid nephrolithiasis are complex. An increase in endogenous acid production and defective urinary ammonium excretion have been implicated in development of unduly acidic urine in this population [33,35]. Defective ammonium excretion was shown in studies of idiopathic uric acid stone formers under controlled metabolic diet (Fig. 3). This defect was further unmasked by administration of an oral acid load (ammonium chloride) to amplify the ammoniagenic defect [35]. This finding was further supported in a study of uric acid stone formers on a random diet, showing lack of a rise of urinary ammonium in association with greater dietary acid intake (sulfate load) [35]. The lack of rise in urinary ammonium was shown to be compensated in uric acid stone formers by increasing excretion of urinary titratable acids (phosphates) and decreased urinary citrate excretion [33,35]. Furthermore, at any given acid load uric acid stone formers demonstrated higher net acid excretion (Fig. 4) [35]. This study suggests that greater endogenous acid production is in part responsible for unduly acid urine in uric acid stone formers. Mechanisms that are responsible for the increase in net acid production in uric acid stone formers are not yet fully understood.

One study in a large cohort has demonstrated increased incidence of kidney stone disease in patients with type 2 diabetes mellitus [36]. However, the nature of the stones in this study was not disclosed. Lately, several investigators have reported an increased association of uric acid stones with diabetes mellitus [37-41]. Furthermore, a recent metabolic study using a hyperinsulinemic-euglycemic clamp procedure has shown the pathophysiologic link between insulin resistance and defective urinary acidification in uric acid stone formers [42]. In this study, urine pH (surrogate marker of renal insulin resistance) was shown to correlate significantly with glucose disposal rate (surrogate marker of peripheral insulin resistance). The result of this metabolic study was further supported in a large cohort of kidney stone formers from two kidney stone registries in the United States [43]. An inverse relationship was shown between body weight and urinary pH in over 3000 patients with kidney stones.

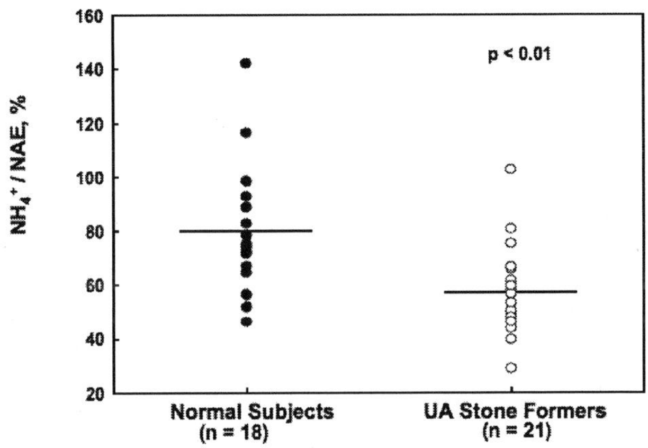

FIGURE 3. Renal acidification in uric acid stone formers.

Experimental *in vitro* studies have shown that insulin enhances renal ammoniagenesis in canine renal proximal tubular cells when incubated with glutamine, the main substrate for renal ammonia production [44]. Moreover, insulin has been shown to activate the Na^+/H^+ exchanger (NHE-3) in a dose-dependent manner, thus stimulating ammonia secretion [45-47]. Metabolic studies using the hyperinsulinemic-euglycemic clamp have shown that insulin causes a significant rise in urinary ammonium excretion in normal subjects [42]. In contrast, ammonium excretion was shown to be blunted under the same metabolic conditions in uric acid stone formers [48].

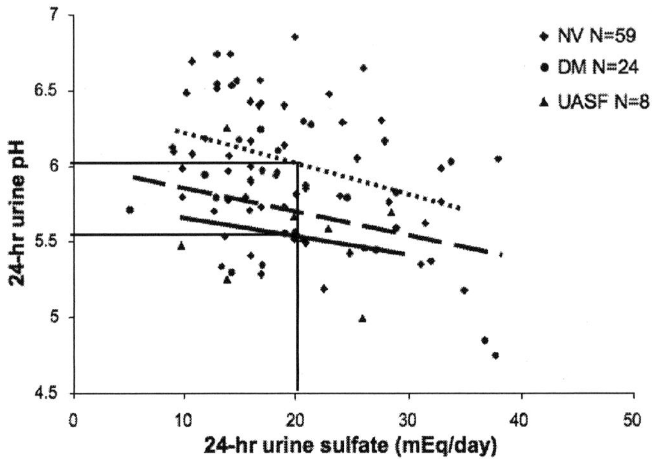

FIGURE 4. Dietary acid load and urinary pH.

It is plausible to suggest that the underlying mechanism of increased acid production in uric acid stone formers and in patients with type 2 diabetes may be linked to insulin resistance. The exact nature of the organic anion responsible for increased acid production in these patients in unknown. However plasma lactate has been shown to increase in type 2 diabetes [49]. This increased level of serum lactate may contribute to increased excretion of titratable acid in this population.

More than one billion adults around the world are overweight and 312,000,000 of them are obese [50]. In parallel, the prevalence of nephrolithiasis in the United States is on the rise [51]. Our recent metabolic studies and population-based epidemiologic studies have shown a link between obesity and uric acid stones. It is possible that the mean urinary pH gradually shifts to lower values as well. Thus, unduly low urinary pH values may arise as one of the components of the metabolic syndrome.

CONCLUSION

Urinary pH is one the most important determinants of both calcium phosphate and uric acid crystallization. The pathophysiologic basis of high urinary pH—except for TPM-induced kidney stones—has not been fully explored. An optimal treatment would be an agent that augments urinary citrate without increasing urinary pH. Low urinary pH in patients with uric acid nephrolithiasis is due to defective ammonium excretion and increased acid production, which may both be linked to renal insulin resistance. The reversal of insulin resistance may ameliorate these defects and increase urine pH.

REFERENCES

1. Kamel KS, Cheema-Dhadli S, Shafiee MA, Halperin ML. Dogmas and controversies in the handling of nitrogenous wastes: excretion of nitrogenous wastes in human subjects. *J Exp Biol.* May 2004;207(Pt 12):1985-1991.
2. Parks JH, Worcester EM, Coe FL, Evan AP, Lingeman JE. Clinical implications of abundant calcium phosphate in routinely analyzed kidney stones. *Kidney Int.* Aug 2004;66(2):777-785.
3. Welch BJ, Graybeal D, Moe OW, Maalouf NM, Sakhaee K. Biochemical and stone-risk profiles with topiramate treatment. *Am J Kidney Dis.* Oct 2006;48(4):555-563.
4. White HS, Brown SD, Woodhead JH, Skeen GA, Wolf HH. Topiramate enhances GABA-mediated chloride flux and GABA-evoked chloride currents in murine brain neurons and increases seizure threshold. *Epilepsy Res.* Oct 1997;28(3):167-179.
5. Zhang X, Velumian AA, Jones OT, Carlen PL. Modulation of high-voltage-activated calcium channels in dentate granule cells by topiramate. *Epilepsia.* 2000;41 Suppl 1:S52-60.
6. Herrero AI, Del Olmo N, Gonzalez-Escalada JR, Solis JM. Two new actions of topiramate: inhibition of depolarizing GABA(A)-mediated responses and activation of a potassium conductance. *Neuropharmacology.* Feb 2002;42(2):210-220.
7. Zona C, Ciotti MT, Avoli M. Topiramate attenuates voltage-gated sodium currents in rat cerebellar granule cells. *Neurosci Lett.* Aug 15 1997;231(3):123-126.
8. Zona C, Ragozzino D, Ciotti MT, et al. Sodium, calcium and late potassium currents are reduced in cerebellar granule cells cultured in the presence of a protein complex conferring resistance to excitatory amino acids. *Eur J Neurosci.* Nov 1 1993;5(11):1479-1484.
9. Gibbs JW, 3rd, Sombati S, DeLorenzo RJ, Coulter DA. Cellular actions of topiramate: blockade of kainate-evoked inward currents in cultured hippocampal neurons. *Epilepsia.* 2000;41 Suppl 1:S10-16.
10. Gryder DS, Rogawski MA. Selective antagonism of GluR5 kainate-receptor-mediated synaptic currents by topiramate in rat basolateral amygdala neurons. *J Neurosci.* Aug 6 2003;23(18):7069-7074.
11. Poulsen CF, Simeone TA, Maar TE, Smith-Swintosky V, White HS, Schousboe A. Modulation by topiramate of AMPA and kainate mediated calcium influx in cultured cerebral cortical, hippocampal and cerebellar neurons. *Neurochem Res.* Jan 2004;29(1):275-282.
12. Abramowicz M. Drugs for epilepsy. *Treatment Guide Medical Letter.* Vol 9; 2003:57-64.
13. Preminger GM, Sakhaee K, Skurla C, Pak CY. Prevention of recurrent calcium stone formation with potassium citrate therapy in patients with distal renal tubular acidosis. *J Urol.* Jul 1985;134(1):20-23.
14. Shorvon SD. Safety of topiramate: adverse events and relationships to dosing. *Epilepsia.* 1996;37 Suppl 2:S18-S22.
15. Nicar MJ, Skurla C, Sakhaee K, Pak CY. Low urinary citrate excretion in nephrolithiasis. *Urology.* Jan 1983;21(1):8-14.
16. Pak CY. Prevention and treatment of kidney stones. Role of medical prevention. *J Urol.* Mar 1989;141(3 Pt 2):798-801.
17. Meyer JL, Smith LH. Growth of calcium oxalate crystals. II. Inhibition by natural urinary crystal growth inhibitors. *Invest Urol.* Jul 1975;13(1):36-39.
18. Sidhu H, Gupta R, Thind SK, Nath R. Inhibition of calcium oxalate monohydrate (COM) crystal growth by pyrophosphate, citrate and rat urine. *Urol Res.* 1986;14(6):299-303.
19. Nicar MJ, Hill K, Pak CY. Inhibition by citrate of spontaneous precipitation of calcium oxalate in vitro. *J Bone Miner Res.* Jun 1987;2(3):215-220.
20. Geller DA, Ostrow JD, Moore EW, Celic L, Nancollas GH. Binding of calcium by organic anions, determined by perturbation of the equilibrium solubility of [^{14}C]calcium oxalate. *Clin Chim Acta.* Jul 14 1989;182(3):255-270.
21. Greischar A, Nakagawa Y, Coe FL. Influence of urine pH and citrate concentration on the upper limit of metastability for calcium phosphate. *J Urol.* Mar 2003;169(3):867-870.

22. Tiselius HG. A simplified estimate of the ion-activity product of calcium phosphate in urine. *Eur Urol.* 1984;10(3):191-195.
23. Coe FL, Strauss AL, Tembe V, Le Dun S. Uric acid saturation in calcium nephrolithiasis. *Kidney Int.* May 1980;17(5):662-668.
24. Sorensen LB. Role of the intestinal tract in the elimination of uric acid. *Arthritis Rheum.* Oct 1965;8(5):694-706.
25. Enomoto A, Kimura H, Chairoungdua A, et al. Molecular identification of a renal urate anion exchanger that regulates blood urate levels. *Nature.* May 23 2002;417(6887):447-452.
26. Pak CY, Holt K, Zerwekh JE. Attenuation by monosodium urate of the inhibitory effect of glycosaminoglycans on calcium oxalate nucleation. *Invest Urol.* Sep 1979;17(2):138-140.
27. Riese RJ, Sakhaee K. Uric acid nephrolithiasis: pathogenesis and treatment. *J Urol.* Sep 1992;148(3):765-771.
28. Moe OW, Abate N, Sakhaee K. Pathophysiology of uric acid nephrolithiasis. *Endocrinol Metab Clin North Am.* Dec 2002;31(4):895-914.
29. Sekine T, Watanabe N, Hosoyamada M, Kanai Y, Endou H. Expression cloning and characterization of a novel multispecific organic anion transporter. *J Biol Chem.* Jul 25 1997;272(30):18526-18529.
30. Cha SH, Sekine T, Fukushima JI, et al. Identification and characterization of human organic anion transporter 3 expressing predominantly in the kidney. *Mol Pharmacol.* May 2001;59(5):1277-1286.
31. Ichida K, Hosoyamada M, Hisatome I, et al. Clinical and molecular analysis of patients with renal hypouricemia in Japan-influence of URAT1 gene on urinary urate excretion. *J Am Soc Nephrol.* Jan 2004;15(1):164-173.
32. Cameron JS, Moro F, Simmonds HA. Gout, uric acid and purine metabolism in paediatric nephrology. *Pediatr Nephrol.* Feb 1993;7(1):105-118.
33. Sakhaee K, Adams-Huet B, Moe OW, Pak CY. Pathophysiologic basis for normouricosuric uric acid nephrolithiasis. *Kidney Int.* Sep 2002;62(3):971-979.
34. Alvarez-Nemegyei J, Medina-Escobedo M, Villanueva-Jorge S, Vazquez-Mellado J. Prevalence and risk factors for urolithiasis in primary gout: is a reappraisal needed? *J Rheumatol.* Nov 2005;32(11):2189-2191.
35. Cameron MA, Maalouf NM, Adams-Huet B, Moe OW, Sakhaee K. Urine composition in type 2 diabetes: predisposition to uric acid nephrolithiasis. *J Am Soc Nephrol.* May 2006;17(5):1422-1428.
36. Taylor EN, Stampfer MJ, Curhan GC. Diabetes mellitus and the risk of nephrolithiasis. *Kidney Int.* Sep 2005;68(3):1230-1235.
37. Pak CY, Sakhaee K, Moe O, et al. Biochemical profile of stone-forming patients with diabetes mellitus. *Urology.* Mar 2003;61(3):523-527.
38. Daudon M, Lacour B, Jungers P. High prevalence of uric acid calculi in diabetic stone formers. *Nephrol Dial Transplant.* Feb 2005;20(2):468-469.
39. Daudon M, Traxer O, Conort P, Lacour B, Jungers P. Type 2 diabetes increases the risk for uric acid stones. *J Am Soc Nephrol.* Jul 2006;17(7):2026-2033.
40. Ekeruo WO, Tan YH, Young MD, et al. Metabolic risk factors and the impact of medical therapy on the management of nephrolithiasis in obese patients. *J Urol.* Jul 2004;172(1):159-163.
41. Daudon M, Lacour B, Jungers P. Influence of body size on urinary stone composition in men and women. *Urol Res.* Jun 2006;34(3):193-199.
42. Abate N, Chandalia M, Cabo-Chan AV, Jr., Moe OW, Sakhaee K. The metabolic syndrome and uric acid nephrolithiasis: novel features of renal manifestation of insulin resistance. *Kidney Int.* Feb 2004;65(2):386-392.
43. Maalouf NM, Sakhaee K, Parks JH, Coe FL, Adams-Huet B, Pak CY. Association of urinary pH with body weight in nephrolithiasis. *Kidney Int.* Apr 2004;65(4):1422-1425.
44. Chobanian MC, Hammerman MR. Insulin stimulates ammoniagenesis in canine renal proximal tubular segments. *Am J Physiol.* Dec 1987;253(6 Pt 2):F1171-1177.
45. Nagami GT. Luminal secretion of ammonia in the mouse proximal tubule perfused in vitro. *J Clin Invest.* Jan 1988;81(1):159-164.
46. Gesek FA, Schoolwerth AC. Insulin increases Na(+)-H+ exchange activity in proximal tubules from normotensive and hypertensive rats. *Am J Physiol.* May 1991;260(5 Pt 2):F695-703.

47. Klisic J, Hu MC, Nief V, et al. Insulin activates Na(+)/H(+) exchanger 3: biphasic response and glucocorticoid dependence. Am J Physiol Renal Physiol. Sep 2002;283(3):F532-539.
48. Cameron MS MN, Abate N, Moe OW, Sakhaee K. The Renal Acidification Response to Insulin Differs Between Uric Acid Stone Formers and Normal Subjects (Abstract). *J Am Soc Nephrol.* 2004;15(abstract issue):518A.
49. Crandall DL, Fried SK, Francendese AA, Nickel M, DiGirolamo M. Lactate release from isolated rat adipocytes: influence of cell size, glucose concentration, insulin and epinephrine. *Horm Metab Res.* Jul 1983;15(7):326-329.
50. Hossain P, Kawar B, El Nahas M. Obesity and diabetes in the developing world--a growing challenge. *N Engl J Med.* Jan 18 2007;356(3):213-215.
51. Stamatelou KK, Francis ME, Jones CA, Nyberg LM, Curhan GC. Time trends in reported prevalence of kidney stones in the United States: 1976-1994. *Kidney Int.* May 2003;63(5):1817-1823.

Hyperoxaluria and Bariatric Surgery

John R. Asplin

Litholink Corporation and University of Chicago, Chicago IL

Abstract. Bariatric surgery as a means to treat obesity is becoming increasingly common in the United States. An early form of bariatric surgery, the jejunoileal bypass, had to be abandoned in 1980 due to numerous complications, including hyperoxaluria and kidney stones. Current bariatric procedures have not been systematically evaluated to determine if they cause hyperoxaluria. Presented here are data showing that hyperoxaluria is the major metabolic abnormality in patients with bariatric surgery who form kidney stones. Further studies are needed to assess the prevalence of hyperoxaluria in all patients with bariatric surgery.

Keywords: Nephrolithiasis, Obesity, Kidney Failure, Oxalate
PACS: 87.19.Xx

INTRODUCTION

Extreme obesity is associated with multiple medical problems and it has been demonstrated that mortality increases significantly when body mass index (defined as height in cm/weight in kg) is above 35 [1]. Medical co-morbidities such as diabetes mellitus, hyperlipidemia, sleep apnea, hypertension and arthritis reduce the quality of life as well as shortening life span. Although many dietary and lifestyle programs have shown success inducing weight loss acutely, there is little data to support that such programs maintain long term weight loss and the expected health benefits for those who use the programs. Bariatric surgery developed in response to the lack of success of diet and lifestyle changes in effectively reducing weight.

The first common bariatric procedure was the jejunoileal (JI) bypass [2]. In this surgery, the proximal 35 cm of the jejunum is anastamosed to the ileum 10 cm from the ileocecal valve, providing very little intestinal surface area for absorption. The altered intestinal physiology did result in significant weight loss, but the accompanying malabsorption of vitamins, bile acids, fats, and other nutrients led to a number of complications. Many subjects suffered from liver disease, arthritis, vitamin deficiencies, bone disease, and kidney stones [3]. Hyperoxaluria was determined to be the etiology of the kidney stones. The malabsorbed fatty acids would bind intestinal oxalate, leaving a greater portion of intestinal oxalate free to be absorbed. In addition, reduced absorption of bile salts in the small intestine delivered abnormal amounts of bile salts to the colon, which damaged the colonic mucosa making it more permeable to oxalate. The combined effect of these two factors led to an increase in absorption of dietary oxalate [4]. Kidney stones were quite common, and hyperoxaluria could be so severe to lead to kidney damage, and in the most extreme cases, kidney failure. Due to

CP900, *Renal Stone Disease, 1st Annual International Urolithiasis Research Symposium,*
edited by A. P. Evan, J. E. Lingeman, and J. C. Williams, Jr.

the significant level of complications, the FDA banned the jejunoileal bypass in 1980. However, 25,000 JI bypasses had been performed prior to the ban and patients continued to present with complications for years after. Many of the bypasses needed to be surgically revised to relieve the side effects [3].

When JI bypass was banned a new bariatric procedure was needed for patients with severe obesity. The Roux-en-y gastric bypass, which had first been introduced as a treatment for obesity by Mason and Ito in 1967, became the new bariatric procedure of choice [5]. Gastric bypass induces weight loss by restricting the size of the gastric reservoir, altering caloric intake by inducing dumping syndrome in response to high carbohydrate meals, and by causing a feeling of anorexia. Later, other bariatric procedures were introduced, some focused on restricting caloric intake by reducing the size of the stomach, such as gastric banding, and other procedures caused some degree of malabsorption, such as the very long limb gastric bypass and the biliopancreatic diversion. However, none of the procedures were felt to lead to the severe degree of malabsorption seen with JI bypass and therefore complication rates were less, and the risk of hyperoxaluria and stone disease were considered small.

Prevalence of obesity has increased dramatically over the last 20 years. Based on data from the NHANES studies, approximately 15% of the population had BMIs in the obese range from 1962 to 1985 [6]. However, in the NHANES study of 1994 and the most recent data from 2000 there was a clear increase in the rate of obesity, reaching 30% of the adult population by the 2000 survey. From 1994 to 2000 there was a 40% increase in the rate of extreme obesity (defined as a BMI >40). As would be expected, as the rate of obesity in the US increased, so has the rate of bariatric surgery. From 1998 to 2002, bariatric surgery increased 3 fold from approximately 20,000 procedures to over 60,000 procedures [7]. Over that time period the most common procedure performed was a gastric bypass, accounting for approximately 80% of bariatric surgery cases. Biliopancreatic diversion and pure restrictive procedures accounted for the rest, being performed at about equal rates.

MODERN BARIATRIC SURGERY AND HYPEROXALURIA

Despite the great increase in bariatric surgery, only one study attempted to measure urine oxalate excretion in patients with bariatric surgery other than JI bypass. In 1981, Hofmann et al reported urine oxalate excretion rates in 22 patients who had undergone biliopancreatic diversions, compared with a set of control patients, all spouses of the patients [8]. Only one surgical met their definition of hyperoxaluria. However, sparse data are provided about the study design, such as gender of the subjects, time from bariatric surgery and any dietary data, nor was any statistical analysis provided as to whether the bariatric surgery patients' urine oxalate excretion was different than the controls. Overall, there is little known about the risk of stone disease after bariatric surgery.

A study from the Mayo clinic was one of the first to suggest a link between bariatric surgery and kidney stones [9]. In 2005 Nelson et al reported on 23 patients who they classified as having enteric hyperoxaluria diagnosed after having bariatric surgery. The series included both patients with the standard Roux-en-Y gastric bypass as well as patients with the very long limb gastric bypass, a procedure felt to result in some degree of malabsorption and more significant weight loss. Twenty one of the twenty three patients presented with kidney stones and the vast majority were found to have hyperoxaluria when urine chemistries were measured. Of those presenting with kidney stones, the mean urine oxalate excretion rate was 85 mg/day. Two of the patients presented with acute kidney failure and were found to have oxalosis on kidney biopsy. This study is a retrospective review of those subjects who presented with renal problems after bariatric surgery. In order to estimate the prevalence of such renal problems in the bariatric surgery population the investigators performed a survey of all subjects who had the very long limb gastric bypass at the Mayo Clinic. Of the 258 subjects they attempted to contact, 73% responded, of which 16% developed kidney stones after the bariatric surgery. This work supports the premise that hyperoxaluria and kidney stones are a complication of gastric bypass surgery and that some of these patients are at risk for kidney damage from severe hyperoxaluria.

We have also undertaken a study to determine if hyperoxaluria may be a complication of modern bariatric procedures [10]. Using a database from a clinical laboratory specializing in measuring urine chemistries in kidney stone patients (Litholink Corporation, Chicago IL), we identified all patients who had reported prior bariatric surgery. 132 patients were identified as having bariatric surgery after 1980. We did not attempt to classify the type of surgery as we were not confident that patients could reliably distinguish the types of surgery. We compared the urine chemistries to normal subjects, routine stone forming patients without a history of bowel disease or intestinal surgery, and patients who had JI bypass surgery. Patients with modern bariatric surgery had urine oxalate excretion nearly double that of non-stone forming subjects and routine stone forming patients (Figure 1), though not quite as high as had been seen with JI bypass procedures. Calcium oxalate supersaturation, the driving force for crystallization, was even higher in patients with modern bariatric surgery than JI bypass, as the modern bariatric patients had slightly higher urine calcium and lower urine volumes.

Since our study only contains post-surgery urine chemistries, it could be possible that hyperoxaluria is a characteristic of patients with severe obesity and that we are incorrect in assigning the cause of the hyperoxaluria to the weight loss surgery. Lemann et al showed that urine oxalate excretion increases with body weight, though none of the subjects in his study had the level of hyperoxaluria we report, nor were they chosen for obesity [11]. Taylor et al have reported that risk of kidney stone disease increases with BMI, though urine chemistry data was not available to determine if hyperoxaluria played a role in this phenomenon [12]. To address this issue, we compared female patients with bariatric surgery (n = 104) to routine female stone formers from the Litholink data base, chosen over a two month period, who weighed more than 100 kg (n = 56). The bariatric surgery group weighed 94 kg on average at the time of the evaluation and had a urine oxalate excretion of 73 mg/d, whereas the obese stone forming patients had an average weight of 120 kg but had a mean oxalate excretion of only 36 mg/d (Figure 2). It seems unlikely that obesity by itself explains the hyperoxaluria seen in the bariatric surgery patients.

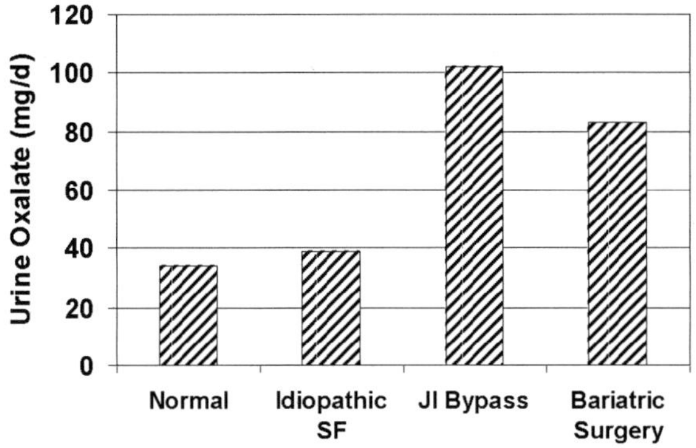

FIGURE 1. Comparison of urine oxalate excretion in normal subjects, idiopathic stone forming patients, patients with jejunoileal bypass and patients with modern bariatric surgery.

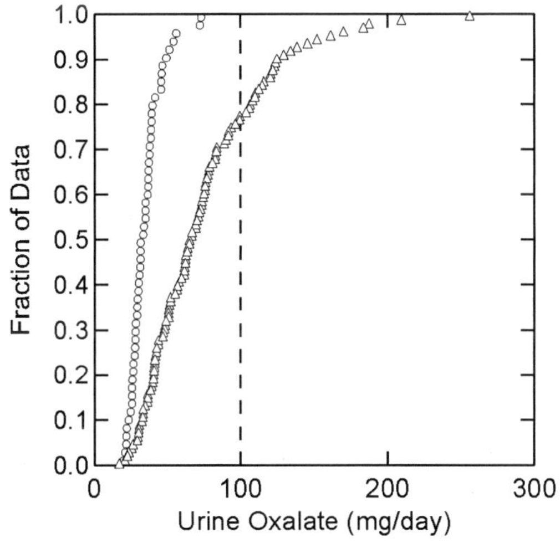

FIGURE 2. Quantile plot of urine oxalate excretion in women with bariatric surgery (triangles) and women with idiopathic kidney stone disease (open circles). Women with bariatric surgery have much higher urine oxalate, with over 20% having a urine oxalate greater than 100 mg/day.

Another way to address the effect of bariatric surgery on urine oxalate excretion would be to determine urine oxalate excretion before and after bariatric surgery. There have been no reports in the literature of oxalate measured pre and post bariatric surgery. Figure 3 shows data from two such patients identified from my own clinical experience. Both patients had a history of kidney stones and had urine chemistries measured as part of routine medical care. Both patients had Roux-en-Y gastric bypass. As can be seen in the figure, both patients had significant and persistent elevations of urine oxalate after their surgery. Stone formation rates also increased after the bariatric surgery.

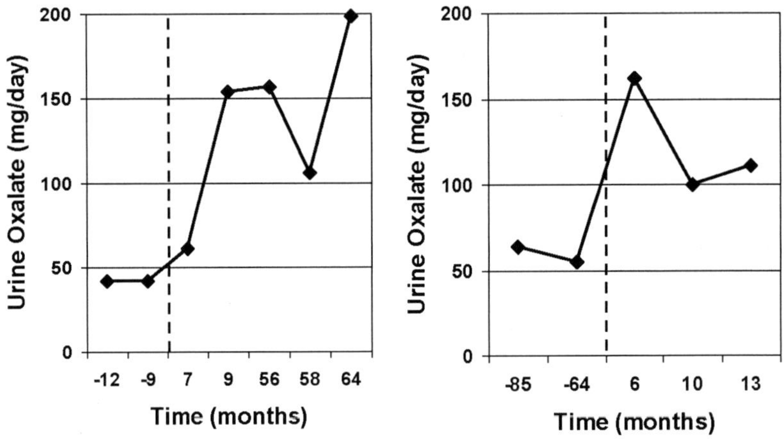

FIGURE 3. Urine oxalate excretion in two patients who had urine oxalate measured prior to gastric bypass surgery and subsequent to the surgery. The vertical dashed line shows the time of the gastric bypass surgery.

DISCUSSION

There are limitations to the data presented here. The studies are retrospective and are subject to bias. The patients included in the studies all presented with either kidney stones or kidney failure, there is not a random sampling of bariatric surgery patients to determine the frequency of hyperoxaluria. Thus, the patients presented may be representative of only a small portion of the total population of bariatric surgery patients. In addition, our data did not allow us to analyze patients based on the type of surgery performed. It seems likely that the different surgical procedures will carry varying degrees of risk for hyperoxaluria. Cross-sectional studies comparing oxalate excretion in patients with various bariatric procedures, as well as prospective studies measuring urine oxalate before and after bariatric surgery are needed to fully delineate the extent of the problem. The data we presented here does supply evidence that there are some patients who develop hyperoxaluria and kidney stones as a result of bariatric surgery. A recent study by Encinosa et al found nephrolithiasis to be the 9th most common cause of emergency room visit in the 6 months post bariatric surgery [13]. Since the rate of bariatric surgery continues to increase, stone rates are likely to increase and more research will be needed to define the extent of this problem.

ACKNOWLEDGMENTS

Fredric L. Coe provided assistance in the analysis of data. Joan Parks and Susan Donahue provided support in the acquisition of the data. This work was supported by NIDDK grant R44DK059086

REFERENCES

1. J. Roth, X. Qiang, S.L. Marban et al. Obes Res 12, 88s-99s (2004)
2. J.H. Payne and L.T. DeWind. Am. J. Surg. 118, 141-147 (1969)
3. J.A. Requarth, K.E. Burchard, T.A. Colacchio, et al. Arch. Surg. 130, 318-325 (1995)
4. J.Q. Stauffer. Am. J. Clin. Nutr. 30, 64-71 (1977)
5. E.E. Mason and C.C. Ito. Surg. Clin. North Am. 47, 1345-1354 (1967)
6. K.M. Flegal, M.D. Carroll, C.L. Ogden and C.L. Johnson. JAMA 288, 1723-1727 (2002)
7. H.P. Santry, D.L. Gillen, D.S. Lauderdale. JAMA 294, 1909-1917 (2005)
8. A.F. Hofmann, G. Schmuck, N Scopinaro. et al. Int. J. Obes. 5, 513-518 (1981)
9. W. K. Nelson, B.A. Scott, S.G. Houghton, et al. Surg Obes Relat Dis 1, 481-485 (2005)
10. J.R. Asplin and F.L. Coe. J. Urol. 177, 565-569 (2007)
11. J. Lemann, J.A. Pleuss, E.M. Worcester et al. Kidney Int. 49, 200-208 (1996)
12. E.N. Taylor, M.J. Stampfer and G.C. Curhan. JAMA 293, 455-462 (2005)
13. W.E Encinosa, D.M. Bernard, CC Chen et al. Medical Care 44:706-712 (2006)

Epidemiologic Insights into Stone Disease as a Systemic Disorder

Gary C. Curhan

Renal Division and Channing Laboratory, Department of Medicine, Brigham and Women's Hospital, Harvard Medical School; and Department of Epidemiology, Harvard School of Public Health; 181 Longwood Avenue, Boston, MA, USA

Abstract. Examining the epidemiology of stone disease can provide insight into etiology. There is a growing body of evidence that stone disease is not simply a disorder of the kidney. In fact, nephrolithiasis is clearly a systemic disorder. Conditions associated with stone disease include the classic ones such as inflammatory bowel disease and primary hyperparathyroidism. More recent studies have demonstrated strong associations with obesity, gout, diabetes and hypertension. Future studies will help uncover the underlying common pathophysiologic abnormalities.

Key words: nephrolithiasis, obesity, diabetes, gout, hypertension, urine composition
PACS: 87.19.Xx

INTRODUCTION

Epidemiology is defined as the study of the distribution and determinants of disease. Examination of these factors may provide insight into the systemic nature of nephrolithiasis.

The distribution of nephrolithiasis is usually quantified in terms of prevalence and incidence. In the US, the prevalence of a history of stone disease increased from 3.8% in NHANES II (1976-80) to 5.2% in NHANES III (1988-1994) [1]. Somewhat surprisingly, a recent study from the Olmstead County Epidemiology Project reported that incidence rates appear to have stabilized or may have fallen over the past two decades [2].

Dietary risk factors

Risk factors for stone disease are usually divided into three main categories: dietary, non-dietary and urinary. It is important to note that the importance of different risk factors varies by age and sex (and likely race).

Dietary factors that have been consistently shown to reduce the risk of stone formation include higher dietary calcium intake and higher fluid intake [3-5]. In older men and women, higher potassium intake is also associated with reduced risk of stone formation. In women, but not in men, higher phytate intake reduces the risk. Sucrose intake is associated with an increased risk of stone formation. In older men, higher

CP900, *Renal Stone Disease, 1st Annual International Urolithiasis Research Symposium,* edited by A. P. Evan, J. E. Lingeman, and J. C. Williams, Jr.

vitamin C intake increases the risk. Other factors such as animal protein and magnesium have not been consistently associated with risk.

Individual beverages may impact risk independent of their effect on urine volume [6, 7]. Beverages that have been associated with a reduced risk of stone formation include milk, coffee, tea, beer and wine, likely by increasing urine flow and reducing urine concentration. Grapefruit juice appears to increase the risk but the mechanism is unknown.

Non-dietary risk factors

A number of systemic conditions have been known to increase the risk of stone formation including inflammatory bowel disease and primary hyperparathyroidism. However, only recently has it been appreciated that more common systemic disorders influence the risk of nephrolithiasis. These conditions include obesity [8], gout [9, 10], and diabetes [11].

Obesity

While obesity has long been believed to be associated with stone formation, evidence was lacking until recently. Taylor and colleagues [8] found in a prospective study of three large cohorts (Nurses' Health Study I, Nurses' Health Study II and the Health Professionals Follow-up Study) that the risk of stone formation increased with increasing weight (Fig. 1); the magnitude of the increase was greater in women than in men.

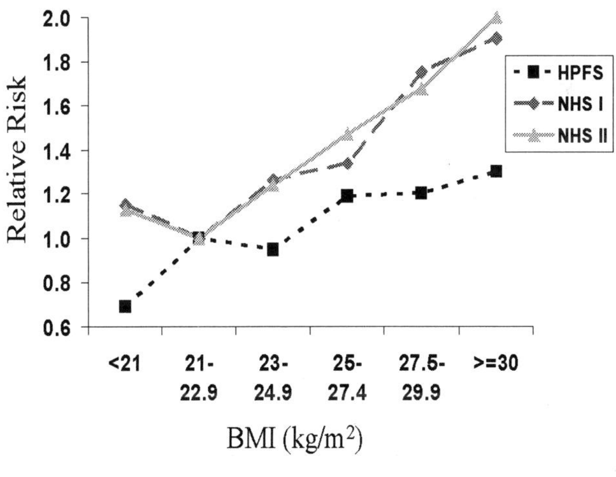

Figure 1. Relative risk of symptomatic kidney stones versus body mass index [8]. HPFS: Health Professionals Follow-up Study. NHS: Nurses' Health Study.

Similar relations were seen when examining other measures of body size such as weight and waist circumference. These associations were independent of age, fluid intake and other dietary risk factors. Thus, it appears that being overweight or obese increases the risk of stone formation independent of dietary factors.

Gout

Gout has long been associated with risk of uric acid stones but may also increase the risk of calcium oxalate stones. Using data from NHANES III, gout was associated with a 46% increased risk of being a stone former in men and 65% increased risk in women [10]. In the one prospective study, men with a history of gout were more than twice as likely as those with no history of gout to subsequently develop a kidney stone, independent of age, dietary factors and body mass index [9].

Diabetes mellitus

Insulin resistance may be one potential explanation for the increased risk of stone formation observed with increasing BMI. The exact roles of insulin and insulin resistance in stone formation remain unclear. The association between a history of type II diabetes mellitus and risk of nephrolithiasis has only recently been studied. In cross-sectional analyses, men and women with a history of diabetes were more likely to also have a history of nephrolithiasis [11]. When examined prospectively, the risk was increased by 58% in younger women and 27% in older women; there was no association in men but this may have been due to the late mean age of onset of diabetes in the male cohort.

Hypertension

A history of nephrolithiasis increases the risk of subsequently developing hypertension [12, 13]. However, a history of hypertension does not appear to increase the risk of stone formation. One possible explanation is that hypertension is more likely to develop as a result of renal damage related the obstruction or treatment of stone disease (e.g. ESWL).

Urinary risk factors

Examination of 24-hour urine results may provide insight into the potential mechanisms that will explain the associations between systemic disorders and nephrolithiasis. To date, two large studies have examined the relation between body size and 24-hour urine composition [14, 15]. Maalouf and colleagues reported an inverse association between urine pH and body weight [15]. Taylor and colleagues reported on all the commonly measured urinary factors [16]. In addition to confirming the inverse association with urine pH, an inverse association was observed for urinary calcium in women. Positive associations were seen for urine oxalate and citrate in women, but not men, and urine uric acid. There was no association with total volume.

The relation between 24-hour urine composition and risk of hypertension has also been studied [17]. Surprisingly, there was no consistent association in a cross-sectional study between history of hypertension and urine excretion of calcium, magnesium, sodium and potassium. However, urine citrate was strongly inversely associated with hypertension. The role of acid-base regulation in the etiology of hypertension deserves further study.

CONCLUSIONS

Nephrolithiasis is clearly a systemic disorder and a variety of factors influence urine composition of lithogenic substances, including the generation of acid and oxalate. Well accepted dietary risk factors, such as dietary calcium, are influenced by age, sex and body mass index. Future studies need to examine how these systemic factors interrelate and should result in improved preventive strategies that can be tailored to the individual patient.

ACKNOWLEDGMENTS

This work was supported by grants from the National Institutes of Health including Grants DK59583, DK73381, CA87969, CA55075, and CA50385.

REFERENCES

1. K. K. Stamatelou, M. E. Francis, C. A. Jones, L. M. Nyberg, and G. C. Curhan, *Kidney Int* 63, 1817-1823, (2003).
2. J. C. Lieske, L. S. Pena de la Vega, J. M. Slezak, E. J. Bergstralh, C. L. Leibson, K. L. Ho, and M. T. Gettman, *Kidney Int* 69, 760-764, (2006).
3. G. C. Curhan, W. C. Willett, E. L. Knight, and M. J. Stampfer, *Arch Intern Med* 164, 885-891, (2004).
4. G. Curhan, W. Willett, F. Speizer, D. Spiegelman, and M. Stampfer, *Ann Intern Med* 126, 497-504, (1997).
5. G. C. Curhan, W. C. Willett, E. B. Rimm, and M. J. Stampfer, *N Engl J Med* 328, 833-838, (1993).
6. G. C. Curhan, W. C. Willett, F. E. Speizer, and M. J. Stampfer, *Ann Intern Med* 128, 534-540, (1998).
7. G. C. Curhan, W. C. Willett, E. B. Rimm, D. Spiegelman, and M. J. Stampfer, *Am J Epidemiol* 143, 240-247, (1996).
8. E. N. Taylor, M. J. Stampfer, and G. C. Curhan, *JAMA* 293, 455-462, (2005).
9. H. J. Kramer, H. K. Choi, K. Atkinson, M. Stampfer, and G. C. Curhan, *Kidney Int* 64, 1022-1026, (2003).
10. H. M. Kramer and G. Curhan, *Am J Kidney Dis* 40, 37-42, (2002).
11. E. N. Taylor, M. J. Stampfer, and G. C. Curhan, *Kidney Int* 68, 1230-1235, (2005).
12. F. Madore, M. J. Stampfer, E. B. Rimm, and G. C. Curhan, *Am J Hypertens* 11, 46-53, (1998).
13. F. Madore, M. J. Stampfer, W. C. Willett, F. E. Speizer, and G. C. Curhan, *Am J Kidney Dis* 32, 802-807, (1998).
14. G. C. Curhan, W. C. Willett, F. E. Speizer, and M. J. Stampfer, *Kidney Int* 59, 2290-2298, (2001).
15. N. M. Maalouf, K. Sakhaee, J. H. Parks, F. L. Coe, B. Adams-Huet, and C. Y. Pak, *Kidney Int* 65, 1422-1425, (2004).
16. E. N. Taylor and G. C. Curhan, *Am J Kidney Dis* 48, 905-915, (2006).
17. E. N. Taylor, D. B. Mount, J. P. Forman, and G. C. Curhan, *Am J Kidney Dis* 47, 780-789, (2006).

III. INSIGHTS INTO HYPERCALCIURIA AND STONE DISEASE

Soluble Adenylyl Cyclase: Potential Role in Mineral Metabolism

Weidong Geng* and Orson W. Moe*†

*Charles and Jane Pak Center of Mineral Metabolism and Clinical Research, and
†Departments of Internal Medicine and Physiology, University of Texas Southwestern Medical Center,
5323 Harry Hines Blvd, Dallas, TX 75390-8885, USA

Abstract. The conversion of a signal of inorganic ion concentration to a second messenger is of fundamental biologic significance. The soluble adenylyl cyclase (sAC) serves such a purpose by transducing divalent cation concentrations and bicarbonate concentrations into intracellular cyclic AMP levels. sAC is widely expressed and may represent a generic bicarbonate sensor providing the afferent pathway to bicarbonate-regulated biologic processes. The best described action of sAC to date is in the mediation of bicarbonate-induced changes in sperm motility. Since a number of processes in mineral metabolism—such as bone formation, bone resorption, intestinal calcium absorption, and renal calcium transport in the distal convoluted tubule—are regulated by bicarbonate, sAC may play a role at multiple levels in mineral metabolism.

Keywords: calcium, second messengers.
PACS: 87.16.Uv

INTRODUCTION

Cyclic adenosine monophosphate (cAMP) is a second messenger that transduces signals to intracellular effectors. Classically, cAMP comes from G protein-coupled transmembrane adenylyl cyclase (tmAC) [1]. In contrast, soluble adenylyl cyclase (sAC) is distinct from the traditional G-protein-regulated transmembrane adenylyl cyclases [2-4]. sAC is soluble and located in the cytoplasm and intracellular organelles [5,6] enabling cAMP to be directly generated inside of the cell and compartmentalized in the vicinity of its targets [5,7]. sAC does not respond to the heterotrimeric G-protein regulators and forskolin, but rather it is stimulated by bicarbonate ion. It is considered a “bicarbonate sensor” in the rat and plays an essential role in mammalian sperm biology [4,6,8,9]. Homozygous sAC-deficient mice are infertile due to a severe sperm-motility defect; a phenotype that can be rescued by provision of cell-permeant cAMP [10]. Besides testis and sperm cells, sAC is also found in kidney, choroid plexus [8] and multiple cell lines [5]. The broad expression pattern of sAC suggests that sAC may subserve a multitude of functions throughout the body, including calcium homeostasis.

Adenylyl cyclase converts ATP to cyclic adenosine monophosphate (cAMP). Nine membrane-bound isoforms (tmAC I–IX) and one sAC have been cloned and characterized [1,11,12]. tmAC has membrane domains and two cytoplasmic catalytic

CP900, *Renal Stone Disease, 1st Annual International Urolithiasis Research Symposium*, edited by A. P. Evan, J. E. Lingeman, and J. C. Williams, Jr.

domains, C1 and C2. Rat sAC has two catalytic domains but no true transmembrane domain. The overall similarity among all ACs is about 60%. Catalytic domains (C1 and C2) have the highest conserved sequences, ranging from 50-90% [11]. All tmACs are stimulated by the stimulatory G-protein ($G_{\alpha s}$) [1]. Except for type IX, all tmACs are stimulated by foskolin [11]. Each tmAC also has a variety of regulatory mechanisms. For example, tmAC-VII is activated by protein kinase C while tmAC-III can be activated by Ca^{2+}/CaM [11].

Reed and coworkers used a genome-wide linkage analysis of three kindreds and mapped a locus and cloned a novel gene linked to idiopathic hypercalciuria, a syndrome characterized by intestinal calcium hyperabsorption, hypercalciuric calcium nephrolithiasis, and low bone mineral density in varying degrees [13,14]. Around the same time, Chen, Buck, Levin and coworkers purified and cloned a soluble adenylyl cyclase from rat testis [7,8]. Human sAC has 33 exons, spans 104 kb and the full-length cDNA from intestine has 5085 nucleotides (GenBank AF331033) (Fig. 1). The polypeptide sequence predicts two AC catalytic sites (Fig. 1). A number of putative functional motifs have been predicted, but only the cyclase sites have been confirmed.

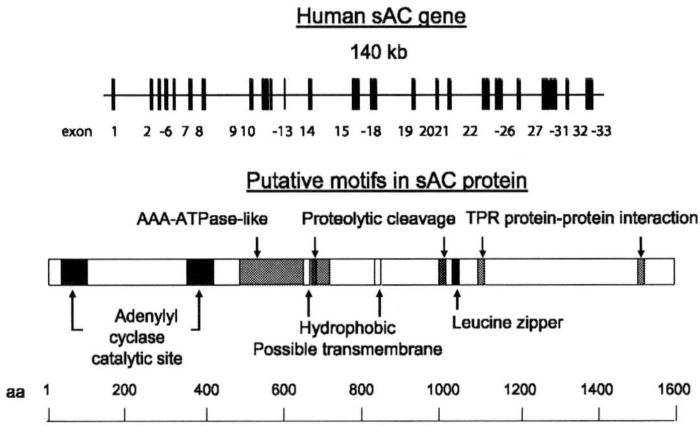

FIGURE 1. Gene and protein structure of human soluble adenylyl cyclase (sAC). Protein functional motifs are predicted from the primary sequence. Only the function of the cyclase domain has been confirmed. Although there is evidence of cleavage of sAC, the predicted proteolytic sites have not been verified.

INORGANIC ION SENSING BY sAC

Adenylyl cyclase needs divalent cations to express its cyclase activity. In addition to divalent cations, sAC also responds to HCO_3^- [15]. Figure 2 shows the dose-response of recombinant hsAC to changes in ambient Mg^{2+}, Mn^{2+}, Ca^{2+}, and HCO_3^-. The patterns are complex. Mg^{2+} stimulates hsAC with first order kinetics ($K_{0.5}$ = 2.4) (Fig. 2A). Mn^{2+} on the other hand, stimulates hsAC to a V_{max} that is 20-fold higher than that of Mg^{2+}. The dose-dependence shows a classic cooperative sigmoidal curve ($K_{0.5}$ = 4.0 mM, Hill coefficient = 2.3) (Fig. 2B). Of special interest is the fact that hsAC is exquisitely sensitive to HCO_3^-. In the presence of Mg^{2+}, cyclase activity is stimulated by HCO_3^- by first order kinetics with a $K_{0.5}$ of 8.7 mM (Fig. 2C). Under maximal stimulation by Mn^{2+}, addition of HCO_3^- inhibits cyclase activity, also with first order kinetics, with a $K_{0.5}$ of 4.0 mM (Fig. 2D). Ca^{2+} is a weak stimulator for adenylyl cyclase activity. To better visualize the dose response of Ca^{2+}, we stimulated the basal level of cyclase activity by adding a small amount of Mg^{2+} and HCO_3^-. In the presence of 2 mM Mg^{2+} and 20 mM HCO_3^-, Ca^{2+} stimulated cyclase activity in a dose-dependent manner from 0.12 to 1.05 mM (Fig. 2E). At more physiological cytosolic concentrations from 2 to 1,200 nM ionized Ca^{2+}, cyclase activity also increased in a dose-dependent manner (Fig. 2F). This suggests that the interaction between HCO_3^- and hsAC is highly complex and depends on whether the enzyme is Mg^{2+}-bound, Mn^{2+}-bound, or Ca^{2+}-bound.

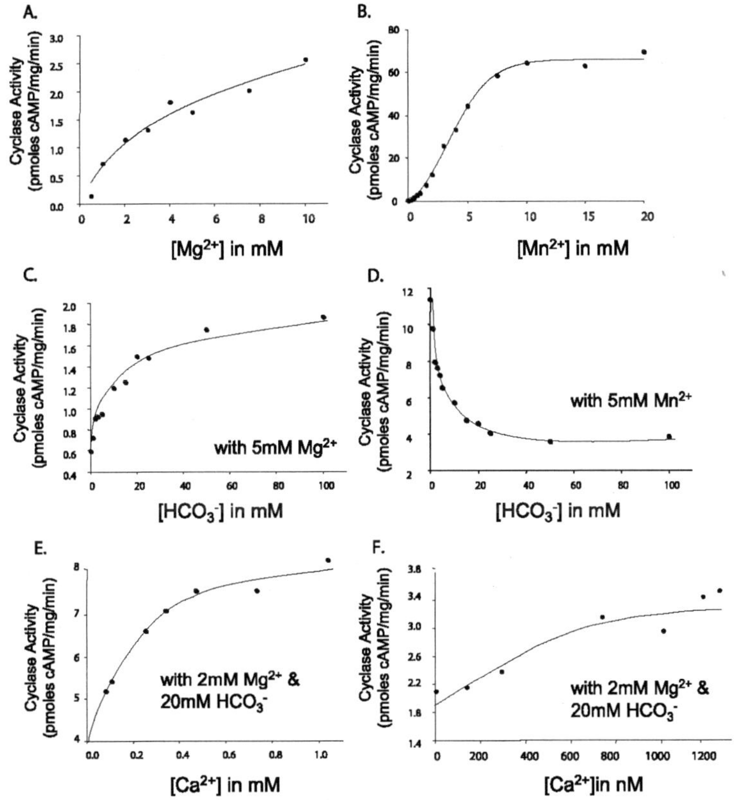

Figure 2. Dose-response curves showing the effect of Mg^{2+}, Mn^{2+}, Ca^{2+}, or HCO_3^- on cyclase activity of purified recombinant $hsAC^{aa1\text{-}483}$. Recombinant $hsAC^{aa1\text{-}483}$ was assayed for adenylyl cyclase activity in the presence of $MgCl_2$ (*A*), $MnCl_2$ (*B*), HCO_3^- plus 5 mM Mg^{2+} (*C*), HCO_3^- plus 5 mM Mn^{2+} (*D*), $CaCl_2$ in millimolar concentrations plus 2mM Mg^{2+} & 20 mM HCO_3^- (E), or $CaCl_2$ in physiological intracellular concentrations plus 2mM Mg^{2+} & 20 mM HCO_3^- (F), at the concentrations shown along the x-axis. In *D*, free Mn^{2+} was clamped at 5 mM as HCO_3^- was varied. For the physiological concentrations in F, ionic Ca^{2+} was manipulated by adding either EGTA or $CaCl_2$.

STRUCTURAL STUDIES OF sAC

Binding sites for the divalent cations and HCO_3^- in human sAC have not been visualized. Putative sites can be predicted by alignment of the amino acid sequence with the known divalent cation binding sites in tmAC (Fig. 3). tmAC contains two sites for cation binding that are referred to as A and B. The crystal structure of tmAC indicates that Mg^{2+} or Zn^{2+} binds to the A-site and Mn^{2+} binds to the B-site [16]. It is interesting to note that Mg^{2+} and Zn^{2+} bind to the same site in tmAC but have opposite effects on cyclase activity. Mg^{2+} stimulates [16] but Zn^{2+} inhibits [17] cyclase activity. Human sAC conserves the same amino acids that could serve as the binding sites for divalent cations (Fig. 3). Steegborn and coworkers first solved the crystal structure of cyanobacterial sAC [18]. D1017, I1018, and D1061 of cyanobacterial sAC coordinate the Ca^{2+} binding site that is equivalent to the B-site of tmAC5. The identified Ca^{2+} binding site, D1061, of cyanobacterial sAC is equivalent to the B site of tmAC5 and D99 of hsAC (Fig. 3).

```
                                                                        B-site
hsAC_C1             MNTPKEEFQDWPIVRIAAHLPDLIVYGHFSPERPFMDYFDGVLMFVDISGFTAMTEKFSS   60
CyaC_S_platensis    --------------------GDLTLD--LRPEPRLIT-----ILFSDIVGFTRMSNALQ- 1029
tmAC_VC1            ---------MEMKADINAKQEDMMFHKIYIQKHDNVS-----ILFADIEGFTSLASQCT-  408
                     .:.... .        :   *: .        :   :   .. ::* ** *** ::.   :

                                                               A-site
hsAC_C1             AMYMDRGAEQLVEILNYHISAIVEKVLIFGGDILKFAGDALLALWRVERKQ--LKNIITV  118
CyaC_S_platensis    -------SQGVAELLNEYLGEMTRAVFENQGTVDKFVGDAIMALYGAPEEMSPSEQVRRA 1082
tmAC_VC1            -------AQELVMTLNELFARFDKLAAENHCLRIKILGDCYYCVSGLPEAR--ADHAHCC  459
                    :   . .:: :.   **   :. :  . .           *: **.   .:     .    .:
```

Figure 3. Alignment of the partial amino acid sequences of the human sAC C1 domain, *S. platensis* cyaC domain, and trans-membrane AC (type V) C1 domain. Equivalent A- and B-sites (in gray color) in hsAC for divalent cation binding are indicated.

Co-crystallization of sAC with HCO_3^- produced no crystals and soaking HCO_3^- into crystals dissolved them. The HCO_3^- binding site was not seen in crystals when an sAC crystal was flash-soaked with HCO_3^- followed by freezing. Based on these findings, the authors proposed a mechanism by which HCO_3^- promotes the closure and metal recruitment of the catalytic active site. Cann and coworkers identified a putative HCO_3^- binding site in bacterial AC (Anabaena cyaB1) [2]. By sequence alignment and comparison of the HCO_3^--sensitive and -insensitive adenylyl cyclases, they found that HCO_3^--sensitive cyclases have a characteristic lysine (K646 in cyaB1) and threonine (T721 in cyaB1) residues (Fig. 4). Similar K and T residues can be found in the 1st and 2nd catalytic sites respectively in both rat and human sAC. When K646 was mutated to A, cyclase activity was reduced by >95% and was refractory to HCO_3^- activation. When T721 was mutated to A, both cyclase activity and HCO_3^- sensitivity were preserved. However, if T721 was mutated to D, the mutant protein retained its cyclase activity but lost HCO_3^- sensitivity.

This data is subject to the following interpretation. The loss of HCO_3^- -sensitivity is difficult to interpret when the V_{max} of the enzyme is reduced from 238 to 2.8 nmole/mg/min. The lysine residue is likely critical for cyclase activity but its role in

HCO_3^- sensing is uncertain. The threonine is unlikely to be critical as T to A mutation fully retains HCO_3^- -sensitivity. However, the introduction of aspartate to replace threonine abolished HCO_3^- -sensitivity. However, the HCO_3^- site is still elusive. Clearly, functional analysis or crystallography studies are needed. The crystal structure of cyanobacterial sAC suggests that HCO_3^- promotes the closure and metal recruitment of the catalytic active site [18]. However, the exact binding site for HCO_3^- is not seen in the cyanobacterial sAC crystals.

```
             aa#                                                            aa#
                                   ↓                              ↓
cyaB1        638 FNYEGT LD  KF I GDALM (59aa) GSH KRMDYT VIGDGVN   728

rsAC C1       87 L I FGGD I L  KFAGDALL (55aa) GDE TRNY FI VIGQAVD  172
rsAC C2      336 FMFD  ------------KGCSFL (51aa) GHT VRHEYT VIGQKVN  407

hsAC C1       87 L I FGGD I L  K FAGDALL (55aa) GDET HSH FLVIGQAVD 172
hsAC C2      345 FMFD  ------------KGCSFL (51aa) GHTV RHEYT VIGQKVN 413
```

C1: 1st catalytic site C2: 2nd catalytic site

Figure 4. Alignment of catalytic sites of HCO_3^--sensitive AC's.

sAC IN ORGAN PHYSIOLOGY

sAC was first cloned and characterized from rat testis [7,8]. sAC is located in the cytoplasm and intracellular organelles, enabling cAMP to be generated inside the cell and compartmentalized in the vicinity of its targets [5,7]. sAC does not respond to heterotrimeric G-protein regulators and forskolin but is stimulated by HCO_3^-. sAC is considered a "HCO_3^- sensor" and plays an essential role in mammalian sperm biology [7-10,19]. In epididymis, luminal pH and HCO_3^- regulate the recycling of V-ATPase in clear cells through the action of sAC [20]. Homozygous targeted disruption of sAC in mice leads to infertility due to a severe sperm-motility defect [10]. Cyclase activity and cAMP content are markedly reduced in the spermatozoa of $sAC^{-/-}$ mice [19]. Sperm developed from $sAC^{-/-}$ mice are unable to fertilize zona-intact eggs due to lack of HCO_3^- induced Ca^{2+} entry, protein tyrosine phosphorylation, and hyperactivated motility that are the necessary steps during capacitation of sperm [19]. Provision of cell-permeate cAMP can rescue this phonotype [10,19]. There are no reported structural abnormalities in testes and epididymides in $sAC^{-/-}$ mice [10]. Kidney and bone function were not reported in these mice. Besides testis and sperm cells, sAC is also found in choroid plexus [8], and multiple cell lines [5].

SPECULATION OF THE ROLE OF sAC IN MINERAL METABOLISM

Human sAC is highly polymorphic with at least 17 sites of allelic sequence variations. The human locus was first identified by linkage in three kindreds with an

LOD score of >10 [13]. Although some of these sequence variations can be found in apparently normal individuals, some of these occur with higher frequency in patients with absorptive hypercalciuria and osteoporosis compared to normal controls and can potentially be pathogenic mutations. The functional significance of these base changes is not yet defined at present. The effect of base changes that alters amino acid sequence in a non-conservative fashion is currently being studied. sAC can potentially affect mineral metabolism in several ways.

Bone turnover is tightly controlled by the balanced actions of osteoblasts and osteoclasts. It is well documented that high HCO_3^- concentration stimulates bone formation and inhibits bone resorption whereas low HCO_3^- concentration inhibits bone formation and stimulates bone resorption via direct physicochemical effects on the bone matrix as well as biologic effects through bone cells. It is not well understood how the ambient HCO_3^- concentration translates to a change in biologic function of osteoblasts and osteoclasts. hsAC may provide the link. hsAC is highly expressed in both osteoblasts and osteoclasts. The relationship between acid-base status and bone is well established. Alkali therapy given to patients with incomplete renal tubular acidosis exhibited increased radial bone mineral density [21]. Using biochemical markers of bone activity, Osther showed increased osteocalcin (bone formation) and decreased hydroxyproline (bone resorption) with alkali therapy [22]. Epidemiologic data have demonstrated a direct association higher alkali content of the diet with higher bone density [23]. Systemic pH and $[HCO_3^-]$ alter bone mineral content by direct physicochemical means or biologically via osteoblasts and osteoclasts [24,25]. In general, high HCO_3^- and alkali pH inhibit, and low $[HCO_3^-]$ and acidic pH stimulate bone resorption. Metabolic alkalosis and acidosis exert reciprocal effects on osteoclasts and osteoblasts [24,26]. Low $[HCO_3^-]$ stimulates and high HCO_3^- inhibits osteoclastic activity [27-30] but the signaling pathway remains unclear. sAC may be the link between ambient $[HCO_3^-]$ concentration and osteoclast function.

The seminal work of Sutton, Wong and Dirks from 1979 [31] demonstrated that distal calcium absorption is inhibited by systemic acidosis and stimulated by alkalosis. Part of this effect may be secondary to the effect of luminal and cellular pH on the apical calcium entry channel TRPV5 [32,33] but the effect of luminal HCO_3^- on calcium transport can conceivably be mediated by sAC which is highly expressed in the distal convoluted tubule.

Gut calcium transport has been shown to be regulated by bicarbonate [34]. Duodenum and ileum from rats fed a low calcium diet absorbs calcium at medium pH 7.4. Reduction in mucosal and serosal medium bicarbonate from 25 to 10 mM (with concomitant reduction in pH) decreased duodenal and ileal net calcium absorption due to a decrease in the mucosal-to-serosal flux. Similar changes in pH induced by changing pCO_2 did not affect calcium transport suggesting that it is HCO_3^- rather than pH that is controlling calcium flux. The role of sAC in this response is yet unexplored.

ACKNOWLEDGMENTS

The authors are supported by the National Institutes of Health (DK-48482, DK-20543) and the Simmons Family Foundation.

REFERENCES

1. Sunahara RK, Taussig R. Isoforms of mammalian adenylyl cyclase: multiplicities of signaling. *Mol Interv* 2:168-184, 2002
2. Cann MJ, Hammer A, Zhou J, Kanacher T. A defined subset of adenylyl cyclases is regulated by bicarbonate ion. *J Biol Chem* 278(37):35033-8, 2003
3. Litvin TN, Kamenetsky M, Zarifyan A, Buck J, Levin LR. Kinetic properties of "soluble" adenylyl cyclase. Synergism between calcium and bicarbonate. *J Biol Chem* 278:15922-6, 2003
4. Wuttke MS, Buck J, Levin LR. Bicarbonate-regulated soluble adenylyl cyclase. *JOP* 2(4 Suppl):154-158, 2001
5. Zippin JH, Chen Y, Nahirney P, Kamenetsky M, Wuttke MS, Fischman DA, Levin LR, Buck J. Compartmentalization of bicarbonate-sensitive adenylyl cyclase in distinct signaling microdomains. *FASEB J* 17:82-84, 2003
6. Zippin JH, Farrell J, Huron D, Kamenetsky M, Hess KC, Fischman DA, Levin LR, Buck J. Bicarbonate-responsive "soluble" adenylyl cyclase defines a nuclear cAMP microdomain. *J Cell Biol* 164(4):527-534, 2004
7. Buck J, Sinclair ML, Schapal L, Cann MJ, Levin LR. Cytosolic adenylyl cyclase defines a unique signaling molecule in mammals. *Proc Natl Acad Sci U S A* 96:79-84, 1999
8. Chen Y, Cann MJ, Litvin TN, Iourgenko V, Sinclair ML, Levin LR, Buck J. Soluble adenylyl cyclase as an evolutionarily conserved bicarbonate sensor. *Science* 289:625-628, 2000
9. Sinclair ML, Wang XY, Mattia M, Conti M, Buck J, Wolgemuth DJ, Levin LR. Specific expression of soluble adenylyl cyclase in male germ cells. *Mol Reprod Dev* 56:6-11, 2000
10. Esposito G, Jaiswal BS, Xie F, Krajnc-Franken MA, Robben TJ, Strik AM, Kuil C, Philipsen RL, van Duin M, Conti M, Gossen JA, Jaiswal BS. Mice deficient for soluble adenylyl cyclase are infertile because of a severe sperm-motility defect. *Proc Natl Acad Sci U S A* 101:2993-2998, 2004
11. Patel TB, Du Z, Pierre S, Cartin L, Scholich K. Molecular biological approaches to unravel adenylyl cyclase signaling and function. *Gene* 269:13-25, 2001
12. Taussig R, Gilman AG. Mammalian membrane-bound adenylyl cyclases. *J Biol Chem* 270:1-4, 1995
13. Reed BY, Heller HJ, Gitomer WL, Pak CY. Mapping a gene defect in absorptive hypercalciuria to chromosome 1q23.3-q24. *J Clin Endocrinol Metab* 84:3907-13, 1999
14. Reed BY, Gitomer WL, Heller HJ, Hsu MC, Lemke M, Padalino P, Pak CY. Identification and characterization of a gene with base substitutions associated with the absorptive hypercalciuria phenotype and low spinal bone density. *J Clin Endocrinol Metab* 87:1476-1485, 2002
15. Geng W, Wang Z, Zhang J, Reed BY, Pak CY, Moe OW. Cloning and characterization of the human soluble adenylyl cyclase. *Am J Physiol Cell Physiol* 288:C1305-1316, 2005
16. Tesmer JJ, Sunahara RK, Johnson RA, Gosselin G, Gilman AG, Sprang SR. Two-metal-Ion catalysis in adenylyl cyclase. *Science* 285:756-760, 1999
17. Klein C, Heyduk T, Sunahara RK. Zinc inhibition of adenylyl cyclase correlates with conformational changes in the enzyme. *Cell Signal* 16:1177-1185, 2004
18. Steegborn C, Litvin TN, Levin LR, Buck J, Wu H.Bicarbonate activation of adenylyl cyclase via promotion of catalytic active site closure and metal recruitment. *Nat Struct Mol Biol* 12:32-37, 2005
19. Xie F, Garcia MA, Carlson AE, Schuh SM, Babcock DF, Jaiswal BS, Gossen JA, Esposito G, van Duin M, Conti M. Soluble adenylyl cyclase (sAC) is indispensable for sperm function and fertilization. *Dev Biol* 296:353-362, 2006

20. Pastor-Soler N, Beaulieu V, Litvin TN, Da Silva N, Chen Y, Brown D, Buck J, Levin LR, Breton S. Bicarbonate-regulated Adenylyl Cyclase (sAC) Is a Sensor That Regulates pH-dependent V-ATPase Recycling. *J Biol Chem* 278:49523-49529, 2003
21. Preminger GM, Sakhaee K, Skurla C, Pak CY. Prevention of recurrent calcium stone formation with potassium citrate therapy in patients with distal renal tubular acidosis. *J Urol* 134:20-23, 1985
22. Osther PJ, Bollerslev J, Hansen AB, Engel K, Kildeberg P. Pathophysiology of incomplete renal tubular acidosis in recurrent renal stone formers: evidence of disturbed calcium, bone and citrate metabolism *Urol Res* 21:169-173, 1993
23. Tucker KL, Hannan MT, Chen H, Cupples LA, Wilson PW, Kiel DP. Potassium, magnesium, and fruit and vegetable intakes are associated with greater bone mineral density in elderly men and women. *Am J Clin Nutr* 69:727-736, 1999
24. Bushinsky DA. Metabolic alkalosis decreases bone calcium efflux by suppressing osteoclasts and stimulating osteoblasts. *Am J Physiol* 271:F216-222, 1996
25. Bushinsky DA. Acid-base imbalance and the skeleton. *Eur J Nutr* 40:238-244, 2001
26. Buclin T, Cosma M, Appenzeller M, Jacquet AF, Decosterd LA, Biollaz J, Burckhardt P. Diet acids and alkalis influence calcium retention in bone. *Osteoporos Int* 12:493-499, 2001
27. Arnett TR, Dempster DW. Protons and osteoclasts. *Bone Miner Res* 5:1099-1103, 1990
28. Goldhaber P, Rabadjija L. H+ stimulation of cell-mediated bone resorption in tissue culture. *Am J Physiol* 253:E90-98, 1987
29. Kraut JA, Mishler DR, Singer FR, Goodman WG. The effects of metabolic acidosis on bone formation and bone resorption in the rat. *Kidney Int* 30:694-700, 1986
30. Krieger NS, Sessler NE, Bushinsky DA. Acidosis inhibits osteoblastic and stimulates osteoclastic activity in vitro. *Am J Physiol* 262:F442-448, 1992
31. Sutton RA, Wong NL, Dirks JH. Effects of metabolic acidosis and alkalosis on sodium and calcium transport in the dog kidney. *Kidney Int* 15: 520-533, 1979
32. Yeh BI, Kim YK, Jabbar W, Huang CL. Conformational changes of pore helix coupled to gating of TRPV5 by protons. *EMBO J* 24:3224-3234, 2005
33. Yeh BI, Sun TJ, Lee JZ, Chen HH, Huang CL. Mechanism and molecular determinant for regulation of rabbit transient receptor potential type 5 (TRPV5) channel by extracellular pH. *J Biol Chem* 278:51044-51052, 2003
34. Favus MJ, Bushinsky DA, Coe FL. Effects of medium pH on duodenal and ileal calcium active transport in the rat. *Am J Physiol* 251(5 Pt 1):G695-700, 1986

TRPV5-mediated Ca^{2+} Reabsorption and Hypercalciuria

Kirsten Y. Renkema, Joost G. J. Hoenderop, and René J. M. Bindels

Department of Physiology, Nijmegen Centre for Molecular Life Sciences, Radboud University Nijmegen Medical Centre, the Netherlands

Abstract. The concerted action of the intestine, kidney and bone results in the maintenance of a normal Ca^{2+} balance, a mechanism that is tightly controlled by the calciotropic hormones vitamin D, parathyroid hormone and calcitonin. Disturbances in the Ca^{2+} balance have been linked to diverse pathophysiological disorders like urolithiasis, hypertension, electroencephalogram abnormalities and rickets. Importantly, the final amount of Ca^{2+} that is released from the body is determined in the distal part of the nephron, where active Ca^{2+} reabsorption occurs. Here, Transient Receptor Potential Vanilloid member 5 (TRPV5), a highly Ca^{2+}-selective channel, has been recognized as the gatekeeper of active Ca^{2+} reabsorption. The *in vivo* relevance of TRPV5 has been further investigated by the characterization of TRPV5 knockout ($TRPV5^{-/-}$) mice, which exhibit severe disturbances in renal Ca^{2+} handling, such as profound hypercalciuria, intestinal Ca^{2+} hyperabsorption and reduced bone thickness. Hypercalciuria increases the risk of kidney stone formation in these mice. This review highlights our current knowledge about TRPV5-mediated Ca^{2+} reabsorption and emphasizes the physiological relevance and the clinical implications related to the $TRPV5^{-/-}$ mice model.

Keywords: calcium reabsorption, TRPV5, active calcium transport, kidney, urolithiasis, TRPV5 knockout
PACS: 87.16.Uv

INTRODUCTION

The maintenance of body Ca^{2+} balance is essential for many vital functions, including intracellular signaling, muscle contraction, neuron excitation and bone mineralization [1]. Ca^{2+} is absorbed in the intestine, reabsorbed in the kidneys and exchanged in bone, which is controlled by calciotropic hormones, including the biologically active form of vitamin D, 1,25-dihydroxyvitamin D_3 ($1,25(OH)_2D_3$), parathyroid hormone (PTH) and calcitonin [2]. Moreover, dietary Ca^{2+} intake can regulate Ca^{2+} transport in a hormone-independent manner [3]. The final amount of Ca^{2+} that is excreted in the urine is determined in the kidneys. In the distal part of the nephron, the epithelial Ca^{2+} channel Transient Receptor Potential Vanilloid member 5 (TRPV5) is expressed, which acts as the gatekeeper of active transcellular Ca^{2+} transport [4]. In the human, disturbances in active Ca^{2+} reabsorption can lead to increased urinary Ca^{2+} loss. Hypercalciuria is an important risk factor in kidney stone formation [5]. This review highlights the physiological and clinical implications of TRPV5-mediated active Ca^{2+} reabsorption.

CP900, *Renal Stone Disease, 1st Annual International Urolithiasis Research Symposium,* edited by A. P. Evan, J. E. Lingeman, and J. C. Williams, Jr.

TRPV5-MEDIATED ACTIVE CA^{2+} REABSORPTION

In healthy individuals, the extracellular Ca^{2+} concentration is tightly controlled by the concerted action of intestine, kidney and bone. In intestine and kidney, Ca^{2+} can (re-)enter the circulation in a paracellular (passive) as well as a transcellular (active) manner [1]. In kidney, the bulk of filtered Ca^{2+} is reabsorbed through the paracellular route in the proximal tubule and, to a lesser extent, the thick ascending limb of Henle (TAL), where it is functionally coupled to Na^+ reabsorption [6]. The fine-tuning of active Ca^{2+} reabsorption takes place in the distal convoluted (DCT) and connecting tubule (CNT), where Ca^{2+} is reabsorbed in a transcellular manner. These latter segments are the main regulatory target for the calciotropic hormones [1, 2, 7]. At the cellular level, active Ca^{2+} reabsorption is accomplished in three steps, depicted in Fig. 1. First, Ca^{2+} enters the cell via the epithelial Ca^{2+} channel TRPV5, after which it is transferred through the cytosol via Ca^{2+}-binding protein calbindin-D_{28K} to the basolateral side of the cell, where Ca^{2+} is finally extruded into the interstitium by the Na^+-Ca^{2+}-exchanger (NCX1) and the plasma membrane Ca^{2+}-ATPase (PMCA1b) [1].

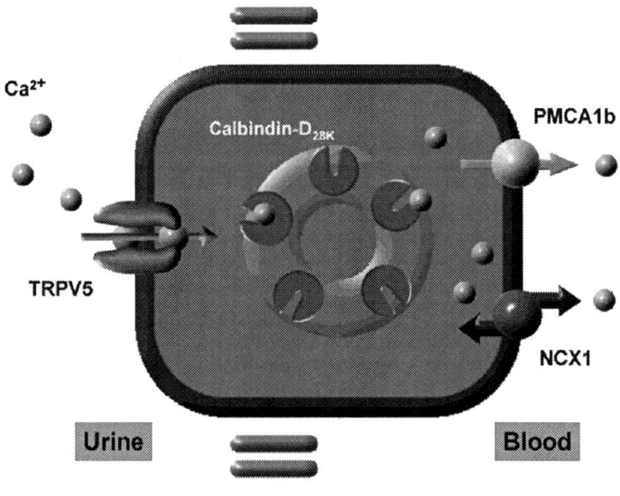

FIGURE 1. Transcellular Ca^{2+} reabsorption in kidney. Schematic representation of transcellular Ca^{2+} reabsorption consisting of apical entry of Ca^{2+} through the epithelial Ca^{2+} channel TRPV5, cytosolic diffusion of Ca^{2+} bound to calbindin-D_{28K} and extrusion across the basolateral membrane by Na^+/ Ca^{2+}-exchanger (NCX1) and plasma membrane Ca^{2+}-ATPase (PMCA1b). Transcellular Ca^{2+} reabsorption occurs in the distal convoluted tubule and connecting tubule in kidney.

REGULATION OF TRPV5 ACTIVITY

A tight control of TRPV5 activity is of major importance for the final amount of Ca^{2+} reabsorbed in the body. TRPV5 regulation occurs at different levels. Here, we outline the long-term transcriptional and translational effects of the calciotropic hormones $1,25(OH)_2D_3$, PTH, calcitonin and estrogen, and dietary Ca^{2+} on active Ca^{2+} transport. Importantly, the Ca^{2+}-sensing receptor (CaSR), present in the epithelium of parathyroid gland cells, senses circulatory Ca^{2+} levels [8]. In response to changes in plasma Ca^{2+} levels, the CaSR is (in)activated, which results in the release of calciotropic hormones in the blood. Hypocalcemia inactivates the CaSR and thereby promotes the secretion of PTH by the parathyroid gland, which stimulates $1,25(OH)_2D_3$ production. In the past, promoter analyses revealed putative $1,25(OH)_2D_3$ responsive elements (VDRE's) in the promoter sequence of TRPV5 [9, 10]. Increased $1,25(OH)_2D_3$ levels activate vitamin D receptor-mediated gene transcription, leading to increased Ca^{2+} transporter expression levels, ultimately increasing intestinal Ca^{2+} absorption and renal Ca^{2+} reabsorption [11]. On the contrary, hypercalcemia leads to the activation of the CaSR, inhibiting PTH-release from the parathyroid glands and stimulating the secretion of calcitonin into the blood from the C-cells of the thyroid gland. This results in a decrease of serum Ca^{2+} levels and inhibition of bone resorption. In more detail, evidence for the regulation of TRPV5 by $1,25(OH)_2D_3$ has been obtained in studies where rats were raised on a vitamin D-depleting diet. Concurrently with the plasma $1,25(OH)_2D_3$ and Ca^{2+} levels, renal TRPV5 mRNA and protein expression decreased in these rats. Furthermore, repletion of $1,25(OH)_2D_3$ via intraperitoneal injection resulted in a significant upregulation of TRPV5 mRNA expression to a similar level as present in control littermates. This was accompanied by a normalization of plasma Ca^{2+} levels [12].

In a similar way, mice genetically ablated from 25-hydroxyvitamin D_3-1α-hydroxylase (1αOHase, the renal enzyme controlling $1,25(OH)_2D_3$ synthesis), demonstrated a significant downregulation of renal TRPV5 mRNA levels with concomitant hypocalcemia. Repletion of these mice with $1,25(OH)_2D_3$ resulted in normalization of both TRPV5 expression and serum Ca^{2+} levels [13]. It is known that estrogen plays an important role in bone mineralization. Estrogen-deficiency after the menopause leads to a negative Ca^{2+} balance and is associated with postmenopausal osteoporosis [14, 15]. Independent of $1,25(OH)_2D_3$, estrogen was identified as a hormone stimulating TRPV5 expression in the kidney. In ovariectomized 1αOHase knockout mice, 17β-estradiol supplementation resulted in elevated renal TRPV5 mRNA and protein levels, accompanied by normalization of the serum Ca^{2+} levels [16]. As for PTH, removal of the parathyroid glands in rats was shown to diminish both serum PTH and Ca^{2+} levels, which was accompanied by decreased renal TRPV5, calbindin-D_{28K} and NCX1 mRNA expression levels. PTH-supplementation of these rats resulted in the rescue of the phenotype and restoration of Ca^{2+} transporter abundance, without changes in blood $1,25(OH)_2D_3$ levels [3]. Together, this suggests that PTH affects renal Ca^{2+} handling through the regulation of the expression of the Ca^{2+} transport proteins, including TRPV5. Additionally, dietary Ca^{2+} can regulate the expression levels of TRPV5. In control mice, high dietary Ca^{2+} content decreased the expression of renal TRPV5 mRNA and protein expression. In 1αOHase knockout mice, the role of dietary Ca^{2+} was investigated in the absence of $1,25(OH)_2D_3$. Feeding these mice a high Ca^{2+} containing diet resulted in the recovery from diminished Ca^{2+} transporter expression levels and hypocalcemia to a significant upregulation of renal and intestinal Ca^{2+} transporters [3, 13]. From these studies, it was concluded that Ca^{2+} transport protein expression and general body Ca^{2+} balance can be regulated by dietary Ca^{2+}, independently of $1,25(OH)_2D_3$.

TRPV5 KNOCKOUT MICE

TRPV5 knockout ($TRPV5^{-/-}$) mice were generated by TRPV5 gene ablation to substantiate the physiological function of this channel in Ca^{2+} reabsorption *in vivo* [17]. $TRPV5^{-/-}$ mice displayed hypercalciuria compared to their wild-type littermates ($TRPV5^{+/+}$ mice), while remaining normocalcemic. Moreover, $TRPV5^{-/-}$ mice demonstrated a significant renal loss of phosphate, predisposing these animals to an increased risk of calcium phosphate precipitation in the urinary tract [18]. Interestingly, urinary acidification and polyuria were consistently detected in $TRPV5^{-/-}$ mice [17]. Polyuria reduces urinary Ca^{2+} concentrations, while a decrease in urinary pH can prevent calcium phosphate precipitation in particular. This suggests compensatory renal mechanisms in an effort to facilitate the excretion of large amounts of Ca^{2+}. Furthermore, $TRPV5^{-/-}$ mice displayed increased serum $1,25(OH)_2D_3$ levels, accompanied by elevated intestinal TRPV6 and calbindin-D_{9K} expression levels and concomitant Ca^{2+} hyperabsorption in comparison with $TRPV5^{+/+}$ micc. This was hypothesized to compensate for the renal Ca^{2+} leak present in $TRPV5^{-/-}$ mice leading to the maintenance of normal plasma Ca^{2+} levels. Recently, $TRPV5^{-/-}$ mice were cross-bred with 1αOHase knockout mice to investigate the effects of exclusion of the increased serum $1,25(OH)_2D_3$ levels in $TRPV5^{-/-}$ mice. TRPV5/1αOHase double knockout mice demonstrated decreased TRPV6 and calbindin-D_{9K} mRNA and protein expression levels, hypocalcemia and severe bone abnormalities. This indicated that hypervitaminosis D in $TRPV5^{-/-}$ mice is responsible for the upregulation of intestinal Ca^{2+} transport proteins and the resulting Ca^{2+} hyperabsorption [19]. Characterization of TRPV5/calbindin-D_{28K} double knockout mice in comparison to calbindin-D_{28K} single knockout and $TRPV5^{-/-}$ mice further substantiated that TRPV5, and not calbindin-D_{28K}, constitutes the rate-limiting step of active Ca^{2+} reabsorption in kidney [20]. Urinary Ca^{2+} excretion, intestinal Ca^{2+} absorption, expression levels of epithelial Ca^{2+} transporters and serum parameters in calbindin-D_{28K} single knockout mice were comparable to wild-type littermates. Moreover, TRPV5/calbindin-D_{28K} double knockout mice did not demonstrate a further disturbance in the Ca^{2+} balance compared to $TRPV5^{-/-}$ mice. In summary, $TRPV5^{-/-}$ mice display renal hypercalciuria with concomitant normocalcemia, due to a severe disturbance in the rate-limiting step of active renal Ca^{2+} reabsorption. The renal Ca^{2+} loss is compensated by intestinal Ca^{2+} hyperabsorption. *In vivo* studies on this unique animal model are of benefit to our knowledge on renal Ca^{2+} loss and are therefore particularly beneficial to individuals with hypercalciuria.

TRPV5 IN BONE

The majority of the body Ca^{2+} content is stored in bone, where the balanced processes of bone formation and resorption maintain bone homeostasis [21]. Bone remodeling is accurately controlled and regulates together with intestinal and renal Ca^{2+} (re)absorption the overall body Ca^{2+} homeostasis [1]. The proteins involved in Ca^{2+} transport processes in bone are largely elusive. Recently, van der Eerden *et al.* investigated the role of TRPV5- mediated Ca^{2+} transport in bone. It was shown that TRPV5, calbindin-D_{28K}, calbindin-D_{9K}, NCX1 and PMCA1b mRNA are present in human and murine bone samples. In osteoclasts, the same Ca^{2+} transporters were detected, whereas TRPV5 and calbindin-D_{9K} were absent in osteoblasts [22]. These results strongly indicated that transcellular Ca^{2+} transport processes are present in bone. In TRPV5$^{-/-}$ mice, bone thickness and mineralization were reduced in comparison to TRPV5$^{+/+}$ mice [17]. Hypothetically, this could be a primary result of TRPV5 ablation, a consequence of the negative Ca^{2+} balance or a direct result of the high serum $1,25(OH)_2D_3$ levels [23]. TRPV5$^{-/-}$ mice display severely disturbed bone resorption as a consequence of malfunctional osteoclasts together with an increased number of osteoclasts [22]. High serum $1,25(OH)_2D_3$ levels were absent in TRPV5/1αOHase double knockout mice, which demonstrated a further decrease in bone mineralization compared to TRPV5$^{-/-}$ mice [19]. This indicated that hypervitaminosis D did not cause the bone degradation in TRPV5$^{-/-}$ mice. As TRPV5 is an essential Ca^{2+} transport protein in osteoclastic bone resorption, alterations in TRPV5 function will likely have implications for metabolic bone diseases and this suggests it as a possible target for therapeutic interventions.

TRPV5 IN CHRONIC METABOLIC ACIDOSIS AND ALKALOSIS

Acid-base homeostasis is known to affect renal Ca^{2+} handling [1, 24, 25]. Metabolic acidosis, which can occur as a result of renal failure or distal renal tubular acidosis, is associated with renal Ca^{2+} loss and an increased risk to Ca^{2+}-containing kidney stone formation. Chronic metabolic acidosis can lead to Ca^{2+} loss from bone and ultimately result in metabolic bone disease [26]. Conversely, chronic metabolic alkalosis is known to decrease urinary Ca^{2+} excretion. Recently, our group demonstrated that systemic acid-base status regulates the expression of proteins involved in active Ca^{2+} reabsorption. Our data showed that metabolic acidosis causes the downregulation of TRPV5 and calbindin-D_{28K} mRNA and protein expression levels in the kidney. Metabolic acidosis did not affect Ca^{2+} excretion in TRPV5$^{-/-}$ mice, in which active Ca^{2+} reabsorption was abolished. Therefore, diminished expression of Ca^{2+} transporters in kidney is responsible for the chronic metabolic acidosis-related renal Ca^{2+} loss. In contrast, the Ca^{2+}-sparing effect of metabolic alkalosis was associated with enhanced TRPV5 and calbindin-D_{28K} abundance. However, the Ca^{2+}-sparing effect persisted in TRPV5$^{-/-}$ mice, suggesting that additional mechanisms, apart from the increase of active Ca^{2+} reabsorption, contribute to the occurrence of hypocalciuria in chronic metabolic alkalosis [27].

TRPV5 IN HYPERCALCIURIA

Hypercalciuria constitutes the main risk factor in kidney stone formation [18, 28]. The identification of an unambiguous causal factor and the establishment of a classification system for idiopathic hypercalciuria are complicated. Currently, a tripartite classification is being used, distinguishing renal, absorptive and resorptive hypercalciuria of which the first two forms are most common [29]. Individuals with a positive family history of nephrolithiasis have an enhanced risk to an episode of kidney stones in life compared to those without a positive history [30]. This is strongly in favor of genetic factors involved in the pathogenesis of hypercalciuria. Because different transport proteins and hormones are involved in the maintenance of the Ca^{2+} balance, defects in Ca^{2+} homeostasis could have many causal factors and, therefore, hypercalciuria could be monogenic as well as polygenic in its etiology. TRPV5 gene ablation in mice leads to severe forms of hypercalciuria, proposing TRPV5 as a candidate gene involved in idiopathic hypercalciuria [17, 31]. In the past, mutation analyses for the TRPV5-encoding gene did not disclose a primary role for TRPV5 in autosomal dominant idiopathic hypercalciuria patients [32]. However, the involvement of TRPV5 Ca^{2+} channels in other subtypes of hypercalciuria cannot be excluded and needs further investigation.

OUTLOOK

TRPV5 ablation in mice leads to hypercalciuria, causing compensatory intestinal Ca^{2+} hyperabsorption and bone abnormalities. These deficiencies have been frequently reported in patients with hereditary idiopathic hypercalciuria. In this perspective, the identification of mutations in genes encoding renal players in active Ca^{2+} (re)absorption constitutes an emerging field in our understanding of hypercalciuria-related kidney stone formation. Although the underlying molecular basis remains unknown, the search for genetic defects related to hypercalciuria is still ongoing.

ACKNOWLEDGMENTS

This work was financially supported in part by grants from the Dutch Kidney Foundation (C03.6017 and C06.2170), the Dutch Organization of Scientific Research (Zon-Mw 016.006.001, NWO-ALW 814.02.001, NWO-CW 700.55.302) and the Dutch Stomach-Intestine–Liver foundation (MWO 03-19). We thank the members of our laboratory for valuable discussion and advice.

REFERENCES

1. J. G. Hoenderop, B. Nilius and R. J. Bindels, *Physiol Rev* **85**, 373-422 (2005).
2. S. Hurwitz, Crit Rev Biochem *Mol Biol* **31**, 41-100 (1996).
3. M. van Abel, J. G. Hoenderop, A. W. van der Kemp, J. P. van Leeuwen and R. J. Bindels, *Am J Physiol Gastrointest Liver Physiol* **285**, G78-85 (2003).

4. J. G. Hoenderop, B. Nilius and R. J. Bindels, *Biochim Biophys Acta* **1600**, 6-11 (2002).
5. J. Y. Clark, I. M. Thompson and S. A. Optenberg, *J Urol* **154**, 2020-2024 (1995).
6. P. A. Friedman, *Exp Nephrol* **8**, 343-350 (2000).
7. J. G. Hoenderop, A. Hartog, M. Stuiver, A. Doucet, P. H. Willems *et al.*, *J Am Soc Nephrol* **11**, 1171-1178 (2000).
8. E. M. Brown and R. J. MacLeod, *Physiol Rev* **81**, 239-297 (2001).
9. D. Muller, J. G. Hoenderop, G. F. Merkx, C. H. van Os and R. J. Bindels, *Biochem Biophys Res Commun* **275**, 47-52 (2000).
10. K. Weber, R. G. Erben, A. Rump and J. Adamski, *Biochem Biophys Res Commun* **289**, 1287-1294 (2001).
11. A. W. Norman, W. H. Okamura, J. E. Bishop and H. L. Henry, *Mol Cell Endocrinol* **197**, 1-13 (2002).
12. J. G. Hoenderop, D. Müller, A. W. Van Der Kemp, A. Hartog, M. Suzuki *et al.*, *J Am Soc Nephrol* **12**, 1342-1349 (2001).
13. J. G. Hoenderop, O. Dardenne, M. Van Abel, A. W. Van Der Kemp, C. H. Van Os *et al.*, *Faseb J* **16**, 1398-1406 (2002).
14. R. L. Prince, *Endocr Rev* **15**, 301-309 (1994).
15. M. M. Young and B. E. Nordin, *Proc R Soc Med* **62**, 242 (1969).
16. M. Van Abel, J. G. Hoenderop, O. Dardenne, R. St Arnaud, C. H. Van Os *et al.*, *J Am Soc Nephrol* **13**, 2102-2109 (2002).
17. J. G. Hoenderop, J. P. van Leeuwen, B. C. van der Eerden, F. F. Kersten, A. W. van der Kemp *et al.*, *J Clin Invest* **112**, 1906-1914 (2003).
18. J. Tessier, M. Petrucci, M. L. Trouve, L. Valiquette, G. Guay *et al.*, *Kidney Int* **60**, 1141-1147 (2001).
19. K. Y. Renkema, T. Nijenhuis, B. C. van der Eerden, A. W. van der Kemp, H. Weinans *et al.*, *J Am Soc Nephrol* **16**, 3188-3195 (2005).
20. D. Gkika, Y. J. Hsu, A. W. van der Kemp, S. Christakos, R. J. Bindels *et al.*, *J Am Soc Nephrol* **17**, 3020-3027 (2006).
21. S. Harada and G. A. Rodan, *Nature* **423**, 349-355 (2003).
22. B. C. van der Eerden, J. G. Hoenderop, T. J. de Vries, T. Schoenmaker, C. J. Buurman *et al.*, *Proc Natl Acad Sci U S A* **102**, 17507-17512 (2005).
23. E. A. Smith, E. P. Frankenburg, S. A. Goldstein, K. Koshizuka, E. Elstner *et al.*, *J Endocrinol* **165**, 163-172 (2000).
24. R. A. Sutton, N. L. Wong and J. H. Dirks, *Kidney Int* **15**, 520-533 (1979).
25. C. C. Marone, N. L. Wong, R. A. Sutton and J. H. Dirks, *Nephron* **28**, 294-296 (1981).
26. J. Lemann, Jr., D. A. Bushinsky and L. L. Hamm, *Am J Physiol Renal Physiol* **285**, F811-832 (2003).
27. T. Nijenhuis, K. Y. Renkema, J. G. Hoenderop and R. J. Bindels, *J Am Soc Nephrol* **17**, 617-626 (2006).
28. S. E. Lloyd, S. H. Pearce, S. E. Fisher, K. Steinmeyer, B. Schwappach *et al.*, *Nature* **379**, 445-449 (1996).
29. C. Y. Pak, F. Britton, R. Peterson, D. Ward, C. Northcutt *et al.*, *Am J Med* **69**, 19-30 (1980).
30. G. C. Curhan, W. C. Willett, F. E. Speizer, D. Spiegelman and M. J. Stampfer, *Ann Intern Med* **126**, 497-504 (1997).
31. S. D. Bianco, J. B. Peng, H. Takanaga, Y. Suzuki, A. Crescenzi *et al.*, *J Bone Miner Res* (2006).
32. D. Müller, J. G. Hoenderop, R. Vennekens, P. Eggert, F. Harangi *et al.*, *Nephrol Dial Transplant* **17**, 1614-1620 (2002).

Idiopathic Calcium Nephrolithiasis And Hypercalciuria: The Role Of Genes

Giovanni Gambaro and Cataldo Abaterusso

Dept. of Biomedical and Surgical Sciences, Division of Nephrology, University of Verona, Verona, Italy.

Abstract. Idiopathic calcium nephrolithiasis and hypercalciuria are multifactorial disease conditions, the pathogenesis of which involves the interaction of environmental and individual factors. Data support a strong role of genes in the pathogenesis of these two conditions. Findings obtained in monogenic disorders characterized by renal calcium stones, and/or hypercalciuria, and/or nephrocalcinosis have proposed a number of genes as candidate genes in the pathogenesis of the common idiopathic calcium nephrolithiasis and hypercalciuria. The physiological role of these genes, and findings in monogenic disorders and idiopathic, multifactorial disorders will be presented.

Keywords: calcium sensing receptor, chloride channel 5, anion exchanger 1, soluble adenylyl cyclase, hypercalciuria, calcium nephrolithiasis.
PACS: 87.19.Xx

INTRODUCTION

Idiopathic calcium nephrolithiasis (ICN) and hypercalciuria (IHC) are multifactorial disease conditions, the pathogenesis of which involves the interaction of environmental and individual factors. The importance of hereditary factors in ICN and IHC has emerged from a number of investigations in families of patients with renal stones and/or hypercalciuria.

A study in monozygotic and dizygotic twins have shown that genetic background explain 56% of the risk of stones, larger than dietary and environmental influences on nephrolithiasis [1].

The excretion in urine of lithogenic substances seems to be under the influence of genetic factors, as Goodman et al [2] observed that in stone formers the relative risks of an abnormal excretion of calcium and citrate, which are partly genetically driven, was 9.18 and 3.79 respectively, far higher than the relative risks for abnormal nutritional intakes [3]. This suggests that the contribution of genetic factors on the risk of stones is much larger than that associated with nutritional exposures.

The analysis of calciuria in families supports the importance of genes since calcium excretion is positively correlated between parents and their progeny and between siblings, but not between spouses [4]. According to findings obtained in parents and offspring, half of the variance of calciuria is due to genetic factors [4]. This conclusion has been recently confirmed in families studied for nephrolithiasis. Evidence for a

CP900, *Renal Stone Disease, 1st Annual International Urolithiasis Research Symposium,* edited by A. P. Evan, J. E. Lingeman, and J. C. Williams, Jr.

major gene explaining 58% of the segregation of hypercalciuria, with an 11% additive polygenic effect has been shown [5].

However, the specific genes involved in ICN and IHC have yet to be identified. Candidate genes have been proposed according to their identification as responsible for Mendelian disorders characterized by calcium stones or allied phenotypes (i.e., hypercalciuria, nephrocalcinosis), or as involved in calcium handling in kidney, bone and intestine. Some are or have been actively investigated and are discussed here, while others have not yet been thoroughly investigated (Table 1).

Calcium-sensing receptor

The calcium-sensing receptor (CaSR) gene, located on chromosome 3q13.3-q21, encodes for a plasma membrane G-protein-coupled receptor that is activated by binding calcium ions to its extracellular domain. It is present in all tissues involved in extracellular calcium regulation, where it controls cellular activity in relation with the plasma calcium concentration [6]. CaSR regulates PTH secretion by parathyroid cells, calcium reabsorption by kidney tubular cells, and influences intestinal calcium absorption and bone remodeling.

Activating mutations of the gene for the CaSR extracellular domain leads to autosomal dominant condition known as familial hypocalcemia with hypercalciuria [7]. Patients belonging to these kindreds have a clinical syndrome mirroring hypoparathyroidism: They have hypocalcemia and normal (i.e. relatively low) serum parathyroid hormone levels. Activating mutations in the CaSR gene causes hypercalciuria and hypocalcemia, because activation of basolateral CaSR in cells of the thick ascending limb of Henle's loop inhibits active and passive calcium reabsorption, and because inhibition of PTH secretion further down-regulates calcium reabsorption in the distal tubule.

The hypothesis for a role of CaSR in hypercalciuria and nephrolithiasis arises from the idea that a mild activation of the CaSR causes the increased intestinal calcium absorption and calcium renal loss observed in IHC with the autosomal inheritance generally observed. The alternative hypothesis is that inactivating mutations of the CaSR cytoplasmic domain cause IHC & ICN in association with border-line/mild hypercalcemia as shown in the very rare familial hypercalcemia with hypercalciuria [8]. However, two studies carried out in subjects with idiopathic stone disease did not support a pathogenetic role of CaSR. In 359 French-Canadian sib pairs of stone formers the CaSR locus was shown by linkage analysis not to be associated with IHC & ICN [9]. In addition, in 9 French families with idiopathic hypercalciuria, no CaSR mutation was discovered [10]. It is not possible to rule out that mutations of CaSR could be found in some other families or other populations, or that mutations of regulatory regions of the gene exist; nevertheless these findings suggest that CaSR mutations do not play a major role in IHC.

The role of CaSR polymorphisms has also been investigated in the Italian population using a case-control design with the hypothesis that polymorphisms may not be neutral in regulating the CaSR gene product activity or its transcription levels, and thus they may increase the risk for hypercalciuria [11]. The association of calciuria with CaSR exon 7 SNPs (G/T at codon 986, G/A at codon 990, and C/G at codon 1011) in normocalciuric control subjects, and in both hypercalciuric and normocalciuric calcium nephrolithiasic patients was evaluated. Although 90% of the hypercalciuric stone formers did not present the 990Gly SNP, it explained a small but significant variance of calciuria. Interestingly, in human embryonic kidney cells transfected with a plasmid containing the CaSR gene, spikes of intracellular calcium concentration induced by increasing the extracellular calcium were much higher in cells with the polymorphic 990Gly SNP receptor than in those with the wild type CaSR [12]. Thus, the 990Gly allele corresponds to an activating SNP and may increase CaSR sensitivity or its response to calcium ions, increasing inhibition of renal calcium reabsorption and eventually increasing calciuria.

Recent findings in over 600 Italian ICN patients indicate that the genotypes of the 5'UTR tract of the CaSR gene and the haplotype of the first block of the CaSR gene characterized by the sequence CATTCA are associated with kidney stone disease [13]. No relationship was observed between the haplotype and measured phenotypes (urinary excretion of calcium, plasma levels of PTH and calcium). Since this sequence comprises the region that regulates CaSR gene transcription, different renal CaSR expression might be expected in stone formers which would favor lithogenesis through an influence on water and/or calcium metabolism in distal and collecting tubule within the papilla.

Chloride channel 5

Nine different chloride channel (ClC) proteins have been described, some of which are plasma membrane channels and others, including the ClC-5, which reside mostly in intracellular membranes.

ClC-5, located in subapical endosomes of kidney tubular cells, contributes to the acidification of the organelles involved in the endocytosis of low molecular-weight proteins by proximal tubules [14]. The channel CLCN5 gene [15] is located on the short arm of the X chromosome (Xp11.22) [16], and encodes a 746-amino acid protein expressed in the renal proximal tubules, the thick ascending loop of Henle, and the α-intercalated cells of the collecting ducts [14]. Mutations of this gene are responsible for Dent's disease, which includes a group of inherited disorders of the renal tubule: X-linked recessive nephrolithiasis with renal failure, X-linked recessive hypophosphatemic rickets and idiopathic low molecular weight proteinuria [17]. These very rare conditions are characterized by medullary nephrocalcinosis, nephrolithiasis, hypercalciuria, low molecular-weight proteinuria and other tubular dysfunctions, renal failure and rickets in variable combinations. CLC5 knockout mice demonstrate severe impairment of receptor-mediated endocytosis, including the endocytotic retrieval of the plasma membrane multiligand megalin and cubilin receptors [18]. Similarly to humans, knockout mice have low molecular weight proteinuria, but do not develop hypercalciuria and nephrolithiasis. So far, the relationship between impaired endocytosis and renal calcium handling remains unclear. It has been proposed that hypercalciuria results from secondary changes in the regulation of calciotropic hormone caused by urinary loss of key hormone-binding proteins.

To date, more than 70 different nonsense or missense mutations, insertions or deletions in the CLCN5 have been reported in the literature [19].

It has been suggested that the disease may occur more commonly than believed, in less overt forms and perhaps without apparent family histories. This hypothesis arose from the observation that in the large pedigree described by Frymoyer et al [20], a man was identified with an inactivating mutation in the CLCN5 gene who did not have low molecular weight proteinuria (together with the other features of the Dent's disease) and in whom the only biochemical abnormality was hypercalciuria [21]. This suggested the theory that mutations in CLCN5 might contribute to the phenotype in patients with the diagnosis of IHC and/or ICN.

Scheinman et al looked for CLCN5 gene mutations in a group of 32 adults and children with idiopathic hypercalciuria, but no CLCN5 gene mutations were observed [21]. An alternative approach to this problem is to search for CLCN5 mutations in groups of patients who may have a high prevalence of mutations, i.e. ESRD patients with previous stones. We have addressed the problem of possible missed diagnosis of Dent's disease by looking for CLCN5 mutations in 24 ESRD patients who had renal stones and found no mutations in the CLCN5 gene, confirming that Dent's disease is really quite rare even in a pool of patients in which it might have been over-represented [22].

To our knowledge, no linkage or polymorphism association study has been performed in IHC and/or ICN looking at the CLCN5 gene.

Anion Exchanger(s)

Several transporters in type α intercalated cells play a role in the transepithelial acid secretion and bicarbonate reabsorption. Among these are the multiple gene products encompassing the vacuolar H^+-ATPase, band 3-AE1, the plasma membrane $Cl/HCO3^-$ exchanger of erythrocytes (SLC4A1), and carbonic anhydrase II [23]. Mutations in one of these components could be responsible for primary distal renal tubular acidosis (dRTA), a hereditary renal tubular disorder, which is characterized by impaired renal acid secretion resulting in metabolic acidosis. Clinical symptoms are nephrocalcinosis, nephrolithiasis, osteomalacia, and growth retardation. Biochemical alterations consist of hyperchloremic metabolic acidosis, hypokalemia with muscle weakness, hypercalciuria, and inappropriately raised urinary pH. dRTA is genetically heterogeneous; however, most frequently the anion exchanger AE1 gene is involved. Mutations in the AE1 gene (on chromosome 17) have been found in both autosomal dominant and recessive dRTA cases [24]. Since it is known that subtle forms of dRTA may present only with hypercalciuria and calcium renal stones, it has been suggested that the dRTA molecular defects may also cause IHC & ICN. We have previously looked for a linkage between the AE1 locus and familial ICN [25]. The association of an anomalous erythrocyte oxalate self-exchange with ICN, which is dependent on an abnormal phosphorylation of the band 3-AE1 exchanger, has been described [26,27]. Physiological and clinical studies support the importance of this defect in ICN; interestingly, partial acidification defects were disclosed in stone formers with the erythrocyte anomaly [28]. In a family study, the abnormal erythrocyte oxalate self-exchange appeared to be genetically determined, segregating as an autosomal dominant trait. However, the 17q21-qter locus containing the AE1 gene and the abnormal oxalate self-exchanger were not in linkage in 2 three-generation families with renal stones [25]. Therefore, most likely the erythrocyte oxalate self-exchanger is an intermediate phenotype, possibly with polygenic determination.

Recently, the physiological role of the anion exchanger SLC26A6 expressed in the apical membrane of mouse proximal tubule and intestinal epithelium has been investigated [29]. It is capable of mediating the exchange of a number of anions: Cl^-/formate, Cl^-/OH^-, Cl^-/HCO_3^-, and also Cl^-/oxalate. Interestingly, knockout mice lacking SLC26A6 develop hyperoxaluria, hyperoxalemia and calcium oxalate renal stones. According to *in vitro* studies, animals lacking SLC26A6 have a defective intestinal secretion of oxalate resulting in enhanced oxalate absorption. This animal model represents a condition of primary intestinal hyperoxaluria, of which the existence in humans is uncertain. Hence, whether such an exchanger (and in particular variants of it) plays a role in human calcium oxalate nephrolithiasis is not known.

TABLE 1. Other Candidate Genes.

Candidate Gene	Abnormality	Disorder	Phenotype Relevant to Stones	Notes
Na^+-K^+-$2Cl^-$ cotransporter (NKCC2) (15q15-q21.1)	Transepithelial NaCl transport across the medullary thick limb of the Henle's loop	Bartter's syndrome type 1	Hypercalciuria, nephrocalcinosis	No investigation in stone patients and families
Luminal potassium channel, (ROMK) (1p36)	Transepithelial NaCl transport across the medullary thick limb of the Henle's loop	Bartter's syndrome type 2	Hypercalciuria, nephrocalcinosis	No investigation in stone patients and families
Claudin16/ Paracellin-1 (3q27)	Tight junctions of the Henle's thick ascending limb, magnesium-calcium reabsorption	Familial hypomagnesaemia with hypercalciuria and nephrocalcinosis	Hypercalciuria, nephrocalcinosis, incomplete dRTA, hypocitraturia	No investigation in stone patients and families
Sodium-phosphate transported tp. 2a (NPT2a) (5q35)	Proximal phosphate reabsorption	Hypophosphatemic nephrolithiasis and osteoporosis	Nephrolithiasis	Only 2 patients have been described. No investigation in stone patients and families [33]
Epithelial Ca2+ channel 1 (ECaC1) (7q35)	Renal and small intestine apical calcium entry	None described	None described	No mutation found in 9 hypercalciuric families [31]

Soluble Adenylyl Cyclase

Intracellular cAMP plays a major role in cell biology because of the modulating activity of a number of activities, including gene transcription. Many different adenylyl cyclase (AC) isoforms have been recognized, but one, the ubiquitously expressed soluble adenylate cyclase (sAC), is particularly interesting in reference to renal stones.

Reed et al [30] have reported linkage of absorptive hypercalciuria to chromosome 1q23-24 in 3 families with familial absorptive hypercalciuric and low vertebral mineral density. Although this region is rather broad, they hypothesized that the sAC gene mutations play a pathogenetic role in this syndrome. Actually sAC mutations/variants were more frequently observed in stone forming patients with absorptive hypercalciuria than in controls. Two studies have addressed the role of a gene belonging to the same locus or of the sAC gene with contradictory results. The 1q23-24 locus was not associated with IHC in 9 European hypercalciuric families [31]. On the contrary, the association between polymorphysm 923C>T of the sAC and hypercalciuria was reported in ICN Italian patients [32].

Since none of the evidence given by Reed et al [30] irrefutably demonstrates that the sAC gene plays a role in absorptive hypercalciuria, whether sAC has a role in ICN is still an open question.

CONCLUSIONS

While research on the role of most of the candidate genes in the common ICN and IHC has produced negative or only marginal results so far, the recent results obtained in Italy from a very large population of ICN patients suggest a special influence of CaSR in the risk (and possibly in the pathogenesis) of renal stones.

Discovering that the CaSR gene or other genes are involved in IHC and ICN may lead to the discovery of new pharmacological targets or tools for diagnosing the risk of ICN, and last, but not least, to advancement in the understanding of the pathogenesis of ICN and IHC.

ACKNOWLEDGMENTS

This study was supported by grant No. 2005063822_004 from the Italian Ministry of University and Research.

REFERENCES

1. D. S. Goldfarb, M. E. Fischer, Y. Keich and J. Goldberg, Kidney Int. 67, 1053-1061 (2005).
2. H .O. Goodman, R. P. Holmes and D. G. Assimos, J. Urol. 153, 301-307 (1995).
3. G. C. Curhan, W. C. Willett, E. B. Rimm and M. J. Stampfer, N. Engl. J. Med. 328, 833-838 (1993).
4. G. Bianchi, G. Vezzoli, D. Cusi, T. Cova, A. Elli, L. Soldati, G. Tripodi, M. Surian, E. Ottaviano, P. Rigatti, S. Ortolani, N. Engl. J. Med. 319,897-901 (1988)

5. J. C. Loredo-Osti, N. M. Roslin, J. Tessier, T. M. Fujiwara, K. Morgan and A. Bonnardeaux, Kidney Int. 68, 966-971 (2005).
6. E. M. Brown, Am. J. Med. 106, 238-253 (1999).
7. S. H. S. Pearce, C. Williamson, O. Kifor, M. Bai, M. G. Coulthard, M. Davies, N. Lewis-Barned, D. McCredie, H. Powell, P. Kendall-Taylor, E. M. Brown and R. V. Thakker, N. Engl. J. Med. 335, 1115-1122 (1996).
8. T. Carling, E. Szabo, M. Bai, P. Ridefelt, G. Westin, P. Gustavsson, S. Trivedi, P. Hellman, E. M. Brown, N. Dahl and J. Rastad. J. Clin. Endocr. Metab. 85, 2042-2047 (2000).
9. M. Petrucci, P. Scott, D. Ouimet, M. L. Trouve, Y. Proulx, L. Valiquette, G. Guay, A. Bonnardeaux. Kidney Int. 58, 38-42 (2000).
10. N. Lerolle, F. Coulet, B. Lantz, F. Paillard, P. Houillier, F. Soubrier, B. Gattegno, X. Jeunemaitre, P. Ronco and E. Rondeau, Nephrol. Dial. Transplant. 16, 2317-2322 (2001).
11. G. Vezzoli, A. Tanini, L. Ferrucci, L. Soldati, C. Bianchin, F. Franceschelli, C. Malentacchi, B. Porfirio, D. Adamo, A. Terranegra, A. Falchetti, D. Cusi, G. Bianchi and M. L. Brandi, J. Am. Soc. Nephrol. 13, 2517-2523 (2002).
12. L. Soldati, A. Terranegra, R. Biasion, T. Arcidiacono, V. Paloschi, S. Giannini, and G. Vezzosi J. Am. Soc. Nephrol. 16, 65A (2005).
13. R. Terranegra, T.Arcidiacono, R. Biasion, V. Paloschi, L. Borghi, M. L. Brandi, E. Croppi, R. Caudarella, A. D'Angelo, G. Gambaro, F. Macciardi, G. Mossetti, P. Strazzullo, A. Trinchieri, D. Cusi, L. Soldati and G. Vezzoli, Nephrol. Dial. Transplant. 21 (suppl 14), iv292 (2006).
14. W. Gunther, A. Luchow, F. Cluzeaud, A. Vandewalle and T. J. Jentsch, Proc. Natl. Acad. Sci. USA. 95, 8075-8080 (1998).
15. S. E. Lloyd, S. H. Pearce, W. Gunther, H. Kawaguchi, T. Igarashi, T. J. Jentsch and R. V. Thakker, J. Clin. Invest. 99, 967-974 (1997).
16. S. J. Scheinman, M. A. Pook, C. Wooding, J. T. Pang, P. A. Frymoyer and R. V. Thakker, J. Clin. Invest. 91, 2351-2357 (1993).
17. R. V. Thakker, Kidney Int. 57, 787-793 (2000).
18. E. I. Christensen, O. Devuyst, G. Dom, R. Nielsen, P- Van der Smissen, P. Verroust, M. Leruth, W. B. Guggino and P. J. Courtoy, Proc. Natl. Acad. Sci. U S A. 100, 8472-8477 (2003).
19. E. Tosetto, G. M. Ghiggeri, F. Emma, G. Barbano, A. Carrea, G. Vezzoli, R. Torregrossa, M. Cara, G. Ripanti, A. Ammenti, L. Peruzzi, L. Murer, I. M. Ratsch, L. Citron, G. Gambaro, A. D'Angelo and F. Anglani, Nephrol. Dial. Transplant. 21, 2452-2463 (2006)
20. P. A. Frymoyer, S. J. Scheinman, P. B. Dunham, D. B. Jones, P. Hueber and E. T. Schroeder, N. Engl. J. Med. 325, 681-686 (1991).
21. S. J. Scheinman, J. P. Cox, S. E. Lloyd, S. H. Pearce, P. V. Salenger, R. R. Hoopes, D. A. Bushinsky, O. Wrong, J. R. Asplin, C. B. Langman, A. G. Norden, and R. V. Thakker, Kidney Int. 57, 232-9 (2000).
22. E. Tosetto, R. Graziotto, L. Artifoni, J. Nachtigal, C. Cascone, C. Conz, M. Piva, R. Dell'Aquila, E. De Paoli Vitali, L. Citron, F. Nalesso, A. Antonello, U. Vertolli, R. Zagatti, A. Lupo, A. D'Angelo, F. Anglani and G. Gambaro, J. Hum. Genet. 51, 25-30 (2006).
23. P. Jarolim, C. Shayakul, D. Prabakaran, L. Jiang, A. Stuart-Tilley, H. L. Rubin, S. Simova, UJ. Zavadil, J. T. Herrin, J. Brouillette, M. J. Somers, E. Seemanova, C. Brugnara, L. M. Guay-Woodford and S. L. Alper, J. Biol. Chem. 273, 6380-6388 (1998).
24. M. A. Devonald, A. N. Smith, J. P. Poon, G. Ihrke and F. E. Karet, Nat. Genet. 33, 125-127, 2003
25. G. Gambaro, A. De Bortoli, G. A. Danieli, A. Borsatti, H. E. Williams, F. Marchini and B. Baggio, "Abnormal erythrocyte self-exchange in idiopathic stone formers is not linked with chromosome 17" in Urolithiasis 2, edited by R. Ryall et al., Plenum Press, NY, 1994, pp.107-108.
26. B. Baggio, G. Gambaro, F. Marchini, E. Cicerello, R. Tenconi, M. Clementi and A. Borsatti, N. Engl. J. Med. 314: 599-604 (1986).
27. B. Baggio, M. Plebani and G. Gambaro, Crit. Rev. Clin. Lab. Sci. 35, 153-187 (1998).
28. G. Gambaro, F. Marchini, M.Bevilacqua, A. Borsatti, and B. Baggio, Kidney Int. 35, 754 (1989).
29. Z. Jiang, J. R. Asplin, A. P. Evan, V. M. Rajendran, H. Velazquez, T. P. Nottoli, H. J. Binder and P. S. Aronson, Nat. Genet. 38, 474-478 (2006).

30. B. Y. Reed, W. L. Gitomer, H. J. Heller, M. C. Hsu, M. Lemke, P. Padalino and C. Y. C. Pak, J. Clin. Endocrinol. Metab. 87, 1476-1485 (2002).
31. D. Muller, J. G. Hoenderop, R. Vennekens, P. Eggert, F. Harangi, K. Mehes, V. Garcia-Nieto, F. Claverie-Martin, C. H. Os, B. Nilius and R. J. M. Bindels, Nephrol. Dial. Transplant. 17, 1614-1620 (2002).
32. T. Lusenti, D. Nicoli, E. Farnetti, B. Casali, V. Franco, N. Tessitore and P. Borgatti P, J. Am. Soc. Nephrol. 4 (suppl 14), 703A (2003).
33. D. Prie, V. Huart, N. Bakouh, G. Planelles, O. Dellis, B. Gerard, P. Hulin, F. Benque-Blanchet, C. Silve, B. Grandchamp and G. Friedlander, N. Engl. J. Med. 347, 983-991 (2002).

Pathophysiology of the Hypercalciuria in the Genetic Hypercalciuric Stone-Forming Rats

David A. Bushinsky

University of Rochester School of Medicine and Dentistry, Division of Nephrology, Department of Medicine, 601 Elmwood Avenue, Box 675, Rochester, NY 14642, USA

Abstract. Given evidence for a genetic cause of hypercalciuria, we screened adult male and female Sprague-Dawley (SD) rats for hypercalciuria and used those with the highest urinary calcium excretion to breed the next generation, followed by subsequent selection and inbreeding of their most hypercalciuric progeny. By the 30th generation, and continuing to the present, the GHS rats (for Genetic Hypercalciuric Stone-forming rats) excrete 8-10 times as much calcium as simultaneously studied control rats The GHS rats were found to have defects in calcium transport in the intestine, kidneys and bone, similar to abnormalities found in many patients with idiopathic hypercalciuria. The GHS rats also form kidney stones. By the conclusion of an 18 wk study, all of the GHS rats formed stones, while there was no stone formation in similarly treated SD controls. The GHS rats, when fed a standard 1.2% calcium diet, form only poorly crystalline apatite stones. However, when 5% hydroxyproline is added to the diet of the GHS rats, they form only calcium oxalate stones.

Keywords: urolithiasis; kidney stones; animal models.
PACS: 87.19.Xx

INTRODUCTION

Nephrolithiasis, with a lifetime incidence of up to 13%, results in significant morbidity as well as substantial economic costs, not only from direct cost of medical treatment but also indirectly through time lost from work [1-10]. Approximately 70% of all kidney stones are composed of calcium (Ca), generally bonded with oxalate (Ox) and/or phosphate (P) [1,3,4,7,9,11-13].

Urine (U) Ca is distributed over a wide range of values in man [1,7,8,12,14-19] and in the rat [15,20-27]. Hypercalciuria is, by far, the most common metabolic abnormality found in patients with Ca nephrolithiasis [1-9,12,28]. Indeed, idiopathic hypercalciuria (IH), defined as excess Ca excretion with no identifiable metabolic cause, is found in approximately 40% of stone-formers [1,3,4,9,29] but has an incidence of fewer than 10% of the overall population [30]. The only consistent abnormality in people who excrete large amounts of UCa is this increased risk of kidney stone formation [1,3,4,6-9,12,14,18,31-34]. The elevation in UCa leads to increased urine supersaturation (SS) with respect to a solid phase, generally CaOx or $CaHPO_4$, which increases the likelihood of developing a kidney stone [12,35,36].

CP900, *Renal Stone Disease, 1st Annual International Urolithiasis Research Symposium,* edited by A. P. Evan, J. E. Lingeman, and J. C. Williams, Jr.

Idiopathic hypercalciuria (IH) is an inherited metabolic abnormality [27,37-39]. In pediatric patients with nephrolithiasis, 73% have a family history of kidney stones in at least one first or second order relative, as opposed to a prevalence of 22% in a control population [40]. Of patients with hypercalciuria, the prevalence of nephrolithiasis in the family history was 69% [40]. Coe *et al.* also found a strong inheritance pattern in patients with nephrolithiasis [41].

In support of a genetic basis for hypercalciuria, we have bred a strain of rats for this disorder. After 70 generations of inbreeding, all of the rats are hypercalciuric; they excrete ~8-10 times as much UCa as control rats and uniformly form kidney stones [13,20-22,24,36,42-57] (reviewed in [27,39,53,58,59]).

Mechanisms of Hypercalciuria [60]

In a normal, non-pregnant, adult, intestinal Ca absorption is precisely balanced by UCa resulting in a constant total amount of body Ca [3,4,9,61,62]. It is logical to assume that IH is caused by dysregulation of Ca transport at sites where large fluxes of Ca must be precisely regulated. These sites are the intestine, kidney and bone [60]. Thus there are three alternative mechanisms, alone or in combination, by which UCa could be increased: 1) increased intestinal Ca absorption either through an increase in effective 1,25$(OH)_2D_3$; 2) decreased renal mineral reabsorption either of Ca or P; and/or 3) enhanced bone resorption.

USE OF THE RAT TO STUDY HYPERCALCIURIA AND STONE FORMATION

Rats exhibit spontaneous hypercalciuria [23] and can be bred to excrete far greater amounts of Ca than normal controls. We have studied the mechanism of hypercalciuria and stone formation in rats in order to better understand hypercalciuria and nephrolithiasis in man. We use the rat to study hypercalciuria for several reasons. The diet of a rat can be precisely controlled and its mineral content reduced (or increased) to levels that are unacceptable in humans. The rat's environment is constant, its excretions can be quantitatively collected and the animal can be sacrificed to study its intestine, kidney or bone. Our findings, summarized below, indicate that hypercalciuria in the rat [13,20-22,24,27,36,39,42-53,58] appears, in large measure, to be analogous to hypercalciuria in man in that, in both, there is increased intestinal Ca absorption, decreased renal Ca reabsorption and enhanced bone demineralization [1,3,4,7,9,10,12,14,19,27,28,35,60].

Mechanism of Hypercalciuria and Stone Formation in the GHS Rat

Given evidence for a genetic cause of hypercalciuria [23,37,41,63], we screened adult male and female Sprague-Dawley (SD) rats for hypercalciuria and used those with the highest UCa to breed the next generation, followed by subsequent selection and inbreeding of their most hypercalciuric progeny [20-22,24,27,36,39,42-

51,53,55,58]. By the 30th generation, and continuing to the present, the GHS rats (for Genetic Hypercalciuric Stone-forming, previously termed IH rats) excrete 8-10 times as much Ca as simultaneously studied control rats [13,20-22,24,27,36,39,42-53,57,58]. While we plot data from female rats, UCa in male GHS rats is also ~8-10-fold greater than UCa in male SD rats. Compared to similarly fed SD rats, the GHS rats remain significantly hypercalciuric (8-10 fold increase in UCa) on a 1.2% Ca diet, on a 0.6% Ca diet, on a 0.02% Ca diet, on a 0.65% P diet and on a 0.14% P diet and in the presence or absence of a thiazide diuretic [20-22,24,36,42-52,55] and the rats remain hypercalciuric whether they are given continual or intermittent access to food.

Intestinal Ca Absorption

Our studies of the GHS rats have shed light on the mechanism of hypercalciuria in this model [20-22,24,27,36,39,42-53,58]. In the 4th generation of GHS rats we found that UCa and intestinal Ca absorption were greater in GHS rats compared to control rats [24]. *In vitro* duodenal net Ca flux was correlated with serum $1,25(OH)_2D_3$; however, with increasing serum $1,25(OH)_2D_3$ there was greater net Ca influx and net Ca absorption in GHS rats than in controls. We studied the 10th generation GHS rats and found that there was a continued increase in UCa and in net Ca flux due to an increase in mucosa-to-serosa flux, with no change in serosa-to-mucosa Ca flux [22]. Thus the hypercalciuria in the GHS rats appears to be due, at least in part, to a primary intestinal overabsorption of dietary Ca.

We utilized a low Ca diet (LCD) to determine if there were mechanisms in addition to increased intestinal Ca absorption responsible for hypercalciuria in the GHS rats [20]. If increased intestinal Ca absorption was the only mechanism responsible for the hypercalciuria then provision of a diet without appreciable Ca would result in an equalization of UCa between the GHS and the controls rats. However, although LCD led to a marked decrease in UCa there was continued hypercalciuria in the GHS rats, leading to negative Ca balance (UCa greater than available dietary Ca), indicating that in addition to enhanced intestinal Ca absorption [24] there must be an additional mechanism of hypercalciuria leading to a loss of bone mineral, the only significant source of Ca in the body [20].

Bone Calcium Resorption

To determine if there is a contribution of bone to the hypercalciuria we studied neonatal bone (calvariae) from GHS and control SD rats. We found that cultured calvariae exhibited greater sensitivity to $1,25(OH)_2D_3$ than did bone from controls [43]. Compared to controls there was significantly greater Ca efflux from the calvariae from GHS rats at 1 and 10 nM $1,25(OH)_2D_3$. In contrast, PTH induced similar bone resorption in control and GHS calvariae. Immunoblot analysis demonstrated a fourfold increase in the level of $1,25(OH)_2D_3$ receptors (VDR), similar to the increased intestinal receptors described previously [22,43,48]. There was no comparable change in VDR RNA levels as measured by slot blot analysis, suggesting the altered regulation of the VDR occurs posttranscriptionally. That both bone and intestine display an increased amount of $1,25(OH)_2D_3$ receptors, suggests that this may be a systemic disorder of Ca regulation in the GHS rat and that enhanced bone resorption may be responsible, in part, for the hypercalciuria in the GHS rat.

To determine the contribution of bone to the increased UCa in the GHS rat *in vivo*, we fed GHS and controls a high Ca diet, then switched them to a low Ca diet. Control and GHS rats in each group were then continued on low Ca diet ± injection of the bone resorption blocker (50μg/kg/24h) [47]. UCa was greater in GHS than in control on high and low Ca diets. With the low Ca diet the GHS rats were in negative Ca balance. Alendronate caused a significant decrease in UCa in GHS, but not in control, rats and brought GHS UCa below Ca intake. Thus on a low Ca diet there is a significant contribution of bone Ca to increased UCa in the GHS rat.

Renal Calcium Reabsorption

To determine if GHS rats have abnormal renal Ca reabsorption we performed ^{14}C-inulin clearance studies [46]. Each rat was parathyroid-ectomized and infused with $CaCl_2$. Both GHS and control rats had similar glomerular filtration rates and the same ultrafiltrable Ca concentrations resulting in similar filtered loads of Ca [46]. The GHS rats had ~3 times the fractional Ca excretion and UCa compared with controls. The results were similar whether the rats were fed a normal or a low Ca diet [46]. Thus, in addition to increased intestinal Ca absorption and increased bone resorption, the GHS rats appear to have a defect in renal Ca reabsorption.

Vitamin D Receptor

The finding of increased intestinal Ca absorption without an elevation in $1,25(OH)_2D_3$ levels led us to hypothesize that alteration of the receptor for vitamin D might be responsible for the abnormal regulation of Ca by enterocytes [22,64]. The magnitude of $1,25(OH)_2D_3$ action correlates with receptor number and saturation [65,66] both in rats *in vivo* [67-69] and in cell culture studies *in vitro* [70,71]. The vitamin D receptor (VDR)-rich cytosolic fractions from GHS rat proximal duodenum bound more $[^3H]1,25(OH)_2D_3$ than similar fractions prepared from controls [22]. Using Serum Catchard analysis we found that this increase in binding of $1,25(OH)_2D_3$ by the VDR was due to an increase in the number of intestinal binding sites rather than enhanced affinity of the VDR for its ligand. Northern analysis of GHS and control mRNA revealed no increased expression of the VDR gene to account for the increase in receptor number. Gene transcription of the VDR was comparable for both groups of rats, as was synthesis of the vitamin D-dependent Ca-binding protein, calbindin D_{9K}. Using western blot analysis, however, more calbindin D_{9K} was detected in intestinal protein from the GHS rats than from controls [22]. The excess number of VDR in the GHS rats would be expected to increase intestinal Ca transport by increasing the action of $1,25(OH)_2D_3$, which would stimulate expression of TRPV5 and calbindin D_{9K}. Increased Ca transport would lead to an increase in serum Ca and thus an increased Filtered load of Ca. The increased serum Ca would also decrease serum PTH [72], a principal regulator of renal tubular Ca reabsorption [61,73]. The combination of an increased filtered load of Ca and reduced PTH would clearly lead to significant hypercalciuria [61,73]. Thus there is an increase in $1,25(OH)_2D_3$ action in GHS rats despite normal serum $1,25(OH)_2D_3$. Further support for the rat model being analogous to IH in humans comes from a recent human study which demonstrated increased VDR in monocytes in patients with idiopathic hypercalciuria [74]. Peripheral blood monocytes (PBM) were obtained from male IH CaOx stone formers and age-matched controls and analyzed for VDR content by immunoblot analysis. Although serum $1,25(OH)_2D_3$ levels were not different between the groups, PBM VDR levels were significantly elevated in the stone-formers.

We then determined that the VDR in the GHS rats hyper-responded to minimal doses of $1,25(OH)_2D_3$ [48] which occurred through an increase in VDR stability without involving alterations in gene transcription, *de novo* protein synthesis or mRNA sequence. $1,25(OH)_2D_3$ administration also led to an increase in duodenal and renal calbindin mRNA levels in GHS rats, whereas levels were either suppressed or unchanged in control rats. Thus the hyper-responsiveness appears to be of functional significance in that it affects VDR-responsive genes in $1,25(OH)_2D_3$ target tissues. The relatively normal serum $1,25(OH)_2D_3$ levels, increased VDR, and normal VDR mRNA suggest that high rates of expression of vitamin D-responsive genes mediate the hypercalciuria in the GHS rats. The mechanism of elevated VDR and state of receptor function are not known.

To determine if degradation of VDR is altered in GHS rats, GHS and control male rats fed a normal Ca diet were injected with $1,25(OH)_2D_3$ or vehicle 24 hr prior to cycloheximide, and then sacrificed after 0 to 8 hr. Duodenal and kidney VDR were increased in GHS versus control rats, and $1,25(OH)_2D_3$ increased VDR or calbindins (D_{9k} and D_{28k}) further in control but not GHS rats. Duodenal VDR half-life was prolonged in the GHS rats. $1,25(OH)_2D_3$ prolonged duodenal VDR half-life in control rats compared to that of untreated GHS rats. This study supports the hypothesis that prolongation of VDR half-life increases VDR tissue levels and mediates increased VDR-regulated genes that result in hypercalciuria. Using real-time PCR, a far more sensitive technique than Northern or slot blot analysis, and western analysis we have confirmed that the VDR mRNA and protein in the kidney, duodenum, jejunum and ileum remains elevated in a recent generation (70th) of the GHS rats compared to normocalciuric SD controls.

Calcium Sensing Receptor

The Ca receptor (CaR) is a seven membrane-spanning protein that is a member of the G-coupled protein family of plasma membrane receptors [75] and is expressed in a wide variety of tissues including parathyroid, kidney and gastrointestinal tract [60,76,77].

As the CaR contains vitamin D response elements in its promoter region [78], and both the GHS rats [56] and human stone formers [74] also have been shown to have elevated VDR, we asked whether there was increased CaR in kidneys of the GHS rats. We determined renal CaR gene expression and regulation in response to $1,25(OH)_2D_3$ in GHS and control rats [54]. Male GHS and control SD rats were fed a diet adequate in Ca (0.6% Ca). Western blotting revealed a marked increase in CaR protein in the GHS rat compared to controls. Northern analysis of extracts of renal cortical tissue revealed a major CaR transcript of 7 kb and a less abundant 4 kb transcript, both of which were present in greater abundance in the GHS rat under basal conditions. The administration of 1,25$(OH)_2D_3$ increased renal CaR mRNA levels in a dose- and time-dependent manner in both GHS and wild-type control rats. However, in GHS rat kidney, 1,25$(OH)_2D_3$ induced a greater and a more sustained elevation of CaR mRNA level. The upregulation of CaR expression in response to 1,25$(OH)_2D_3$ was through both increased gene transcription and stabilization of the mRNA. Along with the hyper-responsiveness of VDR regulation as described above, the enhanced upregulation of the CaR gene in response to 1,25$(OH)_2D_3$ might lead to excess CaR, which then contributes to the hypercalciuria. Thus we found that not only was there increased CaR mRNA and protein in the GHS rat kidney, but also that 1,25$(OH)_2D_3$ increased CaR through both elevated CaR gene expression and prolonged tissue half-life [54].

The calcimimetic, cinacalcet, is a small organic molecule that acts as an allosteric activator of the CaR, increasing the sensitivity of the CaR to Serum Ca and substantially lowering PTH levels [79-81]. In patients with secondary hyperparathyroidism treated with cinacalcet exhibit a substantial reduction of PTH (~50%) and a modest reduction of serum Ca (~10%) [79,81]. The effect of cinacalcet on human UCa and supersaturations with respect to common solid phases responsible for kidney stones has not been reported.

The effects of cinacalcet on renal Ca excretion are complex. A reduction in PTH should increase UCa; in addition, increasing the sensitivity of the renal CaR to Ca should lead to an increase in UCa. However, the lowered filtered load of Ca from cinacalcet-induced hypocalcemia should lower UCa. To determine the effect of cinacalcet on UCa, GHS and SD rats (as controls) were fed a 0.6% Ca diet for 14 days. As expected, UCa was far higher in the GHS rats ($p<0.001$). The addition of cinacalcet did not significantly alter UCa in the GHS rats but increased UCa in the control rats ($p<0.01$). Rats were then placed on a 0.02% Ca diet (LCD). As expected, UCa remained higher in the GHS rats than in the control rats [20]. The addition of cinacalcet led to a significant decrease in UCa in the GHS ($p<0.01$) but not the control rats fed LCD. At the conclusion of the experiment serum Ca fell with cinacalcet with both SD and GHS rats. Interestingly PTH was lower in the GHS rats than in the control rats suggesting that secondary hyperparathyroidism does not contribute to the hypercalciuria in the GHS rats.

The addition of cinacalcet led to a marked fall in PTH and Ca in both groups of rats, indicating that cinacalcet was effective in lowering PTH and appears to reset the level at which serum Ca is regulated as it does in man [79-81]). UCa is significantly greater than dietary Ca intake in the GHS rats on LCD, which means that the source of the additional UCa is bone. That UCa actually fell with cinacalcet in the GHS rats suggests that PTH is necessary to resorb bone mineral and contributes to the hypercalciuria of the GHS rats fed LCD. The control rats fed cinacalcet increased UCa on NCD and did not lower their UCa on LCD with cinacalcet (in spite of a lower filtered load of Ca, creatinines were similar in all rats) suggesting that cinacalcet may have also affected the renal CaR, resulting in a decreased renal tubular Ca reabsorption.

CONCLUSION

Thus the GHS rats were found to have defects in Ca transport in the intestine, kidneys and bone, similar to abnormalities found in many patients with idiopathic hypercalciuria [1-10,12,12,35,60]. The GHS rats also form kidney stones. By the conclusion of an 18 wk study, all of the GHS rats formed stones, while there was no stone formation in similarly treated SD controls. The GHS rats, when fed a standard 1.2% Ca diet, form only poorly crystalline apatite stones [36,42,44,45,47,51]. However, when 5% OH-proline is added to the diet of the GHS rats they form only CaOx stones [49,52].

REFERENCES

1. D. A. Bushinsky, in *Kelly's Textbook of Medicine*, Edited by H. D. Humes (Lippincott Williams & Wilkens, New York, 2000), p. 1243.
2. D. A. Bushinsky, W. R. Parker, K. M. Alexander, and N. S. Krieger, *Am J Physiol (Renal Fluid Electrolyte Physiol)* **281**, F1058-F1066 (2001).
3. D. A. Bushinsky, *J Am Soc Nephrol* **9**, 917 (1998).
4. R. D. Monk and D. A. Bushinsky, in *Comprehensive Clinical Nephrology, 2 ed.*, Edited by R. Johnson and J. Frehally (Mosby, London, 2003), p. 731.
5. Consensus Conference, *JAMA* **260**, 977 (1988).
6. C. Y. C. Pak, in *The Kidney: Physiology and Pathophysiology, 2 ed.*, Edited by D. W. Seldin and G. Giebisch (Raven Press, Ltd., New York, 1992), Chap. 69, p. 2461.
7. F. L. Coe, J. H. Parks, and J. R. Asplin, *N Engl J Med* **327**, 1141 (1992).
8. F. L. Coe, M. J. Favus, and J. R. Asplin, in *The Kidney, 7 ed.*, Edited by B. M. Brenner (W.B. Saunders Company, Philadelphia, 2004), Chap. 39, p. 1819.
9. R. D. Monk and D. A. Bushinsky, in *Williams Textbook of Endocrinology, 10 ed.*, Edited by P. R. Larsen, H. M. Kronenberg, S. Melmed, and K. S. Polonsky (W.B.Saunders, Philadelphia, 2003), Chap. 28, p. 1411.
10. D. A. Bushinsky, *N Eng J Med* **346**, 124 (2002).
11. J. S. Adams, in *Primer on the Metabolic Bone Diseases and Disorders of Mineral Metabolism, 2 ed.*, Edited by M. J. Favus (Raven Press, New York, 1993), Chap. 37, p. 178.
12. F. L. Coe and D. A. Bushinsky, *Am J Physiol (Renal Fluid Electrolyte Physiol)* **247**, F1-F13 (1984).
13. D. A. Bushinsky, in *Primer on the Metabolic Bone Diseases and Disorders of Mineral Metabolism, 6 ed.*, Edited by M. J. Favus (American Society of Bone and Mineral Research, Washington, D.C., 2006), Chap. 81, p. 456.
14. J. H. Parks and F. L. Coe, *Seminars in Nephrology* **16**, 398 (1996).
15. D. A. Bushinsky and N. S. Krieger, in *Disorders of Bone and Mineral Metabolism*, Edited by F. L. Coe and M. J. Favus (Raven Press, New York, 1992), Chap. 18, p. 417.
16. D. A. Bushinsky and N. S. Krieger, in *The Kidney: Physiology and Pathophysiology*, Edited by D. W. Seldin and G. Giebisch (Raven Press, New York, 1992), p. 2395.
17. A. Hodgkinson and L. N. Pyrak, *Br. J. Surg.* **46**, 10 (1958).
18. F. L. Coe and J. H. Parks, in *Nephrolithiasis: Pathogenesis and Treatment, 2 ed.*, Edited by F. L. Coe and J. H. Parks (Year Book Medical Publishers, Inc., Chicago, 1990), Chap. 4, p. 108.
19. F. L. Coe *et al.*, *Am. J. Med.* **72**, 25 (1982).

20. M. Kim *et al.*, *Kidney Int* **43**, 189 (1993).
21. D. A. Bushinsky *et al.*, *Kidney Int* **45**, 58 (1994).
22. X.-Q. Li *et al.*, *J Clin Invest* **91**, 661 (1993).
23. M. J. Favus and F. L. Coe, *Mineral Electrolyte Met* **2**, 150 (1979).
24. D. A. Bushinsky and M. J. Favus, *J Clin Invest* **82**, 1585 (1988).
25. D. A. Bushinsky, M. J. Favus, C. Langman, and F. L. Coe, *Am. J. Physiol.* **251** (*Renal Fluid Electrolyte Physiol.* 20) 251, F17-F24 (1986).
26. D. A. Bushinsky, M. J. Favus, and F. L. Coe, *Am. J. Physiol. (Renal Fluid Electrolyte Physiol. l6)* **247**, F746-F752 (1984).
27. D. A. Bushinsky, *Seminars in Nephrology* **16**, 448 (1996).
28. R. D. Monk and D. A. Bushinsky, in *Kidney Stones: Medical and Surgical Management*, Edited by F. Coe *et al.* (Lippincott-Raven, Philadelphia, 1996), p. 759.
29. F. L. Levy, B. Adams-Huet, and C. Y. Pak, *Am J Med* **98**, 50 (1995).
30. W. G. Robertson and D. B. Morgan, *Clin Chim Acta* **37**, 503 (1972).
31. F. L. Coe, *Kidney Int.* **24**, 392 (1983).
32. G. Maschio *et al.*, *Am. J. Med.* **71**, 623 (1981).
33. F. L. Coe, *Ann. Int. Med.* **87**, 404 (1977).
34. F. L. Coe, J. H. Parks, and Y. Nakagawa, *Seminars in Nephrology* **11**, 98 (1991).
35. D. A. Bushinsky, *J Clin Invest* **111**, 602 (2003).
36. D. A. Bushinsky, W. R. Parker, and J. R. Asplin, *Kidney Int* **57**, 550 (2000).
37. K. Mehes and Z. Szelid, *Eur J Pediatr* **133**, 239 (1980).
38. F. Harangi and K. Mehes, *Eur J Pediatr* **152**, 64 (1993).
39. D. A. Bushinsky, *Current Opinion in Nephrology and Hypertension* **8**, 479 (1999).
40. C. Polito *et al.*, *Pediatr Nephrol* **15**, 211 (2000).
41. F. L. Coe, J. H. Parks, and E. S. Moore, *N Engl J Med* **300**, 337 (1979).
42. D. A. Bushinsky *et al.*, *Kidney Int* **48**, 1705 (1995).
43. N. S. Krieger, V. M. Stathopoulos, and D. A. Bushinsky, *Am J Physiol (Cell Physiol)* **271**, C130-C135 (1996).
44. D. A. Bushinsky *et al.*, *Kidney Int* **55**, 602 (1999).
45. J. R. Asplin *et al.*, *Kidney Int* **51**, 640 (1997).
46. S. Tsuruoka, D. A. Bushinsky, and G. J. Schwartz, *Kidney Int* **51**, 1540 (1997).
47. D. A. Bushinsky, K. J. Neumann, J. Asplin, and N. S. Krieger, *Kidney Int* **55**, 234 (1999).
48. J. Yao, P. Kathpalia, D. A. Bushinsky, and M. J. Favus, *J Clin Invest* **101**, 2223 (1998).
49. A. P. Evan, S. B. Bledsoe, S. B. Smith, and D. A. Bushinsky, *Kidney Int* **65**, 154 (2004).
50. S. J. Scheinman *et al.*, *Kidney Int.* **57**, 232 (2000).
51. D. A. Bushinsky, M. D. Grynpas, and J. R. Asplin, *Kidney Int* **59**, 1415 (2001).
52. D. A. Bushinsky *et al.*, *Kidney Int* **61**, 975 (2002).
53. R. R. Hoopes *et al.*, *J Am Soc Nephrol* **14**, 1844 (2003).
54. J. Yao, A. J. Karnauskas, D. A. Bushinsky, and M. J. Favus, *J Am Soc Nephrol* **16**, 1300 (2005).
55. D. A. Bushinsky and J. R. Asplin, *J Am Soc Nephrol* **16**, 417 (2005).
56. A. J. Karnauskas *et al.*, *J Bone Min Res* **20**, 447 (2005).
57. D. A. Bushinsky, K. LaPlante, and J. R. Asplin, *Kidney Int* **69**, 1586 (2006).
58. D. A. Bushinsky, *Am. J. Kidney Dis.* **36**, 61 (2000).
59. D. A. Bushinsky, K. K. Frick, and K. Nehrke, *Curr Opinion Nephrol Hyperten* **15**, 403 (2006).
60. K. K. Frick and D. A. Bushinsky, *J Am Soc Neph* **14**, 1082 (2003).
61. D. A. Bushinsky, in *Primer on the Metabolic Bone Diseases and Disorders of Mineral Metabolism*, 5 ed., Edited by M. J. Favus (American Society for Bone and Mineral Research, Washington, D.C., 2003), Chap. 15, p. 97.
62. D. A. Bushinsky, in *Primer on Kidney Diseases, 4 ed.*, Edited by A. Greenberg (Academic Press, San Diego, 2005), Chap. 13, p. 120.
63. C. Y. C. Pak *et al.*, *J Urology* **126**, 717 (1981).
64. M. J. Favus, *J Am Soc Nephrol* **5**, S54-S58 (1994).

65. H. A. P. Pols, J. C. Birkenhager, J. P. Schilte, and T. J. Visser, *Biochim Biophys Acta* **970**, 122 (1988).
66. T. A. Reinhardt and R. L. Horst, *J Biol Chem* **264**, 15917 (1989).
67. M. J. Favus *et al.*, *J Clin Invest* **82**, 218 (1988).
68. M. Strom, M. E. Sandgren, T. A. Brown, and H. F. DeLuca, *Proc Natl Acad Sci USA*. **86**, 9770 (1989).
69. M. Sandgren and H. F. DeLuca, *Proc Natl Acad Sci USA*. **87**, 4312 (1990).
70. T. L. Chen, P. V. Hauschka, S. Cabrales, and D. Feldman, *Endocrinology* **118**, 250 (1986).
71. E. M. Costa, M. A. Hirst, and D. Feldman, *Endocrinology* **117**, 2203 (1985).
72. D. A. Bushinsky and R. D. Monk, *The Lancet* **352**, 306 (1998).
73. M. J. Favus, D. A. Bushinsky, and J. Lemann, Jr., in *Primer on the Metabolic Bone Diseases and Disorders of Mineral Metabolism, 6 ed.*, Edited by M. J. Favus (American Society of Bone and Mineral Research, Durham, 2006), p. 76.
74. M. J. Favus, A. J. Karnauskas, J. H. Parks, and F. L. Coe, *J Clin Endocrinol Metab* **89**, 4937 (2004).
75. D. Riccardi *et al.*, *Proc Natl Acad Sci USA* **92**, 131 (1995).
76. W. G. Goodman, *Seminars in Nephrology* **23**, 17 (2004).
77. E. M. Brown and R. J. MacLeod, *Physiol Rev* **81**, 239 (2001).
78. L. Canaff and G. N. Hendy, *J Biol Chem* **277**, 30337 (2002).
79. L. D. Quarles *et al.*, *J Am Soc Neph* **14**, 575 (2003).
80. T. B. Drueke, *Nephrol Dial Transplant* **19**, 20 (2004).
81. G. A. Block *et al.*, *N Eng J Med* **350**, 1516 (2004).

IV. UPDATE OF CRYSTAL-CELL ATTACHMENT, PROTEIN INHIBITORS, AND URINARY DETERMINATES OF CRYSTALLIZATION

Macromolecules Relevant to Stone Formation

Rosemary L. Ryall, Alison F. Cook, Lauren A. Thurgood, and Phulwinder K. Grover

Department of Surgery, Flinders Medical Centre and Flinders University, Adelaide, SA, 5042, AUSTRALIA

Abstract. Despite years of research, no single macromolecule in kidney calculi or in urine has yet been shown to fulfill a specific function in stone pathogenesis. In this paper we briefly review papers investigating the urinary excretion of individual macromolecules, their effects on calcium oxalate (CaOx) crystallization and attachment of crystals to renal epithelial cells, and the influence of lithogenic conditions on their renal expression in cultured cells and animal models. Using prothrombin fragment 1 (PTF1) and human serum albumin as examples, we show the types of patterns resulting from the binding of a fluorescently tagged protein to a specific CaOx monohydrate (COM) crystal face and its incorporation into the crystal structure. Molecular modeling is also used to illustrate how PTF1 can align with the atomic array on a COM crystal surface. We conclude that although many macromolecules are, by strict definition, relevant to stone formation, very few are probably truly influential.

Keywords: macromolecules, proteins, calcium oxalate, urolithiasis, intracrystalline inclusion
PACS: 87.14.Ee

RELEVANCE: A QUESTION OF DEFINITION

In preparing this manuscript, our charter was to review macromolecules relevant to stone formation. But what makes a macromolecule *relevant* to stone formation? Its presence in kidney stones? Its excretion in healthy urine? Alteration of its urinary excretion in stone formers? Its expression in the human kidney? Its induction or suppression by lithogenic conditions *in vivo* or *in vitro?* Formation of kidney stones following ablation of its gene? Its inhibition (or promotion) of crystal nucleation? Growth? Aggregation? Cellular adhesion?

In fact, any macromolecule can be loosely described as relevant to stone formation by virtue of its possession of any of the features listed above. However, that does not necessarily mean that it has any influence whatsoever on the disease process, so our problem becomes one of separating chaff from grain... and yet more questions. Why the interest in macromolecules *at all*, and why in any *particular* macromolecule? Because all stones contain them, and because it has been shown to be present in stones. And that is where we shall start.

CP900, *Renal Stone Disease, 1st Annual International Urolithiasis Research Symposium,* edited by A. P. Evan, J. E. Lingeman, and J. C. Williams, Jr.

PROLEGOMENON

The synthesis of a galaxy of biominerals throughout the phylogenetic tree—from pearls to bone and coral to eggshells—is orchestrated by proteins [1]. Some of these direct mineral ions to the construction site, where they fashion them into crystalline building blocks and assemble them into intricate filigrees, weapons, armory and dwellings. Others act as macromolecular scaffolds that become incorporated into the final mineral fabric, imparting rigidity, texture and elasticity. Kidney calculi, though pathological, are biominerals nonetheless. And like their salubrious counterparts, they contain macromolecules, now known as the organic matrix, whose distribution throughout the stone structure has been documented in numerous ultrastructural studies performed over many years.

The invariable presence of matrix in all calculi has always been, and still is, generally regarded as indicative that its component molecules must have fulfilled some function(s) in their production. Identifying those functions relies on knowing which individual macromolecules perform them. However, unlike healthy biominerals, whose formation is temporally and physically controlled by specific proteins, stones are associated with a range of macromolecules so broad that it would be irrational to assume that they all undertake essential roles in stone pathogenesis.

CHAFF AND GRAIN: MACROMOLECULES IN STONES

Table 1 lists the macromolecules that have been reported to be present in kidney stones composed of calcium oxalate (CaOx) or calcium phosphate.

TABLE 1: **Macromolecules detected in kidney stones**. References to original paper reporting the detection of each macromolecule can be found in [2-5].

PROTEINS	
human serum albumin (HSA)	α and γ-globulins
Tamm-Horsfall glycoprotein (THG)	nephrocalcin (NC)
α-1-microglobulin	haemoglobin
neutrophil elastase	transferrin
osteopontin	α-1-antitrypsin
CD59 protein (protectin)	superoxide dismutase
β-2-microglobulin	α-1-acid glycoprotein
apolipoprotein A1	retinol-binding protein
renal lithostathine	prothrombin fragments 1 & 1+2
porin	inter-α-trypsin inhibitor chains
calprotectin (calgranulin)	
GLYCOSAMINOGLYCANS	
hyaluronan	heparan sulfate

Some of the macromolecules in Table 1 may well regulate one or more of the physicochemical or physiological steps in stone formation, but most are more likely to be chaff—uninvited intruders or ineffectual drop-in visitors that play no defined role and whose presence results simply from their being in the wrong place at the wrong time. Of those, some are probably components of the trail of blood and cellular litter left in the inchoate stone's wake, which then become incorporated into the final structure. Hematuria typically accompanies renal colic, and many of the proteins listed in Table 1, including for example, hemoglobin, transferrin, osteopontin, prothrombin fragments 1 and 1+2, neutrophil elastase, α-1-microglobulin and albumin are present in human blood. They may thus be effects of the stone, though that does not preclude their still having an effect on subsequent events: some of them, as will be seen below, are inhibitors of crystallization. Other components of stone matrix, such as superoxide dismutase, are likely to be released in response to inflammation.

Thus, while the presence of a macromolecule in calculi might make it *relevant* to stone formation, it does not necessarily have a specific *influence* on stone development. The only way that can be assessed is to test its effect on the processes involved in stone pathogenesis, and this has been done for only a handful of the macromolecules in Table 1. It is impossible in this short review to do justice to the huge body of literature devoted to investigating the potential roles of macromolecules in stone formation. Therefore, while we refer to specific papers for some macromolecules, others have featured in too many studies to cite individually. In those instances, reference is made to more comprehensive reviews [2-6] in which details of individual papers can be found.

SEPARATING THE CHAFF FROM THE GRAIN

Several physicochemical phenomena are involved in kidney stone formation. Nucleation of insoluble crystals is crucial, since stones will obviously not form in their absence. However, equally important is the retention of those crystals in the kidney; otherwise they would be harmlessly expelled in the urine. Any process that causes enlargement of crystalline particles to the point where they obstruct the collecting system ("Free Particle" Stone Formation) or which encourages their adhesion to the renal epithelium ("Fixed Particle" Stone formation), will obviously favor stone pathogenesis. Traditionally, therefore, attempts to assign roles to macromolecules have focused on their excretion in urine, their effects on crystallization or adhesion of crystals to renal cells, or factors that affect their molecular synthesis. In the following brief review, we discuss only macromolecules that have been specifically identified immunologically or biochemically, or by amino acid sequence analysis.

Inhibitors of crystallization *in vitro* and *in vivo*

Macromolecules that have been shown to inhibit significantly at least one of the recognized steps in crystallization include the bikunin light chain of inter-α-inhibitor [3,5], prothrombin fragment 1 PTF1 [7,8], α-1-microglobulin [9], fibronectin [10], calgranulin [11], chondroitin sulfate [5,6], heparan sulfate [12,13] and osteopontin (OPN) [3,5]. Tamm-Horsfall glycoprotein (THG) inhibits, promotes or has no influence on CaOx crystallization, depending upon ambient conditions [3,5]. While

THG is a unique macromolecule whose ability to self-associate into macromolecular behemoths can explain its contradictory effects on crystallization, it is also true that the effects of the others are not as consistent as we might like to believe. The inhibition of crystallization by chondroitin sulfate, for instance, which has been reported in some studies, could not be reproduced in others [3]. This is hardly surprising. Macromolecules that inhibit in aqueous solution may have no influence in urine, or may promote when adsorbed on to a surface. There are, therefore, numerous discrepancies in the reported effects of some macromolecules, which can be attributed to differences in their purity or physiological source, their measurement in solutions of varying composition and using a wide range of techniques, and the fact that crystallization is not a single event. Rather, it comprises the separate, but interdependent, processes of crystal nucleation, growth and aggregation, and macromolecules can influence these to different extents [3,14].

Inhibitors and mediators of crystal adhesion and internalization

A number of macromolecules, not all of which have been detected in stones, have been reported to inhibit or mediate the binding of CaOx crystals to cultured renal cells, or the retention of crystals in animal models of nephrolithiasis. Annexin-II, which is present on the surface of MDCKI cells, avidly binds COM crystals [15]. Hyaluronan binds COM crystals [16], as do β-tubulin [17] and a protein related to nucleolin [18], while hyaluronan, CD44 protein, and OPN appear to play a role in the retention of CaOx crystals in a rat model of nephrocalcinosis [19]. Collagen types I and IV, also appear to be potent mediators of crystal binding to renal epithelial cells [20]. OPN [21,22] and fibronectin [20] have been reported to promote and also to inhibit [10,23,24] the adhesion of CaOx crystals to epithelial cells.

Other macromolecular inhibitors of crystal attachment or internalization include chondroitin sulfate A and B, heparan sulfate, hyaluronic acid, OPN [21,23] and bikunin [25]. THG has been reported to have no material effect on binding [23], although its identification in a preparation of whole urinary proteins (which also contained OPN, PTF1+2 and bikunin) has prompted some authors to believe that it does reduce crystal binding [26]. Again, it is clear that recorded effects of macromolecules on the binding of crystals to renal cells are not always reproducible: fibronectin, OPN and hyaluronan produce contradictory effects, which probably result from differences in the use of different cell lines and incubation or culture conditions.

Urinary excretion of macromolecules

The urinary excretion patterns of some macromolecules have been compared in stone formers and healthy controls, but with inconclusive results. This is hardly surprising, perhaps since subjects in those studies were drawn from different ethnic backgrounds; the types of stone formers (e.g., single, multiple, bariatric) were not standardized, and data were not always stratified for age, weight, gender and diet. Thus, the excretions of THG [27] and total and individual GAGs [2,5,6] have been shown to differ, but also to be identical in both groups. Bikunin excretion is raised

[28] and reduced in stone formers [29]. OPN excretion is lower in stone formers [30,31] and the same in stone formers [32,33], both of which seem illogical, given that OPN mRNA and OPN expression *increase* during experimental nephrolithiasis (see below). These inconsistencies would suggest that little is to be gained by measuring urinary concentration or output of THG, GAGs, bikunin and OPN, but measurement of other proteins, which at first might *appear* to be more promising, is no less problematic.

PTF1 levels were shown to be lower in stone formers compared with controls [31], which was used as the basis for regarding it as a urinary marker of the disease [34]. Albumin [33,35] and transferrin [35] excretion is raised in stone formers, while α-1-microglobulin concentration is reduced [9]. At the present time at least, these findings have not been contradicted by other reports. Nonetheless, it is imperative to be circumspect. For instance, a reduced concentration of α-1-microglobulin [9] was used to explain the presence of crystalluria, while a lower excretion of PTF1 and OPN by stone formers was proposed as a reason for stone formation [31]. However, it is no less logical to use the presence of crystalluria or stones as the reason for the lower protein levels, since the concentration of any urinary protein that binds to stone crystals will be significantly underestimated when crystals are excreted in the urine or formed upon later cooling of the specimen. This has been clearly demonstrated for PTF1 [36] and OPN [37] and recognised as a possible explanation for reduced OPN concentration in stone formers' urine [38].

Results will also be inaccurate if the urine contains blood. OPN, PTF1, albumin, transferrin and α-1-microglobulin, for instance, are all present in blood, which is characteristically present in urine from active stone formers. The conclusion that "albumin and transferrin may play a presumptive role in stone formation" [35], because their urinary excretion is raised, is therefore open to doubt. Increased excretion of bikunin, which is a marker of systemic proteolysis [38], may well simply result from inflammation induced by the stone's presence in the urinary tract. It is obvious, therefore, that measurement of individual urinary macromolecules is fraught with insurmountable difficulties—it is impossible to demand that stone formers excrete urine free of crystals and blood!

Changes in mRNA or protein expression

Proteomic, immunological and molecular biological techniques have been used to study changes in the level of expression of some macromolecules or their mRNA in cultured renal cells, or in animal models of nephrolithiasis, following exposure to oxalate or CaOx crystals. mRNA levels of fibronectin [10], matrix Gla protein [39] and OPN [39-41] were reported to increase in kidneys of lithogenic rats, while fibronectin expression was stimulated in MDCK cells challenged with CaOx crystals [10], as was the production of OPN [42]. Heparan sulfate expression also increases in lithogenic rats [43] as does the level of bikunin mRNA [44], which also increases in MDCK cells exposed to oxalate, but not to CaOx crystals [45].

However, as was evident with the studies described above, results have not always been concordant. The THG gene has been reported both to be up-regulated [46] and down-regulated [47] in experimental nephrolithiasis; but the protein's expression is unaffected by exposure to CaOx crystals in cultured cells [48]. Similarly, though one study reported that prothrombin mRNA levels rise in experimental nephrolithiasis in rats [49], a later paper has shown that they fall [50]. But caution is warranted. Lest we assume from such studies that such observations are necessarily significant, it is wise to note that the gene expression of 35 different proteins was altered by more than 2-fold in NRK-52E cells exposed to COM crystals [51] and a whopping one hundred and seventy three genes were at least 2-fold regulated at one or more points during progression of experimental nephrolithiasis in rats [52]. Reason dictates that not all of these proteins are key players in stone formation. In fact, most changes are more likely to result from non-specific inflammatory processes or toxicity caused by the agent used to induce CaOx crystal deposition.

Relevance or influence?

Many years of painstaking work have shown us beyond doubt that various macromolecules are implicated in stone formation, but are they truly *relevant?* Instead, it is probably more appropriate to ask: *What makes a macromolecule* ***influential*** *in stone formation?* When all's said and done, there is one fundamental reason why we have looked at the effects of any particular macromolecule on crystallization or crystal-cell binding, or studied its genetic regulation and expression in cell culture or animal models, or compared its urinary excretion in stone formers and controls—it binds to crystals! By covering the surface of a crystal, a macromolecule can hinder its collision with other crystals, impede the deposition of solute ions, and retard or encourage its binding to an epithelial cell. Binding of a macromolecule to a crystal surface is thus a vital part of stone formation, because it can dictate whether crystal nucleation progresses to stone formation. And it is only in relatively recent times that we have been able to see, close-up, how it actually occurs.

THE IMPORTANCE OF COMPATIBILITY

The intimate relationship between calcium oxalate and PTF1

The function of healthy minerals in living organisms relies, absolutely, on ensuring the consistency of the desired structure—*every time*. Nature achieves this using a stepwise approach, the second stage of which is known as interfacial or molecular recognition [53]. This phenomenon, which guarantees the nucleation of a specific mineral of a defined shape, size, texture and orientation, is orchestrated by genetically determined sites within proteins [54]. These sites exhibit epitaxial alignment, as well as electrostatic, geometric and stereochemical complementarity between the structures of the protein and the crystal lattice [55] at the interface between the two [53,55]. Although formation of crystals in the urinary tract differs from controlled biomineralization, the relationship between macromolecule and mineral, and therefore any effects on crystallization or cellular adhesion, must still rely on compatibility between the physical configuration of the protein and the atomic array on the crystal face.

PTF1 is a powerful inhibitor of CaOx crystal growth and aggregation in undiluted, ultrafiltered human urine [7] and under inorganic conditions [56], properties that must depend upon binding of the molecule to the CaOx crystal surface. But *which* surface? Figure 1 shows the distribution patterns that would result if a protein were to bind irreversibly to one of the three faces of COM and become interred within the structure. The patterns resulting from binding to the side and end faces are known as bowties or intersectoral zoning [57]. The distribution of a macromolecule within a crystal can be determined by growing crystals in solutions containing the macromolecule tagged with a coloured or fluorescent dye [57]. Figure 2 shows the fluorescence patterns of a single inorganic COM crystal that was precipitated from a solution containing PTF1 labelled with fluorescein isothiocyanate (FITC) (green) and HSA labelled with Alexa Fluor 647 (red). The observed patterns are consistent with binding of PTF1 principally to the end face of the COM crystal, and HSA to the side face, as shown diagrammatically in the associated diagrams.

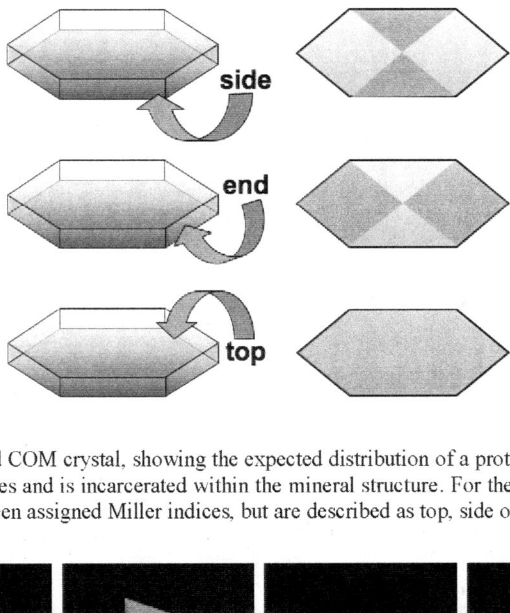

FIGURE 1. A stylised COM crystal, showing the expected distribution of a protein after it binds to one of the three crystal faces and is incarcerated within the mineral structure. For the sake of simplicity, the three faces have not been assigned Miller indices, but are described as top, side or end.

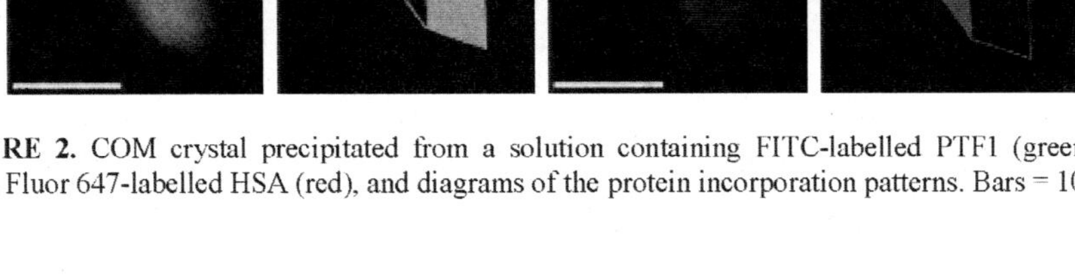

FIGURE 2. COM crystal precipitated from a solution containing FITC-labelled PTF1 (green) and Alexa Fluor 647-labelled HSA (red), and diagrams of the protein incorporation patterns. Bars = 10μm.

Figure 2 shows that individual proteins can bind selectively to different COM faces and will, presumably, thus have different effects on crystal growth and aggregation, and the ability of the crystal to adhere to cells. In parallel with salubrious biomineralization, binding depends upon the molecular configuration of the protein and its structural compatibility with the array of atoms on the crystal surface.

The inhibitory effects of PTF1 are mediated through the N-terminal region of the molecule [58], which contains 10 Gla (γ-carboxyglutamic acid) residues. Gla is renowned for its strong Ca-binding properties. Of the 10 Gla residues in PTF1, only Gla's 15, 20, 21, 26, 30 and 33 are available for bonding to a surface [59]. The shape of the molecule allows only Gla's 15 and 20, 20 and 21, or 26, 30 and 33 to contact a surface together. Thus the highest number that can bond with a flat COM surface at one time is 3. Models of the region of the F1 molecule containing Gla's 26, 30 and 33 against the 3 COM faces were constructed for the best arrangements that could be achieved by eye, using the modelling program Accelrys. Figure 3A shows a ribbon diagram of the complete Ca-stabilized PTF1 molecule, as well as an enlarged view of the Gla domain (Fig. 3B). A closer view of the best arrangement of Gla's 26, 30 and 33, relative to the lattice atoms of the COM end face, are shown in Fig. 3C. This face was chosen because Fig. 2 shows that it is this face to which PTF1 binds.

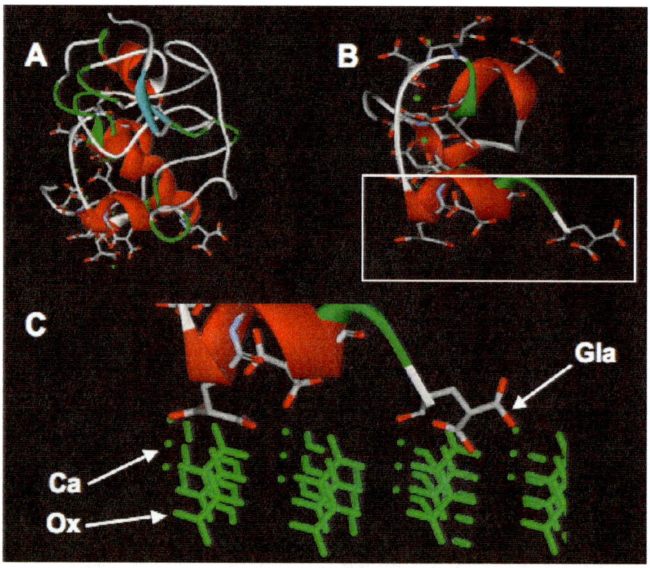

FIGURE 3. A: Three dimensional structure of the entire Ca-stabilized PTF1 molecule. B: Enlarged view of the Gla domain. Ca atoms are depicted as green balls. C: Close up view of the bordered area in B, showing the Gla groups and their relationship to Ca atoms on the end face of COM.

While modeling is useful for understanding interactions between proteins and crystal surfaces, it does not so easily convey the entrapment of PTF1 *inside* the COM crystal [60]—from the point of nucleation. Figure 4 shows a CaOx crystal filtered from urine several minutes after sodium oxalate solution was added to induce CaOx deposition. Organic material is clearly visible on the filtration membrane, as well as interspersed throughout well-defined crystallites comprising the newly formed single crystal: it is impossible to discern where organic and mineral materials begin and end.

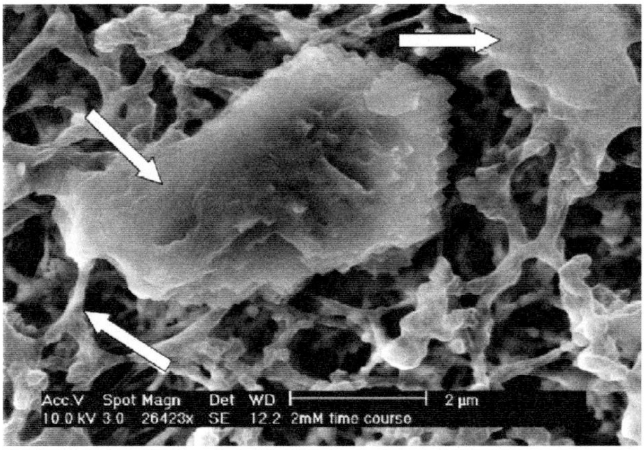

FIGURE 4. A CaOx crystal precipitated from centrifuged and filtered urine by the addition of sodium oxalate solution. The crystal was removed by filtration as soon as practicably possible after addition of the sodium oxalate. Macromolecular material is indicated by arrows. The bar represents 2µm.

We have proposed that the incarceration of macromolecules within CaOx represents a form of protection against urolithiasis [60-63], since after internalization by epithelial cells, crystals riddled with proteins would be more susceptible to lysosomal proteases. These would open channels throughout the mineral architecture and infiltrate into the crystalline core, rendering the structure more vulnerable to eventual dissolution. This hypothesis is supported by studies showing that degradation and dissolution of COM by MDCK cells are increased in crystals containing greater amounts of intracrystalline protein [64,65].

SUMMARY AND CONCLUSIONS

If nothing else, the information presented in this review has demonstrated that macromolecules are obligate participants in stone formation. If they were not, CaOx precipitated within the urinary tract would look and feel identical to the fine white powder available from any commercial source. However, it should be equally clear that a great deal of information generated by years of research has done little to clarify our understanding of the roles of macromolecules in stone formation and prevention. Many have been identified as participants, though only very few have been studied in any detail. More may yet be identified. Others may be shown in the future to be completely irrelevant. Still, on the basis of available knowledge, accumulating information about a select few seems to suggest that their apparent relationships with urolithiasis are not merely chance encounters. It is always dangerous to nominate an individual for an accolade, since it carries the risk of inadvertently omitting a worthy recipient. Time may well prove us wrong, but on the basis of what we now know, we can tentatively predict that in ten years' time, of the many proteins found in stones and urine, osteopontin, prothrombin fragment 1, hyaluronan, Tamm-Horsfall glycoprotein, bikunin and calgranulin will continue to be mentioned regularly in stone dispatches....

...for many are called, but few are chosen [Matthew 22:14].

ACKNOWLEDGEMENTS

We gratefully acknowledge Grant No. NIDDK R01 DK064050-01A1 from the National Institutes of Health, USA. Alison Cook was the recipient of a Flinders University Postgraduate Scholarship.

REFERENCES

1. S. Weiner and L. Addadi, *J. Materials Chem.* **7**, 689-702 (1997).
2. R.L. Ryall, *World J. Urol.* **11**, 59-65 (1997).
3. R.L. Ryall, "Macromolecules and kidney stone formation: Waste of space or space for waste?," In *Stone Disease* Edited by J. Segura et al, Health Publications, Editions 21, 2003, pp. 69-79.
4. R.L. Ryall, *Nephron* **98**, 37-42 (2004).
5. S.R. Khan and D.J. Kok, *Frontiers in Biosc.* **9**, 1450-1482 (2004).
6. R.L. Ryall, *Pediatr. Nephrol.* **10**, 656-666 (1996).
7. R.L. Ryall, P.K. Grover, A.M.F. Stapleton, D.K. Barrell, Y. Tang, R.L. Moritz and R.J. Simpson, *Clin. Sci.* **89**, 533-541 (1995).
8. P.K. Grover, R.L. Moritz, R.J. Simpson and R.L. Ryall, *Eur. J. Biochem.* **253**, 637-644 (1998).
9. S. Tardivel, J. Médétognon, C. Randoux, M. Kébédé, T. Drüeke, M. Daudon, C. Hennequin and B. Lacour, *Urol. Res.* **27**, 243-249 (1999).
10. M. Tsujihata, O. Miyaka, K. Yoshimura, K. Kakimoto, S. Takahara and A. Okuyama, *J. Urol.* **164**, 1718-1723 (2000).
11. S.N. Pillay, J.R. Asplin and F.L. Coe, *Am. J. Physiol.* **275**, F255-F261 (1998).
12. S. Yamaguchi, T. Yoshioka, M. Utsonomiya, T. Koide, M. Osafune, A. Okuyama and T. Sonoda, *Urol. Res.* **21**, 187-192 (1993).
13. K. Suzuki and R.L. Ryall, *Br. J. Urol.* **78**, 15-21 (1996).
14. B. Hess, R.L. Ryall, J.P. Kavanagh, S.R. Khan, D.J. Kok, A.L. Rodgers and H.-G. Tiselius, *Eur. Urol.* **40**, 220-230 (2001).
15. V. Kumar, G. Farell, S. Deganello and J.C.Lieske, *J. Am. Soc. Nephrol.* **14**, 289-297 (2003).
16. C.F. Verkoelen, B.G. van der Boom and J.C. Romjin, *Kidney Int.* **58**, 1045-1054 (2000).
17. H.K. Koul and S. Koul, "β-tubulin is the major cell membrane COM-crystal binding protein in renal epithelial cells", in: *Kidney Stones: Inside and Out*, edited by M.D.I. Gohel and D.W.T. Au, The Hong Kong Polytechnic University, 2004, pp. 123-125.
18. E.A. Sorokina and J.G. Kleinman, *J. Biol. Chem.* **274**, 27492-27496 (1999).
19. M. Asselman, A. Verhulst, M.E. De Broe and C.F. Verkoelen, *J. Am. Soc. Nephrol.* **14**, 3155-3166 (2003).
20. G. Kramer, G.E. Steiner, M. Prinz-Kashani, B. Bursa and M. Marberger, *B.J.U. Int.* **91**, 554-559 (2003).
21. T. Yasui, K. Fujita, A. Kiyofumi and K. Kohri, *Intl. J. Urol.* **9**, 100-109 (2002).
22. T. Yamate, K. Kohri, T. Umekawa, N. Amasaki, N. Amasaki, Y. Isikawa, M. Iguchi and T. Kurita, *Eur. Urol.* **30**, 388-393 (1996).
23. J.C. Lieske, R. Leonard and F.G. Toback, *Am. J. Physiol.* **268**, F604-F612 (1995).

24. M. Tsujihata, K. Yoshimura, K. Tsujikawa, N. Tei and A. Okuyama, *Int. J. Urol.* **13**, 743-746 (2006).
25. S. Ebisuno, M. Nishihata, T. Inagaki, M. Umehara and Y. Kohjimoto, *J. Am. Soc. Nephrol.* Suppl **14**, S436-S440 (1999).
26. V. Kumar, G. Farell and J.C. Lieske, *J. Urol.* **170**, 221-225 (2003).
27. B. Hess, *Miner. Electrolyte Metab.* **20**, 393-398 (1994).
28. K. Suzuki, H. Kobayashi, S. Kageyama, K. Shibata, M. Fujie and T. Terao, *J. Urol.* **166**, 268-274 (2001).
29. J. Médétognon-Benisson, S. Tardivel, C. Hennequin, M. Daudon, T. Drüeke and B. Lacour. *Urol. Res.* **27**, 69-75 (1999).
30. T. Yasui, K. Fujita, Y. Hayashi, K. Ueda, S. Kon, M. Maeda, T. Uede and K. Kohri, *Urol. Res.* **27**, 225-230 (1999).
31. S. Nishio, M. Hatanaka, H. Takeda, T. Iseda, H. Iwata and M. Yokoyama, *J. Am. Nephrol. Soc.* **10**, S394-S396 (1999).
32. D.S. Bautista, J. Denstedt, A.F. Chambers and J.F. Harris, *J. Cell Biochem.* **61**, 402-409 (1996).
33. P.A. Cadieux, D.T. Beiko, J.D. Watterson, J.P. Burton, J.C. Howard, B.E. Knudsen, B.S. Gan, J.K. Mc Cormick, A.F. Chambers, J.D. Denstedt and G. Reid, *J. Clin. Lab. Anal.* **18**, 170-175 (2004).
34. K.J. Bergsland, J.K. Kelly, B.J. Coe and F.L. Coe, *Am. J. Renal Physiol.* **291**, F530-F536 (2006).
35. G. Pourmand, H. Nasseh, A. Sarrafnejad, A Mojtahedi, A. Mehrsai, D.H.Alamdari and K. Nourijelyani, *Urol. Int.* **76**, 163-168 (2006).
36. C.J. Dean, P.J. Macardle and R.L. Ryall, "The effect of the presence of calcium oxalate crystals on the measurement of prothrombin fragment 1 in urine", in: *Urolithiasis 2000*, edited by Rodgers AL et al, University of Cape Town, 2000, pp. 150-152.
37. L.A. Thurgood, P.K. Grover and R.L. Ryall, "A problem protein: Unexpected irregularities in the measurement of urinary osteopontin", in: These Proceedings, pp. 196-199.
38. C. Mizon, F. Piva, V. Queyrel, M. Balduyck, E. Hachulla and J. Mizon, *Clin. Chem. Lab. Med.* **40**, 579-596 (2002).
39. T. Yasui, K. Fujita, S. Sasaki, M. Sato, M. Sugimoto, S. Hirota, Y. Kitamura, S. Nomura and K. Kohri, *Urol. Res.* **27**, 255-261 (1999).
40. T. Umekawa, T. Yamate, N. Amasaki, K. Kohri and T. Kurita, *Urologia Internationalis* **55**, 6-10 (1995).
41. S.R. Khan, J.M. Johnson, A.B. Peck, J.G. Cornelius and P.A. Glenton, *J. Urol.* **168**, 1173-1181 (2002).
42. J.C. Lieske, M.S. Hammes, J.R. Hoyer and F.G.Toback, *Kidney Int.* **51**, 679-683 (1997).
43. S. Iida, M. Inoue, S. Yoshii, T. Yanagaki, S. Chikama, A. Shimada, K. Matsuoka, S. Noda and S.R. Khan, *J. Am. Soc. Nephrol.* **10**, S412-S416 (1999).
44. S. Iida, A.B. Peck, J. Johnson-Tardieu, M. Moriyama, P.A. Glenton, K.J. Byer, and S.R. Khan, *J. Am. Soc. Nephrol.* **10**, 986-996 (1999).
45. S. Iida, A.B. Peck, K.J. Byer and S.R. Khan, *J. Urol.* **162**, 1480-1486 (1999).
46. S. Katsuma, S. Shiojima, A. Hirasawa, K. Takagaki, Y. Kaminishi, M. Koba, Y. Hagidai, M. Muria, T. Ohgi, J.Yano and G. Tsujimoto, *Biochem. Biophys. Res. Commun.* **296**, 544-552 (2002).
47. S.R. Marengo, D.H.-C. Chen, H.-L.C. Kaung, M.I. Resnick and L. Yang, *J. Urol.* **167**, 2192-2197 (2002).
48. O. Miyake, T. Yoshioka, K. Yoshimura, K. Kakimoto, S. Yamaguchi, T. Koide and A. Okuyama, *Br. J. Urol.* **81**, 14-19 (1998).
49. K. Suzuki, T. Tanaka, K. Miyazawa, C. Nakajima, M. Moriyama, K. Suga, M. Murai and J. Yano, *J. Am. Nephrol. Soc.* **10**, S408-S411 (1999).
50. P. Grover, K. Miyazawa, M. Coleman, J. Stahl and R. Ryall, *J. Pathol.* **210**, 273-281 (2006).
51. K. Miyazawa, C. Domiki, M. Moriyama and K. Suzuki, "cDNA macroarray analysis of genes in renal epithelial cells exposed to calcium oxalate crystals", in: *Kidney Stones: Inside and Out*, edited by M.D.I. Gohel and D.W.T. Au, The Hong Kong Polytechnic University, 2004, pp. 130-131.
52. S. Shiojima, S. Hirasawa, K. Tagagaki, Y. Kaminishi, M. Koba, Y. Hagidai, M. Murai, T. Ohgi, J. Jano and G. Tsujimoto, *Biochem. Biophys. Res. Comm.* **296**, 544-552 (2002).

53. S. Mann, D.D. Archibald, J.M. Didymus, T. Douglas, B.R. Heywood, F.C. Meldrum and N.J. Reeves, *Science* **261**, 1286-1292 (1993).
54. A.H. Heuer, D.J. Fink, V.J. Laraia, J.L. Arias, P.D. Calvert, K. Kendall, G.L. Messing, J. Blackwell, P.C. Reike, D.H. Thompson. A.P. Wheeler, A. Veis and I. Caplan, *Science* **255**, 1098-1105 (1992).
55. B.R. Heywood, *Microscopy Res. Tech.* **27,** 376-388 (1994).
56. P.K. Grover and R.L. Ryall, *Eur. J. Biochem.* **263**, 50-56 (1999).
57. B. Kahr and R.W. Gurney, *Chem. Rev.* **101**, 893-951 (2001).
58. P.K. Grover and R.L. Ryall, *Clin. Sci.* **102**, 425-434 (2002).
59. L. Li, T. Darden, C. Foley, R. Hiskey and L. Pedersen (1995) *Protein Science* **4**, 2341-2348 (1995).
60. R.L. Ryall, M.C. Chauvet and P.K. Grover, *Br. J. Urol. Int.* **96**, 654-663 (2005).
61. R.L. Ryall RL, D.E. Fleming, I.R. Doyle, N.A. Evans, C.J. Dean and V.R. Marshall, *J. Struct. Biol.* **134**, 5-14 (2001).
62. D.E. Fleming, A. van Riessen, M.C. Chauvet, P.K. Grover, B. Hunter, W. van Bronswijk and R.L. Ryall, *J. Bone Min. Res.* **18**, 1282-1291 (2003).
63. R.L. Ryall, D.E. Fleming, P.K. Grover, M.C. Chauvet, C.J. Dean and V.R. Marshall, *Mol. Urol.* **4**, 391-402 (2003).
64. M.C. Chauvet, R.L. Ryall, *J. Struct. Biol.* **151**, 12-17 (2005).
65. P.K. Grover, L.A. Thurgood and R.L. Ryall, "Intracrystalline proteins promote dissolution of urinary calcium oxalate crystals in cultured renal epithelial cells", In: These proceedings, pp. 200-203.

Role of Anion Transporter SLC26A6 (CFEX) in Prevention of Hyperoxaluria and Urolithiasis

Peter S. Aronson

Departments of Medicine and of Cellular and Molecular Physiology, Yale University School of Medicine, P.O. Box 208029, New Haven, CT 06520-8029, USA

Abstract. In the proximal tubule of the kidney, a significant fraction of Cl^- is transported by apical membrane Cl^--formate exchange and Cl^--oxalate exchange. Studies to identify the transporter(s) mediating apical membrane Cl^--anion exchange in the proximal tubule led to the characterization of CFEX (SLC26A6). Functional expression of CFEX in *Xenopus* oocytes demonstrated that the transporter is capable of mediating multiple modes of anion exchange including Cl^--oxalate exchange. Comparison of wild-type and CFEX null mice with respect to transport in renal brush border vesicles and microperfused tubules demonstrated that CFEX primarily mediates Cl^--oxalate exchange rather than Cl^--formate exchange in the proximal tubule *in vivo*. CFEX null mice were observed to have a high incidence of calcium oxalate urolithiasis that was attributable to hyperoxaluria. Hyperoxaluria in CFEX null mice was found to result from a defect in oxalate secretion in the intestine, thereby causing increased net absorption of ingested oxalate and elevated plasma oxalate concentration. Thus, by mediating intestinal oxalate secretion, CFEX plays an essential role in preventing hyperoxaluria and calcium oxalate nephrolithiasis.

Keywords: Kidney stones, mouse, membrane transport, brush border membrane vesicles
PACS: 87.16.Uv

INTRODUCTION

The majority of the Na^+ and Cl^- filtered by the kidney is reabsorbed in the proximal tubule. We used brush border membrane vesicles as an experimental system to identify apical membrane transport activities that might mediate Cl^- absorption in this nephron segment. Although we could not detect significant Na^+-Cl^- or Na^+-K^+-$2Cl^-$ cotransport [1], we did demonstrate Cl^--formate exchange and Cl^--oxalate exchange [2,3]. In addition, others found evidence for Cl^--OH^- exchange activity in renal brush border vesicles [4], and for Cl^--OH^- and Cl^--HCO_3^- exchange activities on the apical membrane of intact proximal tubule cells [5].

Cl^--OH^- or Cl^--HCO_3^- exchange in parallel with Na^+-H^+ exchange is a potential mechanism for NaCl entry across the apical membrane of proximal tubule cells, as shown in Fig. 1. But Cl^--formate exchange and Cl^--oxalate exchange can mediate substantial quantities of Cl^- absorption only if there are mechanisms to recycle these organic anions from the lumen back into the cell. Studies using renal brush border vesicles failed to demonstrate direct Na^+-formate cotransport, but instead found that an inward H^+ gradient markedly stimulated formate uptake [2,6]. These findings supported a model by which Cl^--formate exchange could mediate NaCl entry across

CP900, *Renal Stone Disease, 1st Annual International Urolithiasis Research Symposium,* edited by A. P. Evan, J. E. Lingeman, and J. C. Williams, Jr.

the apical membrane of proximal tubule cells [2], as illustrated in Fig. 1. The inward H^+ gradient generated by Na^+-H^+ exchange would drive filtered formate into the cell by H^+-coupled transport, and then the outward formate gradient would drive Cl^- entry by Cl^--formate exchange.

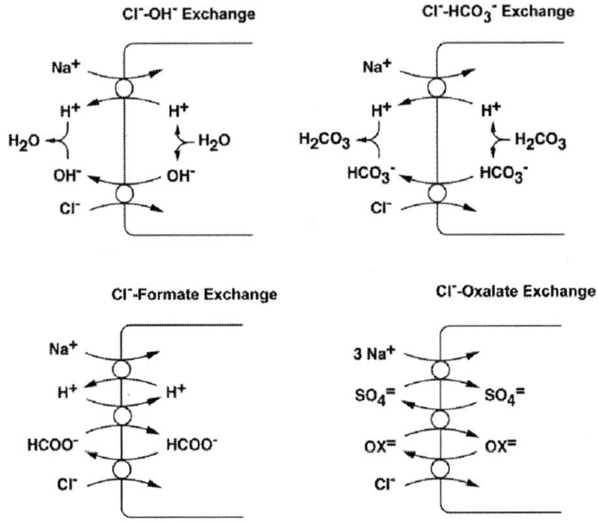

FIGURE 1. Models of apical membrane NaCl entry mediated by different modes of Cl^--base exchange.

Possible mechanisms to recycle oxalate from lumen to cell were similarly evaluated in renal brush border vesicles. Although there was no significant Na^+-oxalate cotransport activity, oxalate-sulfate exchange was found [7], consistent with previously described sulfate-anion exchange activity [8]. These findings supported a model by which Cl^--oxalate exchange could mediate NaCl entry across the apical membrane of proximal tubule cells [7], as also illustrated in Fig. 1. Sulfate absorption by Na^+-sulfate cotransport would generate an outward sulfate gradient that could then drive oxalate uptake by sulfate-oxalate exchange. The resulting cell to lumen oxalate gradient would then drive Cl^- entry by Cl^--oxalate exchange.

The models of NaCl transport shown in Fig. 1 were tested in tubule microperfusion studies. These studies showed that formate and oxalate strongly stimulated the rate of transepithelial NaCl absorption [9]. Moreover, the tubule perfusion experiments supported the proposed mechanisms of formate and oxalate recycling illustrated in Fig. 1 [10]. For example, luminal application of the Na^+-H^+ exchange inhibitor EIPA abolished stimulation of Cl^- absorption by formate, but did not affect stimulation by oxalate. Conversely, deletion of sulfate from the perfusion solutions abolished oxalate stimulation of Cl^- absorption, but did not affect stimulation by formate. These findings were entirely consistent with the models for NaCl transport in Fig. 1, in which formate recycling is dependent on Na^+-H^+ exchange, and oxalate recycling is sulfate-dependent as it occurs by Na^+-sulfate cotransport in parallel with sulfate-oxalate exchange. These models were also supported by the observations that formate-stimulated Cl^- absorption was abolished in NHE3 null mice, whereas oxalate-stimulated transport was not affected [11].

STUDIES ON THE ANION EXCHANGER SLC26

An important advance toward the molecular identification of the apical membrane anion exchanger(s) mediating proximal tubule Cl^- reabsorption was the discovery that pendrin (SLC26A4), a member of the SLC26 "sulfate transporter" family, can actually function as a monovalent anion exchanger and mediate Cl^--formate exchange [12]. We therefore evaluated pendrin as a candidate transporter to mediate apical membrane Cl^--formate exchange in the proximal tubule. Using immunocytochemical methods, we were unable to detect pendrin expression in proximal tubule cells, but instead observed pendrin expression on the apical membrane of some cells in the collecting tubule [13]. Studies by others identified this pendrin-expressing cell population as non-alpha intercalated cells and demonstrated that pendrin mediates HCO_3^- secretion in the cortical collecting tubule [14]. Additional evidence against a role for pendrin in the proximal tubule was that there was no reduction in either brush border membrane Cl^--formate exchange or transepithelial NaCl absorption in pendrin null mice [15].

However, based on the finding that pendrin could mediate Cl^--base exchange, we screened the mouse EST database to try to identify one or more novel homologues of pendrin that might be expressed in the proximal tubule [13]. We successfully identified a cDNA that encoded a pendrin homologue expressed on the brush border membrane in mouse kidney [13]. It proved to be the mouse orthologue of human SLC26A6, which had been independently identified by other groups searching for novel SLC26 gene family members [16,17]. Expression of SLC26A6 was detected widely in both epithelial and non-epithelial tissues including heart, placenta, liver, skeletal muscle, kidney, pancreas, stomach and small intestine [13,16-18]. Immunolocalization studies revealed that SLC26A6 has polarized expression on the apical membrane of cells in many epithelia in addition to the proximal tubule [13,19] including pancreatic duct [16], stomach [20], and small intestine [18].

We performed functional expression studies of mouse SLC26A6 in *Xenopus* oocytes and demonstrated Cl^--formate exchange activity [13]. We therefore called the transporter CFEX [13]. But subsequent functional expression studies by our group and others demonstrated that SLC26A6 has broad anion specificity and can mediate multiple anion exchange reactions involving Cl^-, formate, oxalate, sulfate, HCO_3^- and OH^- as substrates (e.g. Cl^--oxalate exchange, Cl^--HCO_3^- exchange, oxalate-sulfate exchange) [18,21-23]. We found that Cl^--oxalate exchange mediated by CFEX is electrogenic, consistent with exchange of divalent oxalate for monovalent Cl^- [21], similar to the electrogenic Cl^--oxalate exchange activity we had observed in renal brush border vesicles many years earlier [3]. Competition studies indicated that affinity of CFEX for oxalate is appreciably greater than for Cl^-, HCO_3^-, sulfate or formate [21,22]. Moreover, when tested at equal substrate concentrations, transport of oxalate was twice as high as that of sulfate or formate [21], as shown in Fig. 2. These findings underscored the potential role of CFEX as an oxalate transporter.

Studies in CFEX null mice have provided insight into the actual physiological roles of CFEX *in vivo*. For example, as shown in Fig. 3a, the ability of an outward Cl^- gradient to stimulate oxalate influx into renal brush border membrane vesicles was completely abolished in CFEX null mice, demonstrating that CFEX mediates all of the apical membrane Cl^--oxalate exchange activity in proximal tubule cells [24]. In contrast to the complete loss of Cl^--oxalate exchange activity, there was only a very modest partial defect in Cl^--formate exchange in renal brush border membrane vesicles from CFEX null mice [24], as shown in Fig. 3b. The results of tubule microperfusion studies are illustrated in Fig. 3c. Consistent with the predominant role of CFEX as a Cl^--oxalate exchanger rather than a Cl^--formate exchanger, the increment in transepithelial NaCl absorption induced by the addition of oxalate to the luminal perfusate was completely abolished in CFEX null mice, whereas the increment in NaCl absorption induced by formate was only partially inhibited [25].

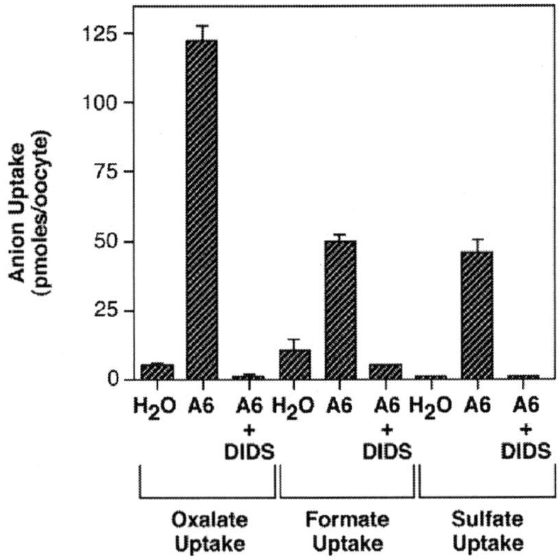

FIGURE 2. Functional expression studies of mouse SLC26A6 in *Xenopus* oocytes [21].

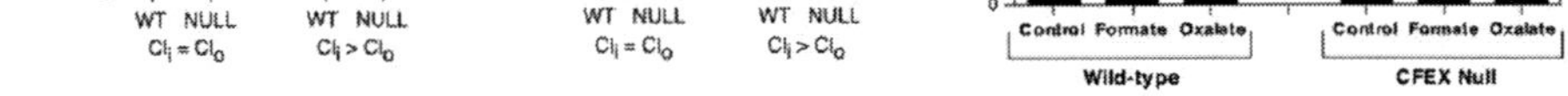

FIGURE 3. Proximal tubule transport defects in CFEX null mice. (a) Cl^--oxalate exchange, and (b) Cl^--formate exchange assayed in renal brush border vesicles from wild-type and CFEX null mice [24]. (c) Effects of formate and oxalate on volume absorption (J_V), a measure of transepithelial NaCl transport, by proximal tubules microperfused *in situ* in wild-type and CFEX null mice [25].

In view of this evidence for the role of CFEX as an oxalate transporter, a striking phenotype observed in CFEX null mice was a high frequency of calcium oxalate urolithiasis [24]. We found calcium oxalate stones in the bladders of many null mice, as shown in Fig. 4a, and detected calcium oxalate deposits in the kidneys of CFEX null mice, as illustrated in Fig. 4b.

The propensity toward calcium oxalate urolithiasis was attributable to severe hyperoxaluria in CFEX null mice [24], as shown in Fig. 5a. Moreover, as illustrated in Fig. 5b, plasma oxalate was greatly elevated in CFEX null mice [24], thereby explaining hyperoxaluria on the basis of enhanced filtration of oxalate rather than a primary renal leak of oxalate due to impaired tubular reabsorption. The high levels of plasma and urine oxalate in CFEX null mice were greatly reduced when mice were fed an oxalate-free diet [24], as also shown in Figs. 5a and 5b. These observations demonstrated that dietary oxalate must be the source of most of the excess oxalate appearing in the urine and plasma of CFEX null mice. Thus, CFEX null mice appeared to represent a genetic model of enteric hyperoxaluria in which there is enhanced net absorption of dietary oxalate.

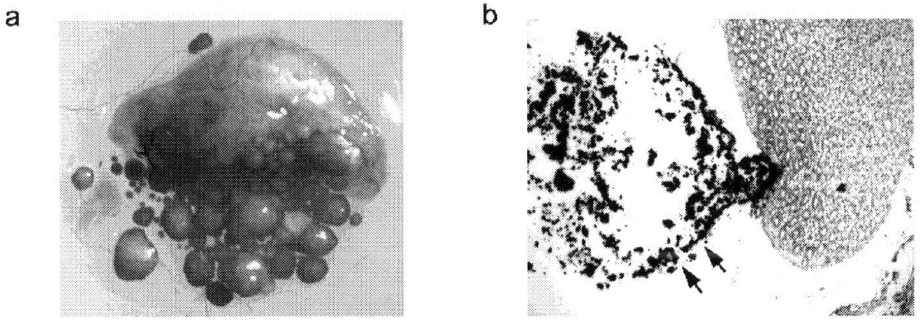

FIGURE 4. Calcium oxalate urolithiasis in CFEX null mice [24]. (a) Stones found in the bladder of a CFEX null mouse. (b) Calcium oxalate mass in the urinary space of a CFEX null mouse.

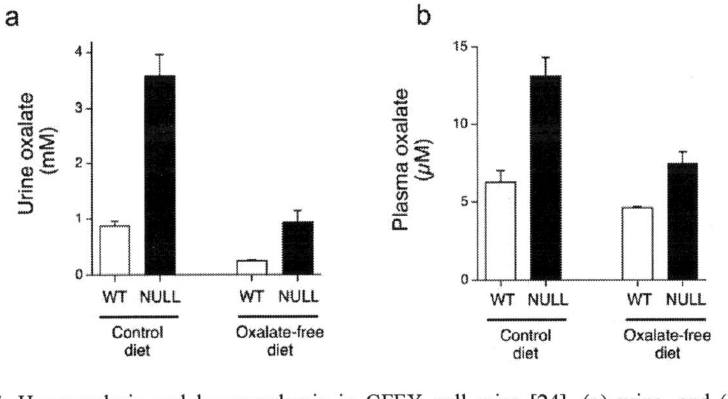

FIGURE 5. Hyperoxaluria and hyperoxalemia in CFEX null mice [24]. (a) urine, and (b) plasma oxalate concentrations in wild-type and CFEX null mice fed a control oxalate-containing diet or an oxalate-free diet.

As described earlier, CFEX is expressed on the apical membrane in many gastrointestinal tissues including the pancreas and small intestine [16,18]. Moreover, many years ago we had observed Cl^--oxalate exchange activity in brush border membrane vesicles isolated from small intestine [26]. Given the relatively high concentration of Cl^- in the lumen of the small intestine, it would be expected that Cl^--oxalate exchange would function in the direction of mediating Cl^- absorption and oxalate secretion, as in the proximal tubule. To directly assess if CFEX mediates oxalate secretion in the small intestine, we measured unidirectional absorptive and secretory fluxes of radiolabeled oxalate across strips of duodenal epithelium mounted in Ussing chambers *in vitro* [24]. We found that duodenal tissue from CFEX null mice has a major defect in the serosa to mucosa secretory flux of oxalate, resulting in conversion of net oxalate transport from secretion to absorption [24]. As additional evidence for the concept that CFEX plays a major role in intestinal oxalate secretion, we observed a significant reduction in fecal oxalate concentration in CFEX null mice *in vivo* [24].

Hatch and colleagues similarly reported hyperoxaluria in an independent line of CFEX null mice generated by Soleimani [27]. They measured unidirectional oxalate fluxes across ileal epithelium *in vitro*, and also demonstrated conversion of net oxalate transport from secretion to absorption in intestinal tissue from CFEX null mice [27]. Moreover, they demonstrated a specific defect in Cl^--dependent oxalate secretion in CFEX null mice, consistent with the role of CFEX as a Cl^--oxalate exchanger [27].

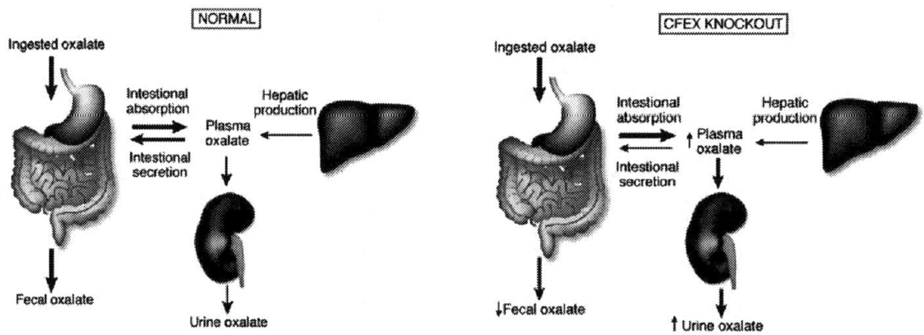

FIGURE 6. Oxalate homeostasis in normal and CFEX knockout mice [28]. The primary defect in CFEX null mice is a greatly reduced secretory flux of oxalate in the intestine, leading to increased net absorption of ingested oxalate, elevated plasma oxalate concentration, and increased renal oxalate excretion.

Oxalate homeostasis in wild-type and CFEX knockout mice are contrasted schematically in Fig. 6 [28]. Under normal conditions there is net absorption of a small fraction of ingested oxalate [29]. As indicated by the results of feeding an oxalate-free diet in Fig. 5, the absorption of ingested oxalate is the source of most of the plasma and urine oxalate even in wild-type mice. The components of plasma and urine oxalate that remain in mice fed an oxalate-free diet reflect endogenous hepatic production. We propose that net absorption of ingested oxalate in wild-type mice is maintained at a low level due to the large secretory backflux of oxalate mediated by CFEX in the intestine, as illustrated in Fig. 6. In CFEX null mice, this secretory flux is defective, leads to greatly augmented net absorption of oxalate, and results in hyperoxalemia and hyperoxaluria, as also shown in Fig. 6. Thus, according to this model, CFEX has a major constitutive role in limiting net intestinal absorption of oxalate, thereby preventing hyperoxaluria and calcium oxalate urolithiasis.

CONCLUSIONS

These studies suggest that inherited or acquired defects in function or regulation of CFEX are potential molecular mechanisms causing hyperoxaluria and calcium oxalate urolithiasis. For example, the increased incidence of hyperoxaluria and nephrolithiasis in patients with small bowel disease or resection [30] has been attributed to the direct and indirect effects of increased luminal levels of bile salts and fatty acids to stimulate enteric oxalate absorption [31]. The studies of oxalate homeostasis in CFEX null mice raise the possibility that loss of CFEX-mediated oxalate secretion in the small intestine may also contribute to enteric hyperoxaluria.

ACKNOWLEDGMENTS

Work in the author's laboratory has been supported by National Institutes of Health grants R01-DK37933 and P01-DK17433.

REFERENCES

1 J. L. Seifter, R. Knickelbein, and P. S. Aronson, *Am J Physiol* 247 (5 Pt 2), F753 (1984).
2 L. P. Karniski and P. S. Aronson, *Proc Natl Acad Sci USA* 82 (18), 6362 (1985).
3 L. P. Karniski and P. S. Aronson, *Am J Physiol* 253 (3 Pt 2), F513 (1987).
4 D. G. Warnock and V. J. Yee, *J Clin Invest* 67 (1), 103 (1981).
5 I. Kurtz, G. Nagami, N. Yanagawa et al., *J Clin Invest* 94 (1), 173 (1994); J. N. Sheu, R. Quigley, and M. Baum, *Am J Physiol* 268 (5 Pt 2), F847 (1995).
6 A. M. Saleh, H. Rudnick, and P. S. Aronson, *Am J Physiol* 271 (2 Pt 2), F401 (1996).
7 S. M. Kuo and P. S. Aronson, *J Biol Chem* 271 (26), 15491 (1996).
8 J. B. Pritchard, *Am J Physiol* 252 (2 Pt 2), F346 (1987).
9 L. Schild, G. Giebisch, L. P. Karniski et al., *J Clin Invest* 79 (1), 32 (1987); T. Wang, G. Giebisch, and P. S. Aronson, *Am J Physiol* 263 (1 Pt 2), F37 (1992); M. Wareing and R. Green, *Journal of Physiology* 477 (Pt 2), 347 (1994).
10 T. Wang, A. L. Egbert, Jr., T. Abbiati et al., *Am J Physiol* 271 (2 Pt 2), F446 (1996).
11 T. Wang, C. L. Yang, T. Abbiati et al., *Am J Physiol Renal Physiol* 281 (2), F288 (2001).
12 D. A. Scott, R. Wang, T. M. Kreman et al., *Nature Genetics* 21 (4), 440 (1999); D. A. Scott and L. P. Karniski, *Am J Physiol Cell Physiol* 278 (1), C207 (2000).
13 F. Knauf, C. L. Yang, R. B. Thomson et al., *Proc Natl Acad Sci U S A* 98 (16), 9425 (2001).
14 I. E. Royaux, S. M. Wall, L. P. Karniski et al., *Proc Natl Acad Sci U S A* 98 (7), 4221 (2001).
15 L. P. Karniski, T. Wang, L. A. Everett et al., *Am J Physiol Renal Physiol* 283, F952 (2002).
16 H. Lohi, M. Kujala, E. Kerkela et al., *Genomics* 70 (1), 102 (2000).
17 S. Waldegger, I. Moschen, A. Ramirez et al., *Genomics* 72 (1), 43 (2001).
18 Z. Wang, S. Petrovic, E. Mann et al., *Am J Physiol Gastrointest Liver Physiol* 282 (3), G573 (2002).
19 R. B. Thomson, T. Wang, B. R. Thomson et al., *Proc Natl Acad Sci U S A* 102 (37), 13331 (2005).
20 S. Petrovic, Z. Wang, L. Ma et al., *Am J Physiol Gastrointest Liver Physiol* 283 (5), G1207 (2002).
21 Z. Jiang, Grichtchenko, II, W. F. Boron et al., *J Biol Chem* 277 (37), 33963 (2002).
22 Q. Xie, R. Welch, A. Mercado et al., *Am J Physiol Renal Physiol* 283 (4), F826 (2002).
23 H. Lohi, G. Lamprecht, D. Markovich et al., *Am J Physiol Cell Physiol* 284 (3), C769 (2003).
24 Z. Jiang, J. R. Asplin, A. P. Evan et al., *Nat Genet* 38 (4), 474 (2006).
25 Z. Wang, T. Wang, S. Petrovic et al., *Am J Physiol Cell Physiol* 288 (4), C957 (2005).
26 R. G. Knickelbein, P. S. Aronson, and J. W. Dobbins, *J Clin Invest* 77 (1), 170 (1986).
27 R. W. Freel, M. Hatch, M. Green et al., *Am J Physiol Gastrointest Liver Physiol* 290 (4), G719 (2006).
28 P. S. Aronson, *Kidney Int* 70 (7), 1207 (2006).

29 R. P. Holmes and D. G. Assimos, *Urol Res* 32 (5), 311 (2004).
30 L. H. Smith, H. Fromm, and A. F. Hofmann, *N Engl J Med* 286 (26), 1371 (1972); E. M. Worcester, *Endocrinol Metab Clin North Am* 31 (4), 979 (2002).
31 M. Hatch and R. W. Freel, *Urological research* 33 (1), 1 (2005).

SLC5 Sodium-Anion Cotransporters and Renal Urate Transport

David B. Mount[*†], Charles Y. Kwon[*], Consuelo Plata[‡], Michael F. Romero[§], and Kambiz Zandi-Nejad[*]

[*]*Renal Division, Brigham and Women's Hospital:Room 542, Harvard Institutes of Medicine, 4 Blackfan Circle, Boston, MA 02115*
[†]*Division of General Internal Medicine, VA Boston Healthcare System*
[‡]*Departamento de Nefrología y Metabolismo Mineral*
Instituto Nacional de Ciencias Médicas y la Nutrición Salvador Zubirán, Mexico City, Mexico
[§]*Department of Physiology and Biomedical Engineering, Mayo Clinic College of Medicine, Rochester, MN*

Abstract. Renal urate transport plays a key role in determining the concentration of circulating uric acid. The reabsorption of filtered urate by the renal proximal tubule appears to require apical sodium-dependent anion transport and the apical URAT1 urate-anion exchanger, in that sodium-dependent transport of lactate, ketoacids, nicotinate, and pyrazinoate (PZA) increases the intracellular concentration of substrates for the subsequent exchange with luminal urate. We have identified SLC5A8 and SLC5A12 as candidates for the sodium-anion cotransporter that collaborates with URAT1. Both transporters function as sodium-dependent nicotinate/monocarboxylate/PZA transporters. Localization studies reveal serial co-expression of these transporters with URAT1, with Slc5a12 in the early proximal tubule and Slc5a8 in S2 and S3 segments. Renal urate excretion is conceivably affected by changes in the activity of SLC5A8, SLC5A12, and/or URAT1, with implications for the pathogenesis of hyperuricemia, nephrolithiasis, and related disorders.

Keywords: hyperuricemia; URAT1, urate transporter-1; SLC5, solute carrier family 5; PZA. Pyrazinoate; nicotinate; probenicid; benzbromarone.
PACS: 87.16.Uv

INTRODUCTION

Renal uric acid transport is of relevance to an increasing number of disorders. In particular, hyperuricosuria is an evident risk factor for calcium-oxalate stones [1]; affected patients generally have a urine pH that is >5.0, with urinary supersaturation of sodium-urate and calcium oxalate due to concomitant increases in urinary calcium and sodium [1,2]. A reduced renal excretion of urate [3] is in turn the underlying pathophysiology in the majority of gouty patients with an "under-excretor" phenotype [4]; notably, however, it is the associated reduction in urinary pH that leads to the formation of uric acid stones in these patients [5,6]. There is also an increasing interest in the role of uric acid in hypertension [7] and progressive renal disease [8], as reviewed elsewhere [7,9]. Uric acid is furthermore acquiring provocative roles in

CP900, *Renal Stone Disease, 1st Annual International Urolithiasis Research Symposium*, edited by A. P. Evan, J. E. Lingeman, and J. C. Williams, Jr.

inflammation [10,11], cardiovascular disease [12], heart failure [13,14], and the metabolic syndrome [15-17].

Considerable strides have recently been made in the molecular physiology of renal uric acid transport, beginning with the identification of URAT1, an apical anion exchanger that is essential for reabsorption of filtered urate by the proximal tubule [18]. This brief review focuses on the mechanisms of renal urate transport and on the identification and characterization of SLC5A8 and SLC5A12, candidates for the sodium-anion transporter that collaborates with URAT1 in proximal urate reabsorption.

Renal Urate Transport

In the majority of mammalian species, uric acid generated from purine metabolism undergoes oxidative degradation via the uricase enzyme, producing soluble allantoin. However, in humans and other primates, the uricase gene is crippled by two mutations that introduce premature stop codons [19]. This genetic inactivation of uricase, combined with extensive reabsorption of filtered urate, results in urate levels in human plasma that are approximately ten times that of most other mammals [20].

Approximately one third of urate elimination occurs in the gastrointestinal tract, with the remainder excreted in the urine [21]. In plasma, uric acid circulates primarily as urate and is freely filtered by renal glomeruli. Bidirectional transport along the nephron results in either net reabsorption (humans, primates, rats, and dogs) or secretion (pigs and rabbits); notably, pigs and rabbits [22,23] lack the apical urate-anion exchanger that is found in all the "reabsorptive" species, presumably due to genetic inactivation the URAT1 anion exchanger (see below). The bulk of renal urate transport occurs within the proximal tubule, with minimal or non-existent contributions from the distal nephron [24]. Both reabsorption and secretion can be detected in reabsorptive species, such as the dog [24].

The dominant model of renal urate excretion has for decades consisted of four steps, the so-called "4-component model": glomerular filtration, reabsorption from the glomerular ultrafiltrate, subsequent secretion, and then "post-secretory reabsorption" [25]. The key assumption underlying this model is that the anti-uricosuric agent pyrazinamide inhibits proximal tubular secretion. In the typical "pyrazinamide suppression test" [26] the oral administration of 2-3 grams results in a marked decrease in the fractional excretion of urate; this effect is mediated by pyrazinoate (PZA), the de-amidated metabolite [27]. Dog experiments had revealed that pyrazinamide abolished the secretory peak of ^{14}C-labeled urate injected into the renal artery; given that the initial urinary bolus of radioactive urate preceded that of ^{14}C-inulin, the primary source of this urinary ^{14}C-urate peak was thought to be tubular secretion rather than glomerular ultrafiltration. By extension, the anti-uricosuric effect of pyrazinamide was attributed to an inhibition of urate secretion [28]. The pyrazinamide suppression test was thus adopted as a pharmacological method to quantify renal tubular urate secretion [26].

The 4-component model was developed to explain the interactions between pyrazinamide and uricosuric agents such as probenecid and benzbromarone

[25,29,30]. Specifically, when these drugs are administered after pyrazinamide there is a striking attenuation of their uricosuric effect [21]. Uricosuric agents were thus postulated to have a dominant effect on "post-secretory reabsorption", since their ability to increase urate excretion was blunted when putative secretion was inhibited with pyrazinamide. It follows that these processes would occur serially, in anatomically separate segments of the proximal tubule; indeed, just such a progression is incorporated in current textbook models of renal urate transport. Notably, however, physiological studies in reabsorptive species indicate a *co-existence* of reabsorption and secretion along the entire length of the proximal tubule [35].

The possibility that PZA does not inhibit secretion, but rather stimulates urate *reabsorption*, was considered and rejected during the initial formulation of the initial formulation of the 4-component model [26,31]. However, a seminal observation in 1985 by Guggino and Aronson suggested that PZA does indeed stimulate tubular reabsorption [32]; the same investigators had previously reported analogous data for lactate [22]. Using brush border membrane vesicles (BBMV) from renal cortex it was demonstrated that Na^+-dependent uptake of PZA or lactate resulted in a marked stimulation of vesicular urate uptake via the brush-border urate-anion exchanger (URAT1). Urate reabsorption by the proximal tubule thus appears to involve collaboration between an apical Na^+-dependent cotransporter and apical urate-anion exchange (see Fig. 1).

URAT1, the Apical Urate-Anion Exchanger

An apical urate-anion exchange activity was first described in renal cortical brush border membrane vesicle preparations (BBMV) from rats and dogs [22,33-35]. This anion exchanger accepts various monovalent organic anions, including urate, p-aminohippurate (PAH) and lactate, in addition to chloride (Cl^-) and hydroxyl (OH^-) [22]. Apical urate-anion exchange activity is absent in species with net urate secretion [22,36], whereas it is present and highly sensitive to uricosuric agents in urate-reabsorbing species [33,34]. A similar urate exchanger has been demonstrated in BBMV from human kidney, albeit with some important distinctions; in particular, PAH and OH^- are not substrates [37].

The URAT1 protein was recently identified as the dominant apical urate exchanger of human proximal tubule [18]. URAT1 is encoded by the *SLC22A12* gene, a member of the large SLC22 family of organic ion transporters. Loss-of-function mutations in SLC22A12 cause a hereditary form of hypouricemia, definitive genetic proof of the importance of this transporter in renal urate reabsorption. URAT1 is part of the organic anion transporter (OAT) branch of the SLC22 gene family; other subgroups include organic cation transporters and organic cation transporter novel type / carnitine transporters [38]. URAT1 is the human ortholog of RST (renal-specific transporter), cloned from murine kidney several years ago [39]. Immunohistochemistry reveals URAT1 protein at the apical membrane of proximal tubules in both human [18] and mouse [40] kidney. Heterologous expression in *Xenopus* oocytes indicates that human URAT1 is capable of urate transport (^{14}C-labeled urate uptake), with a K_m of 371 ± 28 μM. Uricosuric drugs such as probenecid are potent inhibitors of URAT1; this indicates that their effect on serum urate is mediated through inhibition of urate reabsorption, rather than an activation of renal secretion. URAT1 has the highest affinity for aromatic organic anions, such as nicotinate and PZA, followed by lactate, β-hydroxybutyrate, acetoacetate, and inorganic anions such as Cl^- and nitrate. These relative affinities are manifest by a marked activation ("*trans*-stimulation") of ^{14}C-urate uptake in URAT1-expressing oocytes that have been individually microinjected with PZA, nicotinate, and lactate (i.e., "in-*trans*" to the ^{14}C-urate); the relative response fits with the *trans*-stimulation of urate exchange in human BBMV Na^+-dependent transport of these monovalent anions [41] (see also below). The same anions are capable of "*cis*-inhibiting" the uptake of ^{14}C-urate when present in the extracellular medium, another operative characteristic of the anion exchanger.

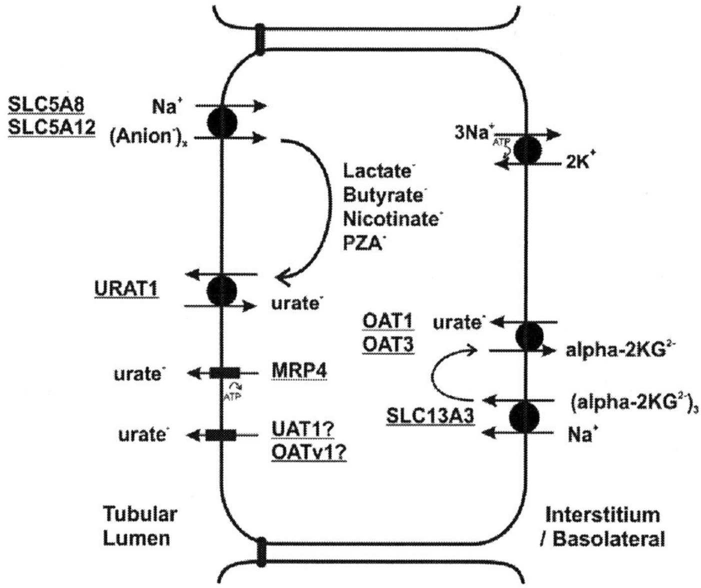

FIGURE 1. Urate transport mechanisms in the proximal tubule. Sodium-dependent entry of monovalent anions by the SLC5A8 and SLC5A12 cotransporters stimulates the absorption of luminal urate via the anion exchanger URAT1. Apical secretion of urate may occur through an ATP-driven efflux pathway (MRP4 63) or through voltage-sensitive electrogenic pathways (OATv1 64 and/or UAT1 65). Basolateral entry of urate during urate secretion by the proximal tubule is stimulated by sodium-dependent uptake of the divalent anion α-ketoglutarate via SLC13A3, leading to urate-α-ketoglutarate exchange via OAT1 (SLC22A6) and/or OAT3 (SLC22A8) 66-68. The identity of the exit pathway(s) for urate during urate reabsorption is not as yet known.

Sodium-Dependent Anion Transport and Renal Urate Reabsorption

URAT1 reabsorbs urate from the glomerular ultrafiltrate by exchanging luminal urate with monovalent intracellular anions such as PZA and lactate. The intracellular concentration of these anions is largely determined by Na^+-dependent absorption from the same glomerular ultrafiltrate; this generates a *secondary* Na^+-dependency of urate reabsorption, increasing proximal urate reabsorption via subsequent anion exchange. The nephron is thus "primed" for urate reabsorption by the Na^+-dependent loading of proximal tubule cells with anti-uricosuric anions such as PZA.

Overlapping studies from several labs have suggested that a single cotransport activity in renal BBMV is responsible for the Na^+-dependent uptake of PZA, nicotinate, lactate, pyruvate, β-hydroxybutyrate, and acetoacetate [42-44]; urate is not a direct substrate. Notably, these anions are all substrates for URAT1 and share a tendency to increase serum uric acid *in vivo*. By extension from the BBMV data [32,41], increased plasma concentrations of anti-uricosuric anions result in increased glomerular filtration, increased delivery to the proximal tubule, and increased intracellular concentration in tubular epithelial cells. Increases in intracellular activity of these anions in turn induce urate reabsorption and hyperuricemia, via "*trans*-stimulation" of URAT1 from inside the cell.

Several clinical scenarios illustrate the physiological importance of this relationship. Hyperuricemia is thus a well-recognized concomitant of the increased concentration of β-hydroxybutyrate and acetoacetate found in diabetic ketoacidosis [45,46]. Increases in lactic acid, as seen in alcohol intoxication [47], result in hyperuricemia due to increased urate reabsorption [48]; transient increases in lactate and/or keto-acids may contribute to the association between gout and alcohol [49]. The effects of keto-acids and lactate do not appear to secondary to the respective acidoses, given that the experimental infusion or ingestion of these anions can also lead to urate retention [45,50,51]. Finally, the treatment of hypercholesterolemia with nicotinic acid (niacin) can be complicated by hyperuricemia [52], as can the treatment of tuberculosis with pyrazinamide [53,54].

Patients with "renal hypouricemia" and loss-of-function mutations in URAT1 have been found to lack a response to both pyrazinamide and uricosurics [55]. This provides genetic confirmation of the linkage between PZA and urate reabsorption; as predicted by the model shown in Fig. 1, a functional urate exchanger is necessary for the anti-uricosuric effect of PZA. Furthermore, BBMV urate exchange is not detectable in animal species that secrete urate in the absence of significant reabsorption [22]; presumably the *SLC22A12* gene is inactivated in these species, much as the uricase gene is inactivated in humans and other hominoids. Again, PZA has no effect on urate transport in species in which secretion predominates [21]. These observations all tend to refute the 4-component model, since PZA appears to require a functioning *reabsorptive* transporter for its anti-uricosuric effect.

Characterization of SLC5A8 and SLC5A12

The most prominent missing information in the molecular physiology of renal urate transport has been the molecular identity of the sodium-dependent anion cotransporter(s) that collaborates with URAT1. We utilized a bioinformatics approach to identify SLC5A8 and SLC5A12, novel members of the SLC5 gene family of sodium-dependent solute transporters, as candidates for this transport activity. We initially identified a number of novel SLC5 transporters via *tblastn* searches of genomic databases in both HTGS (NCBI) and the Celera Discovery System. Two of the novel SLC5 genes, on chromosomes 12q22-24 (SLC5A8) and 11p14 (SLC5A12), encode proteins with ~50% identity to the Na^+-iodide transporter (SLC5A5); this homology suggested that these novel paralogs encode sodium-anion cotransporters. Of note, several expressed sequence tags (ESTs) from renal cDNA libraries were identified for mouse Slc5a8 and Slc5a12; as putative sodium-anion cotransporters expressed in kidney, these SLC5 paralogs were potential candidates for the sodium-PZA/anion cotransporter(s).

Full-length cDNAs were isolated for mouse and human orthologs of both transporters, using a combination of EST characterization and RT-PCR. These cDNAs were assembled in the *Xenopus* expression vector pGEMHE. We generated cRNA from these constructs and injected *Xenopus laevis* oocytes as described [56,57], followed by measurement of ^{14}C-labeled nicotinate and butyrate transport. Oocytes injected with cRNA for all four transporters (mouse and human SLC5A8/Slc5a8 and SLC5A12/Slc5a12) mediated considerable Na^+-dependent nicotinate and butyrate uptake (K.Z. *et al.*, manuscript submitted). Cis-inhibition studies revealed that both SLC5A8 and SLC5A12 transport lactate, pyruvate, PZA, and ketoacids (K.Z. *et al.*, manuscript submitted). Kinetic characterizations revealed Michaelis-Menten constants of 296 and 417 mM for SLC5A8 and SLC5A12, respectively. Measurement of membrane potential in Slc5a8-expressing cells revealed Na^+-dependent depolarization (+28 to +46 mV) in the presence of 1 mM butyrate, PZA or nicotinate; no such activity has been detected in SLC5A12-expressing cells. Notably, prior evidence had suggested both electrogenic [58] and electroneutral [43,59] modalities for BBMV Na^+-dependent monocarboxylate and/or nicotinate/PZA transport. Using Na^+-sensitive electrodes and measurement of membrane potential, Plata *et al.* recently demonstrated that zebrafish Slc5A8 is electrogenic, whereas Slc5a12 from this species is clearly electroneutral [60]. Zebrafish Slc5a12 is a lower affinity, high capacity Na^+-monocarboxylate cotransporter, while Slc5a8 is a high affinity, low capacity Na^+-monocarboxylate cotransporter [60]. Both of these transporters are found in the early portion of the embryonic kidney. Therefore, it seems likely that SLC5A8 mediates the electrogenic transport activity in mammalian kidney, whereas SLC5A12 mediates electroneutral Na^+-dependent monocarboxylate/nicotinate/PZA transport.

Mouse Slc5a8 transcript is detectable by RT-PCR in kidney, colon, stomach, ovaries, thyroid, and placenta; Slc5a12 transcript is detectable in kidney, small intestine, and ovaries. Notably, however, quantitative RT-PCR reveals that transcripts for both transporters are the most abundant in kidney. Murine *in situ* hybridization reveals expression of Slc5a12 in proximal tubules in the superficial cortex; immunfluorescence with a peptide-specific antibody confirms expression in S1 segments. In contrast, Slc5a8 transcript and protein appear restricted to S2 and S3 segments. Immunofluorescence with a URAT1-specific antibody reveals expression along the entire length of the proximal tubule, with lesser signal in S1 segments than in S3. In *Xenopus* oocytes co-expressing Slc5a8 with URAT1, pre-loading with PZA in the presence of Na^+ results in a considerable increase in urate uptake, versus control cells (water-injected cells or cells expressing URAT1 alone).

Perspectives

In summary, SLC5A8 and SLC5A12 have the expected functional characteristics of the renal Na^+-dependent monocarboxylate/nicotinate/PZA transporters detected in renal BBMV preparations [42-44]. SLC5A8 is likely responsible for the previously observed electrogenic transport [58], whereas SLC5A12 is likely responsible for electroneutral Na^+-dependent monocarboxylate and/or nicotinate/PZA transport in cortical BBMV preparations [43,59]. SLC5A12 is expressed in the early proximal tubule, with SLC5A8 in S2 and S3 segments; consistent with this expression pattern, SLC5A12 appears to function as a lower affinity nicotinate transporter than SLC5A8. Both paralogs are co-expressed with URAT1, and urate transport is potentiated by Na^+-PZA loading in oocytes expressing SLC5A8 with URAT1. Therefore, SLC5A8 and SLC5A12 appear to collectively encode the Na^+-anion cotransport mechanism that collaborates with URAT1 in the reabsorption of urate from the glomerular ultrafiltrate.

These findings have several implications for the physiology and pathophysiology of urate homeostasis. First, given the longstanding observations that increases in circulating ketoacids, lactate, nicotinate, or PZA lead to hyperuricemia, hyperuricemia conceivably ensues from overactivity of either SLC5A8, SLC5A12, and/or URAT1 itself. A corollary is that SLC5A8 and/or SLC5A12 are likely required for renal urate reabsorption; clarification of the degree to which this is the case will ultimately require characterization of the relevant single and double knockout mice. Second, urate reabsorption by the kidney evidently parallels that of Na^+-Cl^- [61], such that Na^+-avid states are characterized by hyperuricemia and often complicated by gout [62]. Again, it is conceivable that anti-natriuretic stimuli such as angiotensin-II increase renal urate reabsorption by acting on either SLC5A8, SLC5A12, and/or URAT1.

ACKNOWLEDGMENTS

Supported by NIH grants DK-57708 (DBM), DK-56218 (MFR), and DK60845 (MFR), an Advanced Research Career Development Award from the Veterans Administration (DBM), a Pediatric Scientist Development Award from the NIH (CYK), American Heart Association Postdoctoral Fellowship Award 0225706T (KZ), and a Genzyme Renal Innovations Grant (KZ).

REFERENCES

1. Sorensen, C.M. & Chandhoke, P.S. Hyperuricosuric calcium nephrolithiasis. *Endocrinol Metab Clin North Am* 31, 915-25 (2002).
2. Pak, C.Y., Poindexter, J.R., Peterson, R.D., Koska, J. & Sakhaee, K. Biochemical distinction between hyperuricosuric calcium urolithiasis and gouty diathesis. *Urology* 60, 789-94 (2002).
3. Rieselbach, R.E., Sorensen, L.B., Shelp, W.D. & Steele, T.H. Diminished renal urate secretion per nephron as a basis for primary gout. *Ann Intern Med* 73, 359-66 (1970).
4. Boss, G.R. & Seegmiller, J.E. Hyperuricemia and gout. Classification, complications and management. *N Engl J Med* 300, 1459-68 (1979).

5. Maalouf, N.M., Cameron, M.A., Moe, O.W. & Sakhaee, K. Novel insights into the pathogenesis of uric acid nephrolithiasis. *Curr Opin Nephrol Hypertens* 13, 181-9 (2004).
6. Sakhaee, K., Adams-Huet, B., Moe, O.W. & Pak, C.Y. Pathophysiologic basis for normouricosuric uric acid nephrolithiasis. *Kidney Int* 62, 971-9 (2002).
7. Johnson, R.J. et al. Is there a pathogenetic role for uric acid in hypertension and cardiovascular and renal disease? *Hypertension* 41, 1183-90 (2003).
8. Nakagawa, T. et al. Hyperuricemia causes glomerular hypertrophy in the rat. *Am J Nephrol* 23, 2-7 (2003).
9. Sanchez-Lozada, L.G. et al. Hormonal and cytokine effects of uric acid. *Curr Opin Nephrol Hypertens* 15, 30-33 (2006).
10. Shi, Y., Evans, J.E. & Rock, K.L. Molecular identification of a danger signal that alerts the immune system to dying cells. *Nature* 425, 516-21 (2003).
11. Martinon, F., Petrilli, V., Mayor, A., Tardivel, A. & Tschopp, J. Gout-associated uric acid crystals activate the NALP3 inflammasome. *Nature* (2006).
12. Waring, W.S., Webb, D.J. & Maxwell, S.R. Uric acid as a risk factor for cardiovascular disease. *Qjm* 93, 707-13 (2000).
13. Hare, J.M. & Johnson, R.J. Uric acid predicts clinical outcomes in heart failure: insights regarding the role of xanthine oxidase and uric acid in disease pathophysiology. *Circulation* 107, 1951-3 (2003).
14. Anker, S.D. et al. Uric acid and survival in chronic heart failure: validation and application in metabolic, functional, and hemodynamic staging. *Circulation* 107, 1991-7 (2003).
15. Fam, A.G. Gout, diet, and the insulin resistance syndrome. *J Rheumatol* 29, 1350-5 (2002).
16. Bonora, E. et al. Prevalence of insulin resistance in metabolic disorders: the Bruneck Study. *Diabetes* 47, 1643-9 (1998).
17. Nakagawa, T. et al. A Causal Role for Uric acid in Fructose-induced Metabolic Syndrome. *Am J Physiol Renal Physiol* (2005).
18. Enomoto, A. et al. Molecular identification of a renal urate anion exchanger that regulates blood urate levels. *Nature* 417, 447-52 (2002).
19. Wu, X.W., Lee, C.C., Muzny, D.M. & Caskey, C.T. Urate oxidase: primary structure and evolutionary implications. *Proc Natl Acad Sci U S A* 86, 9412-6 (1989).
20. Hediger, M.A. Kidney function: gateway to a long life? Nature 417, 393, 395 (2002).
21. Roch-Ramel, F. & Guisan, B. Renal Transport of Urate in Humans. *News Physiol Sci* 14, 80-84 (1999).
22. Guggino, S.E., Martin, G.J. & Aronson, P.S. Specificity and modes of the anion exchanger in dog renal microvillus membranes. *Am J Physiol* 244, F612-21. (1983).
23. Martinez, F., Manganel, M., Montrose-Rafizadeh, C., Werner, D. & Roch-Ramel, F. Transport of urate and p-aminohippurate in rabbit renal brush-border membranes. *Am J Physiol* 258, F1145-53 (1990).
24. Weiner, I.M. Urate transport in the nephron. *Am J Physiol* 237, F85-92 (1979).
25. Diamond, H.S. & Paolino, J.S. Evidence for a postsecretory reabsorptive site for uric acid in man. *J Clin Invest* 52, 1491-9 (1973).
26. Steele, T.H. Urate secretion in man: the pyrazinamide suppression test. *Ann Intern Med* 79, 734-7 (1973).
27. Weiner, I.M. & Tinker, J.P. Pharmacology of pyrazinamide: metabolic and renal function studies related to the mechanism of drug-induced urate retention. *J Pharmacol Exp Ther* 180, 411-34 (1972).
28. Davis, B.B., Field, J.B., Rodnan, G.P. & Kedes, L.H. Localization And Pyrazinamide Inhibition Of Distal Transtubular Movement Of Uric Acid-2-C14 With A Modified Stop-Flow Technique. *J Clin Invest* 44, 716-21 (1965).
29. Steele, T.H. & Boner, G. Origins of the uricosuric response. *J Clin Invest* 52, 1368-75 (1973).
30. Lemieux, G., Vinay, P., Gougoux, A. & Michaud, G. Nature of the uricosuric action of benziodarone. *Am J Physiol* 224, 1440-9 (1973).

31. Gutman, A.B., Yu, T.F. & Berger, L. Tubular secretion of urate in man. *J Clin Invest* 38, 1778-81 (1959).
32. Guggino, S.E. & Aronson, P.S. Paradoxical effects of pyrazinoate and nicotinate on urate transport in dog renal microvillus membranes. *J Clin Invest* 76, 543-7 (1985).
33. Blomstedt, J.W. & Aronson, P.S. pH gradient-stimulated transport of urate and p-aminohippurate in dog renal microvillus membrane vesicles. *J Clin Invest* 65, 931-4. (1980).
34. Kahn, A.M. & Aronson, P.S. Urate transport via anion exchange in dog renal microvillus membrane vesicles. *Am J Physiol* 244, F56-63 (1983).
35. Kahn, A.M., Branham, S. & Weinman, E.J. Mechanism of urate and p-aminohippurate transport in rat renal microvillus membrane vesicles. *Am J Physiol* 245, F151-8 (1983).
36. Werner, D., Martinez, F. & Roch-Ramel, F. Urate and p-aminohippurate transport in the brush border membrane of the pig kidney. *J Pharmacol Exp Ther* 252, 792-9 (1990).
37. Roch-Ramel, F., Werner, D. & Guisan, B. Urate transport in brush-border membrane of human kidney. *Am J Physiol* 266, F797-805. (1994).
38. Koepsell, H. & Endou, H. The SLC22 drug transporter family. *Pflugers Arch* (2004).
39. Mori, K. et al. Kidney-specific expression of a novel mouse organic cation transporter-like protein. *FEBS Lett* 417, 371-4 (1997).
40. Hosoyamada, M., Ichida, K., Enomoto, A., Hosoya, T. & Endou, H. Function and localization of urate transporter 1 in mouse kidney. *J Am Soc Nephrol* 15, 261-8 (2004).
41. Roch-Ramel, F., Guisan, B. & Schild, L. Indirect coupling of urate and p-aminohippurate transport to sodium in human brush-border membrane vesicles. *Am J Physiol* 270, F61-8 (1996).
42. Garcia, M.L., Benavides, J. & Valdivieso, F. Ketone body transport in renal brush border membrane vesicles. *Biochim Biophys Acta* 600, 922-30 (1980).
43. Manganel, M., Roch-Ramel, F. & Murer, H. Sodium-pyrazinoate cotransport in rabbit renal brush border membrane vesicles. *Am J Physiol* 249, F400-8 (1985).
44. Boumendil-Podevin, E.F. & Podevin, R.A. Nicotinic acid transport by brush border membrane vesicles from rabbit kidney. *Am J Physiol* 240, F185-91 (1981).
45. Goldfinger, S., Klinenberg, E., Jr. & Seegmiller, J.E. Renal Retention of Uric Acid Induced by Infusion of Beta-Hydroxybutyrate and Acetoacetate. *N Engl J Med* 272, 351-5 (1965).
46. Padova, J. & Bendersky, G. Hyperuricemia in diabetic ketoacidosis. *N Engl J Med* 267, 530-4 (1962).
47. Lieber, C.S., Jones, D.P., Losowsky, M.S. & Davidson, C.S. Interrelation of uric acid and ethanol metabolism in man. *J Clin Invest* 41, 1863-70 (1962).
48. Fanelli, G.M., Jr., Bohn, D. & Stafford, S. Functional characteristics of renal urate transport in the Cebus monkey. *Am J Physiol* 218, 627-36 (1970).
49. Choi, H.K., Atkinson, K., Karlson, E.W., Willett, W. & Curhan, G. Alcohol intake and risk of incident gout in men: a prospective study. *Lancet* 363, 1277-81 (2004).
50. Gibson, H.V. & Doisy, E.A. A note on the effect of some organic acids upon the uric acid excretion of man. *J Biol Chem* 55, 605-610 (1923).
51. Michael, S.T. The relation of uric acid excretion to blood lactic acid in man. *Am J Physiol* 141, 71-74 (1944).
52. Gershon, S.L. & Fox, I.H. Pharmacologic effects of nicotinic acid on human purine metabolism. *J Lab Clin Med* 84, 179-86 (1974).
53. Shapiro, M. & Hyde, L. Hyperuricemia due to pyrazinamide. *Am J Med* 23, 596-9 (1957).
54. Akalin, E., Chandrakantan, A., Keane, J. & Hamburger, R.J. Normouricemia in the syndrome of inappropriate antidiuretic hormone secretion. *Am J Kidney Dis* 37, E8 (2001).
55. Ichida, K. et al. Clinical and molecular analysis of patients with renal hypouricemia in Japan-influence of URAT1 gene on urinary urate excretion. *J Am Soc Nephrol* 15, 164-73 (2004).
56. Mount, D.B. et al. Cloning and characterization of KCC3 and KCC4, new members of the cation-chloride cotransporter gene family. *J Biol Chem* 274, 16355-16362 (1999).
57. Xie, Q., Welch, R., Mercado, A., Romero, M.F. & Mount, D.B. Molecular characterization of the murine Slc26a6 anion exchanger, functional comparison to Slc26a1. *Am J Physiol* 283, F826-F838 (2002).

58. Barac-Nieto, M., Murer, H. & Kinne, R. Lactate-sodium cotransport in rat renal brush border membranes. *Am J Physiol* 239, F496-506 (1980).
59. Barbarat, B. & Podevin, R.A. Stoichiometry of the renal sodium-L-lactate cotransporter. *J Biol Chem* 263, 12190-3 (1988).
60. Plata C, Sussman CR, Sindic A, Liang JO, Mount DB, Josephs ZM, Chang M-H, and Romero MF. A novel electroneutral sodium monocarboxylate transport (SMCTn) is present in zebrafish: A comparison to the electrogenic SMCT (SMCTe/Slc5a8). *J Biol Chem*: 10.1074/jbc.M609313200, 2007 Jan 25; [Epub ahead of print] (2007).
61. Steele, T.H. Hyperuricemic nephropathies. *Nephron* 81 Suppl 1, 45-9 (1999).
62. Aronoff, A. Acute gouty arthritis precipitated by chlorothiazide. *N Engl J Med* 262, 767-9 (1960).
63. Van Aubel, R.A., Smeets, P.H., Van Den Heuvel, J.J. & Russel, F.G. Human Organic Anion Transporter MRP4 (ABCC4) is an Efflux Pump for the Purine End Metabolite Urate with Multiple Allosteric Substrate Binding Sites. *Am J Physiol Renal Physiol* (2004).
64. Jutabha, P. et al. Identification of a novel voltage-driven organic anion transporter present at apical membrane of renal proximal tubule. *J Biol Chem* 278, 27930-8 (2003).
65. Lipkowitz, M.S., Leal-Pinto, E., Rappoport, J.Z., Najfeld, V. & Abramson, R.G. Functional reconstitution, membrane targeting, genomic structure, and chromosomal localization of a human urate transporter. *J Clin Invest* 107, 1103-15 (2001).
66. Sweet, D.H. et al. Organic anion transporter 3 (Slc22a8) is a dicarboxylate exchanger indirectly coupled to the Na+ gradient. *Am J Physiol Renal Physiol* 284, F763-9 (2003).
67. Aslamkhan, A., Han, Y.H., Walden, R., Sweet, D.H. & Pritchard, J.B. Stoichiometry of organic anion/dicarboxylate exchange in membrane vesicles from rat renal cortex and hOAT1-expressing cells. *Am J Physiol Renal Physiol* 285, F775-83 (2003).
68. Bakhiya, A., Bahn, A., Burckhardt, G. & Wolff, N. Human organic anion transporter 3 (hOAT3) can operate as an exchanger and mediate secretory urate flux. *Cell Physiol Biochem* 13, 249-56 (2003).

Lessons from a Stone Farm

John P. Kavanagh and P. Nagaraj Rao

Department of Minimally Invasive Urology and Stone Management, South Manchester University Hospitals Foundation Trust, Manchester, M23 9LT, UK

Abstract. The stone farm is a system for measuring macroscopic stone growth of 12 calcium stones simultaneously. It is based on mixed suspension, mixed product removal continuous crystallization principles and the stones are grown continuously for about 500 hours or more. The growth of the stones follows a surface area dependent pattern and the growth rate constants are very similar irrespective of whether the stating materials are fragments of human stone or pieces of marble chip. Increasing citrate from 2mM to 6mM caused a significant growth inhibition which persisted in the presence of urinary macromolecules. Phytate was a very effective inhibitor (about 50% at sub-μM concentrations) but the effective concentration was increased by an order of magnitude in the presence of urinary macromolecules. The effective concentration for inhibition in a crystallization assay was a further two orders of magnitude higher. Urinary macromolecules or almost whole urine were also strongly inhibitory although neither human serum albumin nor bovine mucin had any great effect. The relationship between the size distribution of crystals in suspension and the stone enlargement rate suggests that the primary enlargement mechanism for these *in vitro* stones is through aggregation. The stone farm is a powerful tool with which to study crystallization inhibitors in a new light. Some differences between inhibition of crystallization and inhibition of stone growth have emerged and we have obtained quantitative evidence on the mechanism of stone enlargement *in vitro*. Our findings suggest that the interface between crystals in suspension and the stone surface is the key to controlling stone enlargement.

Keywords: Urolithiasis, calcium oxalate, crystallization, calculi
PACS: 81.10.Dn

INTRODUCTION

Crystallization studies have been the mainstay of *in vitro* urolithiasis research with the underlying assumption that what is learnt from these investigations is applicable to stone formation and growth *in vivo*. With a view to bridging the gap between these two extremes, we have developed a system for growing multiple calcium stones *in vitro*. This is a continuous flow system, based on mixed suspension mixed product removal (MSMPR) principles. Fresh feed solutions are provided on a daily basis while the stones are growing and we refer to the system as a stone farm.

Our goal was to achieve macroscopic stone growth in an urine like environment which might be analogous to a residual fragment enlarging in the renal spaces. We found that this could be achieved by placing a small stone fragment in the small scale MSMPR crystallization chamber which we have previously developed to study

CP900, *Renal Stone Disease, 1st Annual International Urolithiasis Research Symposium*, edited by A. P. Evan, J. E. Lingeman, and J. C. Williams, Jr.

crystallization kinetics in nearly whole urine [1]. In our pilot studies we grew individual stones [2] and while this proved the possibility of achieving our goal, the system was not suitable for making quantitative comparisons between different growth conditions. We therefore scaled the system up to grow 12 stones at once [3] and here we review our experience and findings with the stone farm.

MATERIALS AND METHODS

The Stone Farm

The details of the construction and operation of the stone farm have been given elsewhere [3]. Here we describe the system with the focus on incidental details. Twelve stone fragments (≈100mg) are separately suspended in twelve identical crystallization chambers, each with a working volume of 20ml, maintained at 37°C by external water circulation and stirred by PTFE coated magnetic fleas rotating at 400rpm. These chambers are organised as six pairs, one pair of which is shown in Fig. 1. The surfaces in contact with the feed solutions are glass, stainless steel or PTFE. It was not practicable to maintain a completely closed system throughout the experimental period so the following precautions against infection were used. Freshly purified water was filtered (0.22μm) before being used to make up the salt solutions. Once fully dissolved and made up to the correct volume these were dispensed into sterile bottles, again through 0.22μm filters and in a sterile atmosphere. The artificial urine (AU) solutions were stored at 4°C for up to 5 days. In use, the air inlets to the feed solution bottles were protected by 0.22μm filters. The likelihood of contamination is greatest in the crystallization chambers which are opened daily. We therefore include 0.04% NaN_3 in one of the feed solutions. We never saw any evidence of infection such as cloudiness of stock solutions or unexpected changes in pH of the mixed suspension in the crystallization chambers. Details of the composition of the feed solutions making up the AU urine are described elsewhere [3] but our standard conditions give rise to 6mM Ca and 1.2mM oxalate, pH 6.0 in the crystallization chamber (before any precipitation takes place). The flow rate through each pair of crystallizers was approximately 1 litre per day. Because of the large volumes being prepared, we measured the added water to the salts gravimetrically, taking into account the specific volume of the included salts. Where additions to the feed solutions for half the crystallization chambers were made, we did this by dividing batches of feed solutions in two and then making the addition, rather than preparing separate feed stocks. Feed solutions were replenished each day. At this point the stones and their supports were removed and the tubing and chambers were cleaned by flushing with 0.1M HCl followed by copious purified water. In-line syringes are fitted to enable purging of the lines and priming of the crystallization chambers with fresh feed solutions. Stone masses were measured every two or three days; they were carefully placed and rolled on absorbent paper and allowed to air dry for 15 minutes before being weighed. Between different experiments all tubing was replaced and the crystallization chambers and stone supports were cleaned with chromic acid.

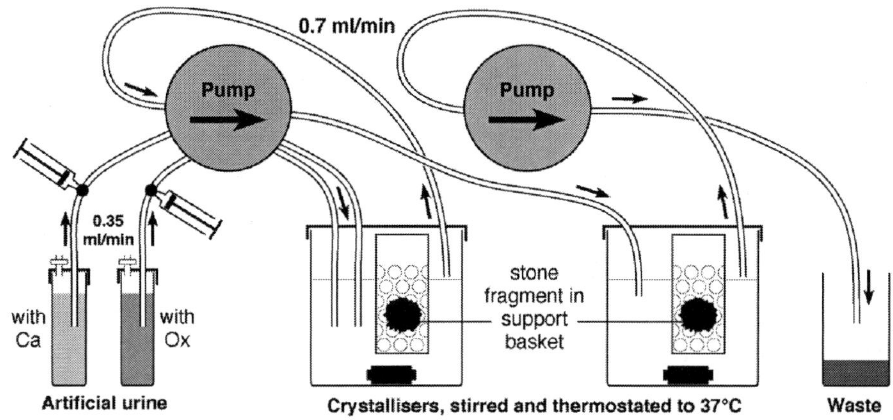

FIGURE 1. One pair of crystallization chambers. Reprinted from figure 1of reference [3] with kind permission of Springer Science and Business Media.

In initial experiments the stone fragments used as the core of the growing stones were derived from human stone fragments. In later experiments we used pieces of marble chips ($CaCO_3$). All the cores were ground to about 100mg with abrasive paper. Their initial masses were obtained after soaking in AU for one hour before being dried as described above. Most stone growth experiments were conducted with the stones in 3 of the pairs of crystallizers receiving control feed solutions and the other 3 pairs receiving the same solutions supplemented with a test agent. In some cases the solutions feeding each set of 3 crystallizers was changed during the course of the experiment. In all cases the primary outcome was considered to be the comparison between the 6 control stones and the 6 supplemented stones while being grown simultaneously. As will be shown below, the growth followed in a surface-dependent manner and the results from the 6 stones growing under identical conditions were averaged and fitted to a growth equation, mass = k * time$^{3/2}$ + c (where k is a growth rate constant and c is the initial mass). These are shown in the figures as ±95% confidence intervals (c.i.), derived from the curve fitting procedure (performed with FigSys, Biosoft, Cambridge, UK).

Urinary Macromolecules And Nearly Whole Urine

When urinary macromolecules (UMM) were used, these were obtained by tangential diafiltration across a filter with a nominal cut-off of 5kD. Urine was reduced in volume to 25% of its starting volume and then diafiltered with purified water until the conductivity was ≤1mS/cm [4]. This was stored frozen at -20°C until required. For use, sufficient UMM for one day was thawed and pooled and this was combined 1:1 with a feed solution (containing calcium) made up in half its usual volume. In this way, UMM are included at approximately their native concentration (without making allowance for any processing losses) and without the concentration of the major ions being altered.

When nearly whole urine was used it was stored at -20°C immediately after collection. For use, that sufficient for one day was thawed, centrifuged briefly (2000g for 5 minutes) and passed through a nylon sieve (20μm). Its pH was adjusted to 6.0 and its calcium adjusted to 6.67mM and 0.02% NaN_3 added. This urine was fed into the crystallizer chambers at 90% of the total flow, while the remainder of the flow was delivered by a 12mM oxalate solution in calcium deficient AU.

Crystal Size Distribution

The size distribution of crystals in suspension around the growing stones was examined just prior to changing feed solutions each day. A Coulter Multisizer was used with a 100μm orifice tube. The system was calibrated with 14μm diameter latex beads. Three consecutive readings of 1ml aspirations were averaged for each of the crystallization chambers. The particle number versus particle diameter data was transformed to ln(particle no.) versus particle size and the best fit straight line fitted to the data. The growth rate and nucleation rates were calculated from the slope and intercept of this line respectively [5].

RESULTS

The Surface

The raw data for the growth of twelve stones in one experiment are shown in Fig. 2A and the average for each arm of the same experiment in Fig. 2B. It is clear that the growth is not linear but gently accelerates. Analysis of the growth of 8 individual stones had previously led us to conclude that the growth is surface area dependent (i.e. mass = k * $time^{3/2}$ + c) [2]. This was based on comparing the goodness of fit of the data to a linear model (constant deposition, mass = k * time + c), a linear growth in diameter model (mass = k * $time^3$ +c) and the surface area growth model. We have repeated this analysis using the control data from 10 experiments (i.e. growth of 60 stones). The correlation coefficients for the surface area model were consistently higher than that of growth versus time or $time^3$ (R^2 = 0.99 vs 0.96 or 0.93 respectively). The best fits to the data from Fig. 2A are shown in Fig. 2C and the fits of the three different models to the control data are shown in Fig. 2D.

The growth of control stones in AU was relatively consistent between experiments when the core material was human stone fragments and even more so when marble chips were used as the core (Fig. 3). The slightly lower and more consistent growth with marble chips can probably be explained by their being slightly smaller and smoother than the human stone fragments.

While we had considered the possibility that the composition of the core material might influence the outcome of these experiments it has become clear that once an initial coating has been laid down, the central material no longer plays any part in the subsequent growth.

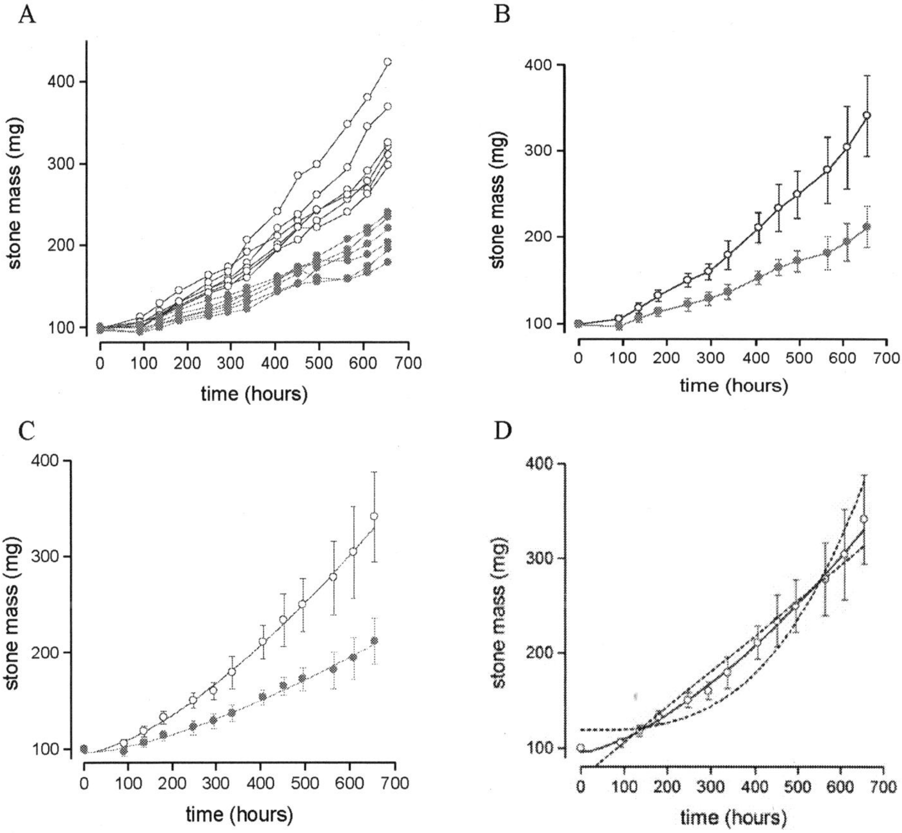

FIGURE 2. Open circles are control data (artificial urine); closed circles have 0.25μM phytate included. **A**, raw data, showing all 12 growth profiles; **B**, means ± s.d.; **C**, mean data with best fit to the surface area model; **D**, control data with best fits to surface area model (solid line) compared to linear growth and constant deposition models (dashed lines).

Citrate

The control AU contains 2mM citrate. When this was increased to 6mM there was significant inhibition and this was also the case when UMM from stone formers or healthy controls were also included (Table 1) and see [4] for more details.

TABLE 1. Growth rate constants (mg/h$^{3/2}$ ± 95% c.i.) for artificial urine (AU) with 2mM citrate and 6mM citrate. (UMM, urinary macromolecules; MC, male controls; MSF, male stone formers).

	2mM citrate	**6mMcitrate**
AU	0.01078 ± 0.00058	0.00230 ± 0.00024
AU + UMM (MC)	0.00405 ± 0.00025	0.00143 ± 0.00013
AU + UMM (MSF)	0.00271 ± 0.00011	0.00107 ± 0.00008

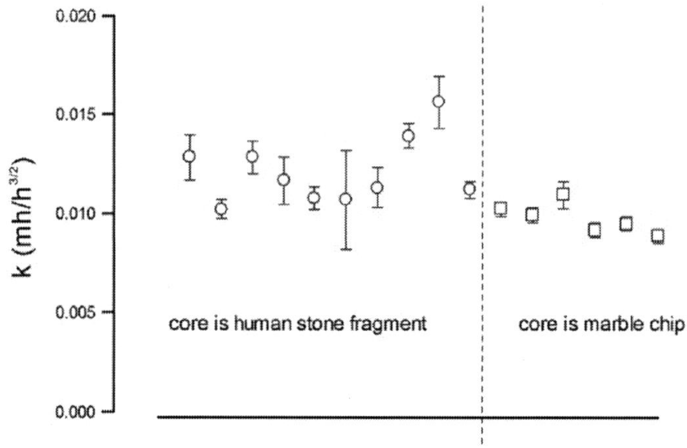

FIGURE 3. Growth rate constants (± 95 c.i.) from 10 control series of stones (artificial urine) grown on human stone fragments and 6 control series grown on marble chips.

Phytate

Inositol hexaphosphate (phytate) is reported to be an effective calcium oxalate and calcium phosphate crystallization inhibitor, *in vitro* and in simple salt solutions [6-9]. Based on these reports, we chose 5μM as our starting concentration to test phytate in the stone farm. This gave almost complete inhibition in AU. Reducing the phytate to 2.5μM also gave nearly 100% inhibition and only by decreasing the concentration to 0.25μM did we begin to see a dose dependent effect with the inhibition being 51% and 55% in two separate experiments (Fig. 4). When we performed an experiment with 0.25μM phytate in AU in which UMM from healthy male controls was included, we found no evidence of any inhibition of stone growth and it was only by increasing the phytate to 2.5μM that we saw evidence of growth inhibition. This amelioration of the inhibition of phytate by UMM was not simply a non specific protein effect as 0.25μM phytate was almost equally effective in the presence of albumin at 100μg/ml (40% inhibition) as with artificial urine alone (Fig. 4). Similarly, we also found that, in an *in vitro* crystallization assay [10], the effective concentration of phytate in artificial urine was about one order of magnitude lower than in human urine [11]. Interestingly, the concentration required for equivalent effects on stone growth and crystallization activity was about 2 orders of magnitude lower for both stone growth in artificial urine and stone growth in artificial urine plus UMM (compared to human urine) [11].

Macromolecules

Human serum albumin and mucin at 100μg/ml and UMM at approximately native concentrations, all in AU and 90% human urine were tested in a series of eight stone farm experiments; in each case the contemporaneous control was artificial urine. This showed that neither albumin nor mucin had any significant effect, while UMM and nearly whole urine almost completely abolished stone growth (Fig. 5). In six other experiments, macromolecules in artificial urine were used as control arms of experiments testing, for example, the effects of citrate or phytate. The results of these reinforce the above conclusion, especially when taking into account another six AU control experiments (Fig. 5).

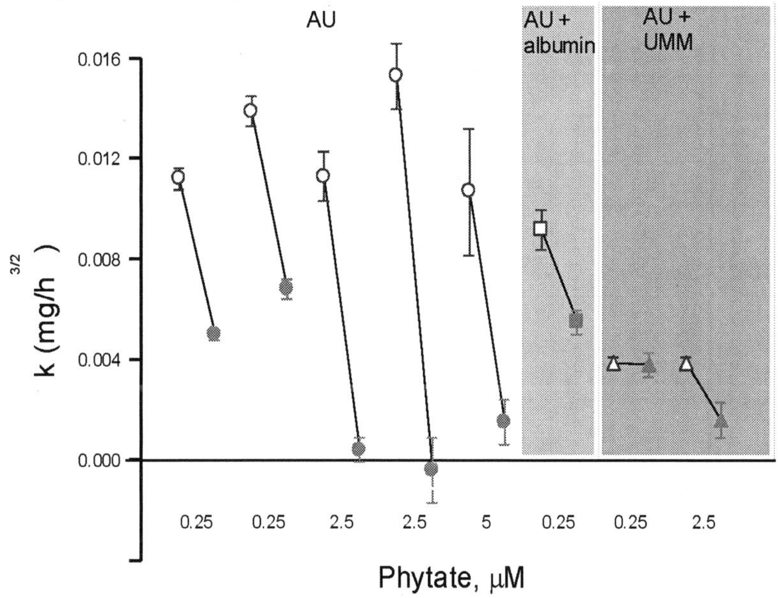

FIGURE 4. Growth rate constants (± 95% c.i.) for control stones grown in AU (open circles) and with added phytate (closed circles). UMM are urinary macromolecules.

Enlargement Mechanism

There are essentially two mechanisms by which stones could enlarge (or by a combination of both). These are through direct crystal growth at the stone surface or by aggregation and incorporation of crystals which developed in suspension [12]. If the first of these were the principal mechanism then it might be expected that, when conditions favor crystal growth, then there will be a lower nucleation rate [5, 13] and crystal growth at the surface would be high and stone enlargement maximised. Conversely, if conditions favor low growth rate (and a high nucleation rate) of suspended crystals, then the crystal growth at the surface would also be slow. Under either of these circumstances we would expect to observe a positive correlation between stone growth rate and crystal growth rate and a negative correlation between stone growth rate and nucleation rate. If the second of these mechanisms (i.e. aggregation) predominates, then the opposite would be expected, namely that the stone growth rate would be positively correlated to the nucleation rate and inversely correlated to the crystal growth rate.

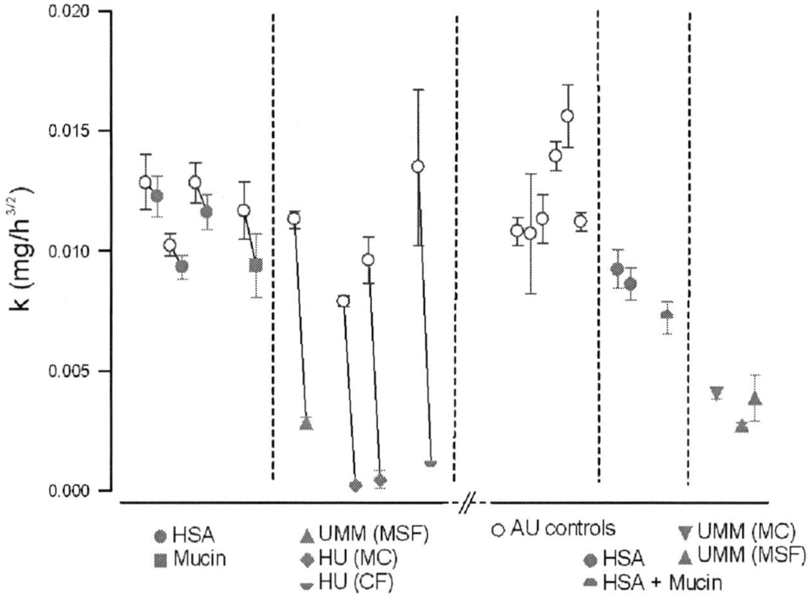

FIGURE 5. Growth rate constants (± 95% c.i.) for control stones grown in artificial urine (AU) (open circles) and with added macromolecules (solid symbols). HSA is human serum albumin, HU is human urine, MC are male controls, MSF are male stone formers, CF are cystic fibrosis patients and UMM are urinary macromolecules.

In order to try to discriminate between these two mechanisms we have examined the relationships between stone growth rate, crystal growth rates and crystal nucleation rates over a period of 26 different growth periods. These involved a series of AU experiments in which control stones were grown with 6mM calcium and 1.2mM oxalate as the input concentrations and test stones were grown with various lower calcium and oxalate concentrations. Although not all of these experiments were contemporaneous, they were all carried out with marble chips as the core material, with which the inter-experimental variability is relatively small. We knew from previous work [5] that changing the input concentrations of calcium and oxalate would bring about a variation in the crystal size distribution of the suspended crystals which, in turn, would correspond to different crystal growth and nucleation rates. We observed significant negative correlation between nucleation rate and crystal growth rate (p<0.001) (Fig. 6A), consistent with our previous findings [5, 13] and a significant positive correlation between stone growth rate and crystal nucleation rate

($p<0.001$) and a significant negative correlation between stone growth rate and crystal growth rate ($p=0.02$) (Fig. 6B and C).

This suggests that the primary enlargement mechanism for stones grown in the stone farm is through aggregation rather than direct surface growth.

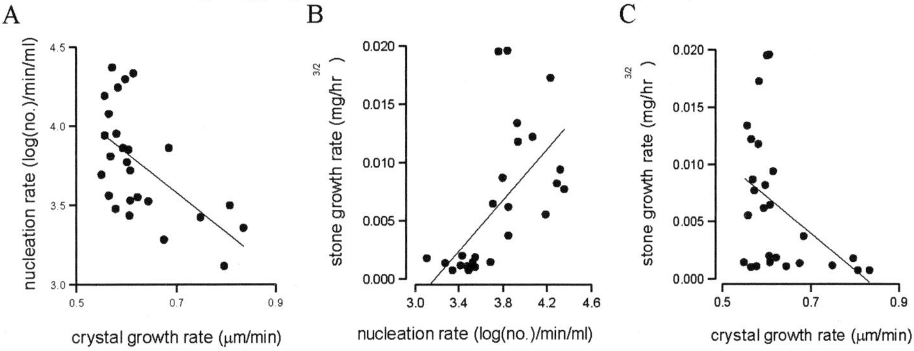

FIGURE 6. Relationships between crystal nucleation rates, crystal growth rates and stone growth rates. Stones were all grown on marble chips in artificial urine with varying calcium and oxalate concentrations in the feed solutions.

CONCLUSIONS AND IMPLICATIONS

For the first time, we are in a position to grow calcium stones reproducibly, *in vitro*, under controlled conditions. The stone farm is suitable for making quantitative measurements and comparisons and we can use the system with nearly whole urine or incorporate urinary macromolecules. In the sense that it operates as a continuous flow system, with a realistic flow rate and solution supersaturation, it is a representative model of the renal system. On the other hand, the residence times are longer than would be the case in a kidney (because the volume of the crystallization chamber is larger than the renal spaces) and the input amount of oxalate is above what would normally be found in urine. Whatever its strengths and weaknesses, it is only an *in vitro* model and any conclusions must be tempered by this recognition. Nevertheless it does act as bridge between purely *in vitro* crystallization systems and the *in vivo* pathological process we are trying to probe.

While the stone farm findings with citrate confirmed the inhibitory activity of citrate they did not reveal any particularly new insights. The results with UMM, nearly whole urine, albumin and mucin are also broadly in line with expectations derived from crystallization experiments, but it is worth noting just how difficult it is to get significant stone enlargement with urinary constituents present. Taken together with other findings from the stone farm and MSMPR crystallization studies we can conclude that this inhibition is effective at the stone surface in addition to any solution/suspension effects.

Our results on the dependence of the enlargement rate on the surface area and the primary importance of aggregation over growth as the accretion mechanism complement each other and are consistent with a two stage aggregation process of collision and consolidation. The likelihood of collisions will be governed by the suspension crystal density and the exposed surface area of the stone, while the efficiency of converting collisions into consolidated material will reflect the ability to form a mechanical bridge [14, 15]. In previous MSMPR crystallization studies under very similar conditions to the stone farm with nearly whole urine, there was a significant crystal density despite the strong inhibition compared to AU [5, 13]. The almost complete elimination of stone enlargement by nearly whole urine therefore suggests that macromolecules from urine prevent suspended crystals that come into contact with the stone from permanently fusing to the surface.

We can similarly argue that the pronounced stone growth inhibition by phytate is also achieved by reducing the efficiency of consolidating suspended crystals into the stone, rather than being simply a consequence of crystallization inhibition. This conclusion follows from our observation that crystallization inhibition requires a much higher concentration of phytate than is effective in inhibiting stone enlargement [11]. A simple explanation for the amelioration of the response to phytate by UMM also follows from the concept that both phytate and UMM are effective because they are active at the interface between colliding crystals from the suspension and the stone surface. If the UMM are sufficient to partially or nearly saturate all available sites, then a much higher phytate concentration will be required for further effective inhibition than if the UMM were absent.

These *in vitro* stone growth experiments demonstrate that stone enlargement, while necessarily involving crystallization, is not simply a direct reflection of that crystallization activity. Stone enlargement is also critically dependent on the interaction at the interface between suspended crystals and the stone surface.

ACKNOWLEDGMENTS

We would like to thank K Ananth, K Chow, J Dixon, S Gilpin, K Saw and RC Walton for their practical assistance in carrying out these experiments and Kidney Research (UK) and The Oxaluria and Hyperoxaluria Fund for supporting these studies.

REFERENCES

1. S. Nishio, J. P. Kavanagh, J. Garside J, *Chemical Engineering Science* **46**, 709-711 (1991)
2. K. Ananth, J. P. Kavanagh, R. C. Walton, *et al.*, *BJU International* **90**, 939-944 (2002)
3. K. Chow, J. Dixon, S. Gilpin, *et al.*, *Urological Research* **32**, 55-60 (2004)
4. K. Chow, J. Dixon, S. Gilpin, *et al.*, *Kidney International* **65**, 1724-1730 (2004)
5. J. P. Kavanagh, L. Jones, P. N. Rao, *Urological Research* **27**, 231-237 (1999)
6. F. Grases, P. March, *Journal Of Crystal Growth* **96**, 993-995 (1989)
7. F. Grases, M. Ramis, A. Costa-Bauza, *Urological Research* **28**, 136-140 (2000)
8. Grases F, Costa-Bauza A: Phytate (IP6) is a powerful agent for preventing calcifications in biological fluids: Usefulness in renal lithiasis treatment. *Anticancer Research* 19:3717-3722, 1999
9. A. Costa-Bauza, B. Isern, J. Perello, *et al.*, *Scand. Journal Of Urology And Nephrology* **39**, 194-199 (2005)
10. J. P. Kavanagh, L. Jones, P.N. Rao, *Clinical Science* **98**, 151-158 (2000)

11. N. K. Saw, K. Chow, J.P. Kavanagh, *et al.*, *Journal Of Urology* In press, (2007)
12. J. P. Kavanagh, *Journal Of Endourology* **13**, 605-610 (1999)
13. Kavanagh JP, Nishio S, Garside J, *et al.*, *Journal Of Urology* **149**, 614-617 (1993)
14. Hounslow MJ, Mumtaz HS, Collier AP, *et al.*: A micro-mechanical model for the rate of aggregation during precipitation from solution. *Chemical Engineering Science* 56:2543-2552, 2001
15. David R, Espitalier F, Cameirao A, *et al.*: Developments in the understanding and modeling of the agglomeration of suspended crystals in crystallization from solution. *KONA* 21:40, 2001

Are Phosphatonins Relevant in the Pathogenesis of Nephrolithiasis?

Aisha Shaikh[*‡] and Rajiv Kumar[*†‡¶]

[*]*Division of Nephrology and Hypertension;* [†]*Endocrinology, Metabolism, Diabetes and Nutrition;* [‡]*Departments of Internal Medicine and* [¶]*Biochemistry and Molecular Biology, 1-120 Medical Sciences, Mayo Clinic College of Medicine, 200 First Street SW, Rochester, MN 55905, USA*

Abstract. Hypercalciuria is the single most important risk factor for stone disease and renal phosphate excretion is a recognized cause of absorptive hypercalciuria. The recent identification of "phosphatonins" that increase renal phosphate excretion has raised the possibility that these factors might be responsible for the phosphaturia seen in some patients with absorptive hypercalciuria. It is important to recognize that both parathyroid hormone and phosphatonins are phosphaturic, but they have opposite effects on $1,25(OH)_2D_3$ regulation. Serum concentrations of fibroblast growth factor-23, one of the phosphatonins, have been shown to be increased in some stone formers suggesting a pathogenic role. Future studies are needed to define the exact role of phosphatonins in nephrolithiasis.

Keywords: nephrolithiasis, phosphatonins and fibroblast growth factor-23
PACS: 87.19.Xx

INTRODUCTION

Nephrolithiasis is a significant health related problem which carries a lifetime risk of 10-15% in the developed countries [1,2]. An increase in the prevalence of nephrolithiasis over the past twenty years [2] makes it exceedingly important to understand the pathogenesis of this disorder. Hypercalciuria is the single most important risk factor for stone disease [3,4] and an increase in renal phosphate (Pi) excretion is often associated with absorptive hypercalciuria [5,6]. Therefore, it is imperative to explore potential mechanisms that lead to renal Pi wasting and kidney stone formation. Additionally, patients with renal sodium-phosphate IIa cotransporter (NPIIa) mutations often have increased renal Pi excretion and renal calculi [7]. The identification of the phosphatonins has opened new avenues of research for disorders of Pi regulation [8]. In this article we will discuss the potential role of phosphatonins in the pathogenesis of nephrolithiasis.

Hypercalciuria

Seventy percent of all kidney stones are composed of calcium-oxalate and calcium-phosphate [9,10]. Hypercalciuria often occurs in patients with calcium nephrolithiasis [3,4] and has been identified as the most important risk factor for stone disease.

CP900, *Renal Stone Disease, 1st Annual International Urolithiasis Research Symposium,* edited by A. P. Evan, J. E. Lingeman, and J. C. Williams, Jr.

Hypercalciuria is caused by diverse group of disorders. Pathophysiologically hypercalciuria is not a single entity and can be due to defects in the kidney, the bone and the intestine. The term 'idiopathic hypercalciuria' is used when no cause of hypercalciuria is identified. Renal hypercalciuria results from defects in renal reabsorption of calcium [11] whereas resorptive hypercalciuria is due to excessive bone resorption [12]. In absorptive hypercalciuria intestinal hyperabsorption of calcium is responsible for the increase in renal calcium excretion [13].

Absorptive Hypercalciuria

Absorptive hypercalciuria is the most common cause of kidney stones accounting for more than half of the reported cases [13] though it rarely appears in pure form and is frequently accompanied by other metabolic derangements [14,15]. There are several proposed mechanisms to explain this entity. Patients with absorptive hypercalciuria absorb a greater fraction of dietary calcium compared to normal subjects [16]. The enhanced intestinal calcium absorption may be dependent or independent of vitamin D. In some patients, the serum $1,25(OH)_2D_3$ concentrations are elevated, and the observation that administration of $1,25(OH)_2D_3$ to normal subjects promotes development of a metabolic picture similar to absorptive hypercalciuria [17] supports the notion that increased calcitriol concentrations contribute to the pathology of absorptive hypercalciuria. It is important to recognize that absorptive hypercalciuria can occur in the absence of $1,25(OH)_2D_3$ elevation, in which case increased end organ sensitivity to $1,25(OH)_2D_3$ is postulated to be present [18]. The exact etiology of the increase in serum $1,25(OH)_2D_3$ concentrations is still a matter of debate, and studies have suggested that a renal phosphate (Pi) leak leads to an increase in $1,25(OH)_2D_3$ production [5,6].Genetically engineered mice with deletions of the NPIIa cotransporter have renal Pi wasting and elevated $1,25(OH)_2D_3$ concentrations [19]. Therefore, it is important to examine whether factors that lead to renal Pi wasting are altered in absorptive hypercalciuria. For several years parathyroid hormone (PTH) was the only known phosphaturic hormone. It is important to recognize that both PTH and phosphatonins are phosphaturic, but they have opposite effects on $1,25(OH)_2D_3$ regulation.

We will briefly review the biology of phosphatonins and then discuss their potential role in nephrolithiasis.

Phosphatonins

Phosphatonins were first identified in a patient with tumor-induced osteomalacia (TIO), in whom the biochemical abnormalities, including hypophosphatemia, hyperphosphaturia and decreased $1,25(OH)_2D_3$ concentrations, resolved after removal of the tumor [8]. This led to the discovery of phosphatonins, which are defined as factors that cause hyperphosphaturia and hypophosphatemia by reducing the activity of the NPIIa cotransporter protein in the proximal tubule of the kidney, reducing $1,25(OH)_2D_3$ concentrations by inhibiting 25-hydroxyvitamin D 1-hydroxylase activity, and inhibiting bone mineralization.

In addition to TIO, X-linked hypophosphatemic rickets (XLH), and autosomal dominant hypophosphatemic rickets (ADHR) are pathological conditions in which serum Pi levels are reduced without significant changes in the serum concentrations of calcium and PTH, and inappropriately low $1,25(OH)_2D_3$ concentrations [20-22]. Genomic and proteomic strategies have led to identification of factors associated with one or more of these syndromes. Fibroblast growth factor-23 (FGF-23), secreted frizzled related protein-4 (sFRP-4), matrix extracellular phosphoglycoprotein (MEPE) and fibroblast growth factor-7 (FGF-7), each possess some or all of the properties associated with phosphatonins [23-25].

FGF-23 is the most widely studied phosphatonin and will be the focus of our discussion.

Effect Of Phosphatonins On Phosphate And Vitamin D

FGF-23 has been implicated in the pathogenesis of TIO, XLH and ADHR [26-28]. Both *in vivo* and *in vitro* experiments have contributed to our understanding the role FGF-23 plays in physiologic and pathologic states.

Administration of FGF-23 in normal mice induces phosphaturia by causing internalization of NPIIa cotransporters in the proximal tubules [29]. In addition, the FGF-23 transgenic mice have hypophosphatemia secondary to increased renal Pi clearance resulting from decreased renal expression of the NPIIa cotransporter genes 30. The role of FGF-23 in Pi regulation is further strengthened by the observation that FGF-23 null mice display significantly high serum Pi levels along with increased renal Pi reabsorption [31]. FGF-23 inhibits 25-hydroxyvitamin D-1α-hydroxylase and blocks the compensatory rise in $1,25(OH)_2D_3$ concentrations, expected as a result of hypophosphatemia. Implantation of FGF-23 expressing Chinese Hamster ovary cells into athymic nude mice, resulted in decreased $1,25(OH)_2D_3$. Likewise, FGF23-null mice showed elevated $1,25(OH)_2D_3$ levels due to the enhanced expression of renal 25-hydroxyvitamin D-1α-hydroxylase [31].

In short, these observations suggest that FGF-23 is phosphaturic but inhibits synthesis of $1,25(OH)_2D_3$. This raises the question, Does FGF-23 play a role in stone formation by virtue of causing increased urinary Pi excretion?

Sodium-Phosphate IIa Cotransporters (NPIIa) And Phosphatonins

Recent observations suggest that renal Pi leak could be due to defects in renal sodium-phosphate IIa cotransporters (NPIIa) [7,32,33]. The NPIIa cotransporter is critical for renal Pi reabsorption and is expressed in the apical membrane of the proximal tubular cells. The absence of this transporter results in renal Pi wasting and hypophosphatemia. It has been observed that NPIIa-/- mice have increased urinary Pi excretion, hypercalciuria and nephrolithiasis [32]. Prie *et al.* studied 20 patients with urolithiasis or osteoporosis with idiopathic hypophosphatemia and phosphaturia [7]. They identified two distinct mutations (A48F and V147M) in the NPIIa gene in two patients. They further substantiated their findings by injecting the mutant mRNA into Xenopus oocytes, which induced significant reduction in Pi uptake. However, some authors have acknowledged the limitations of this study [34]. First, the A48F and V147M mutations were only recognized in a single patient with recurrent kidney stones and idiopathic bone demineralization respectively. Second, the pedigrees of these patients were not studied and no data was obtained on the prevalence of these mutations in a cohort of stone formers or osteoporotic patients. A recent study in a large cohort of hypercalciuric pedigrees did not find genetic polymorphisms at the NPIIa locus to be associated with renal Pi leak [35].

Both PTH and FGF-23 exert phosphaturic effects by internalization of the NPIIa cotransporter from the apical membrane of the proximal tubular cells, though it is likely that both these hormones act via different signal transduction pathways. The question remains as to whether hyperphosphaturia caused by FGF-23 is sufficient to promote formation of stones.

Renal Phosphate Leak And Phosphatonins

Some studies have shown renal Pi leak to be the dominant cause of absorptive hypercalciuria [6,36]. However, these findings have not been supported by other studies. In fact in a study involving 1270 recurrent stone formers, hypercalciuria was present in 60% patients but renal Pi leak was found in only 2-4% subjects [37]. This suggests that renal Pi leak is an important phenomenon but accounts for hypercalciuria in a small number of stone formers. It is postulated that renal Pi leak leads to increase in $1,25(OH)_2D_3$ production which secondarily increases intestinal calcium absorption and bone resorption. It has been suggested that hyperphosphaturia in itself is not sufficient to induce stone formation, but in fact it is the resultant increase in $1,25(OH)_2D_3$ that leads to hypercalciuria and nephrolithiasis. This concept is demonstrated in certain Pi wasting disorders, such as TIO, XLH and ADHR, which are not characterized by nephrolithiasis despite renal Pi wasting and hypophosphatemia. What distinguishes these diseases from other Pi wasting disorders is the absence of $1,25(OH)_2D_3$ elevation which is attributed to the presence of FGF-23. On the other hand, a recent study Bushinsky *et al.* showed that reduction in urine Pi excretion in genetic hypercalciuric stone forming (GHS) rats led to elimination of stone formation [38]. In this study GHS rats were fed low, medium and high Pi diet for 18 weeks. It was observed that urine Pi excretion progressively declined with decreasing Pi intake. On the other hand, urine calcium excretion progressively increased with decreasing Pi intake. Interestingly a significant number of rats that were fed high Pi diet developed nephrolithiasis whereas none of the rats fed low or medium Pi diets developed kidney stones. This study concluded that lowering Pi in the diet reduces urine Pi excretion, and despite the associated increase in urine calcium excretion, the overall decline in urine supersaturation decreases the propensity to stone formation. Based on these findings it is plausible to suggest that phosphatonins, due to their phosphaturic properties, may play a role in stone formation. To date only one study has analyzed the association between phosphatonins and stone disease [39].

FGF-23 And Nephrolithiasis

A recent study by Rendina *et al.* explored the association between FGF-23 and nephrolithiasis [39]. In this study, FGF-23 concentrations were measured in normal subjects and in recurrent stone formers. Stone formers had prior history of two or more calcium-oxalate (78.2%) or calcium-phosphate (21.8%) stones on different occasions over the preceding 4 years. Prior to commencement of the study, all subjects were placed on a fixed diet containing 1000 mg calcium, 100 mEq sodium, 900 mg Pi, 300 g carbohydrates and 70 g proteins (2200 calories) daily for 7 days. Renal Pi leak was identified by reduction in maximal tubular renal phosphate reabsorption normalized for glomerular filtration rate (TmPi/GFR). Among the 110 stone formers, 22 (20%) were noted to have renal Pi leak whereas 88 (80%) patients had normal Pi excretion. None of the normal subjects were noted to have hypophosphatemia or renal Pi leak. FGF-23 concentrations (measured by a carboxy-terminal assay) were found to be elevated in stone formers with renal Pi wasting compared to stone formers without Pi wasting and normal subjects. Serum FGF-23 concentration inversely related to serum Pi concentration. In addition, $1,25(OH)_2D_3$ concentrations were normal in normal subjects and in stone formers with or without renal Pi leak . The authors concluded that FGF-23 plays a role in the pathogenesis of nephrolithiasis. However, there are several limitations of this study. First, among the stone formers, an unusually large proportion of subjects were noted to have renal Pi leak. As discussed earlier, in most studies less than 5% of stone formers exhibit increased urinary Pi excretion. Second, patients with increased Pi wasting typically have high or high normal $1,25(OH)_2D_3$ concentrations and patients with hyperphosphaturia due to the presence of phosphatonins have low $1,25(OH)_2D_3$. In this study, presence of normal $1,25(OH)_2D_3$ is not readily explainable. It is possible that some other factor is influencing $1,25(OH)_2D_3$ regulation. Therefore, findings of this study are difficult to generalize to our typical nephrolithiasis population.

CONCLUSIONS

FGF-23 may potentially play a role in stone formation due to its inherent phosphaturic property. However, FGF-23 decreases $1,25(OH)_2D_3$ formation and serum concentrations which in turn would prevent hypercalciuria. Future studies are needed to define the exact role of phosphatonins in nephrolithiasis. It will be important to assess the association of not only FGF-23, but other phosphatonins as well, in a population of stone formers. It is possible that different phosphatonins have differential effects on $1,25(OH)_2D_3$ regulation, which would explain normal $1,25(OH)_2D_3$ concentrations in some stone formers with renal Pi leak. At this juncture there is insufficient data to implicate phosphatonins in the pathogenesis of stone formation.

REFERENCES

1 D. A. Bushinsky, *Journal of the American Society of Nephrology* **9** (5), 917 (1998).
2 K. K. Stamatelou, M. E. Francis, C. A. Jones *et al.*, *Kidney International* **63** (5), 1817 (2003).
3 C. Y. Pak, *Current Therapy in Endocrinology & Metabolism* **6**, 572 (1997).
4 F. L. Coe and D. A. Bushinsky, *American Journal of Physiology* **247** (1 Pt 2), F1 (1984).
5 P. Bordier, A. Ryckewart, J. Gueris *et al.*, *American Journal of Medicine* **63** (3), 398 (1977).
6 C. P. Williams, D. F. Child, P. R. Hudson *et al.*, *Journal of Clinical Pathology* **49** (11), 881 (1996).
7 D. Prie, V. Huart, N. Bakouh *et al.*, *New England Journal of Medicine* **347** (13), 983 (2002).
8 Q. Cai, S. F. Hodgson, P. C. Kao *et al.*, *New England Journal of Medicine* **330** (23), 1645 (1994).
9 F. L. Coe, J. H. Parks, and J. R. Asplin, *New England Journal of Medicine* **327** (16), 1141 (1992).
10 C. Y. Pak, J. R. Poindexter, B. Adams-Huet *et al.*, *American Journal of Medicine* **115** (1), 26 (2003).
11 K. Sakhaee, M. J. Nicar, D. C. Brater *et al.*, *J Clin Endocrinology & Metabolism* **61** (5), 825 (1985).
12 J. E. Zerwekh, B. Y. Reed-Gitomer, and C. Y. Pak, *Endocrinology & Metabolism Clinics of North America* **31** (4), 869 (2002).
13 C. Y. Pak, F. Britton, R. Peterson *et al.*, *American Journal of Medicine* **69** (1), 19 (1980).
14 F. Pietschmann, N. A. Breslau, and C. Y. Pak, *J Bone & Mineral Research* **7** (12), 1383 (1992).
15 R. Pacifici, M. Rothstein, L. Rifas *et al.*, *J Clinical Endocrinology & Metabolism* **71** (1), 138 (1990).
16 E. M. Brown, G. Gamba, D. Riccardi *et al.*, *Nature* **366** (6455), 575 (1993).
17 A. E. Broadus, S. B. Erickson, J. M. Gertner *et al.*, *Journal of Clinical Endocrinology & Metabolism* **59** (2), 202 (1984).
18 D. A. Bushinsky and M. J. Favus, *Journal of Clinical Investigation* **82** (5), 1585 (1988).
19 H. M. Hoag, J. Martel, C. Gauthier *et al.*, *Journal of Clinical Investigation* **104** (6), 679 (1999).
20 R. Kumar, Bone 27 (3), 333 (2000).
21 M. J. Econs and P. T. McEnery, *Journal of Clinical Endocrinology & Metabolism* **82** (2), 674 (1997).
22 M. K. Drezner, *Kidney International* **57** (1), 9 (2000).
23 T. Berndt, T. A. Craig, A. E. Bowe *et al.*, *Journal of Clinical Investigation* **112** (5), 785 (2003).
24 T. O. Carpenter, B. K. Ellis, K. L. Insogna *et al.*, *Journal of Clinical Endocrinology & Metabolism* **90** (2), 1012 (2005).
25 P. S. Rowe, P. A. de Zoysa, R. Dong *et al.*, *Genomics* **67** (1), 54 (2000).
26 K. B. Jonsson, R. Zahradnik, T. Larsson *et al.*, *New England Journal of Medicine* **348** (17), 1656 (2003).
27 A. E. Bowe, R. Finnegan, S. M. Jan de Beur *et al.*, *Biochemical & Biophysical Research Communications* **284** (4), 977 (2001).
28 Adhr Consortium, *Nature Genetics* **26** (3), 345 (2000).
29 T. Shimada, S. Mizutani, T. Muto *et al.*, *Proceedings of the National Academy of Sciences of the United States of America* **98** (11), 6500 (2001).
30 T. Larsson, R. Marsell, E. Schipani *et al.*, *Endocrinology* **145** (7), 3087 (2004).
31 T. Shimada, M. Kakitani, Y. Yamazaki *et al.*, *Journal of Clinical Investigation* **113** (4), 561 (2004).
32 L. Beck, A. C. Karaplis, N. Amizuka *et al.*, *Proceedings of the National Academy of Sciences of the United States of America* **95** (9), 5372 (1998).
33 H. Chau, S. El-Maadawy, M. D. McKee *et al.*, *Journal of Bone & Mineral Research* **18** (4), 644 (2003).
34 L. V. Virkki, I. C. Forster, N. Hernando *et al.*, *Journal of Bone & Mineral Research* **18** (12), 2135 (2003).
35 J. Y. Lapointe, J. Tessier, Y. Paquette *et al.*, *Kidney International* **69** (12), 2261 (2006).
36 R. W. Gray, D. R. Wilz, A. E. Caldas *et al.*, *Journal of Clinical Endocrinology & Metabolism* **45** (2), 299 (1977).
37 F. L. Levy, B. Adams-Huet, and C. Y. Pak, *American Journal of Medicine* **98** (1), 50 (1995).
38 D. A. Bushinsky, W. R. Parker, and J. R. Asplin, *Kidney International* **57** (2), 550 (2000).
39 D. Rendina, G. Mossetti, G. De Filippo *et al.*, *Journal of Clinical Endocrinology & Metabolism* **91** (3), 959 (2006).

Origin of Urinary Oxalate

Ross P. Holmes, John Knight and Dean G. Assimos

Department of Urology, Wake Forest University School of Medicine, Winston-Salem NC USA

Abstract. Urinary oxalate is mostly derived from the absorption of ingested oxalate and endogenous synthesis. The breakdown of vitamin C may also contribute small amounts to the urinary oxalate pool. The amount of oxalate absorbed is influenced by the oxalate content of the diet, the concentrations of divalent cations in the gut, the presence of oxalate-degrading organisms, transport characteristics of the intestinal epithelium, and other factors associated with the intestinal environment. Knowledge of pathways associated with endogenous oxalate synthesis is limited. Urinary oxalate excretion can be modified using strategies that limit dietary oxalate absorption and the ingestion of oxalogenic substrates such as hydroxyproline.

Keywords: dietary oxalate, oxalate synthesis, intestinal absorption, ascorbate.
PACS: 82.39.-k

INTRODUCTION

Urinary oxalate is derived from 3 sources: the diet, endogenous synthesis, and the breakdown of ascorbic acid. In the absence of any disease that enhances oxalate excretion (primary hyperoxaluria, enteric diseases, bariatric or intestinal surgery), the amount of oxalate excreted in the urine may vary from 5 to 60 mg per day, and the concentration from 0.04 to 0.75 mM. There may be slight differences in excretion due to gender [1], while the impact of age and race are not well defined. Oxalate is not metabolized in the body and is removed from the body principally by urinary excretion. Under certain conditions related to the gradient of oxalate across the intestinal epithelium, secretion of oxalate into the intestine may occur [2].

ASCORBIC ACID BREAKDOWN

Ascorbic acid can breakdown non-enzymatically to produce oxalate. This process is accelerated at alkaline pH. Initial experiments suggested that this breakdown was a significant source of oxalate, but a close scrutiny of the procedures indicated that the breakdown occurred due to processing urine at a high pH [3]. Two studies have examined the effects of 2 g of supplemental ascorbic acid in normal and stone forming subjects who consumed diets controlled in oxalate and other nutrients [4,5]. They showed increases in urinary oxalate excretion of 7.5 to 21.5% in normal subjects and 16.4 to 32.6% in stone forming subjects. An analysis of the diets of 1473 men who formed stones also indicated that the ingestion of more than 1000 mg of ascorbate per day was a risk factor for stone disease [6]. These results suggest that to avoid

CP900, *Renal Stone Disease, 1st Annual International Urolithiasis Research Symposium,*
edited by A. P. Evan, J. E. Lingeman, and J. C. Williams, Jr.

unnecessary contributions to urinary oxalate excretion, stone formers should be advised to ingest no more than 400 mg of ascorbic acid per day [7].

DIETARY OXALATE

The contribution of dietary oxalate to urinary oxalate excretion varies considerably when individuals consume a self-selected diet. A number of factors most likely contribute to this variability due to their influence on oxalate absorption. They include the oxalate content of the diet, the bioavailability of the oxalate, divalent cations in the intestinal stream, oxalate degradation in the gut, intestinal transit times, intestinal physiology, and other intestinal substances or organisms that can influence any one of these parameters. In a small number of individuals (n = 5), we observed that the mean oxalate intake was 150 mg/day. Several studies indicate that normally 1 to 15% of the ingested oxalate is absorbed [8-10]. Hesse and colleagues have suggested that absorptions above 15% of a soluble oxalate load represent a hyperabsorption of oxalate [10]. High absorptions of oxalate will lead to transitory oxalate loads on the kidney and will increase the supersaturation of urine with calcium oxalate. Thus, oxalate hyperabsorption could be a risk factor for stone disease and Voss et al have confirmed this in a case-control study using soluble $^{13}C_2$-oxalate to monitor absorption [10].

The amount of calcium ingested appears to have a strong influence on intestinal oxalate absorption. A prospective study in male health professionals showed that there was an inverse dose effect of dietary calcium on stone formation [11]. In another prospective study, Borghi et al showed that calcium intake was partially responsible for limiting stone formation in a cohort of stone formers [12]. An experimental group with a high calcium intake had a diminished oxalate excretion, as well as a reduced stone recurrence in comparison to a group with a low calcium intake. Both of these prospective studies suggest that the effect of a high calcium intake is to bind to oxalate in the gut and limit its absorption. This effect of dietary calcium on oxalate absorption and urinary oxalate excretion was confirmed by von Unruh et al [13].

Of the other factors that may influence oxalate absorption, there is current interest in the role of the oxalate-degrading organism, *Oxalobacter formigenes* (OxF), in decreasing the amount of intestinal oxalate available for absorption and of the oxalate transporter SLC26A6, which is present in much of the human intestine. Preliminary data suggest that stone formers have a lower colonization rate with OxF than non-stone formers and that this may increase their urinary oxalate excretion [14]. Experiments with control of dietary oxalate, calcium and other nutrients are required to confirm and quantify the effects of OxF on oxalate absorption. The role of SLC26A6 in oxalate transport became apparent after studies in mice in which this gene had been knocked out [15,16]. These mice were hyperoxaluric. Surprisingly, flux experiments on isolated epithelium indicated that intestinal oxalate secretion was defective, suggesting that significant cycling of oxalate occurs across the luminal membrane in this tissue. These results further suggest that another process (tranporter?) is responsible for oxalate influx into enterocytes. It is possible that either the absorptive or secretory components of this cycling process are altered in individuals who hyperabsorb oxalate. A more complete analysis of the transport processes underlying oxalate absorption and an accurate phenotyping of the absorptive characteristics of individuals is required.

ENDOGENOUS OXALATE SYNTHESIS

All tissues can apparently synthesize oxalate as measurable levels of glycolate, glyoxylate, oxalate, glyoxylate reductase and lactate dehydrogenase are found throughout the body. These metabolites and enzymes are centrally involved in the terminal steps of oxalate biosynthesis [17]. The liver, the major metabolic organ in the body, is the main site of oxalate production. The carbon sources utilized for oxalate synthesis are only partially identified [17]. Such sources include the amino acids, hydroxyproline, glycine, phenylalanine and tyrosine. However, their relative contributions have not been accurately quantified and some may be of only minor significance. Carbohydrates can also be converted to oxalate via pathways that result in xylulose-5-phosphate formation. Aldolase can catalyze the breakdown of xylulose-5-phosphate to glycolaldehyde and eventually to oxalate. Carbohydrates known to be converted to oxalate include glucuronate, xylitol and xylulose. The pathway associated with the metabolism of these sugars was demonstrated when patients in Australia and Germany developed oxalosis and organ dysfunction after being infused with large doses of xylitol [18].

To identify pathways that lead to oxalate synthesis we have utilized HepG2 cells, a hepatoma cell line that retains many hepatocyte functions including the synthesis of oxalate, glycolate and glyoxylate [19]. The metabolism of glycine and hydroxyproline by HepG2 cells to glycolate and oxalate is shown in Fig.1.

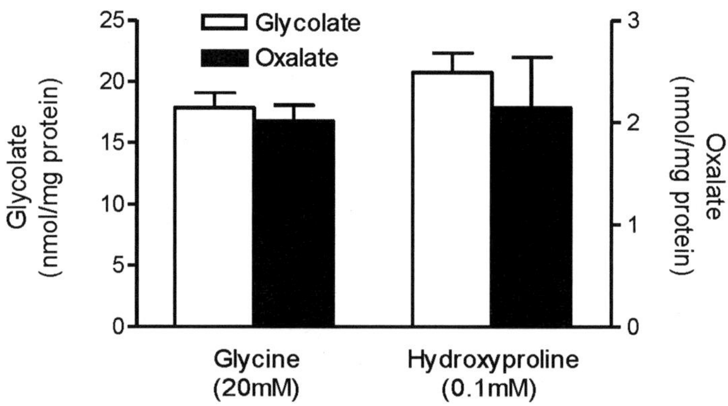

FIGURE 1. Increased glycolate and oxalate synthesis from supplemental glycine and hydroxyproline after 48 hrs incubation in low glucose medium. $^{13}C_2$-glycine was used to trace the metabolism of glycine to $^{13}C_2$-glycolate and $^{13}C_2$-oxalate. Basal amounts of glycolate and oxalate synthesis were 6.1±1.1 nmoles and 1.9±1.0 nmoles/mg protein, respectively.

These results show that HepG2 cells possess pathways to metabolize both hydroxyproline and glycine to glycolate and oxalate, but much more is produced from hydroxyproline as the concentration used was 1/200 that of glycine. The daily turnover of glycine in the body, however, may be 200 times that of hydroxyproline. There is a single catabolic pathway for hydroxyproline degradation where one mole of the amino acid results in the formation of one mole of glyoxylate. This glyoxylate can subsequently be converted to glycolate, oxalate and glycine. In contrast, glycine has numerous metabolic fates, including a decarboxylation, a conversion to serine and utilization in protein synthesis as well as oxidation to glyoxylate. The formation of $^{13}C_2$-oxalate and $^{13}C_2$-glycolate, but not any $^{13}C_1$-oxalate or $^{13}C_1$-glycolate from glycine suggests that $^{13}C_2$-glyoxylate is an intermediate and is formed through the activity of the peroxisomal enzyme, D-amino acid oxidase. A 10-fold differential in the amounts of glycolate and oxalate formed from hydroxyproline and glycine apparently occurs regardless of the subcellular compartmentation of the site of glyoxylate formation (mitochondria for hydroxyproline and peroxisome for glycine). A limited conversion of glycine to glyoxylate and oxalate was observed in isolated peroxisomes, consistent with the limited conversion by HepG2 cells of glycine to glycolate (~0.01%) and oxalate (~0.001%) [20]. A more extensive conversion of glycine to oxalate has been reported *in vivo* (0.05%) [21], suggesting that more extensive metabolism occurs *in vivo* in comparison to that observed *in vitro*. Alternatively, the methodology used in the 1960 publication may not have been accurate. To clarify these issues, the metabolism of glycine to oxalate *in vivo* should be re-evaluated.

The metabolism of hydroxyproline can potentially make an important contribution to oxalate synthesis as collagen turnover leads to the metabolism of 240 to 420 mg of hydroxyproline each day. Hydroxyproline may be also ingested either as collagen in meats and meat products or as gelatin. We have recently shown that the ingestion of gelatin leads to significant increases in urinary oxalate and glycolate excretion [22]. Quantitative estimates of the contribution of hydroxyproline breakdown to endogenous oxalate synthesis are yet to be determined.

The data previously discussed illustrate that the metabolic pathways that lead to oxalate synthesis are still poorly defined. Such information is clinically relevant as it could lead to possible enzymatic targets for drug therapy or dietary strategies that could limit oxalate synthesis. Decreasing endogenous oxalate synthesis could be important in the treatment of the primary hyperoxalurias and calcium oxalate stone disease [23]. The development of knockout mouse models for the primary hyperoxalurias should provide important insights into the biochemical pathways that result in oxalate synthesis, and lead to better strategies for limiting the conversion of glyoxylate to oxalate.

OXALATE-FREE DIETS

The use of oxalate-free diets is one tool we have used to quantify endogenous oxalate synthesis. These studies have also provided an insight into inter- and intra-individual variability in the parameter. A limitation of the approach is that the diet could potentially influence the amount of endogenous synthesis. The composition of the diet mirrors that of the commercially available product, Ensure®, and was made from the base ingredients to eliminate all sources of oxalate [24]. The response of 14 individuals to this diet is shown below in Fig. 2.

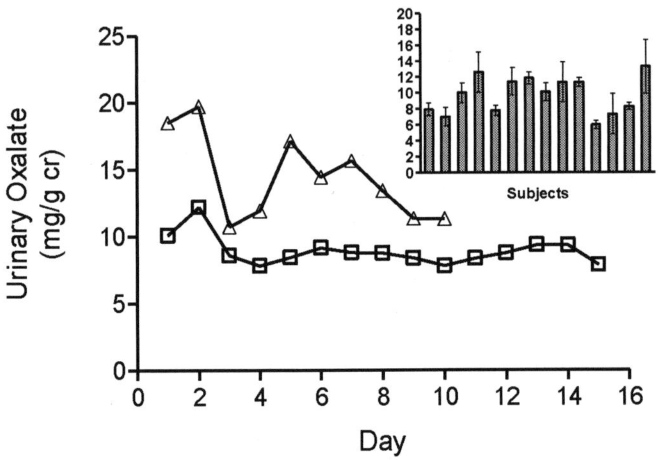

FIGURE 2. Urinary oxalate excretion of two normal subjects on an oxalate-free formula diet. Data in the inset show the mean (± SD) oxalate excretion of 14 subjects on days 3 to 5 of the diet.

Urinary oxalate excretion on an oxalate-free diet is substantially reduced from that observed on controlled oxalate diets [25]. The pattern of oxalate excretion over a 10 to 15 day period is shown for 2 individuals in Fig. 2. The mean 24 hr excretions of 14 other individuals on days 3 to 5 of the diet are shown in the inset. The results show that there is substantial inter- and intra-subject variability in endogenous oxalate synthesis. The mean intra-individual coefficient of variation (CV) was 15.8% and the mean inter-individual CV was 23.5%. Factors that may underlie this variability are unknown. We have shown that glucagon modifies oxalate synthesis in guinea pigs [26], indicating that variations in the levels of metabolic hormones may have an important role.

MODIFICATION OF URINARY OXALATE

Whereas the amount of calcium excreted in urine can be reduced with thiazide drugs, there is no such medical therapy available for reducing urinary oxalate excretion. A subset of individuals with primary hyperoxaluria type 1 respond to pyridoxine therapy with a decreased urinary oxalate excretion [27], but other individuals do not appear to respond to pyridoxine [28]. Dietary therapy is, however, one available option and there are several steps that can be taken to modify the diet without much difficulty, thus enhancing compliance. Reducing oxalate intake is the first step that should be taken. It should be possible with a judicious choice of foods to decrease oxalate intake to less than 75 mg/day. The second step is to ensure that calcium intake is at least 1200 mg/day. Hesse et al illustrated the importance of calcium intake by showing that increasing calcium intake from 1211 to 3858 mg offsets the hyperoxaluria associated with a diet containing 2200 mg oxalate/day [29]. Urinary calcium did increase with the high calcium diet by 20%, but there was no increase in calcium oxalate crystallization indices. The response of individuals with hypercalciuria to calcium intakes above 1200 mg/day remains to be investigated. The third step is to balance calcium and oxalate intakes throughout the day to maintain a molar excess of calcium over oxalate with each meal or snack.

Modifying endogenous oxalate synthesis requires a more complete understanding of the biosynthetic pathways involved. Clearly, excessive ingestion of collagen or gelatin should be avoided to limit hydroxyproline metabolism to oxalate. Some individuals take large doses of these proteins as can be ascertained by an internet search for collagen or gelatin supplements and their uses. Other dietary components or supplements that contribute to oxalate synthesis also warrant consideration.

ACKNOWLEDGMENTS

Our research on dietary oxalate and the endogenous production of oxalate has been supported by NIH grants DK50466, DK62284, DK73732 and MO1 RR07122.

REFERENCES

1. Holmes, R. P., Goodman, H. O., Hart, L. J., and Assimos, D. G. (1993) Kid Intl 44, 366-372
2. Hatch, M., Cornelius, J., Allison, M., Sidhu, H., Peck, A., and Freel, R. W. (2006) Kid Intl 69, 691-698
3. Lemann, J., Hornick, L. J., Pleuss, J. A., and Gray, R. W. (1989) Clin Chem 35, 2107-2110
4. Massey, L. K., Liebman, M., and Kynast-Gales, S. A. (2005) J Nutr 135, 1673-1677
5. Traxer, O., Huet, B., Poindexter, J., Pak, C. Y. C., and Pearle, M. S. (2003) J Urol 170, 397-401
6. Taylor, E. N., Stampfer, M. J., and Curhan, G. C. (2004) J Am Soc Nephrol 15, 3225-3232
7. Levine, M., Conry-Cantilena, C., Wang, Y., Welch, R. W., Washko, P. W., Dhariwal, K. R., Park, J. B., Lazerev, A., Graumlich, J. F., King, J., and Cantilena, L. R. (1996) Proc Natl Acad Sci 93, 3704-3709
8. Prenen, J. A. C., Boer, P., and Mees, E. J. D. (1984) Amer J Clin Nutr 40, 1007-1010
9. Unruh, G. E. v., Voss, S., Sauerbruch, T., and Hesse, A. (2003) J Urol 169, 687-690
10. Voss, S., Hesse, A., Zimmerman, D. J., Sauerbruch, T., and Unruh, G. E. v. (2006) J Urol 175, 1711-1715
11. Curhan, G. C., Willett, W. C., Rimm, E. B., and Stampfer, M. J. (1993) New Engl J Med 328, 833-838
12. Borghi, L., Schianchi, T., Meschi, T., Guerra, A., Allegri, F., Maggiore, U., and Novarini, A. (2002) N Engl J Med 346, 77-84
13. Unruh, G. E. v., Voss, S., Sauerbruch, T., and Hesse, A. (2004) J Am Soc Nephrol 15, 1567-1573
14. Troxel, S. A., Sidhu, H., Kaul, P., and Low, R. K. (2003) J Endourol 17, 173-176
15. Freel, R. W., Hatch, M., Green, M., and Soleimani, M. (2006) Amer J Physiol 290, G719-G728
16. Jiang, Z., Asplin, J. R., Evan, A. P., Rajendran, V. M., Velazquez, H., Nottoli, T. P., Binder, H. J., and Aronson, P. S. (2006) Nat Genet 38, 474-478

17. Holmes, R. P., and Assimos, D. G. (1998) J Urol 160, 1617-1624
18. Conyers, R. A. J., Bais, R., and Rofe, A. M. (1990) Clin Chem 36, 1717-1730
19. Baker, P. R., Cramer, S. D., Kennedy, M., Assimos, D. G., and Holmes, R. P. (2004) Amer J Physiol 287, C1359-C1365
20. Poore, R. E., Hurst, C. H., Assimos, D. G., and Holmes, R. P. (1997) Amer J Physiol 272, C289-C294
21. Elder, T. D., and Wyngaarden, J. B. (1960) J Clin Invest 39, 1337-1344
22. Knight, J., Jiang, J., Assimos, D. G., and Holmes, R. P. (2006) Kid Intl 70, 1929-1934
23. Coulter-Mackie, M. B. (2006) Kid Intl 70, 1891-1893
24. Holmes, R. P., Goodman, H. O., and Assimos, D. G. (1995) Scan Microsc 9, 1109-1120
25. Holmes, R. P., Goodman, H. O., and Assimos, D. G. (2001) Kid Intl 59, 270-276
26. Holmes, R. P., Hurst, C. H., Assimos, D. G., and Goodman, H. O. (1995) Amer J Physiol 269, E568-E574
27. Monico, C. G., Rossetti, S., Olson, J. B., and Milliner, D. S. (2005) Kid Intl 67, 1704-1709
28. Kaelin, A., Casez, J.-P., and Jaeger, P. (2004) Urol Res 32, 61-68
29. Hess, B., Jost, C., Zipperle, L., Takkinen, R., and Jaeger, P. (1998) Nephrol Dial Transplant 13, 2241-2247

JESS: What Can It Teach Us?

Allen L. Rodgers, Shameez Allie-Hamdulay, Graham E. Jackson

Department of Chemistry, University of Cape Town, South Africa

Abstract. Knowledge of the chemical complexes (speciation) in urine can be extremely important in evaluating the risk of crystallization of stone forming salts. In order to determine the speciation, a database of thermodynamic constants for the wide variety of complexes that might form from the known components in urine, is required. JESS (Joint Expert Speciation System) is a software package that has such a database. In the present study, some of its applications in urolithiasis research were explored. To illustrate the effect of therapeutic complexing agents on the risk of calcium oxalate and calcium phosphate (brushite) stone formation, tetracycline was introduced into the urine model. Speciation calculations showed that the risk decreased with increasing tetracycline concentration and increasing pH. In a second application, the saturation index (equivalent to the relative supersaturation) of calcium oxalate and brushite were independently calculated while precipitation of these salts was modeled. This revealed that in mixed calcium oxalate-brushite stones, the former salt is more likely to be the nucleus than the latter. It is suggested that JESS is a powerful tool for obtaining deep insights into the sophisticated crystallization processes which govern stone pathogenesis.

Keywords: urinary complexes, urine modeling, stone formation risk, crystallization, calcium oxalate stones
PACS: 82.39.-k; 81.10.Dn

INTRODUCTION

JESS is a software program for calculating the chemical speciation in a chemical solution [1,2]. JESS itself is an acronym for "Joint Expert Speciation System". The authors have chosen these terms intentionally. They have used the word "Joint" to convey the notion that operation of the system requires explicit interaction between the operator and the program's database. The term "Expert" signals that the operator will need to make informed decisions in implementing the program and, as such, will require a fundamental understanding of the physicochemical characteristics of the species under investigation. The term "Speciation" refers to the form and concentration of all the chemical species which are present in the solution under consideration.

JESS has been widely used in medicine to model metal-ligand equilibria in biological systems [3,4] and to model industrial processes under widely different conditions [1]. It has also been used to predict the solubility of calcium oxalate hydrates at different pH in artificial urine solutions [5]. Recently, it was applied in urolithiasis research for the first time by ourselves [6]. On the other hand, EQUIL is a well known speciation program which has been extensively used in the field of kidney

CP900, *Renal Stone Disease, 1st Annual International Urolithiasis Research Symposium,* edited by A. P. Evan, J. E. Lingeman, and J. C. Williams, Jr.

stone research for calculating the relative supersaturation of urinary salts [7]. We believe that JESS can play an even greater role than EQUIL in understanding the physicochemical processes involved in stone formation. The present paper reviews some of the results which we obtained using JESS and which we have reported previously [6], and explores the potential use of this powerful software program in kidney stone research.

JESS Overview

Jess has an extensive database comprising over 70 000 chemical reactions involving 200 000 physicochemical constants related to enthalpy, entropy, Gibbs free energy, solubility products and redox potentials. Obviously, the vast majority of these reactions are not required for urine modeling. However, there are several of these which are indeed relevant and (importantly) are not included in EQUIL's database.

The program processes a wide variety of reactions including metal-ligand complexation, ligand-ligand associations and ternary and quaternary complexation. Identification and characterization of multi-ligand complexes in urine is a particularly exciting capability, as it is not offered by EQUIL. An example is our recently identified calcium-phosphate-citrate complex $[CaCitPO_4]^{-4}$ which had not been previously implicated in calcium oxalate stone pathogenesis and management [6].

Because JESS allows its database to include reported values of the same constant from multiple sources in the literature, it interrogates its database and flags discrepancies and outliers for the operator's attention. As stated earlier, the latter then selects which value of the particular constant should be used in the modeling process.

JESS offers the option of varying the ionic strength of the solution and also offers the option of allowing precipitation of specified salts to occur. Neither of these options are offered by EQUIL. In the latter program, calculations are based on the notion that precipitation does not occur, thereby culminating in supersaturation. While JESS does the same, it offers the additional option of calculating the equilibrium speciation after precipitation.

JESS's database can be continually updated. New reactions and their associated thermodynamic constants can be introduced routinely at any stage. This is an extremely useful feature, as it is not offered by EQUIL in which constants are hard-wired into the program.

Another extremely useful feature in JESS is its automatic scanning facility in which urinary parameters can be systematically varied over ranges specified by the operator. The program calculates the effect that such variations have on the chemical speciation. Because several parameters can be simultaneously varied, synergistic effects can be investigated.

Finally, JESS allows chemical equilibrium calculations to be coupled with chemical kinetics equations. Both EQUIL and JESS are equilibrium (i.e., thermodynamic) based systems, but the latter's capability to introduce kinetic factors is a major advantage that could be exploited in urolithiasis research.

What has JESS taught us about stone disease thus far?

In a previous study we investigated the effects of the oral administration of a citrate preparation on urinary stone-forming risk factors [8].Our results were in agreement with those reported in several other studies, namely increases in urinary citrate and pH and decreases in urinary calcium and the relative supersaturation of calcium oxalate. In general, stone researchers have always attributed these effects somewhat glibly to the notion that "citrate binds calcium" without rigorously interrogating this concept. However, in a follow-up study, we used JESS to determine the calcium speciation in the urine of our subjects pre- and post- citrate administration [6]. This showed that after citrate administration, the percentage of $[Ca^{2+}]$ and all calcium-containing complexes decreased, as expected, except for a new complex, previously unreported in urolithiasis research, $[CaCitPO_4]^{-4}$ which showed a highly significant increase. In our paper we drew attention to the fact that it is this ternary complex which accounts for the decrease in the percentage of free $[Ca^{2+}]$ (and hence the ultimate decrease in the relative supersaturation of calcium oxalate), rather than some non-defined binary complex involving calcium and citrate [6].

We then employed JESS's scan facility to identify the urinary factors which influence the concentration of this new complex. To our surprise, varying the calcium, oxalate and citrate concentrations had no effect. However, the concentration of this complex was found to increase with increasing pH. We were therefore able to conclude that the therapeutic action of citrate is due to an increase in urinary pH rather than an increase in urinary citrate concentration *per se.*

JESS has thus taught us that identification and physicochemical characterization of the chemical speciation in urine can lead to a sophisticated understanding of the crystallization processes in kidney stone formation

What can JESS teach us about stone disease henceforth?

Urinary speciation in stone formers and healthy controls

An obvious application of JESS is to identify and compare the chemical speciation in the urine of stone formers and healthy controls with a view to establishing whether particular complexes are absent or present in either group. The next step would be to investigate which of these complexes influence the supersaturation of stone forming salts and the chemical conditions (such as pH or concentration of other species) under which such influences are exerted. In order to perform this exercise, a substantial, well defined urine database is needed as input for JESS.

Administration of therapeutic complexing agents.

As stated earlier, JESS allows researchers to model speciation based on the addition of any agent to the solution under investigation. In the case of urine (and urolithiasis), complexing substances such as magnesium, EDTA, tartrate and tetracyclines (among many others) are of interest. All of these are worth exploring. After the modeling has been completed, JESS's predictions can be tested in *in vitro* crystallization experiments.

In the present study, theoretical modeling involving a complexing agent was demonstrated using tetracycline which is excreted unmetabolized in urine and for which relevant constants are stored in JESS's database. In the first instance, JESS was asked to calculate the saturation index of calcium oxalate and brushite as a function of tetracycline concentration at a fixed pH of 6.40. (The saturation index (SI) is equivalent to the relative supersaturation index produced by EQUIL. If log SI = 0, the solution is saturated. On the other hand, if log SI > 0, the solution is supersaturated. Finally, values of log SI < 0, indicate that the salt is undergoing dissolution). The results of this modeling exercise are shown in Fig. 1.

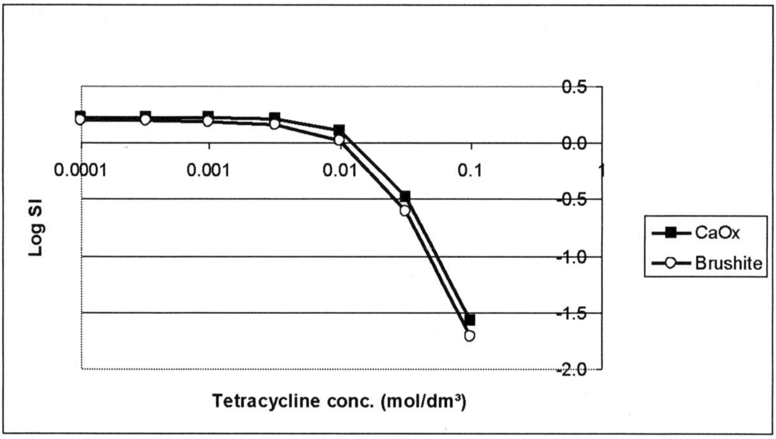

FIGURE 1. SI values as a function of tetracycline concentration at pH 6.0.

It is noted that at tetracycline concentrations > 0.01 mol dm^{-3}, calcium oxalate and brushite both dissolve. In order to identify the complex (or complexes) which cause this effect, a scan of calcium speciation as a function of tetracycline concentration was performed. The results for those complexes whose concentrations changed are shown in Fig. 2.

It is seen that the concentration of [Ca^{2+}] decreases as expected, due to complexation by tetracycline. It is noted that the concentrations of the calcium-containing complexes decrease, except that of [CaH_2(tetracycline)$_2$]. The latter is thus the key complex for utilization of the free Ca^{2+} ions.

In a second application, pH was varied. The percentage of free Ca^{2+} ions was calculated as a function of tetracycline concentration at pH 5.50, 6.40 and 7.50. The concomitant log SI values were also calculated. Results are shown in Figs. 3 and 4, respectively. These show that the risk of calcium oxalate stone formation decreases with increasing concentration of tetracycline and pH.

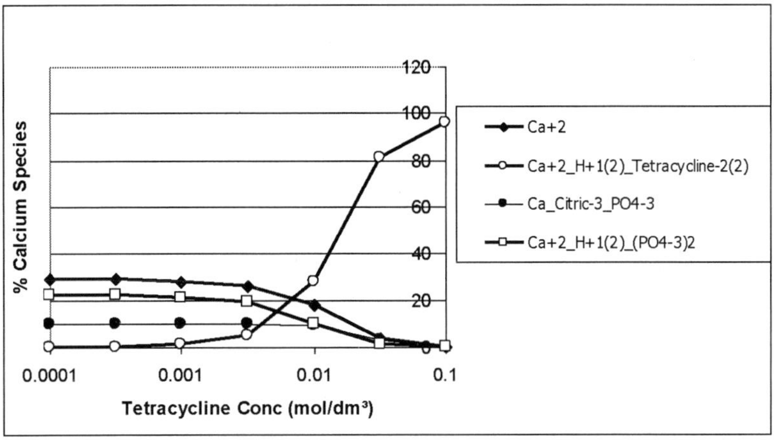

FIGURE 2. Speciation of calcium as a function of tetracycline concentration.

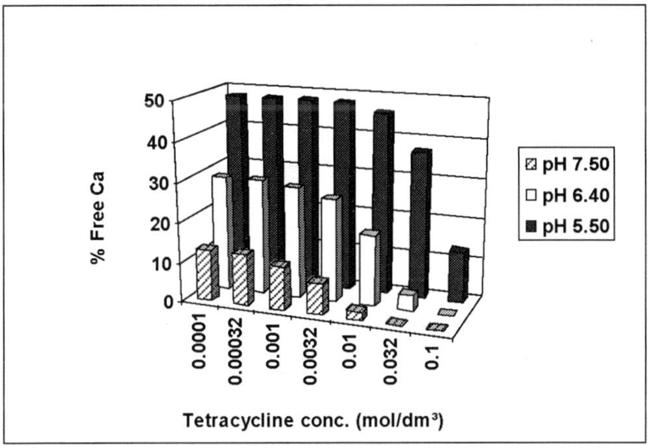

FIGURE 3. Free calcium as a function of pH and tetracycline.

Modeling precipitation processes

JESS can teach us aspects of the crystallization process in urine by predicting the nature of the speciation before and after precipitation of specified salts. For this type of modeling, urine data from stone formers or healthy controls (or both) can be used. Alternatively, the composition of a well-defined synthetic urine could be used. To illustrate the application of JESS in this context in the present study, we modeled the precipitation of calcium oxalate and brushite in independent calculations, using urinary data from healthy controls. In Fig. 5, the pair of bars on the left shows the values of log SI for calcium oxalate when precipitation of brushite occurs as well as when it does not. It is seen that the saturation index of calcium oxalate drops dramatically when brushite precipitates. The pair of bars on the right shows log SI values for brushite when calcium oxalate precipitates as well as when it does not. Here it is seen that precipitation of calcium oxalate has no effect on the saturation index of brushite. Interpretation of these results suggests that during brushite stone formation, the co-precipitation of calcium oxalate is less likely than the co-precipitation of brushite during calcium oxalate stone formation. This is tantamount to saying that in mixed calcium oxalate-brushite stones, the former salt is likely to be more frequently at the nucleus than the latter.

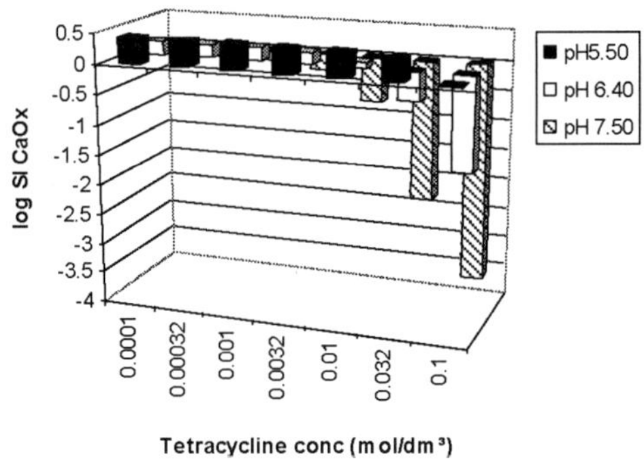

FIGURE 4. Supersaturation index of calcium oxalate as a function of pH and tetracycline.

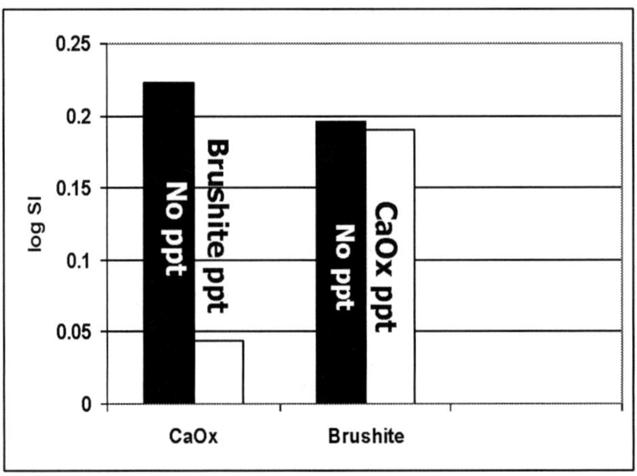

FIGURE 5. Effect of precipitation of brushite and calcium oxalate on supersaturation index.

Modeling kinetic processes

As stated earlier, one of the major shortcomings of EQUIL (and other speciation programs) is that it is based on the assumption that the system is at thermodynamic equilibrium. However, in modeling stone formation, this is not necessarily true. EQUIL predicts the final relative supersaturation rather than the instantaneous value. JESS is able to remedy this shortcoming by incorporating rate constants into its calculations. This facility therefore provides exciting opportunities for predicting the rate of crystallization of stone forming salts in given solutions (real and synthetic urines) under a variety of physicochemical conditions, or to model the rate of absorption of an agent of interest. An obvious follow-up to such computations would be to test the model in *in vitro* experiments involving the widely used MSMPR (mixed suspension, mixed product removal) crystallizer [9] or the stone farm version thereof [10]. The recently advocated urinary depletion effect [11] could also possibly be integrated into a JESS speciation calculation.

Validation of JESS

Having extolled the virtues of JESS, it is important to assess its validity for speciation calculations in urine. In order to achieve such an assessment, comparisons were made with the widely used and highly respected program EQUIL.

Indirect validation

Figure 6 shows the variation in the relative supersaturation (RS) and saturation index (SI) of calcium oxalate as a function of pH, as determined by EQUIL and JESS respectively. The data used for these determinations were those obtained in our previous study [8], except pH values outside the empirically determined range (6.40 - 7.40) were included in the calculations.

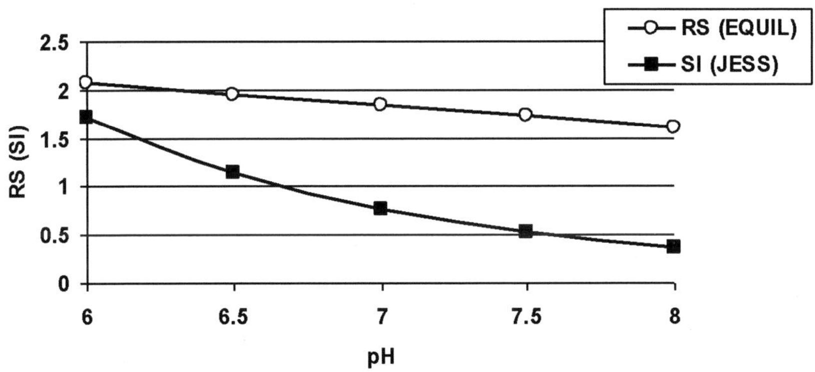

FIGURE 6. Relative supersaturation and saturation index values as calculated by EQUIL and JESS, respectively.

Figure 6 shows that for all pH values, RS (EQUIL) > SI (JESS). There is thus conflict between the outputs of the two programs. Accepting that this discrepancy probably arises as a consequence of differences in the determination of the calcium speciation, we used JESS to scan the calcium speciation as a function of pH (Fig. 7). This showed that besides $[Ca^{2+}]$ and $[CaCitPO_4]^{-4}$, there is another species $[Ca_2H_2(PO4)_2]$ which is influenced by pH. However, more importantly, like $[CaCitPO_4]^{-4}$, EQUIL does not have this complex in its database. We therefore hypothesized that the presence of these two complexes in JESS was the cause of the discrepancy in the output of the two programs. To test this hypothesis, we omitted both complexes from the JESS model, and recalculated the SI values. The results (Fig. 8) confirmed our hypothesis. This confirmation was interpreted by ourselves as an indirect validation of JESS.

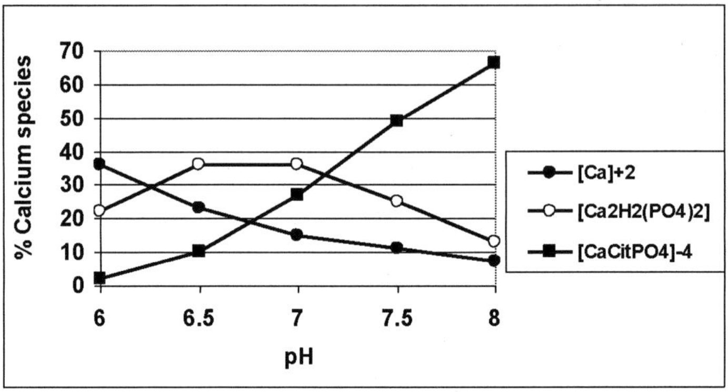

FIGURE 7. Scan of calcium speciation as a function of pH.

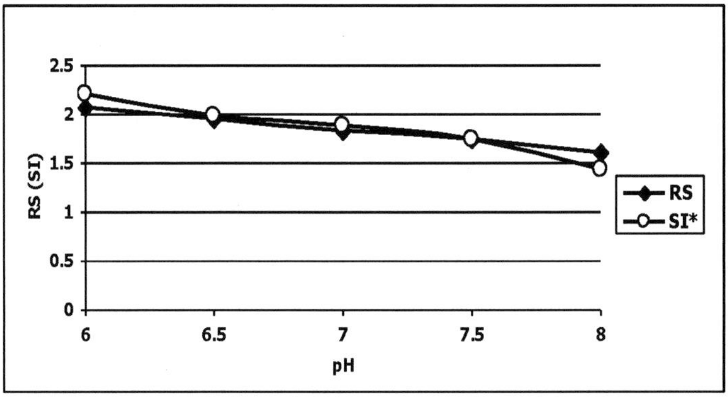

FIGURE 8. Relative supersaturation and saturation index values as calculated by EQUIL and JESS, respectively, as a function of pH, after elimination of the two species thought to have led to differences in the predictions of the two programs.

Direct validation

An artificial urine comprising 320mmol/l sodium chloride, 50mmol/l sodium phosphate, 4.8mmol/l sodium citrate, 1.20mmol/l calcium chloride and 50mmol/l sodium oxalate was prepared [12]. The pH was altered systematically by titration with 0.1mmol/l hydrochloric acid. The concentration of free $[Ca^{2+}]$ was measured using a calcium ion selective electrode. Using the composition of the artificial urine as input data, RS and SI values for calcium oxalate were calculated using EQUIL and JESS respectively. The results (Fig. 9) show that the JESS output is closer to the experimental values than that of EQUIL. We believe that this demonstrates the validity of JESS

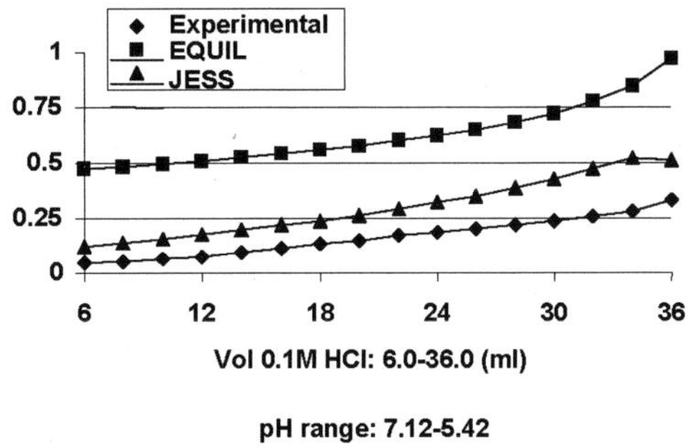

FIGURE 9. Experimental and calculated values for free calcium concentration.

CONCLUSION

JESS is a powerful speciation program with many features which are of direct and significant interest to kidney stone researchers. Its full potential in this field is yet to be explored. There is a reasonable expectation that application of this package to extensive urine databases will reveal much deeper insights into the sophisticated physicochemical processes which influence stone formation than was previously possible.

ACKNOWLEDGMENTS

The authors wish to gratefully acknowledge the financial support of the South African National Research Foundation, the South African Medical Research Council, the South African Urological Association and the University of Cape Town.

REFERENCES

1. P.M.May and K.Murray, *Talanta* **38**, 1409-1417 (1991)
2. P.M.May and K.Murray, *Talanta* **38**,1419-1426 (1991)
3. N.K.Bakar, D.M.Taylor and D.R.Williams, *Chem Spec Bioavailab* **11**, 95-101 (1999)
4. L.M.Webb, D.M.Taylor and D.R.Williams, *Radiat Prot Dosim* **79**, 219-222 (1998)
5. J.Streit, L.C.Tran-Ho and E.Konisberger, *Monatsh Chem* **131**, 1225-1236 (1998)
6. A.Rodgers, S.Allie-Hamdulay and G.Jackson, *Nephrol Dial Transplant* **21**, 361-369 (2006)
7. P.G.Werness, C.M.Brown,L.H.Smith and B.Finlayson, *J Urol* **134**, 1242-1244 (1985)
8. S.Allie-Hamdulay and A.Rodgers, *Urol Res* **33**, 116-124 (2005)
9. J.P.Kavanagh, S.Nishio, J Garside and N.J.Blacklock, *J Urol* **149**, 614-619 (1993)
10. K.Chow, J.Dixon, S.Gilpin, J.P.Kavanagh andP.N.Rao, *Urol Res* **32**, 55-60 (2004)
11. N.Laube, M.Pullmann, S.Hergarten and A.Hesse, *Clin Chem* **49**, 281-285 (2003)
12. R.C.Walton, J.P.Kavanagh, B.R.Heywood and P.N.Rao, *Biochim Biophys Acta* **1723**, 175- 183 (2005)

Calcium Stone Growth in Urine from Cystic Fibrosis Patients and Healthy Controls

Anita McSorley*, Andrew M. Jones*, A. Kevin Webb*, P. Nagaraj Rao† and John P. Kavanagh†

*Manchester Adult Cystic Fibrosis Centre, South Manchester University Hospitals NHS Foundation Trust, Wythenshawe Hospital, Manchester M23 9LT, UK

†Department of Minimally Invasive Endourology and Stone Management, South Manchester University Hospitals NHS Foundation Trust, Wythenshawe Hospital, Manchester M23 9LT, UK

Abstract. Cystic fibrosis patients have an increased risk of renal stone disease. There is some evidence that this may be related to a different excretory pattern of stone risk factors, but an alternative hypothesis, that the urine of cystic fibrosis patients is deficient in urinary inhibitors of crystallization and stone formation has not been tested. Here we have grown calcium stones, *in vitro* , in the presence of urine from healthy controls and compared this with growth in the presence of urine from cystic fibrosis patients. A stone farm was used to grow twelve calcium stones simultaneously, firstly in artificial urine for about 200 hours and then in 90% whole human urine for another 500 hours. Six of the stones received urine from healthy controls and six received urine from adult cystic fibrosis patients. There were no significant differences in stone mass at any of the key time points or in the overall growth pattern ($p>0.05$) between stones destined for, or treated with, urine from CF patients and the controls. Human urine greatly inhibited stone growth *in vitro* but there was no difference in the growth rate in urine from healthy controls and CF patients. This refutes the hypothesis that a tendency for a higher prevalence of urinary stones in CF patients is related to a deficiency in inhibitory activity.

Keywords: Cystic fibrosis, urolithiasis, calcium oxalate.
PACS: 81.10.Dn

INTRODUCTION

Cystic fibrosis (CF) is one of the most common lethal autosomal recessive genetic diseases in the Caucasian population, with a frequency of about 1 in 3000 live births. CF is due to a mutation in the cystic fibrosis transmembrane conductance regulator (CFTR) gene encoding the CFTR protein, a cAMP-regulated chloride channel localized in the apical membrane of epithelial cells [1]. Clinically, the condition manifests as a multi-system disease, but the principal problems are chronic suppurative pulmonary disease, exocrine pancreatic insufficiency and malabsorption. Since its recognition as a distinct disease in 1938, the life expectancy of affected individuals has increased from 6 months to a median survival greater than 30 years [2]. The majority (approximately 90%) of adults with CF have exocrine pancreatic insufficiency, and associated fat malabsorption [3]. This intestinal malabsorption is

CP900, *Renal Stone Disease, 1st Annual International Urolithiasis Research Symposium,* edited by A. P. Evan, J. E. Lingeman, and J. C. Williams, Jr.

severe and of early onset, the main cause being deficiency of pancreatic enzymes. However appropriate pancreatic enzyme replacement therapy can achieve normal or near-normal absorption in most people with cystic fibrosis [4].

As the prognosis of CF patients has improved, it is becoming clear that, as they enter adulthood, these individuals have a higher incidence of renal stone disease than is found in the general population. A variety of metabolic abnormalities have been suggested to account for this, low urine volume, hyperoxaluria, hypercalciuria, hyperuricosuria and hypocitraturia [5-8]. An alternative hypothesis, that these patients lack crystallization inhibitors, has not been explored.

Here we compare the growth of calcium stones *in vitro* in the urine from healthy controls and from cystic fibrosis patients.

MATERIALS AND METHODS

Patients with CF were defined as those with 2 copies of a known genetic mutation consistent with CF or a single copy of a CF gene and features pathognomonic of CF. Urine was collected from 19 patients [mean (s.d.) age 31.6 (14.5), BMI 23.2 (3.5), sex ratio 6M:13F]. 5 patients had a history of renal stones and one had a family history of renal stones. All were on long term oral antibiotics and 13 had additional courses of intravenous antibiotics within the last year. Twelve patients had exocrine pancreatic insufficiency. None of the controls had any personal or family history of stones or any type of kidney disease. Their mean (s.d.) age was 30.1 (9.9) and the sex ratio was 5F:9M. 24 hour urines were collected and stored at -20°C until used.

Twelve stones were grown simultaneously in a stone farm for about 700 hours. This system is a continuous flow method in which approximately 1 liter of urine or artificial urine (AU) passes each stone per day. It is based on twelve individual mixed suspension, mixed product removal, continuous crystallizers [9,10] and is described in detail elsewhere [10]. In order to accommodate the use of nearly whole urine in this study the flow rates and feed solution compositions were changed. Instead of two solutions flowing at equal flows, we have here used one solution flowing at 90% of the total (about 0.63ml/min) and the other at 10% of the total (0.07ml/min). This was achieved by using different pump tubing diameters from the original specification [10]. With artificial urine the composition of the feed solutions was adjusted, so that the solution at 90% flow contained calcium and that at 10% contained oxalate, and when combined they had the same composition as used previously [10]. When human urine was used this was allowed to thaw, pooled, sieved (20μm nylon net, Millipore) and centrifuged (2000g, 5 minutes). The pH was adjusted to between 5.9 and 6.0, 0.02%NaN_3 added and the calcium concentration measured and adjusted to 6.67mM by addition of a small volume of concentrated $CaCl_2$. This urine was used as 90% of the total flow and the same oxalate solution as before used at 10%. The starting material for each stone was a piece of marble chip ($CaCO_3$), of about 100mg. Twelve stones were grown in artificial urine for about 200 hours, at which time the 90% feed solution was changed to human urine. Six stones received urine from CF patients and six from healthy controls and the stones were grown for about another 500 hours.

RESULTS

The mean growth profiles of the six control stones and the six stones that were treated with CF urine are shown in Fig. 1. The weights of the control stones and the CF urine treated stones were not different at 0, 200 or 700 hours ($p > 0.05$). The growth rate constants for the two groups of six stones when grown in artificial urine were 0.0094 ± 0.0021 and 0.0113 ± 0.0048 ($mg/h^{3/2}$ ± 95% confidence intervals, based on surface area dependent growth [11]). These are not significantly different from each other and they are also consistent with the growth of control stones grown in artificial urine on marble chips when the feed solutions were pumped at a ratio of 50:50 (0.0098 $mg/h^{3/2}$ (n=6)) rather than 90:10. On application of human urine there was a period of consolidation with a slight loss of mass before growth restarted. This corresponds to a period in which the stone surface becomes more robust and less friable. The growth in the presence of urine was negligible, just a few mg in about 10 days. The growth rate constants are not significantly different from each other (0.00023 ± 0.00010 in control urine and 0.00059 ± 0.00033 in CF urine; $mg/h^{3/2}$ ± 95% confidence intervals).

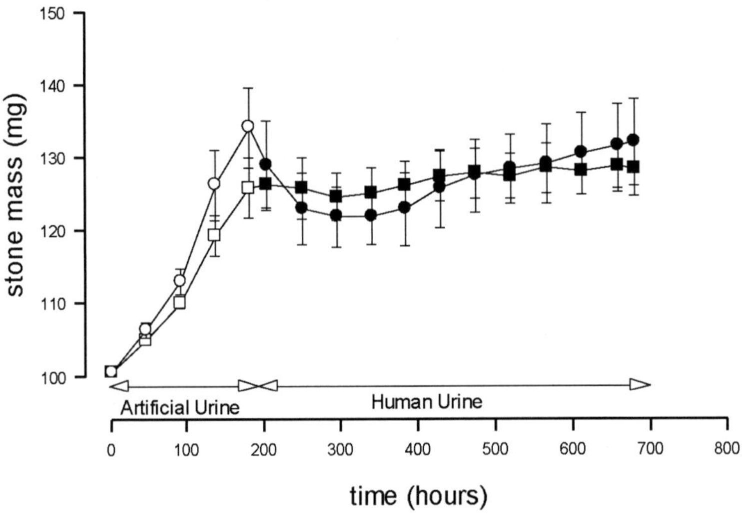

FIGURE 1. Mean mass of 6 stones (± s.e.), open symbols are with artificial urine; filled symbols are with human urine; squares are controls; circles are stones grown with urine from CF patients.

CONCLUSIONS

Various mechanisms have been proposed to account for recurrent idiopathic calcium stone disease and, in respect of stone enlargement (as opposed to stone initiation), the most important are likely to be related to solution chemistry and supersaturation and the role of macromolecules and crystallization inhibitors. In our model, we measure stone enlargement under conditions where the urine pH and calcium are the same in each experimental arm and the oxalate will be approximately the same. The results demonstrate the very powerful effect of whole urine in inhibiting the enlargement of calcium stones. The absence of any inhibitory difference between control urine and that from CF patients suggests that any higher risk of calcium stones in the patients is not due to any deficiency in crystallization inhibitors.

ACKNOWLEDGMENTS

We would like to thank J Dixon, S Gilpin, for their practical assistance in carrying out these experiments and Kidney Research (UK) and The Oxaluria and Hyperoxaluria Fund for supporting these studies.

REFERENCES

1. B. Marcet and J. M. Boeynaems, *Pharmacology & Therapeutics* 112, 719-732 (2006).
2. P. B. Davis, *American Journal Of Respiratory And Critical Care Medicine* 173, 475-482 (2006).
3. C. W. Imrie and A. S. Whyte, *Br J Surg* 62, 490-494 (1975).
4. J. M. Littlewood, S. P. Wolfe, and S. P. Conway, *Pediatric Pulmonology* 41, 35-49 (2006).
5. M. Terribile, M. Capuano, G. Cangiano et al., *Nephrology Dialysis Transplantation* 21, 1870-1875 (2006).
6. E. M. Gibney and D. S. Goldfarb, *American Journal of Kidney Diseases* 42, 1-11 (2003).
7. R. von der Heiden, A. P. G. Balestra, M. G. Bianchetti et al., *Clinical Nephrology* 59, 160-163 (2003).
8. M. R. Perez-Brayfield, D. Caplan, J. M. Gatti et al., *Journal of Urology* 167, 480-484 (2002).
9. S. Nishio, J. P. Kavanagh, and J. Garside, *Chemical Engineering Science* 46, 709-711 (1991).
10. K. Chow, J. Dixon, S. Gilpin et al., *Urological Research* 32, 55-60 (2004).
11. K. Ananth, J. P. Kavanagh, R. C. Walton et al., *BJU International* 90, 939-944 (2002).

A Problem Protein: Unexpected Analytical Irregularities in the Measurement of Urinary Osteopontin

L.A. Thurgood, P.K. Grover, and R.L. Ryall

Department of Surgery, Flinders Medical Centre, Adelaide, SA, 5042, AUSTRALIA

Abstract. Reported mean urinary values of osteopontin (OPN) have varied widely, from <1μg/mL to more than 20 times that value. Since OPN binds to calcium oxalate (CaOx) crystals, the presence of crystals in urine may cause underestimation of its urinary levels. We measured urinary OPN levels in the presence of endogenous or exogenous CaOx monohydrate (COM) and dihydrate (COD) crystals. OPN concentrations decreased in the presence of endogenous and exogenous CaOx crystals, but never below 2μg/mL. Increasing the urinary calcium concentration decreased detectable osteopontin levels, which is likely due to changes in the 3D-confirmation shape of the protein. The value of measuring OPN as a diagnostic marker of urolithiasis must therefore be seriously questioned.

Keywords: osteopontin, enzyme linked immunosorbent assay (ELISA), calcium oxalate
PACS: 87.14.Ee

BACKGROUND AND AIMS

Although osteopontin (OPN) may be important in urolithiasis, urinary concentrations measured using enzyme linked immunosorbent assays (ELISAs) have varied widely [1-5]. Discrepancies might result from the protein's susceptibility to proteolytic cleavage [5], conformational changes induced by calcium [6], or other factors, including crystalluria, storage conditions, and interactions with other urinary components. Urinary prothrombin fragment 1 (PTF1) levels decrease in the presence of COM crystals [7]. Since OPN binds to CaOx, the presence of CaOx crystals in urine (formed *in vivo* or *in vitro*) prior to determination could reduce measurable amounts of the protein and cause underestimation of its urinary concentration and excretion. The aims of this study were to examine the effect of exogenous and endogenous COM and COD crystals on the measurement of urinary OPN.

MATERIALS AND METHODS

Urine (100ml) from healthy volunteers (4 women, 2 men) was collected over 0.1% thimerosal, pooled, centrifuged (10,000 x g), filtered (0.22μm) and divided into 4 samples. The Ca concentration of 2 samples was adjusted to 2mM, and that of the others, to 8 mM. Increasing amounts of exogenous inorganic COM [8] and COD [9]

CP900, *Renal Stone Disease, 1st Annual International Urolithiasis Research Symposium,*
edited by A. P. Evan, J. E. Lingeman, and J. C. Williams, Jr.

crystals were added to separate 3mL aliquots of one 2mM and one 8mM Ca urine sample, at final concentrations of 0, 0,025, 0.5, 0.1, 0.5, 1.0, 5 and 10 mg/mL, and incubated with shaking at 37°C for 2 hours. Crystals were removed by filtration and OPN concentration in the supernatant fluid was measured using an ELISA kit (IBL Hamburg, Germany). Endogenous crystals were precipitated from the remaining 2mM and 8mM Ca urine samples by increasing the oxalate concentration stepwise from 0 to 0.75 μmoles/mL above the measured metastable limit (MSL) [10]. The urines were incubated and filtered, and the OPN concentration measured as described above. Light microscopy confirmed that crystals deposited at 2mM and 8mM Ca were principally COM and COD, respectively.

RESULTS

Increasing amounts of inorganic COM and COD caused wide fluctuations in measured OPN values, but these never fell below ~2μg/mL. COM and COD crystals decreased the overall OPN level by 41.2% and 23.1%, respectively. In almost every case, measured values of OPN concentration were greater at 2mM Ca than at 8mM. At low amounts of added oxalate, formation of endogenous COM and COD crystals increased the measured OPN concentration, which declined and stabilized above the MSL at ~ 2μg/mL.

Formation of endogenous COM crystals caused an overall 57.6% decrease in the OPN level, compared to a drop of 32.3% following formation of COD. Since OPN values were again consistently higher at 2mM calcium than at 8mM, the effects of Ca concentration on OPN concentration were examined in another urine specimen. OPN concentration was unaffected by increasing the calcium concentration to 2mM from the native value of 1mM, but fell between 2mM and 4mM. Further increases to 10mM had no effect on measured OPN levels.

DISCUSSION

Measured urinary OPN concentrations decreased in the presence of COM and COD, irrespective of the quantity of crystals added or formed. However, the final urinary level never dropped below ~2μg/mL, suggesting that a significant proportion of OPN in human urine is detected by the ELISA assay but does not bind to CaOx crystals. The binding sites of the *coating* and *labeled* ELISA antibodies contained in the ELISA kit are different from the two major calcium binding domains on the OPN molecule (Fig. 1). The protein is also vulnerable to serine proteases in urine, where it exists as several fragments [5]. One or more of these may contain the ELISA *coating* and *labeled* antibody binding sites, but not the Ca-binding motifs, and will therefore be detected by the ELISA, but will not bind to CaOx crystal surface.

COM crystals reduced the measured OPN concentration more than did COD. This suggests that the protein binds to and is incorporated into COM more easily than into COD. However, OPN binds to the surface of growing inorganic COM crystals, but is not internalized into the structure [10]; neither is it incorporated into COM crystals

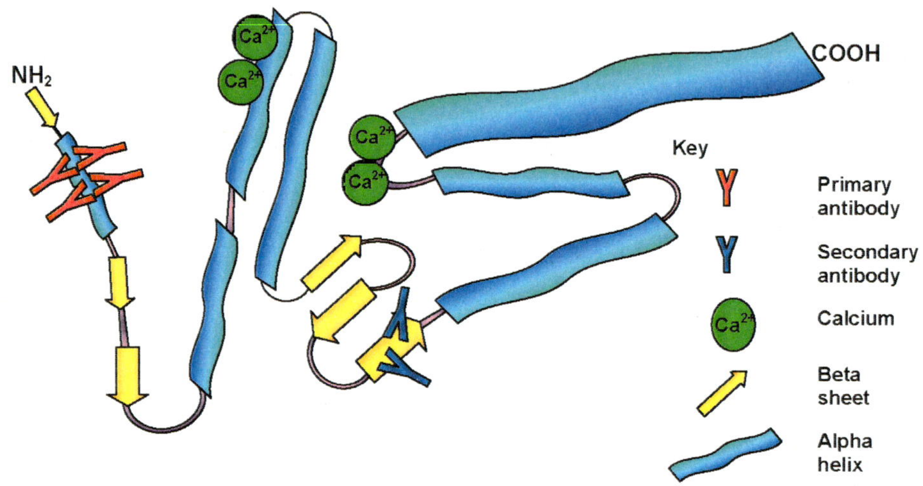

FIGURE 1. Hypothetical structure of OPN, as described in (http://www.cmb.lu.se/ctb/html/OPN.htm) showing the position of the two putative calcium binding motifs, as indicated by the attached calcium ions. Also shown are the attachment sites of the coating and labeled antibodies, as detailed in the literature supplied with the OPN ELISA kit.

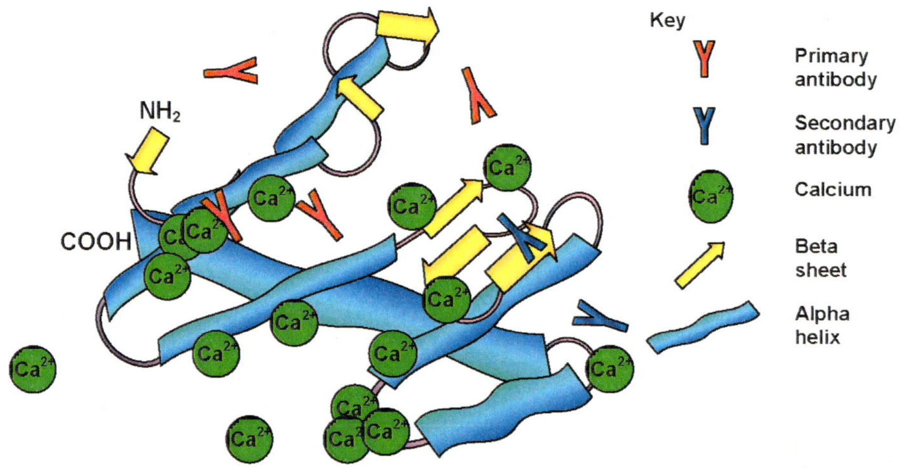

FIGURE 2: Speculative model, based on that presented in Fig 1, showing possible effects of high calcium concentrations on the folding of the OPN molecule. Consequent alterations to the protein's 3-dimensional structure prevent the ELISA antibodies from attaching to their binding sites on the OPN backbone, thereby causing underestimation of the protein's urinary concentration.

precipitated from urine [11]. Therefore, the fall in OPN must have resulted fromattachment of the protein only to the crystal *surfaces*. The decline in OPN concentration with COD formation probably resulted from inclusion of OPN into the mineral [10]. The greater reduction elicited by COM, compared with COD, may have been caused by a greater surface area, as well as its precipitation in larger quantities upon addition of oxalate to urine.

Urinary calcium concentrations greater than 2mM reduced the concentration of OPN by ~25%, perhaps as a result of binding of calcium to OPN. OPN has two major putative calcium binding motifs (Fig. 1), as well as numerous Ca-binding amino acid residues. At low calcium concentrations (1-2mM) only half of OPN's ~50 potential Ca-binding sites are occupied [12], which may allow easy access of the ELISA *coating* and/or *labeled* antibodies to their binding domains. Calcium levels greater than 2mM might alter the protein's 3-dimensional conformation, which is exquisitely sensitive to calcium concentration [6], and obscure or bury the antibody sites, preventing them from docking to the OPN molecule (Fig 2).

SUMMARY AND CONCLUSION

The measurement of urinary OPN concentration is significantly affected by the prevailing calcium concentration (which is typically greater in the urine of stone formers) and the presence of CaOx crystals (which are increased in the urine of stone formers). A significant proportion (~50%) of total urinary OPN does not bind to either inorganic or urinary CaOx crystals and is therefore unlikely to play a role in stone formation. We conclude that the measurement of urinary OPN concentration is unlikely to be of any benefit in the investigation of stone formers.

ACKNOWLEDGEMENT

We gratefully acknowledge support from the National Institutes of Health, USA (Grant No. NIDDK R01 DK064050-01A1).

REFERENCES

1. S. Nishio, M. Hatanaka, H. Takeda, K. Aoki, T. Iseda, H. Iwata and M. Yokoyama, *Mol. Urol.* **4**, 383-389 (2000).
2. J.R. Hoyer, R.A. Pietrzyk, H. Liu, P.A. Whitson, *J. Am. Soc. Nephrol.* **10**, S389-S393 (1999).
2. J.R. Asplin, D. Arsenault, J.H. Parks, F.L. Coe and J.R. Hoyer, *Kidney Int.* **53**, 194-199 (1998).
3. W. Min, H. Shiraga, C. Chalko, S. Goldfarb, G.G. Krishna and J.R. Hoyer, *Kidney Int.* **53**, 189-193 (1998).
5. D.S. Bautista, J. Denstedt, A.F. Chambers and J.F. Harris, *J. Cell. Biol.* **61**, 402-409 (1996).
6. L.W. Fisher, D.A. Torchia, B. Fohr, M.F. Young and N.S. Fedarko, *BBRC* **280**, 460-465 (2001).
7. Dean CJ, Macardle PJ, Ryall RL, "The effect of the presence of calcium oxalate crystals on the measurement of prothrombin fragment 1 in urine." in *Urolithiasis 2000*, edited by Rodgers AL et al, University of Cape Town, 2000, pp 150-152.
8. M.C. Chauvet, R.L. Ryall, *J. Struct. Biol.* **151**, 12-17 (2005).
9. R.C. Walton, J.P. Kavanagh, B.R. Heywood, *J. Struct. Biol.* **143**(1), 14-23 (2003).
10. S.R. Qiu, A. Wierzbicki, C.A. Orme, A.M. Cody, J.R. Hoyer, G.H. Nancollas, S. Zepeda, J.J. De Yoreo, *Proc. Natl. Acad. Sci.* **101**, 1811-1815 (2004).
11. R.L. Ryall, M.C. Chauvet, P.K. Grover, *BJU Int.* **96**, 654-663 (2005).
12. Y. Chen, B.S. Bal, J.P. Gorski, *J. Biol. Chem.* **267**, 24871-24878 (1992).

Intracrystalline Proteins Promote Dissolution of Urinary Calcium Oxalate Crystals in Cultured Renal Epithelial Cells

Phulwinder K. Grover*, Lauren A. Thurgood*, David E. Fleming[¶], Wilhelm van Bronswijk[¶] and Rosemary L. Ryall*

** Department of Surgery, Flinders Medical Centre, Adelaide, SA 5042, AUSTRALIA*
[¶]Department of Applied Chemistry, Curtin University of Technology, Western Australia, AUSTRALIA

Abstract. We have proposed that internalized calcium oxalate (CaOx) crystals containing intracrystalline proteins would be vulnerable to intracellular dissolution. The aims of this study were (1) to measure non-uniform strain and crystallite size in CaOx monohydrate (COM) crystals containing increasing amounts of intracrystalline crystal matrix extract (CME) and (2) to compare the rates of crystal dissolution in Madin-Darby canine kidney (MDCKII) cells. CME was isolated by demineralization of COM crystals generated from human urine. Cold and ^{14}C-oxalate-labelled COM crystals were precipitated from ultrafiltered urine containing CME at final concentrations of 0-5mg/L. Non-uniform strain and crystallite size were determined using synchrotron X-ray diffraction with Rietveld whole-pattern peak fitting and profile analysis, and the protein content of the crystals was analyzed using SDS-PAGE and Western blotting for prothrombin fragment 1. Radiolabeled crystals were added to MDCKII cells and dissolution was expressed as radioactive label released into the medium relative to that in the crystals at zero time. Non-uniform strain increased and crystallite size decreased proportionally with rising CME concentration, reaching saturation between approximately 1 and 5 mg/L, and demonstrating unequivocally the inclusion of increasing quantities of proteins in the crystals. This was confirmed by SDS-PAGE and Western blotting. Crystal dissolution also followed saturation kinetics. These findings were confirmed by field emission scanning electron microscopy (FESEM), which showed that the degree of crystal degradation increased relative to CME concentration. We conclude that intracrystalline proteins enhance intracellular dissolution of CaOx crystals and thus may provide a natural defense against stone pathogenesis.

Keywords: Calcium oxalate, dissolution, urine, calculogenesis, nephrolithiasis.
PACS: 87.14.Ee

INTRODUCTION

The possible roles of proteins in calculogenesis have been intensely studied since they were first detected in the matrix of stones. We have proposed that after cellular attachment and internalization, CaOx crystals containing intracrystalline proteins would be vulnerable to proteases, which would open channels throughout the mineral and facilitate dissolution [1-3]. In previous studies we have shown qualitatively that the amount of prothrombin fragment 1 (PTF1) and osteopontin (OPN) incorporated into urinary CaOx monohydrate (COM) and dihydrate (COD) crystals, respectively, is

CP900, *Renal Stone Disease, 1st Annual International Urolithiasis Research Symposium,*
edited by A. P. Evan, J. E. Lingeman, and J. C. Williams, Jr.

proportional to the concentration of CME in the urine from which the crystals are precipitated [1] and COM crystals precipitated from centrifuged and filtered urine are more susceptible to degradation after adhesion to Madin-Darby canine kidney (MDCKII) cells than those generated from ultrafiltered urine [2].

The aims of this investigation were (a) to measure non-uniform strain and crystallite size in COM crystals containing increasing amounts of CME and (b) to compare rates of dissolution of COM crystals containing increasing amounts of CME after attachment to MDCKII cells.

MATERIALS AND METHODS

Preparation of CME

CME was prepared from CaOx crystals generated in pooled centrifuged and filtered urine as described earlier [1].

Generation of urinary CaOx crystals containing increasing amounts of CME

24-hour urines collected from six healthy laboratory colleagues were pooled, centrifuged and filtered (CF: 10,000 x g; 0.22μm) and ultrafiltered (UF: 10kDa). CME was added at final concentrations of 0, 0.5, 1.0, 2.0, and 5.0mg/L to separate samples of the treated urine. ^{14}C-oxalate-labelled (hot) and non-radiolabeled (cold) urinary COM crystals were then prepared from these samples as described previously [2]. Crystals were sterilized with ethylene oxide, suspended in CaOx-saturated phosphate buffered saline (PBS: pH 7.2) and sonicated. COM crystal morphology was confirmed by bright field and polarized light microscopy. Incorporation of increasing amounts of CME was demonstrated by SDS-PAGE and Western blotting.

Field emission scanning electron microscopy

Using cold COM crystals, parallel incubations were performed with cells cultured in dishes containing sterile 13mm Thermanox Plastic coverslips. At the times specified above, the coverslips and attached cells were removed, mounted on aluminum stubs and processed for FESEM analysis as described previously [1]. Ten fields were randomly selected on each membrane and the length and breadth of 10 individual crystals were measured in each field. A good approximation of surface area in contact with the cell layer was obtained simply from assuming that crystals were rectangular, and multiplying length by breadth.

SDS-PAGE, Western Blotting, and Synchrotron X-ray diffraction

SDS-PAGE and Western Blot analysis were performed as described previously [1]. Synchrotron X-ray diffraction patterns were collected as detailed earlier [3].

Cell culture and measurement of crystal dissolution

High-density quiescent cultures of MDCKII cells were prepared as described by Lieske et al [4]. Crystals (400μg), suspended in CaOx-saturated PBS were added to the cells, which had been washed with the same PBS solution, and incubated at 37°C in a humidified incubator for 60 minutes and re-washed. Growth medium was then added and the cells incubated for 2 minutes and 3, 6, 24 and 48hrs. Dissolution was expressed as ^{14}C-label released into the medium relative to that in the crystals at zero time. Reciprocals of the slopes of plots of T/D *vs* T (where D = % dissolution and T = time), were used to calculate an index of the initial dissolution rate.

Statistical analysis

Each experiment was performed in triplicate and data are plotted as means ± SE. An absence of error bars means that errors are smaller than the symbol used to designate the means. Comparisons were performed using Student's t-test; a P value <0.05 was considered statistically significant.

RESULTS AND DISCUSSION

Crystals consisted principally of birefringent COM, irrespective of the CME concentration. Average surface areas of the crystals were 52.8μm^2 for the crystals generated in the UF urine and 52.2, 49, 50 and 48.4 μm^2 for those precipitated in the presence of 0.5, 1.0, 2.0 and 5.0 mg/L of CME, respectively. These values were not statistically different. Western blots of the demineralized matrix of the crystals grown in UF urine containing 0.5, 1.0, 2.0 and 5.0 mg/L of CME, showed that UPTF1 was absent from the UF urine, but present in increasing amounts in proportion to CME concentration. Non-uniform strain increased and crystallite size decreased proportionally with rising CME concentration, reaching saturation between approximately 1 and 5 mg/L, and demonstrating unequivocally the inclusion of increasing quantities of proteins in the crystals.

Regardless of CME concentration, the rate of dissolution was greatest in the first 6 hours, with saturation occurring after that time. Both the initial rate and final extents of dissolution were proportional to CME concentration. Fig 1 shows the % dissolution data presented as plots of T/D *vs* T. The slopes decreased indirectly with increasing CME concentration and calculated initial dissolution rates increased from 13.4% in the absence of CME to 13.7 ($p<0.01$), 15.2 ($p<0.001$), 18.6 ($p<0.001$) and 18.9% ($p<0.001$) at final CME concentrations of 0.5, 1, 2 and 5mg/L, respectively. These differences were unaffected by adjusting the values for the slight differences in crystal surface area.

FESEM showed that the degree of crystal erosion after incubation for 24 hours was proportional to the CME concentration. In the absence of added CME, only slight etching was visible, but the degree of degradation increased with rising CME concentration. Crystals precipitated at a CME concentration of 5.0mg/L showed extreme erosion, with only their peripheries remaining intact. Destruction of all crystals characteristically began in the centre of the large 100 face, and progressed from there to the rim. Because only ~20% of crystal mineral had dissolved by 24 hours, the extensive excavation shown must have resulted primarily from removal of intracrystalline proteins.

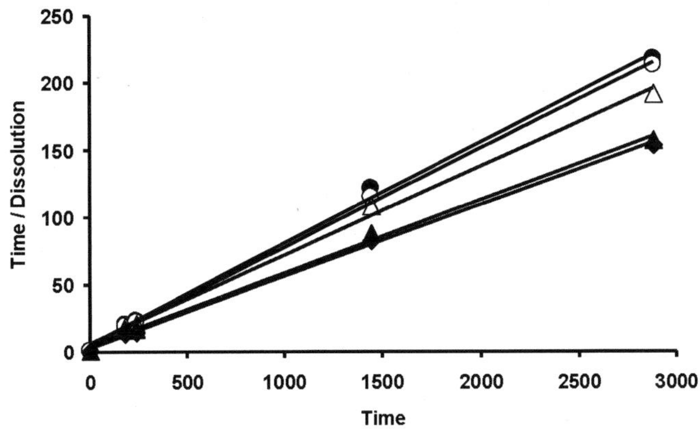

FIGURE 1. Time course of dissolution of crystals precipitated from urine containing CME at final concentrations of 0 (●), 0.5 (○), 1.0 (Δ), 2.0 (▲), and 5.0 (♦) mg/L plotted as T/D vs T.

CONCLUSION

In this model, intracrystalline proteins enhanced intracellular dissolution of CaOx crystals in a dose-response manner. Under physiological conditions intracrystalline proteins, which are present within all crystals precipitated within the renal tubules, will facilitate degradation and dissolution of the crystals following their attachment to, and internalization by epithelial cells in the nephron. Intracrystalline proteins may thus constitute a form of routine natural defense against stone pathogenesis.

ACKNOWLEDGEMENTS

This study was supported by grant No. NIDDK R01 DK064050-01A1 from the National Institutes of Health, USA.

REFERENCES

1. R. L. Ryall, M. C. Chauvet, P. K. Grover, *BJU Int.* **96**, 654-663 (2005).
2. M. C. Chauvet and R. L. Ryall, J. Struct. Biol. 151, 12-17 (2005).
3. D. E. Fleming, A. van Riessen, M. C. Chauvet, P. K. Grover, B. Hunter, W. van Bronswijk, R. L. Ryall, J. Bone Min. Res. 18, 1282-1291 (2003).
4. J. C. Lieske, R. Leonard, F. G. Toback, Am. J. Physiol. 268, F604-F612 (1995)

V. NEW TECHNOLOGIES FOR TREATING STONE DISEASE

Improvements in Intracorporeal Lithotripters for Percutaneous Nephrolithotomy

Ramsay L. Kuo

The International Kidney Stone Institute and Indiana University School of Medicine
Indianapolis, Indiana, USA

Abstract. Percutaneous nephrolithotomy (PNL) is an effective minimally invasive surgical approach for the treatment of large renal stone burden. Intracorporeal lithotripters (ICL) are utilized during PNL to fragment calculi, with some devices capable of concurrently removing fragments as well. Much progress has been made in the design of ICL devices, resulting in potentially more efficient treatment of nephrolithiasis.

Keywords: percutaneous nephrolithotomy, intracorporeal lithotripter.
PACS: 87.54.Hk

INTRODUCTION

Percutaneous nephrolithotomy, a well accepted minimally invasive surgical procedure for the treatment of large volume nephrolithiasis, was first described by Fernstorm and Johannsen in 1976 [1]. This technique involves the establishment of an access tract, or passage, from the flank surface directly into the renal collecting system. The surgeon then inserts a nephroscope into the access tract to allow direct visualization within the kidney. Typically, rigid nephroscopes are utilized for the majority of the treatment process, as they incorporate large caliber working channels enabling insertion of large fragmentation or extraction instruments. In addition, rigid scopes allow delivery of more irrigant and also provide optimal visualization of the collecting system through a rod lens.

Flexible nephroscopes, which incorporate fiber-optic technology, are other important adjunctive instruments for PNL. Visualization with these instruments can be limited at times because of the “honeycomb” effect produced by the fiber-optic bundles. Although the image resolution of fiber-optic endoscopes can be improved by the use of digital filtering technology [2], it does not match that of rigid nephroscopes. The flexibility of these instruments is crucial to allow access to all peripheral calices within the collecting system, but this feature also limits the working channel size such that only smaller, flexible devices such as baskets or laser fibers can be employed. Therefore, flexible nephroscopy is used primarily to treat and extract small residual stones after the main portion has been removed.

Once the stone has been reached percutaneously, ICL devices are utilized in conjunction with nephroscopes to treat the stone burden. A variety of intracorporeal

CP900, *Renal Stone Disease, 1st Annual International Urolithiasis Research Symposium,*
edited by A. P. Evan, J. E. Lingeman, and J. C. Williams, Jr.

devices are available for clinical use. The simplest units provide a means to fragment stones. As technology has advanced, subsequent devices not only comminute stones but also allow for the concurrent removal of fragments. The latest ICLs combine clinically preferred fragmentation modalities while still providing the means for fragment removal. These newer devices have the potential to greatly improve PNL efficiency.

TRADITIONAL INTRACORPOREAL LITHOTRIPTERS

Ultrasonic lithotripter

Ultrasonic lithotripters typically incorporate a handpiece containing a piezoelectric crystal, which is excited by electrical energy. This creates a high frequency vibration of up to 27,000 hertz (Hz) [3]. The vibrational energy is transmitted through a hollow probe which is brought into contact with the stone surface, resulting in fragmentation. Ultrasonic lithotripter handpieces have a central lumen which is contiguous with that of the ultrasonic probe, thus allowing suction to be applied through the device.

The major advantage of the ultrasonic lithotripter lies in its overall clinical efficiency in treating stones. The large caliber probes (ranging from 3.3 to 3.8 Fr), are inserted through rigid nephroscopes. Stones treated with this modality can be simultaneously broken and removed from the collecting system. Ultrasonic probes are also relatively atraumatic, resulting in little effect on the collecting system surface with short periods of direct contact. Because of these favorable characteristics, ultrasonic lithotripsy is often the preferred modality for PNL.

The only clinical disadvantage of this device is its decreased effectiveness when treating very large stones with a hard and dense composition. In these cases, the probe will often "polish" the stone surface without achieving comminution. In these cases, it is often advantageous to initially utilize a separate pneumatic lithotripter to break up the stone into smaller portions which can then be further fragmented and cleared by the ultrasonic unit.

Pneumatic lithotripter

The pneumatic, or ballistic, lithotripter is perhaps the simplest ICL currently available. The main component of this device, which is powered by an external compressed air source, consists of a hollow handpiece containing a metal pellet. A solid blunt probe, with a diameter typically ranging from 2 to 3.2 mm, is secured to the handpiece and the probe tip brought into direct contact with the stone surface. When the handpiece is activated, the pellet in the handpiece is driven forcibly against the solid probe. This "jackhammer" effect enables breakage of the stone into smaller fragments. Denstedt *et al* reported on the initial use of this device and found that it was effective in fragmenting 94% of treated calculi [4].

There are many advantages of the pneumatic lithotripter. First, it is very effective in breaking apart stones. From a clinical standpoint, it is most useful for quickly fragmenting very large stone burden or hard calculi, such as those comprised of calcium oxalate monohydrate or brushite (calcium hydrogen phosphate). This device is also very safe, as the blunt tip of the solid probe will not damage the urothelium of the collecting system. The minimal tissue effects of pneumatic lithotripsy have been demonstrated in a swine model where no pathologic change was seen in areas of the urinary tract treated directly with pneumatic probes after 6 weeks of follow-up [5].

The main disadvantage of the pneumatic lithotripter is that one cannot simultaneously remove stone fragments from the collecting system during treatment. For removal, the surgeon must insert separate grasping forceps or an extraction basket through the nephroscope to extract fragments piecemeal. This can be a cumbersome process when dealing with a large stone.

Holmium laser

The holmium laser has been available since the mid 1990s and presently is widely utilized for the treatment of nephrolithiasis. This laser produces a wavelength of 2140 nm and works through a photothermal mechanism [6]. Laser energy is delivered with flexible quartz fibers ranging from 200 to 1000 microns in diameter. Unlike the older Candela laser, which would only treat pigmented calculi, the holmium laser is effective for fragmenting calculi of all compositions [7]. Because the photothermal effect of the holmium laser results in a vaporization of stone material, it tends to produce smaller fragments during lithotripsy than the pneumatic lithotripter. This has been shown in an *in vitro* experiment utilizing calculi of varying compositions obtained from a stone laboratory[8].

Despite the fact that the holmium laser is commonly used for ureteroscopic lithotripsy, most urologists do not use this device as a first-line ICL during PNL. This is mainly because of the inefficiency of the laser with large stones. Although investigators have utilized the holmium laser during PNL and found it to be an effective lithotrite, its inefficiency in treating large stones has been noted [9].

In addition, concurrent fragment removal when utilizing the holmium laser remains an issue. Cuellar and Averch have reported on the use of a suction probe device through which a holmium laser fiber can be inserted. This adjunctive device facilitates fragment removal during holmium laser PNL, but has not been widely adopted [10].

Lastly, the holmium laser's unique properties also allow it to cut tissue cleanly while maintaining superior hemostasis. As such, this laser can also be utilized for applications such as treating benign prostatic hyperplasia [11]. When treating stones, however, the laser fiber must be in contact with the stone surface at all times to prevent injury or perforation to adjacent urothelial tissue. The potential for tissue injury during stone treatment was demonstrated by Santz-Cruz *et al* in an *ex vivo* porcine ureter experiment, where the holmium laser produced the fastest perforation time of any tested energy modality when activated within 0.5 mm of the ureteral wall [12]. However, the laser was not able to produce acute perforation when the fiber was held 2 mm away from the wall.

Electrohydraulic lithotripter

The electrohydraulic lithotripter (EHL) produces stone fragmentation through acoustic shockwave and cavitation effects generated by a spark at the end of a probe which is typically placed in near contact with the stone surface. Although it is effective in stone fragmentation, EHL can be a traumatic energy modality which may lead to mucosal soft tissue injury. Like the holmium laser and pneumatic lithotripters, EHL lacks a reliable method of concurrent stone fragment removal during PNL. This modality has been superseded by the aforementioned devices.

In summary, most urologists performing PNL with traditional ICLs will use either the ultrasonic or pneumatic lithotripters, as these devices are simple to utilize, effective, and are inserted through rigid nephroscopes that optimize stone visualization. When dealing with very large and hard stones, these devices can be used sequentially, employing the pneumatic unit initially to quickly break up the stone into smaller chunks and then using the ultrasonic unit to finish fragmenting and concurrently removing the smaller pieces. Although effective, the sequential use of these devices, with removal and reinsertion of the respective instruments, can be tedious and time consuming.

EVALUATION OF ICL EFFICIENCY

In the past, with ultrasonic lithotripters becoming the preferred modality for stone fragmentation during PNL, many manufacturers introduced units for clinical use. From the urologist's standpoint, it was difficult to ascertain which units were truly the most efficient. As such, many groups devised testing methods to compare and contrast commercially available ultrasonic ICL devices.

Liatsikos *et al* tested four ultrasonic lithotripter units utilizing Plaster of Paris stone phantoms [13]. In this study, the stone phantoms were placed into a container with water. The probes of each ultrasonic unit were positioned into a rigid nephroscope and continuous irrigation applied through the scope. The stone phantoms were then treated with each ultrasonic device, with the end point being complete fragmentation of each phantom. The inherent weakness of this study is that stone fragmentation was performed by hand. As a result, operator bias could have significantly affected the results of this study.

Haupt designed an *in vitro* system to test ultrasonic lithotripter devices which fixed the handpieces and probes such that the probes pointed downward and were positioned within a water basin [14]. An elaborate weight and fulcrum system then brought a stone phantom, which had been placed within the basin, against the probe tip with a constant force. While eliminating potential operator bias, this complex system would hinder reproducibility of results.

Our group devised another novel *in vitro* hands-free testing system in which the ultrasonic handpieces and probes were secured upright [15]. This system (Fig. 1) utilized an irrigation sheath through which probes were inserted and allowed for continuous tap water irrigation to surround the probes to prevent overheating. An acrylic sheath was then fashioned to fit over the irrigation sheath such that the tip of the probe could be seen.

An Ultracal-30 (U-30) gypsum stone model, which had been shown to provide reproducible fragmentation outcomes in prior *in vitro* shock wave lithotripsy experiments, was chosen for this study [16]. A U-30 stone was placed atop the probe tip once it had been secured within the irrigation and acrylic sheaths, and finally a weighted rod was positioned over the stone to provide a constant pressure keeping the stone in contact with the probe. The advantages of this system included the elimination of user variability, production of reproducible results, and also the simple mechanism of maintaining a constant force against the probe tip/stone interface.

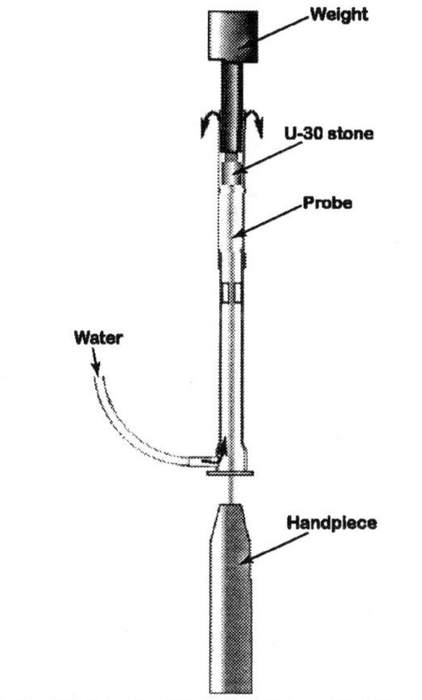

FIGURE 1. Hands-free testing apparatus for the evaluation of ultrasonic lithotripter units [15]. The handpiece and probe combination is secured in an upright fashion, with the probe placed through the irrigation sheath. Irrigant is then run through the irrigation sheath during testing. A test stone is placed atop the probe tip, which is visible through an acrylic cylinder fitted on the end of the irrigation sheath. The weighted rod is then placed atop the test stone, providing a constant force against the test stone.

This system was first utilized to evaluate the efficiency of 5 pure ultrasonic lithotripter devices. These units were the Olympus LUS-1 and LUS-2 (Olympus, Melville, NY), the Circon-ACMI USL-2000 (Circon-ACMI, Southborough, MA), the Karl Storz Calcuson (Karl Storz, Culver City, CA), and Richard Wolf model 2271.004 (Richard Wolf, Vernon Hills, IL). The endpoint of this study was to determine the mean penetration times achieved by each ultrasonic unit in treating groups of U-30 stones.

TABLE 1. Summary of Ultrasonic Lithotripter efficiency ratios

Ultrasonic lithotripter	Efficiency ratio (Mean ± SD)*
Olympus LUS-2	1.0 ± 0.1
Circon-ACMI USL-2000	1.1 ± 0.3
Karl Storz Calcuson	1.4 ± 0.3
Olympus LUS-1	2.1 ± 0.5
Richard Wolf 2271.004	3.6 ± 0.8

* Lower numbers translate to higher efficiency. Data from reference 15.

In this study, all units were utilized at 100% output (power). The Olympus LUS-2 produced the fastest overall mean penetration time of 28.8 ± 2.7 seconds. When this value was used to normalize all other mean penetration times into efficiency ratios, the results are summarized in Table 1.

The results showed that the Olympus LUS-2 and Circon-ACMI USL-2000 units performed at an essentially equivalent efficiency, with all other differences statistically significant by ANOVA using the Tukey-Kramer HSD test.

THE DEVELOPMENT OF NEW COMBINATION ICL DEVICES

To overcome the aforementioned disadvantages of traditional ultrasonic and pneumatic devices, newer ICL devices have attempted to combine these modalities to provide better efficiency of stone treatment. The first of these devices is termed the Lithoclast Ultra (Boston Scientific Corporation, Natick, MA). The other device is called the Cyberwand (Gyrus/ACMI, Southborough, MA).

Lithoclast Ultra

This device combines both pneumatic and ultrasonic lithotripsy through the use of a combination handpiece, which is actually two separate handpieces connected together. The first portion of this combination handpiece is a traditionally designed pneumatic handle with a smaller diameter solid probe which is 1 mm in diameter. The ultrasonic handle, while still driven by a piezoelectric mechanism, is modified to allow insertion of the pneumatic probe through it and then subsequent anchoring of the pneumatic handle. As such, the pneumatic probe is positioned within the hollow ultrasonic probe lumen. Each energy modality can be activated either separately or concurrently during stone treatment, which theoretically allows the quick ballistic fragmentation of a large bulk of stone and then treatment completion with concurrent removal of fragments with the ultrasonic probe.

Because of the wide variety of ultrasonic power and pneumatic frequency settings available with the Lithoclast Ultra device, the testing apparatus designed and utilized by our group for the evaluation of ultrasonic lithotripters was used to assess the efficiency of various setting combinations [17]. Ultrasonic output (power) settings of 40, 70, and 100% were used in concert with pneumatic frequency settings of 1, 4, 8, and 12 Hz. Again, the endpoint used was the mean penetration time achieved using each setting combination with groups of U-30 stones. The pneumatic probe was positioned flush with the end of the ultrasound probe for this study.

The results showed that the setting combination with both the highest ultrasonic output and pneumatic frequency (100% and 12 Hz) produced the fastest mean penetration time of 8.9 ± 1.1 seconds. Notably, the mean penetration times achieved with any combination setting was still faster than the most efficient pure ultrasonic lithotripter, the Olympus LUS-2. Mean penetration times were also compared with ANOVA. As shown in Fig. 2, the analysis revealed that incremental increases in ultrasonic output as well as pneumatic frequency resulted in statistically significant reductions in penetration times (p=0.001 and p<0.001, respectively). However, the pneumatic modality produced the greatest reductions in penetration times.

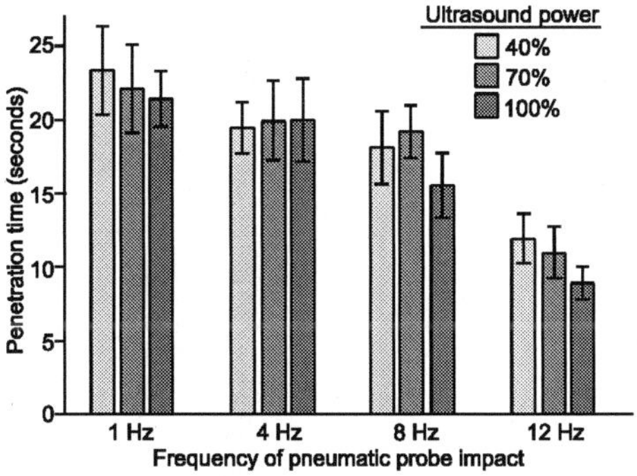

FIGURE 2. Summary of mean penetration times (seconds) achieved with Lithoclast Ultra unit on *y axis* with pneumatic frequency settings on *x axis* and ultrasonic output settings of 40% in green, 70% in orange, and 100% in red. Using ANOVA, increases in pneumatic frequency settings had a much greater proportional effect on decreasing mean penetration times compared to increases in ultrasound output, though each modality produced statistically significant effects.

Pietrow, *et al* have evaluated the efficacy of the Lithoclast Ultra device in a clinical setting in a prospective, randomized trial in 20 consecutive PNL patients comparing treatment and clearance times achieved with the Ultra to those using the Olympus LUS-2 ultrasonic lithotripter [18]. In this trial, the mean stone areas and locations were similar in both patient groups, with the Ultra patients having a mean stone area of 809.2 mm^2 and the LUS-2 patients an area of 795.5 mm^2. The mean stone clearance times were 21.1 minutes for the Ultra, compared to 43.7 minutes for the LUS-2. This translated to a stone clearance rate of 39.5 mm^2/min for the Ultra and 16.8 mm^2/min for the LUS-2. Clearance differences were statistically significant.

Despite the apparent clinical advantages provided by the Lithoclast Ultra, a number of characteristics can detract from the clinical experience with this device. First of all, the combination handpiece can be quite heavy and cumbersome to use. In addition, with the pneumatic probe within the lumen of the ultrasonic probe, fragments can sometimes clog the unit. In addition, the ballistic effect of the pneumatic probe can propel stone fragments away, counteracting the suction of the ultrasonic probe. A new, modified combination handle is in development and may address some of these issues.

Cyberwand

The Cyberwand is a unique device which utilizes a dual probe configuration to deliver both vibrational and ballistic energy to treat stones. This unit has been recently evaluated *in vitro* by Kim *et al* [19]. Unlike the Lithoclast Ultra, this unit utilizes a single handpiece powered through a piezoelectric mechanism. Vibrational energy at approximately 21,000 Hz from the handpiece is transmitted directly through the inner probe in the same manner as a traditional ultrasonic lithotripter. However, the vibrational energy conveyed to the outer probe is dampened through the use of a free mass and spring loaded mechanism which essentially reduces the vibrational frequency to 1,000 Hz and allows limited excursion of the outer probe tip to produce the ballistic "jackhammer" effect on a stone's surface.

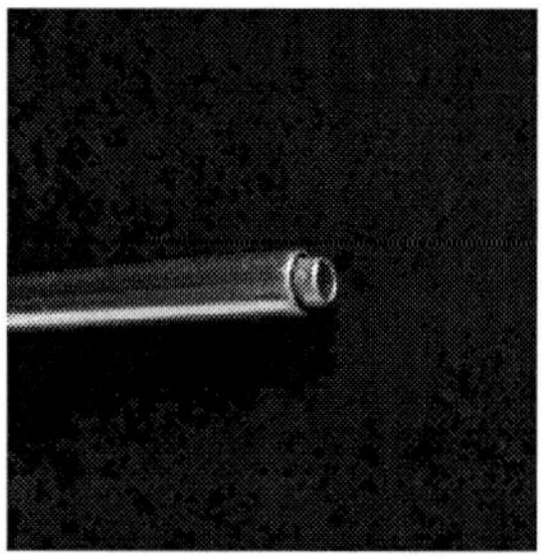

FIGURE 3. Image of the tip of the Cyberwand device. Note the dual probe configuration. The inner, high-frequency probe extends approximately 1 mm beyond the outer, low-frequency probe, at rest.

Our group's *in vitro* ICL testing system has been used to compared penetration efficiency of the Cyberwand with the Lithoclast Ultra device [19]. In this study, which again used groups of U-30 stones, mean stone penetration times with both devices were determined and then compared with unpaired Student t-tests. The mean penetration time achieved by the Cyberwand was 4.8±0.6 seconds, compared to 8.1±0.6 seconds (p<0.0001) for the Lithoclast Ultra.

From a clinical standpoint, a multi-center, randomized, prospective trial is currently underway to compare the treatment efficiency of the Cyberwand device to the Olympus LUS-2 device during PNL.

CONCLUSIONS

Intracorporeal lithotripters are important devices utilized for the treatment of stones during PNL. Improvements in ICL design are ongoing and have resulted in new and potentially more efficient devices. The *in vitro* testing system utilized by our group has provided objective, reproducible results which have been useful in evaluating the efficiency of ICL devices. Prospective, randomized clinical trials continue to be important to confirm the findings from *in vitro* experiments.

ACKNOWLEDGMENTS

The author would like to acknowledge Ryan F. Paterson, M.D., Tiberio M. Siqueira, Jr., M.D., Samuel C. Kim, M.D., Erin K. Hatt, David Lounsbery, Philip Blomgren, James A. McAteer, Ph.D., James C. Williams, Jr., Ph.D., Andrew P. Evan, Ph.D., and James E. Lingeman, M.D. for their contributions to our group's ICL testing system.

REFERENCES

1. I. Fernstrom and B. Johansson, Scand *J Urol Nephrol* 10 (3), 257 (1976).
2. P. Aslan, R. L. Kuo, K. Hazel et al., *J Endourol* 13 (4), 251 (1999).
3. J. W. Segura and A. J. LeRoy, *Urology* 23 (5 Spec No), 7 (1984).
4. J. D. Denstedt, P. M. Eberwein, and R. R. Singh, *J Urol* 148 (3 Pt 2), 1088 (1992).
5. J. D. Denstedt, H. A. Razvi, E. Rowe et al., *J Urol* 153 (2), 535 (1995).
6. G. J. Vassar, K. F. Chan, J. M. Teichman et al., *J Endourol* 13 (3), 181 (1999).
7. M. Grasso, *Urology* 48 (2), 199 (1996).
8. J. M. Teichman, G. J. Vassar, J. T. Bishoff et al., *J Urol* 159 (1), 17 (1998).
9. Y. C. Jou, J. H. Shen, M. C. Cheng et al., Urology 65 (3), 454 (2005).
10. D. C. Cuellar and T. D. Averch, *J Endourol* 18 (8), 780 (2004).
11. R. L. Kuo, S. C. Kim, J. E. Lingeman et al., *J Urol* 170 (1), 149 (2003); R. L. Kuo, R. F. Paterson, T. M. Siqueira, Jr. et al., Urology 62 (1), 59 (2003).
12. R. W. Santa-Cruz, R. J. Leveillee, and A. Krongrad, *J Endourol* 12 (5), 417 (1998).
13. E. N. Liatsikos, C. Z. Dinlenc, J. D. Fogarty et al., *J Endourol* 15 (9), 925 (2001).
14. G. Haupt and A. Haupt, J Urol 170 (5), 1731 (2003).
15. R. L. Kuo, R. F. Paterson, T. M. Siqueira, Jr. et al., *J Urol* 170 (4 Pt 1), 1101 (2003).
16. J. A. McAteer, J. C. Williams, Jr., R. O. Cleveland et al., *Urol Res* 33 (6), 429 (2005).
17. R. L. Kuo, R. F. Paterson, T. M. Siqueira, Jr. et al., *J Endourol* 18 (2), 153 (2004).
18. P. K. Pietrow, B. K. Auge, P. Zhong et al., *J Urol* 169 (4), 1247 (2003).
19. S. C. Kim, B.R. Matlaga., W. Tinmouth et al., *J Urol* In press (2007).

Update On Erbium:YAG lithotripsy

Joel M.H. Teichman*, Hyun Wook Kang[+], Randolph D. Glickman[#], and Ashley J. Welch[+]

Division of Urology, Providence Healthcare, and Department of Urological Sciences, University of British Columbia, Vancouver, British Columbia, Canada, Department of Ophthalmology, University of Texas Health Science Center, San Antonio, TX[#], and Biomedical Optics Program, Department of Biomedical Engineering, University of Texas, Austin, TX[+]*

Abstract. The Holmium:YAG laser fragments stones by a photothermal mechanism. It produces tiny fragments compared to short pulse duration lasers which fragment stones by laser induced shockwave lithotripsy. Holmium:YAG lithotripsy fragments stones of all compositions, but fragments stones slowly. In an effort to achieve photothermal lithotripsy more efficiently, Erbium:YAG lithotripsy has been tested. The Erbium:YAG laser fragments stones up to 5 times more efficiently than the Holmium:YAG laser. Its principal limitation is that it is not transmitted well by currently available fibers. Erbium:YAG lithotripsy is more efficient than Holmium:YAG lithotripsy but it is not yet practical for clinical use with current technology.

Keywords: Erbium:YAG; Holmium:YAG; laser lithotripsy.
PACS: 42.62.–b; 79.20.Ds

INTRODUCTION

The Holmium:YAG laser (λ= 2100 nm) is the dominant tool used currently for intracorporeal laser lithotripsy.[1] It fragments stones of all compositions, is transmitted with small caliber low-OH silica fibers permitting its use in flexible ureteroscopy, and achieves high success rates clinically.[1,2,3,4] Holmium:YAG differs from a prior generation of laser lithotripsy devices (pulsed dye, alexandrite, and Q-switched lasers generally with pulse durations < 1.2 μsec) in that the Holmium:YAG laser has a relatively long pulse duration (generally 250-350 μsec). Short pulse duration lasers fragment stones by a photomechanical (or photoacoustic) mechanism whereas long pulse duration lasers fragment stones by a photothermal mechanism.[5] Increased understanding of the photothermal mechanism of Holmium:YAG lithotripsy has allowed researchers to consider alternate wavelengths that may fragment stones more efficiently than Holmium:YAG. The Erbium:YAG laser (λ=2900 nm) has been studied as it may provide some theoretical advantages over Holmium:YAG lithotripsy. In this paper, the mechanisms and limitations of Holmium:YAG and Erbium:YAG lithotripsy are reviewed.

CP900, *Renal Stone Disease, 1st Annual International Urolithiasis Research Symposium,* edited by A. P. Evan, J. E. Lingeman, and J. C. Williams, Jr.

METHODS, RESULTS AND DISCUSSION

Short Pulse Duration Lasers

Prior experience with short pulse duration lasers (less than 1 μsec) showed that stones fragment as a result of photomechanical effects.[5,6] With such short pulse durations, the laser pulse duration is shorter than the time it takes the acoustic wave to propagate out of the irradiated target volume (water or stone), so that laser-induced stresses accumulate. Stresses are confined when the target volume is relatively incompressible. Under such stress confinement, a cavitation bubble is produced. The cavitation bubble expands spherically in front of the optical fiber tip, collapses to a single focus, and releases a high intensity pressure wave in water as a result of the symmetric bubble collapse. The energy stored and released in the cavitation bubble is proportional to the third power of the maximum bubble radius. Thus, a large cavitation bubble expansion produces a correspondingly larger acoustic transient after the bubble collapses, especially in the case of spherical bubbles, in which the collapse energy is released nearly instantaneously.

Alexandrite and Q-switched lasers (pulse durations generally $\leq$ 500 nsec) produce such high peak powers (as a result of their ultrashort pulse durations) that the energy produces optical breakdown (plasma). Plasma formation requires an extremely high irradiance of $>10^{10}$ W/cm^2 and pulse durations less than 1 μs.[7,8] In either cavitation or plasma formation, the dominant mechanism is LISL.[6,9] Plasma formation is less effective than cavitation bubble collapse for lithotripsy. Depending on the exact pulse duration, a combination of plasma and cavitation may occur.[9]

Experiments with LISL show that when the cavitation bubble is not constrained by a boundary (such as a stone), large spherical bubbles are produced, and as a result of the r^3 relationship between bubble size and collapse pressure, a large shock wave is produced.[9] Conversely, when LISL is performed with the fiber in contact with the stone (and bubble expansion constrained by the stone), a lower collapse pressure, and less lithotripsy is produced. In unconstrained expansion of the cavitation bubble, LISL produces a shock wave that propagates in all directions away from the collapse focus. Thus, the fiber may be positioned in various orientations to the stone surface and still produce fragmentation. A common observation in LISL is that stone fragmentation is heterogeneous (Fig. 1), and often produces large fragment pieces.[6,9] When LISL is compared for irradiation of stones in water versus dry stones in air, greater fragmentation occurs in water, because the water is required for the cavitation bubble to occur. In contrast, LISL in the absence of water can fragment stones by plasma, but less efficiently than cavitation.[9] Because the pulsed dye laser fragments stones as a result of the acoustic transient produced by the collapse of the cavitation bubble, fragmentation does not occur during the bubble stage.[9] Stone fragmentation occurs easily for stones of some compositions (calcium oxalate dehydrate and struvite) and poorly if at all for stones of other compositions (calcium oxalate monohydrate, brushite, and cystine).[10] Recent observations with the frequency doubled

Neodymium:YAG (FREDDY) laser show similar phenomena, as one would expect given its short pulse duration.[11]

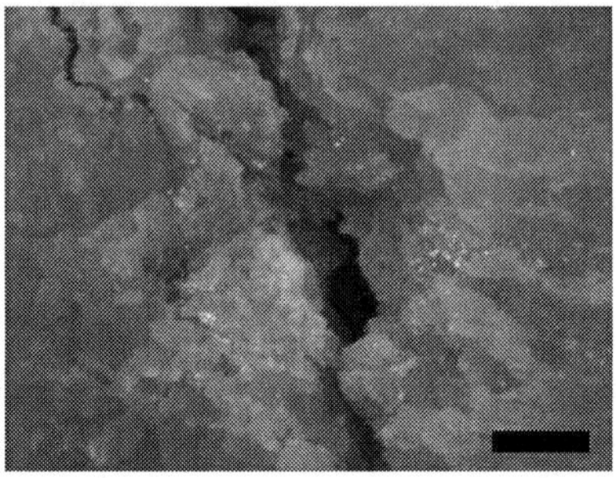

FIGURE 1. Irregular, heterogeneous fragmentation fissure created by Q-switched Nd:YAG laser (λ=1064 nm), pulse duration 6 ns, 30 pulses on surface of cystine stone, radiant exposure 15 J/cm^2. Bar represents 1 mm. (Photo from Kang HW, Teichman JMH, Welch AJ: unpublished data.)

Long Pulse Holmium:YAG Laser Lithotripsy

From its initial clinical use, the Holmium:YAG laser appeared to work differently than the short pulse duration lasers. The Holmium:YAG laser fragments stones of all compositions, including calcium oxalate monohydrate, brushite, and cystine.[2,3,12] It produces smaller fragments than short pulse duration lasers.[3] It produces symmetrical ablation craters on the stone surface (Fig. 2), in contrast to the asymmetric fragmentation seen with short pulse duration lasers.[12,13]

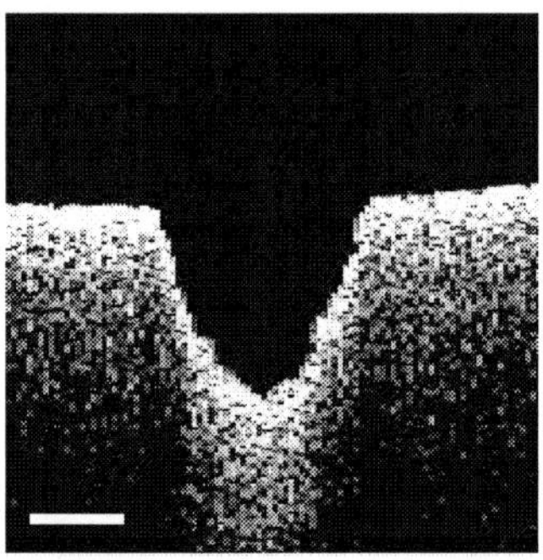

FIGURE 2. Optical computed tomography (OCT) image of cross-section of stone surface after Holmium:YAG irradiation (pulse duration 150 μs, pulse energy 800 mJ, single pulse, 273 μm fiber). In contrast to LISL (Fig. 1), the crater is symmetric and regular, and fragments are smaller [3]. The bar (lower left) represents 200 μm. (Photo from Kang HW, Teichman JMH, Welch AJ: unpublished data.)

Several groups have documented the paucity of photomechanical effects from the long pulse Holmium:YAG laser.[14,15] In a set of experiments, Vasser et al. demonstrated the photothermal mechanism of Holmium:YAG lithotripsy.[16] Ablation of stones of uniform composition was studied in several conditions: hydrated stones irradiated in a water bath, hydrated stones irradiated in air, or dehydrated stones irradiated in air. The greatest stone loss was observed for dehydrated stones irradiated in air implying direct irradiation as the most efficient means to fragment the stone, exactly the opposite findings observed for LISL. High-speed imaging showed that fragmentation begins to occur approximately 60 μsec into the 250 μsec pulse duration, implying direct irradiation as the mechanism of lithotripsy, in contrast to the time sequence of bubble collapse and subsequent fragmentation with the pulsed dye laser. The orientation of the fiber in relation to the stone surface was also tested. When the fiber was positioned tangential to the stone surface (90° laser incident angle, or 0° angle as it appears in parallel with the stone surface), a large vapor bubble was produced, but no lithotripsy occurred on the stone surface either during or after vapor bubble expansion and collapse. In contrast, when the fiber was oriented at a right angle to the stone surface (0° laser incident angle), a smaller vapor bubble occurred (because vapor bubble expansion is limited by the stone) and fragmentation occurred, implying that fluence on the stone surface correlates with lithotripsy, in contrast to LISL where the largest vapor bubble produces the most fragmentation. Greater mass loss was seen when stones at room temperature were irradiated compared to irradiation of stones at -70° C. Photothermal breakdown products were recovered for all stone compositions. Pressure transients were also negligible (generally < 20 bars, Fig. 3). These experiments demonstrate that Holmium:YAG lithotripsy occurs by direct irradiation of the stone, and is a photothermal process, without LISL. Other groups have reported similar findings.[14,17] The photothermal mechanism helps to explain the symmetric and consistent ablation craters (Fig. 2).[2,12,13]

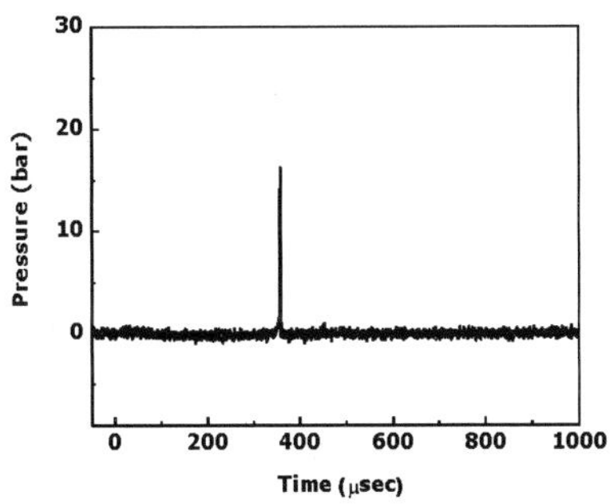

FIGURE 3. Collapse pressure transients during Holmium:YAG lithotripsy (pulse duration 150 μs, pulse energy 800 mJ). The pulsed dye laser, in contrast, generates a pressure transient over 300 times greater magnitude than Holmium:YAG laser.[13] (Photo from Kang HW, Teichman JMH, Welch AJ: unpublished data.)

The difference between laser lithotripsy devices that use photomechanical and photothermal mechanisms is derived primarily from the pulse duration, and not from differences in wavelength. When an experimental Holmium:YAG laser with variable pulse duration was set at 500 nsec (ultrashort pulse duration), a spherical vapor bubble was produced, and after collapse of the vapor bubble, ripples in the water occurred as evidence of photomechanical effects.[18] In contrast, when the same experimental

Holmium:YAG laser was set to a pulse duration of 260 μsec, a pear-shaped vapor bubble occurred (Fig. 4), with multiple collapse loci, and no significant ripples or mechanical effects observed. In contrast to a spherical bubble, an asymmetric bubble produces a small shock wave, because the bubble takes longer to collapse and releases its energy over a longer time frame.[9] This experiment demonstrates that the same wavelength can produce photomechanical or photothermal effects, based on the pulse duration. The wavelength (2100 nm) is close to the peak absorption of water, so that Holmium:YAG lithotripsy is clinically safe as excess energy is well absorbed in water surrounding the target stone.[19]

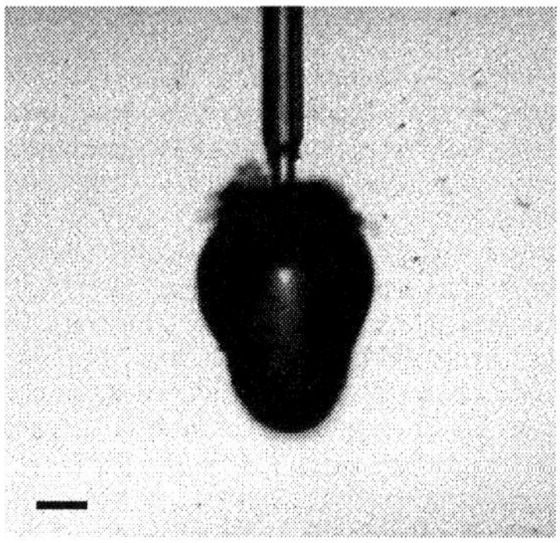

FIGURE 4. Holmium:YAG (pulse duration 260 μs, pulse energy 1.2 J, 365 μm fiber) vapor bubble in advance of the optical fiber. The fiber is positioned in still water (no stone). The vapor bubble is pear-shaped, with an asymmetric collapse, multiple collapse loci, and minimal pressure transients. The bar (lower left) represents 365 μm. (Photo from Kang HW, Teichman JMH, Welch AJ: Unpublished data.)

Lasers using photomechanical or photothermal lithotripsy mechanisms differ in several clinical aspects (Table 1). Holmium:YAG lithotripsy is highly directional, whereas LISL may fragment stones in multiple fiber-stone orientations. The photothermal effect of the Holmium:YAG laser follows the laser range equation, with maximal ablation achieved at a normal incident angle, and no ablation achieved at a 90° incident angle.[16] Moreover, at normal incident angle, there is minimal pressure transients (due to limitation of bubble expansion from the stone) whereas at 90° incident angle there are greater pressure transients. In effect, Holmium:YAG fragmentation occurs when no pressure transients occur, but in the presence of pressure transients and absence of direct irradiation no lithotripsy occurs, because direct optical absorption is the critical factor in lithotripsy.[16] This point was demonstrated in a comparison of Holmium:YAG and pulsed dye lasers where laser fibers were tested near a stone. The pulsed dye laser generated a shockwave 332 times more intense than the Holmium:YAG laser. Holmium:YAG lithotripsy was shown to occur independent of shockwaves.[15] Ablation efficiency of the Holmium:YAG lithotripsy correlates with the incident angle, consistent with its photothermal mechanism.[20,21,22] Holmium:YAG lithotripsy produces symmetric ablation craters with tiny "powderized" fragments whereas LISL produces asymmetric, large fragments.[2,3] Holmium:YAG lithotripsy fragments all stone compositions whereas

LISL often fails to fragment calcium oxalate monohydrate, brushite, and cystine stones.[10,11] Holmium:YAG lithotripsy is most efficient with no separation distance between the fiber tip and stone surface, whereas LISL is most efficient with a small separation distance (1-2 mm) to permit cavitation bubble expansion.[9,16]

The main limitation of Holmium:YAG lithotripsy is that the small ablation craters and "powderized" fragments translate to a slow (inefficient) lithotripsy process. Whereas a few pulses of the pulsed dye laser may fragment a stone into multiple "chunks", Holmium:YAG lithotripsy requires a longer duration of irradiation as the stone is "resected". Pyroelectric imaging of the output from the fibers shows that Holmium:YAG laser output conforms closely to a nearly Gaussian distribution of photons emerging from the fiber tip.[23] This near-Gaussian distribution mirrors the configuration of the ablation craters. Moreover, the size of the ablation craters correlates with the irradiation energy.[24] The more energy delivered to the stone, the larger the ablation craters are. As noted, Holmium:YAG lithotripsy is most efficient with the optical fiber in contact with the stone surface, as direct irradiation produces lithotripsy, contrasted to LISL where fiber stone separation permits maximum cavitation bubble expansion and high collapse pressures. However, even with a modest separation distance between the fiber tip and stone surface Holmium:YAG lithotripsy still occurs. With the fiber not in contact, the Holmium:YAG vapor bubble expands until a vapor channel bridges the gap between fiber and stone surface, and then efficient transmission of Holmium:YAG energy occurs between the fiber and the stone surface through a vapor window (the "Moses" effect).[6,15,18] Figure 4 shows the "Moses" effect can extend nearly 2 mm.

One strategy to make Holmium:YAG lithotripsy more efficient is to ramp up the power settings on the laser to deliver the maximal energy possible into the stone [22]. The problem with this strategy is that high pulse energy reduces the safety profile, increases stone retropulsion, and is associated with fiber tip degradation above 1.0 J.[25] Retropulsion occurs from various mechanisms. With the Holmium:YAG laser, both vapor bubble expansion and fragment ejection play causative roles. Retropulsion increases with pulse energy density, but paradoxically increases with fiber diameter.[24] One would have predicted that retropulsion should decrease with fiber diameter, as energy density is greatest with small caliber fibers.[2] However, plume ejection off the stone surface always occurs at a right angle to the incident laser angle.[24] The inference is that large diameter fibers produce wide, shallow craters compared to small diameter fibers that produce narrow, deep craters. Fragments ejecting off a relatively flat crater surface (as occurs with large diameter fibers) will therefore produce more recoil momentum compared to fragments ejecting off a narrow deep crater.[24] Retropulsion can be reduced using the longest pulse duration available on variable pulse Holmium:YAG laser units.[26,27] Less retropulsion means that the urologist does not need to chase the stone and that each pulse transmits more efficiently directly into the stone rather than wasting some energy into the water because of the separation distance produced from retropulsion.

Erbium:YAG Lithotripsy

Another strategy to make photothermal lithotripsy more efficient is to use efficient wavelengths.[28] Chan et al. irradiated calcium oxalate monohydrate, uric acid, struvite, and cystine stones with a Free Electron Laser.[29] For stones composed of >95% pure uric acid, cystine, calcium oxalate monohydrate, and struvite, more efficient energy absorption occurred at 2.9-3.1 μm compared to 2.1 μm. This increased efficiency was attributed to higher optical absorption coefficients in the stone matrices at the longer wavelengths. The threshold fluence to initiate lithotripsy was lower at 2.9 μm versus 2.1 μm wavelengths by factors of 5.6 for cystine, 15.7 for calcium oxalate monohydrate, and 20.8 for uric acid. The ablation depths were greater for 2.9 μm versus 2.1 μm wavelengths. Less energy is required to initiate lithotripsy at 2.9 μm wavelength compared to the 2.1 μm wavelength, so that relatively more of the 2.9 μm energy goes towards fragmentation. Since the Erbium:YAG laser emits at 2.9-2.94 μm, it was a logical choice for laser lithotripsy.

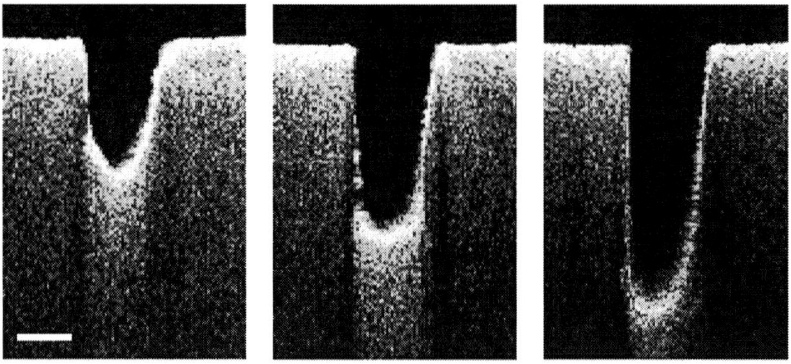

FIGURE 5. OCT cross-sectional images of uric acid stones after 5 pulses of Erbium:YAG lithotripsy (pulse duration 275 μs, 365 μm fiber.) The pulse energy shown is 170 mJ/pulse (left), 294 mJ/pulse (center), and 487 mJ/pulse (right). Bar in lower left corner of left image represents 300 μm. The crater geometries are symmetric and regular, consistent with photothermal lithotripsy. The increased crater size for increased pulse energy is similar to Holmium:YAG lithotripsy. (Photo from Kang HW, Teichman JMH, Welch AJ: unpublished data.)

Erbium:YAG lithotripsy (pulse duration 275 μsec) produces bubble dynamics similar to those of the long pulse Holmium:YAG laser (Fig. 6).[30] In still water, Erbium:YAG produces a vapor bubble that expands more torpedo-like or cigar-shaped, compared to the pear-shaped Holmium:YAG vapor bubble. The expansion time and asymmetric collapse are similar to Holmium:YAG. As evidence of increased photothermal lithotripsy efficiency compared to Holmium:YAG, plume ejection from the stone surface occurs as early as 10 μsec into the Erbium:YAG pulse duration (compared to 60 μsec for Holmium:YAG) (Fig. 7).

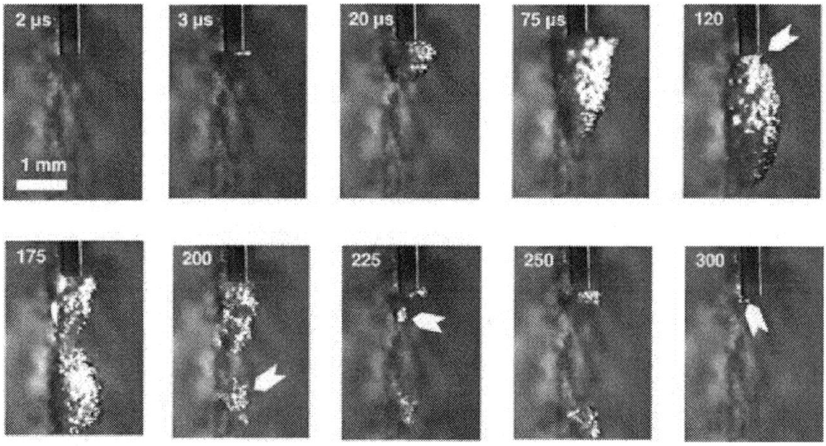

FIGURE 6. Erbium:YAG vapor bubble dynamics. Optical fiber is seen at top of each image immersed in still water. Initial bubble formation and expansion occur at 3 µsec. There are primary, secondary, and tertiary bubble collapses seen at 120, 220 to 225 and 300 µsec, respectively (arrows) From [30], used with permission.

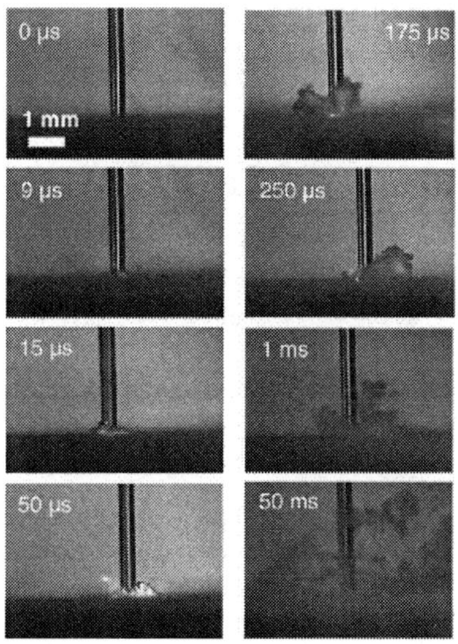

FIGURE 7. Vapor bubble dynamics with 425 µm sapphire optical fiber in contact with stone surface. Fiber is oriented perpendicular to stone surface. Fragment ejection (lithotripsy) occurs as early as 15 µsec. The boundary created by the stone surface constrains bubble expansion. In contrast, in still water unconstrained bubble expansion occurs (Fig. 6). From [30], used with permission.

Like Holmium:YAG, Erbium:YAG vapor bubbles produce a paucity of photomechanical effects (Fig. 8). Moreover, Erbium:YAG irradiation of multiple stone compositions produces consistently symmetrical ablation craters, with no evidence of fracture, consistent with a photothermal mechanism and lack of LISL (Fig. 5).[31]

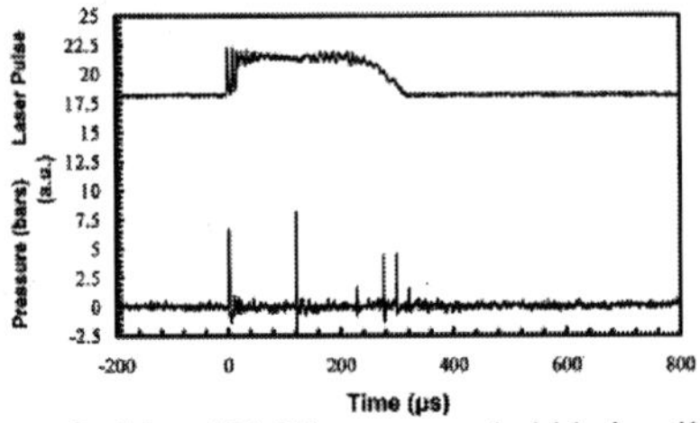

FIGURE 8. Acoustic transients of erbium:YAG laser vapor bubble in still water. Note initial expansion wave and collapse waves at bubble collapses at 120, 220 and 300 μsec. Erbium:YAG bubble collapse does not produce photoacoustic fragmentation. From [30], used with permission.

A head to head comparison between Erbium:YAG and Holmium:YAG lithotripsy was conducted. In one comparison, both lasers were set at 50 mJ pulse energy settings and delivered with a 425 μm sapphire optical fiber.[32] Erbium:YAG achieved greater fragmentation compared to Holmium:YAG for both calcium oxalate monohydrate and cystine stones. Fragment sizes were slightly larger for Erbium:YAG compared to Holmium:YAG lithotripsy. In a second comparison, stones were irradiated with a total of 100 J energy from either the Erbium:YAG laser (50 mJ pulse setting, 425 μm sapphire fiber) or the Holmium:YAG laser (500 mJ pulse setting, 365 μm low-OH silica fiber). Fragmentation still favored Erbium:YAG but the differences were not as great as in the first comparison. Thus, joule for joule, Erbium:YAG is more efficient for lithotripsy than Holmium:YAG energy. A less powerful Erbium:YAG laser would also suffice for lithotripsy compared to the power needs of a Holmium:YAG laser. But clinically, one can easily ramp up the energy settings on the Holmium:YAG laser in order to produce roughly comparable fragmentation as with the Erbium:YAG laser, e.g., the Holmium:YAG laser at 500 mJ pulse energy and 10 Hz (5W) approximates the ablation produced by the Erbium:YAG laser delivering 200 mJ pulse energy at 10 Hz (2W). In fact, since most urologists use a pulse energy of 0.6 – 1.0 J pulse energy, Holmium:YAG lithotripsy achieves faster ablation speed than a putative Erbium:YAG laser, even if the energy characteristics of the Erbium:YAG laser are more efficient than Holmium:YAG, joule for joule.

For Holmium:YAG lithotripsy, low OH- silica fibers are readily available and relatively inexpensive. These fibers attenuate energy transmission above 1700 nm, but still have acceptably low absorption of optical energy at 2100 nm. But above 2500 nm, energy is not well transmitted by low OH- silica fibers. For Erbium:YAG applications, current available fiber choices are germanium or sapphire fibers. Both fibers have some limitations. Sapphire appears to be the better choice as germanium fibers show degradation with 50% reduction in transmission with as few as 50 pulses at 100 mJ pulse energy (Fig. 9). But even using the more robust sapphire fibers, Erbium:YAG energy transmission does not transmit well above 200 mJ pulse energy.

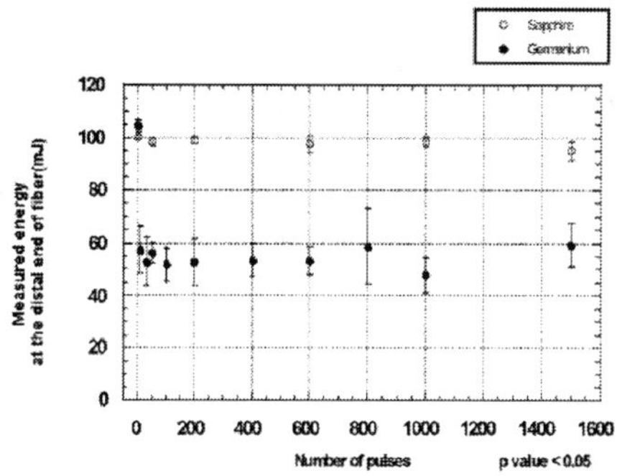

FIGURE 9. Degradation of 450 µm germanium versus 425 µm sapphire fibers for Erbium:YAG lithotripsy. Fibers were placed in contact with >95% pure struvite stone in water and Erbium:YAG laser set at 275 µs pulse duration, 100 mJ pulse energy. (Photo from Kang HW, Teichman JMH, Welch AJ: Unpublished data.)

Does Erbium:YAG have any lithotripsy advantages over Holmium:YAG energy? To answer this question, Erbium:YAG and Holmium:YAG laboratory lasers were tested on stones, with laser beam transmission focused via a lens through an air window onto the stone surface.[29] The laser beams were calibrated and shown to be virtually identical for focal length, beam width, beam profile, and energy density. Pulse energies were varied between 0.2 J and 1.0 J. Thus, any differences in fragmentation between lasers could be attributed to differences in wavelength and not to delivery systems. For all stone compositions and all pulse energies, single pulse Erbium:YAG lithotripsy produced crater volumes roughly 5 times greater than for single pulse Holmium:YAG lithotripsy. When five successive pulses were directed at the same stone surface, the crater volumes were roughly 3 times greater for Erbium:YAG lithotripsy compared to Holmium:YAG lithotripsy. This diminution may reflect debris shielding, where the ejected fragment plume acts as a shield and absorbs some of the subsequent incoming laser energy. This debris shielding may be minimized using irrigation.

TABLE 1. Contrast between short and long pulse duration lasers for lithotripsy

	Short pulse duration lasers	**Long pulse duration laser**
Examples (pulse duration)	Pulsed dye (1.2 µsec), alexandrite (500 ns)	Holmium:YAG (250 µsec), Erbium:YAG (275 µsec)
Bubble geometry	Spherical, symmetrical	Pear-shaped, asymmetrical
Lithotripsy mechanism	Cavitation, plasma, LISL	photothermal
Lithotripsy occurs...	After bubble collapse	During bubble
Lithotripsy most efficient in...	Water	Air
Fiber tip best positioned...	1 mm separation from stone	In contact with stone
Pressure transients	> 600 bars	< 20 bars
Fragments...	Some compositions	All stone compositions
Fragment size	Large chunks	Small fragments (<1 mm)

The clinical challenge is therefore to find a fiber delivery system for Erbium:YAG lithotripsy. As discussed already, sapphire appears to be more robust than germanium, but still does not transmit energy at sufficiently high pulses to be clinically practical. Moreover, sapphire fibers are not commercially available in diameters small enough for use in flexible ureteroscopy. Recent experiments using a hollow waveguide show promise. The hollow waveguide can be produced in small caliber fibers for flexible ureteroscopy, although transmission at the fiber tip has been occasionally problematic, with evidence of hot spots and irregular ablation craters. Until a laser delivery system is developed that overcomes the technical challenges of efficient transmission of mid-infrared wavelengths, and ability to conduct high power laser pulses without damage, the Erbium:YAG laser will not be practical for lithotripsy.

CONCLUSIONS

Lasers can fragment urinary calculi using either photomechanical or photothermal mechanisms, dependent primarily on the laser pulse duration. Holmium:YAG and Erbium:YAG lasers have a relatively long pulse duration and fragment stones by a photothermal mechanism. Erbium:YAG lithotripsy is more efficient than Holmium:YAG lithotripsy, but lithotripsy speed can easily be increased with Holmium:YAG lasers given the efficient transmission of energy using low OH- silica fibers. Erbium:YAG lithotripsy is not yet practical given current technology.

ACKNOWLEDGMENTS

Figures 6-8 are reprinted from *Journal of Urology*, Volume 168, Chan KF, Lee H, Teichman JMH, Kamerer A, McGuff HS, Vargas G, Welch AJ: "Erbium:YAG laser lithotripsy mechanism", pages 436-441, copyright 2002, with permission from American Urological Association.

REFERENCES

1. Sofer M, Watterson JD, Wollin TA, Nott L, Razvi H, Denstedt JD: Holmium:YAG laser lithotripsy for upper tract urinary calculi in 598 patients. *J Urol* **167**: 31-4 (2002).
2. Vassar GJ, Teichman JMH, Glickman RD: Holmium:YAG lithotripsy efficiency varies with energy density. *J Urol* **160**: 471-6 (1998).
3. Teichman JMH, Vassar GJ, Bishoff JT, Bellman GC: Holmium:YAG lithotripsy yields smaller fragments than Lithoclast, pulsed dye or electrohydraulic lithotripsy. *J Urol* **159**: 17-25 (1998).
4. Grasso M, Ficazzola M: Retrograde ureteropyeloscopy for lower pole caliceal calculi. *J Urol.* **162**:1904-8 (1999).
5. Jacques SL: Laser-tissue interactions. Photochemical, photothermal, and photomechanical. *Surg Clin North Am.* **72**:531-58 (1992).
6. Chan KF, Pfefer TJ, Teichman JMH, Welch AJ: A perspective on laser lithotripsy: the fragmentation processes. *J Endourol.* **15**:257-73 (2001).
7. Fradin DW, Bloembergen N and Letellier JP: Dependence of laser-induced breakdown field strength on pulse duration. *Appl Phys Lett* **22**: 635-637 (1973).

8. Doukas AG, Zweig AD, Frisoli JK, Birngruber R and Deutsch TF: Noninvasive determination of shock wave pressure generated by optical breakdown. *Appl Phys B* **53**: 237-245 (1991).
9. Rink K, Delacretaz G, Salathe RP: Fragmentation process of current laser lithotriptors. *Lasers Surg Med.* **16**:134-46 (1995).
10. Dretler SP: An evaluation of ureteral laser lithotripsy: 225 consecutive patients. *J Urol.* **143**: 267-72 (1990).
11. Dubosq F, Pasqui F, Girard F, Beley S, Lesaux N, Gattegno B, Thibault P, Traxer O: Endoscopic lithotripsy and the FREDDY laser: initial experience. *J Endourol.* **20**: 296-9 (2006).
12. Teichman JMH, Vassar GJ, Glickman RD: Holmium:yttrium-aluminum-garnet lithotripsy efficiency varies with stone composition. *Urology* **52**: 392-7 (1998).
13. Teichman JMH, Rao RD, Rogenes VJ, Harris JM: Ureteroscopic management of ureteral calculi: electrohydraulic versus Holmium:YAG lithotripsy. *J Urol* **158**:1357-61 (1997).
14. Schmidlin FR, Beghuin D, Delacretaz GP, Venzi G, Jichlinksi P, Rink K, Leisinger H-J, Graber P: Laser lithotripsy with the Ho:YAG laser: fragmentation process revealed by time-resolved imaging. *SPIE* **3245**.123S (1998).
15. Zhong P, Tong HL, Cocks FH, Pearle MS, Preminger GM: Transient cavitation and acoustic emission produced by different laser lithotripters. *J Endourol.* **12**:371-8 (1998).
16. Vassar GJ, Chan KF, Teichman JM, Glickman RD, Weintraub ST, Pfefer TJ, Welch AJ: Holmium:YAG lithotripsy: photothermal mechanism. *J Endourol.* **13**:181-90 (1999).
17. Schafer SA, Durville FM, Jassemnejad B, Bartels KE, Powell RC: Mechanisms of biliary stone fragmentation using the Ho:YAG laser. *IEEE Trans Biomed Eng.* **41**:276-83 (1994).
18. Jansen ED, Asshauer T, Frenz M, Motamedi M, Delacretaz G, Welch AJ: Effect of pulse duration on bubble formation and laser-induced pressure waves during Holmium laser ablation. *Lasers Surg Med.* **18**:278-93 (1996).
19. Jansen ED, van Leeuwen TG, Motamedi M, Borst C, Welch AJ: Temperature dependence of the absorption coefficient of water for midinfrared laser radiation. *Lasers Surg Med* **14**:258-68 (1994).
20. Freiha GS, Glickman RD, Teichman JMH: Holmium:YAG laser-induced damage to guidewires: experimental study. *J Endourol.* **11**:331-6 (1997).
21. Teichman JMH, Rogenes VJ, McIver BJ, Harris JM: Holmium:yttrium-aluminum-garnet laser cystolithotripsy of large bladder calculi. *Urology* **50**:44-8 (1997).
22. Teichman JMH, Rao RD, Glickman RD, Harris JM: Holmium:YAG percutaneous nephrolithotomy: the laser incident angle matters. *J Urol.* **159**:690-4 (1998).
23. Lee H, Ryan RT, Teichman JMH, Landman J, Clayman RV, Milner TE, Welch AJ : Effect of lithotripsy on Holmium:YAG optical beam profile. *J Endourol.* **17**:63-7 (2003).
24. Lee H, Ryan RT, Teichman JMH, Kim J, Choi B, Arakeri NV, Welch AJ: Stone retropulsion during Holmium:YAG lithotripsy. *J Urol.* **169**:881-5 (2003).
25. Spore SS, Teichman JMH, Corbin NS, Champion PC, Williamson EA, Glickman RD: Holmium: YAG lithotripsy: optimal power settings. *J Endourol.* **13**:559-66 (1999).
26. Finley DS, Peterson J, Abdelshehid C, Ahlering M, Chou D, Borin J, Eichel L, McDougall E, Clayman RV: Effect of Holmium:YAG laser pulse width on lithotripsy retropulsion in vitro. *J Endourol.* **19**:1041-4 (2005).
27. Kang HW, Lee H, Teichman JMH, Oh J, Kim J, Welch AJ: Dependence of calculus retropulsion on pulse duration during Ho: YAG laser lithotripsy. *Lasers Surg Med.* **38**:762-72 (2006).
28. Daidoh Y, Arai T, Komine Y: Determination of optimum wavelength for laser photofragmentation of urinary stones. *J Endourol.* **5**: 245-9 (1991).
29. Chan KF, Hammer DX, Choi B, Teichman JMH, McGuff HS, Pratisto H, Jansen ED, Welch AJ: Free electron laser lithotripsy: threshold radiant exposures. *J Endourol.* **14**: 161-7 (2000).
30. Chan KF, Lee H, Teichman JMH, Kamerer A, McGuff HS, Vargas G, Welch AJ: Erbium:YAG laser lithotripsy mechanism. *J Urol.* **168**: 436-41 (2002).
31. Lee H, Kang HW, Teichman JMH, Oh J, Welch AJ: Urinary calculus fragmentation during Ho: YAG and Er:YAG lithotripsy. *Lasers Surg Med.* **38**:39-51 (2006).
32. Teichman JMH, Chan KF, Cecconi PP, Corbin NS, Kamerer AD, Glickman RD, Welch AJ: Erbium:YAG versus Holmium:YAG lithotripsy. *J Urol.* **165**: 876-9 (2001).

HOLMIUM LASER: PULSE DURATION

Demetrius H. Bagley[*] and Allyson C. Berent[†]

[*]*Jefferson Medical College, Department of Urology, 1025 Walnut Street, Room 1108, Philadelphia, PA 19107, USA*
[†]*Mathew J. Ryan Veterinary Hospital at the University of Pennsylvania, 3900 Delancey Street, Philadelphia, PA 19104-6010, USA*

Abstract. The addition of a variable pulse duration to lasers used for stone removal adds another factor which can modify the effect of the holmium laser on stone fragmentation. More complex combinations of variables with the other adjustable features of the laser may provide more effective stone fragmentation clinically.

Keywords: Urolithiasis
PACS: 79.20.Ds

INTRODUCTION

The holmium laser has become a standard and nearly essential device in endoscopic urologic practice. This laser can be used to fragment calculi and ablate or incise tissue. The laser energy is effectively delivered through flexible fibers in an aqueous medium.

There are relatively few variables which have been employed to alter the efficiency of stone fragmentation with the holmium laser. Each individual laser has controls to vary the energy per pulse and the frequency of the pulses. There are also options in fiber size adapted to each machine. Some more recent laser units also allow variation in the duration of the pulse.

These parameters alter the laser's effect on the target. They affect the fragmentation of calculi and the movement of the calculus during treatment. They also affect the ability to coagulate or to ablate or cut tissue. These effects also can be modified by variations in endoscopic technique and with positioning of the laser fiber relative to the target.

ENERGY DENSITY

The efficiency of holmium YAG laser lithotripsy varies with the density of the energy applied to the calculus. This effect was demonstrated in an *in vitro* study by Vassar *et al.* [1] which applied a range of energies per pulse to calcium oxalate monohydrate calculi through different fibers varying in size from 272 to 940 microns. Overall, the width of the crater produced on the surface of the stone increased with the pulse energy applied [1,2]. For any specific fiber, the stone loss increased with increasing energy per pulse. For any single energy studied, the loss of stone from the

CP900, *Renal Stone Disease, 1st Annual International Urolithiasis Research Symposium,* edited by A. P. Evan, J. E. Lingeman, and J. C. Williams, Jr.

surface increased with a smaller fiber size from 940 to 365 microns. This effect did not extend to the smallest fiber (272 microns) predominantly because of the degradation of the fiber itself.

STONE MOVEMENT

Stone movement increases with a higher pulse energy and also with increasing fiber size [2,3]. In the first study, White *et al.* [2] examined retropulsion of a stone model composed of silicate with a ferrous coating. Three variables—energy, frequency and fiber diameter—were studied. Movement of the model was determined in a clear rigid tube filled with saline. The maximum net retropulsion was examined. The consistent finding was increased movement with 365 and 550 micron fibers.

Lee *et al.* [3] studied this phenomenon more specifically using calculus phantoms composed of plaster of Paris. Their hypothesis that retropulsion occurred as the result of ejected stone debris was confirmed. They found that retropulsion increased as fiber diameter increased and as pulsed energy increased. They also noted that the crater geometry varied with fiber diameter. It was wide and shallow for the larger fibers and narrow and deeper for small fibers. The authors concluded that the crater geometry and the ejected plume of stone debris during fragmentation explained the retropulsion seen with larger optical fibers. They recommended that lithotripsy should be performed with smaller optical fibers to limit retropulsion.

THE "POPCORN" EFFECT

This effect of the laser, causing movement of the calculus, can be employed to maximize the efficiency of stone fragmentation and to reduce the size of multiple fragments of stone trapped within a calyx. Chawla *et al.* demonstrated these phenomena *in vitro* [4]. The authors used sodalime stone phantoms positioned within a test tube as the target. The laser fibers were directed at the fragments, in proximity but not touching them. The laser was then activated at specific settings, using 1 or 1.5 joules per pulse and 20, 30 or 40 hertz. Residual stone fragments were weighed to demonstrate the loss of stone. An increasing loss of weight was seen with higher frequencies (Fig. 1).

However, when the percent weight change was corrected by using the ratio to the kJ employed, the 1 joule setting appeared more efficient than the 1.5 joule and the greatest loss appeared at 20 hertz (Fig. 2). This study demonstrated that the clinically employed "popcorn" effect did, in fact, reduce the volume of stone. It also suggested an optimal setting of 1 joule and 20 Hz for clinical application.

PULSE DURATION

Most holmium lasers are set with a single pulse duration, usually either 250 or 350 microseconds. With a longer pulse duration, there is a lower peak energy delivered since the same total amount of energy is delivered over a longer time. At least two manufacturers have designed their lasers to offer a choice of a shorter or longer pulse duration. (Table 1).

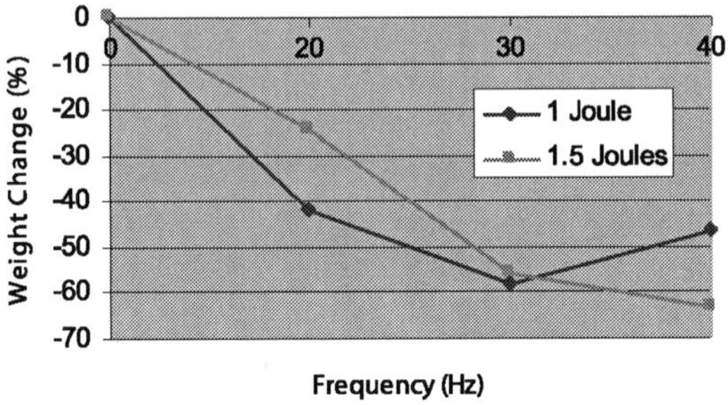

FIGURE 1. Percentage change in weight versus laser settings. From [4], used with permission.

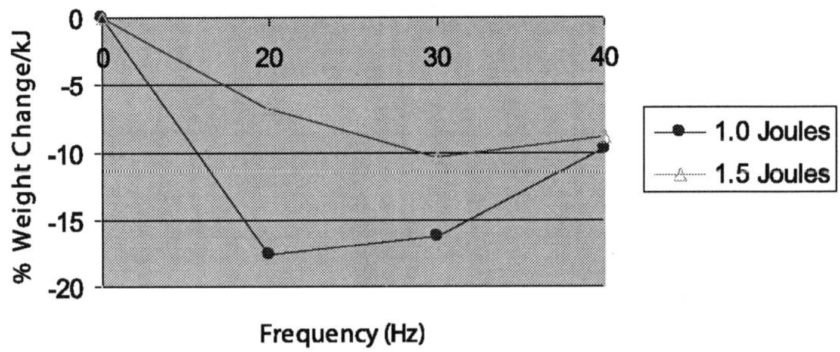

FIGURE 2. Efficiency of laser settings. From [4], used with permission.

Table 1. Variable pulse width Ho:YAG lasers

Manufacturer	Model	Duration (μsec)
Convergent°	Odyssey	350 or 700
LISA§	Sphinx	150 or 800

°Convergent Laser Technologies, 1660 S. Loop Road, Alameda, CA 94502; §LISA Laser Products OHG, Max-Planck-Str. 1, D-37191 Katlenburg-Lindau, Germany

Two studies have examined the effect of pulse duration on stone movement during fragmentation. Both were *in vitro* studies, one looking at the progression of stone along a tube and the other measuring the specific movement of phantoms. Finley *et al.* [5] applied a holmium laser at 1 joule and 10 Hz to a 10 mm plaster cast in a tube using two different fibers and two different pulse durations. They measured the time it took for the phantom to traverse the 8 cm tract in the model. For each size fiber, it took a shorter time to traverse the model with the 350 microsecond pulse duration. Thus, there was more movement with the shorter pulse duration.

In the second model in that study, ceramic phantom calculi were fragmented in a wire mesh calyx which minimized movement. The laser was applied during a 5 minute period with two different fibers at each pulse width. Fragmentation efficiency as measured by stone removal was similar for either pulse width using a 200 micron fiber. With the larger, 400 micron fiber, there was a significant increase in fragmentation efficiency with the longer pulse width.

Kalra *et al.* [6] also used two models to evaluate the effect of pulse width on the movement of objects *in vitro* during holmium activation. In the first model, a metal ball bearing lying within a saline-filled plastic tube was activated with a single laser pulse through either a 200 or 400 micron fiber. Two different pulse widths, 350 and 700 microseconds were employed. There was increased movement at the shorter pulse duration with both the 200 and 400 micron fibers. This effect was more apparent at higher energy settings. The movement increased with an increased energy per pulse. There was minimal effect of the energy setting seen with the 700 microsecond pulse duration (Figs. 3 and 4).

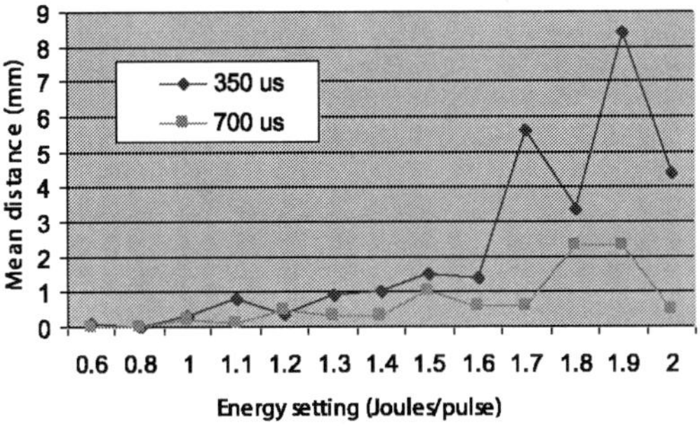

FIGURE 3. Ball bearing displacement after one pulse using a 200 μm fiber. From [6], used with permission.

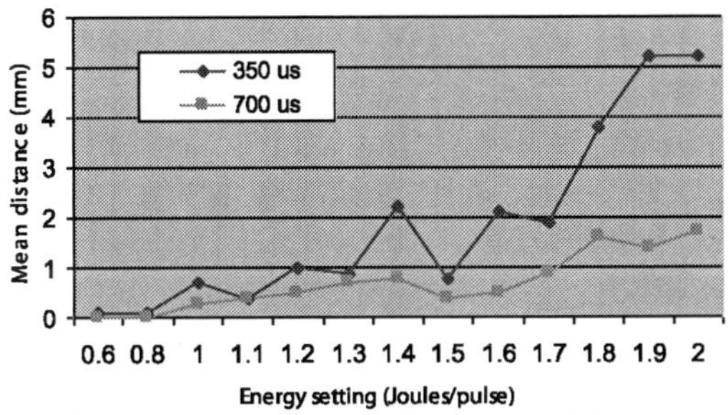

FIGURE 4. Ball bearing displacement after one pulse using a 400 μm fiber. From [6], used with permission.

In the second model employed in this study, sodalime phantoms were positioned in a horizontal plastic tube within saline. The laser was activated against the model until there was 2 mm of movement. At that point, the phantom had migrated out of contact with the fiber. The total energy delivered before movement of the phantom beyond the effective range was then calculated. Significantly, more energy could be delivered using the longer pulse width prior to phantom displacement. Inversely, there was more movement with the shorter pulse duration (Fig. 5).

In summary, in two studies in 4 different models, there was less movement of a targeted stone phantom with a longer pulse duration of the holmium laser. This effect was more apparent at higher energies per pulse. The specific clinical significance of this observation was not tested.

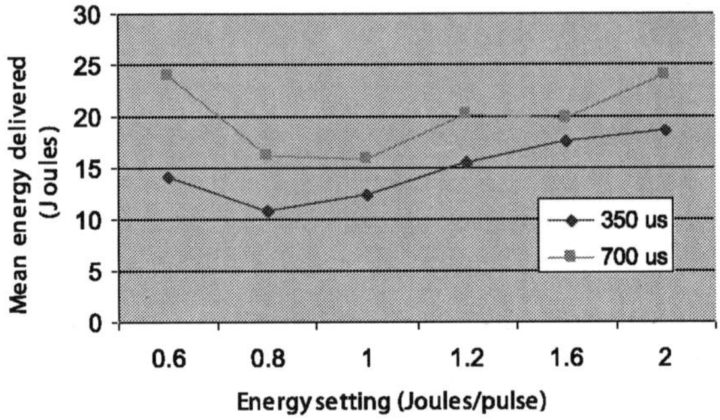

FIGURE 5. Total energy delivered to sodalime phantom prior to displacement. From [6], used with permission.

TISSUE EFFECT

There is no experimental information available regarding the effect of pulse width on cutting or ablation of tissue with the holmium YAG laser. Clinically, there appears to be better coagulation with the longer pulse duration (700 versus 350 microseconds). This requires confirmation in a quantifiable model.

CONCLUSION

The addition of a variable pulse duration adds another factor which can modify the effect of the holmium laser on stone fragmentation. More complex combinations of variables with the other adjustable features of the laser may provide more effective stone fragmentation clinically.

REFERENCES

1. Vassar GJ, Teichman JMH and Glickman RD: Holmium:YAG lithotripsy efficiency varies with energy density. *J Urol* 160: 471-476, 1998.
2. White MD, Moran ME, Calvano CJ, Borhan-Manesh A and Mehlhaff B: Evaluation of retropulsion caused by holmium:YAG laser with various power settings and fibers. *J Endourol* 12 (2) 183-186, 1998.
3. Lee H, Ryan RT, Teichman JMH, Kim J, Choi B, Arakeri N and Welch AJ: Stone retropulsion during holmium:YAG lithotripsy. *J Urol* 169: 881-885, 2003.
4. Chawla SM, Chang MF, Chang A, LeNoir J and Bagley DH: Efficacy of high frequency holmium:YAG laser stone fragmentation: "The Popcorn Effect". *J Endourol* 2007 (in press).
5. Finley DS, Petersen J, Abdelshehid C, Ahlering M, Chou D, Borin, J, Eichel L, McDougall E and Clayman R: Effect of Holmium:YAG laser pulse width on lithotripsy retropulsion in vitro. *J Endourol* 19 (8) 1041-1044, 2005.
6. Kalra P, Le N-B and Bagley DH: Effect of pulse width on object movement in-vitro using the holmium:YAG laser. *J. Endourol* 2007 (in press).

Percutaneous Access: Acute Effects on Renal Function and Structure in a Porcine Model

Rajash K. Handa[*†], Lynn R. Willis[*], Andrew P. Evan[†§], Bret A. Connors[†], Jun Ying[‡], William Fat-Anthony[*], Kelli R. Wind[*], Cynthia D. Johnson[*], Philip M. Blomgren[†], Mark C. Estrada[¶], Ryan F. Paterson[§], Ramsay L. Kuo[§], Samuel C. Kim[§], Brian R. Matlaga[§], Nicole L. Miller[§], Stephanie L. Watkins[§], Shelly E. Handa[§], and James E. Lingeman[§]

Depts of [*]Pharmacology & Toxicology, [†]Anatomy & Cell Biology, and [‡]Medicine, Indiana University School of Medicine, 635 Barnhill Drive, Medical Sciences Bldg, Indianapolis, IN 46202, USA

[¶]Indiana Radiology Partners, 714 North Senate Avenue, Suite 205, Indianapolis, IN 46202, USA

[§]Methodist Hospital Institute for Kidney Stone Disease, 1801 North Senate Boulevard, Suite 220, Indianapolis, IN 46202, USA

Abstract. Percutaneous nephrolithotomy (PCNL) involves gaining access into the urinary collecting system to remove kidney stones. Animal studies demonstrated that a reduction in renal filtration and perfusion in both kidneys, and a decline in tubular organic anion transport in the treated kidney characterizes the acute (hours) functional response to unilateral percutaneous access. The acute morphologic and histological changes in the treated kidney were consistent with blunt trauma and ischemia. Only tubular organic anion transport remained depressed during the late (3-day) response to the access procedure. Human studies revealed an acute decline in glomerular function and bilateral renal vasoconstriction following unilateral PCNL. Therefore, percutaneous access is not a benign procedure, but is associated with acute functional and structural derangements.

Keywords: Percutaneous access; percutaneous nephrolithotomy; tract dilation; kidney function.
PACS: 01.30.Cc

INTRODUCTION

Percutaneous nephrolithotomy (PCNL) has replaced open surgery as the preferred method to treat complex kidney stone disease. The procedure involves needle puncture from the skin surface into the urinary collecting system, which is then dilated and stabilized for the introduction of instrumentation that can view and remove stones. PCNL is associated with high stone free rates, low re-treatment rates, low incidence of complications and morbidity, as well as shorter durations in surgery and convalescence compared to open stone surgery [1-6]. Consequently, PCNL is regarded as a safe and efficient method for the treatment of nephrolithiasis.

Postoperative measurements of renal function have generally been taken several weeks, months or years after PCNL, and indicate that renal function is well preserved

CP900, *Renal Stone Disease, 1st Annual International Urolithiasis Research Symposium,*
edited by A. P. Evan, J. E. Lingeman, and J. C. Williams, Jr.

[7-10]. However, the immediate effects on renal function are unknown, and it is unclear whether surgical procedures—independent of stone removal—alter kidney function acutely. Nor is it known whether the two most common methods of dilating the percutaneous access tract—balloon and serial dilators—have similar or differing effects on renal function and structure. We have begun to address these and other issues in a pig model and in patients, and provide the reader with some of our findings.

ANIMAL STUDIES: ACUTE FUNCTIONAL EFFECTS OF PERCUTANEOUS ACCESS

Adult farm swine (70 kg) were anesthetized and prepared for renal function measurements using inulin and *para*-aminohippuric acid (PAH) clearance methods as previously described [11]. Experienced urologists gained percutaneous access to a lower pole calyx using procedures identical to that performed on patients [12]. Tract dilation was achieved with either balloon or serial semi-rigid dilator systems, followed by placement of a 30 French working-sheath.

Access with either dilator system had similar effects on renal function (Fig. 1). There was an initial fall in glomerular filtration rate (GFR) and renal plasma flow (RPF) of ~50% that remained depressed during the entire post-surgery observation period (Fig. 1A-B). The renal extraction of PAH from the blood (EPAH) was also significantly reduced following the percutaneous access procedure (Fig. 1C). PAH is largely extracted from the blood into the lumens of renal tubules by specific and selective organic anion transporters located on the membranes of renal tubular epithelial cells [13-15], and provides one measure of proximal tubule transport activity. Hence, the decrease in EPAH suggests that percutaneous access is associated with a reduction in the elimination of organic anions by the kidney.

There were also effects on the contralateral, untreated kidney, i.e., reduced GFR and RPF, but not EPAH (Fig. 1D-F). The mechanism(s) involved in mediating the hemodynamic changes in the untreated kidney are unknown, but similar bilateral renal effects have been observed after unilateral shock wave lithotripsy and largely involved renal sympathetic nerves [16].

Therefore, unilateral percutaneous access results in bilateral renal vasoconstriction and unilateral reduction in tubular organic anion transport.

ANIMAL STUDIES: ACUTE STRUCTURAL EFFECTS OF PERCUTANEOUS ACCESS

At the completion of functional measurements (see "Animal Studies: Acute Functional Effects of Percutaneous Access"), kidneys were perfusion fixed *in vivo* and removed for routine histopathology or whole-kidney serial sectioning for morphological analysis [17].

Balloon and semi-rigid dilator systems resulted in similar effects on renal morphology and histology. The access procedure created an open channel (asterisk)

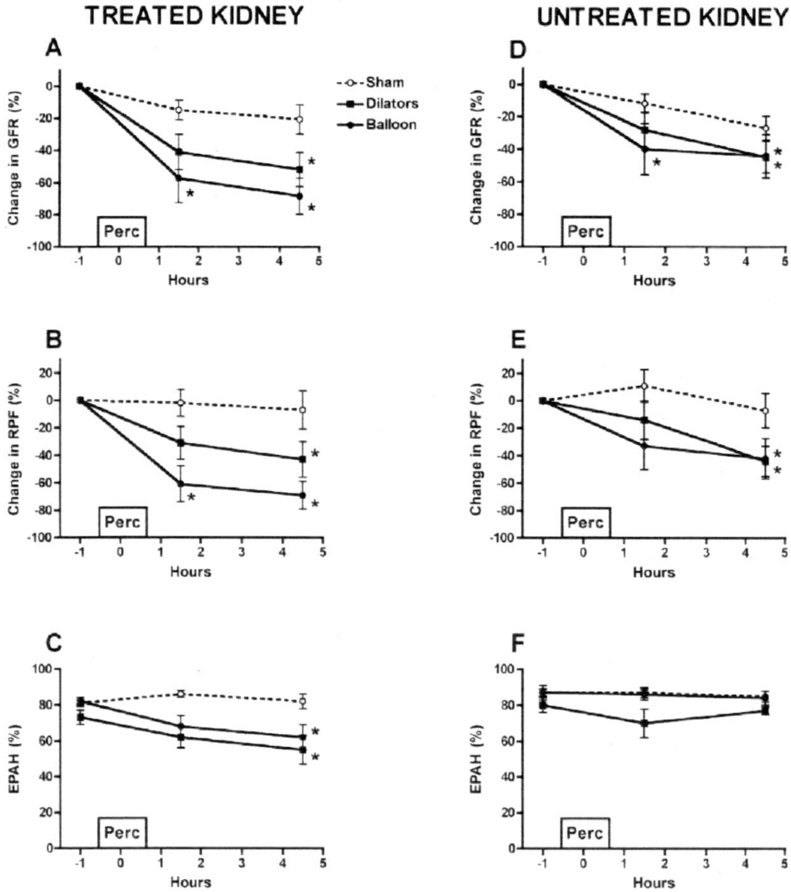

FIGURE 1. Unilateral percutaneous access (Perc) on bilateral renal function in pigs subjected to sham dilation (n = 8), serial semi-rigid dilators (n = 8) or balloon dilation (n = 7). Data are presented as means ± SEM. * = P<0.05 from pre-Perc value using mixed-effect models.

from the renal surface to the papillary tip. The channel was surrounded by an irregular zone of injured parenchyma (arrows) that was on average 2-fold larger in area than the size of the tract (Fig. 2).

Vascular injury included congestion of peritubular capillaries and intraparenchymal hemorrhage resulting from lacerated arcuate veins and arteries. Cellular injury included apical blebbing, vacuolization and necrosis. There was also protein present in the tubules (tubular casts), which reflects injury to the glomerular filtration barrier. All the morphological and histological changes were indicative of blunt trauma and ischemia [18].

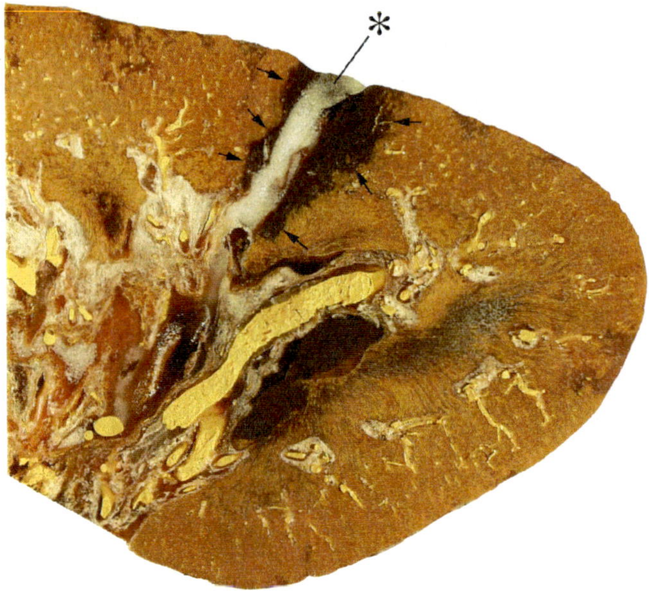

Figure 2. Kidney section showing access site and associated tissue injury.

ANIMAL STUDIES: SHORT-TERM RECOVERY PROFILE AFTER PERCUTANEOUS ACCESS

Renal hemodynamic and tubular function was measured following 3 days of recovery from percutaneous access surgery. This time frame was chosen, in part, because the status of renal function is unknown at a time when urologists may regain access through the existing tract to remove any residual stones. Animals were anesthetized and renal function measurements were performed before and 1 hour after percutaneous access with a balloon dilator. Animals were allowed to regain consciousness and were then anesthetized 3 days later for final measurements of renal function, including sampling of renal venous blood for measurement of EPAH and calculation of RPF.

A decrease in GFR and effective RPF (ERPF) occurred in the instrumented kidney immediately following percutaneous access and returned to pre-operative levels within 3 days (Fig. 3A-B); EPAH remained depressed in the treated kidney at the 3-day measurement (Fig. 3C). We presume that the reduced EPAH is reflective of the destruction, injury and trauma to the renal tubules following surgery.

ERPF is determined by measuring renal PAH clearance and provides an approximation of RPF with the assumption that all of the PAH is removed from the blood in one passage through the kidney. To obtain a true value of RPF, the fractional removal of PAH from the arterial blood must be determined, i.e. EPAH, and the renal

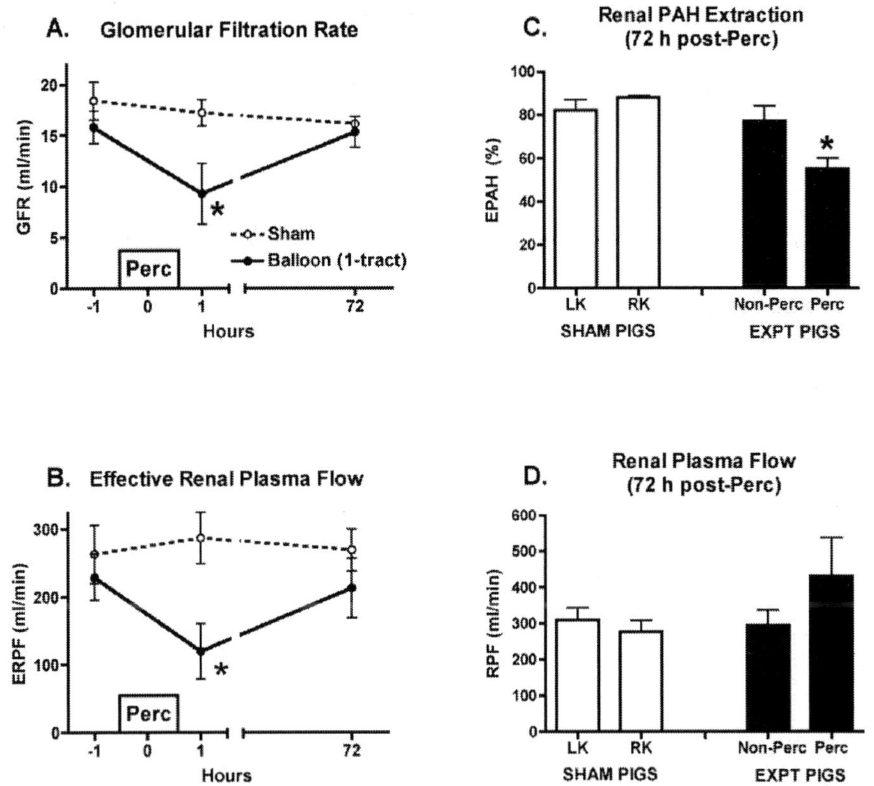

FIGURE 3. Short-term (72-hour) recovery profile of renal function after Perc. Pigs per group = 4-8.

clearance of PAH appropriately corrected [19]. RPF calculations indicate that renal perfusion in the treated kidney tended to be ~50% higher than in the contralateral untreated kidney, or sham-treated kidneys at the 3-day measurement (Fig. 3D). Although the increase in RPF did not reach a level of statistical significance, it suggests that there is a trend for the treated kidney to be in a state of hyperperfusion 3 days after percutaneous access. A direct measurement of regional renal perfusion rates will establish whether this is indeed the case, and also if the elevated perfusion is global or focal to the site of injury.

HUMAN STUDIES: ACUTE RENAL EFFECTS OF PCNL

We performed a retrospective analysis of stone formers who underwent unilateral PCNL with single access at our institution between July 2002 and May 2004. A total of 196 patients with normal pre-operative serum creatinine (Cr) of ≤ 1.5 mg/dL were included in this analysis. Urologists gained access in the operating room using a technique that has been previously described [12]. Tract dilation was accomplished and maintained with a balloon dilating system and a 30 French working-sheath, respectively. Both rigid and flexible nephroscopy with intracorporeal lithotripsy were employed for stone removal. A 10 French Cope loop nephrostomy tube was routinely placed at the end of the procedure. Serum Cr was measured pre-operatively and 1 day post-PCNL to assess renal glomerular function.

Figure 4 shows the patient-distribution curve of the Cr response to PCNL. Serum Cr increased from 0.97 ± 0.02 mg/dL to 1.11 ± 0.02 mg/dL (Δ = 0.14 ± 0.02 mg/dL, $P<0.001$) following PCNL in all patients. Breakdown of the responses revealed that some patients experienced a decline (33/196), no change (37/196) or a rise (126/196) in serum Cr. The latter cohort of patients exhibited ~28% higher serum Cr values after PCNL compared to their pre-operative level of 0.95 ± 0.02 mg/dL. Therefore, PCNL produced an acute decline in renal glomerular function in most patients. Although, these results do not inform whether one or both kidneys contributed to the rise in serum Cr, they do support our findings in animals that the PCNL procedure results in an acute decline in renal glomerular function.

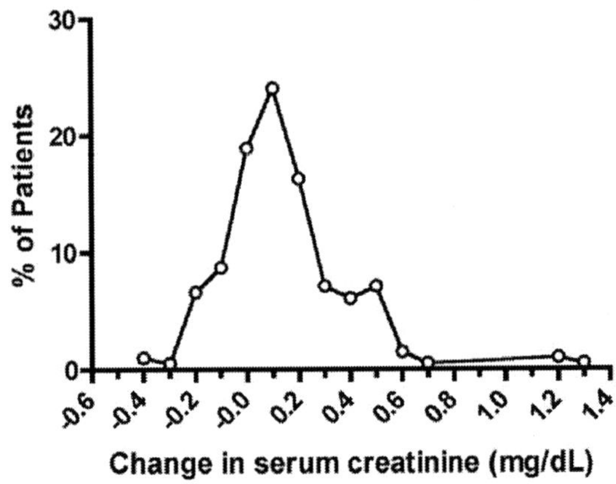

FIGURE 4. Change in 24-hour serum creatinine levels after unilateral PCNL.

Figure 5 shows nuclear renographs from a 29-year-old female patient who underwent unilateral PCNL with single access to remove kidney stones. Renal imaging of intravenously administered 99mTc-mecaptoacetyl triglycine (MAG3) to estimate ERPF was performed before (Fig. 5A) and immediately after PCNL (Fig. 5B), and 30 days post-surgery (Fig. 5C). Split renal function measurements obtained about 2 hours after PCNL revealed that ERPF fell from pre-operative values by 56% and 22% in the PCNL-treated right kidney (radionuclide-filled nephrostomy tube can be seen on image) and untreated left kidney, respectively. At 30 days post-PCNL, ERPF was at normal values in the untreated kidney and approximately 83% recovered in the PCNL-treated kidney. Therefore, the acute response to unilateral PCNL in this patient was bilateral renal vasoconstriction, similar to what we had previously observed in our animal model.

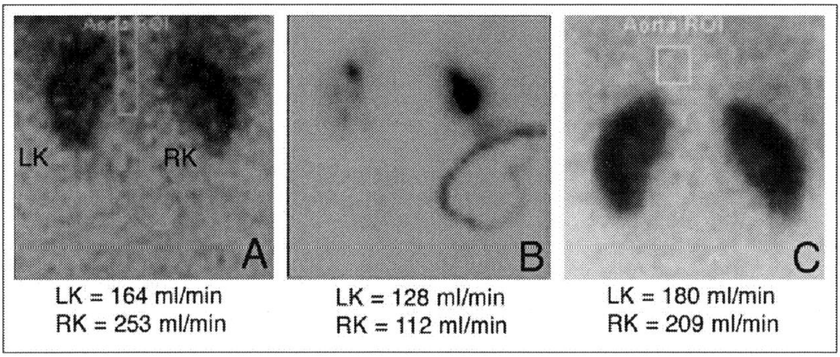

FIGURE 5. Renal perfusion imaging of patient's left (LK) and right (RK) kidney. **A:** pre-PCNL. **B:** immediately after PCNL. **C:** 30 days after PCNL. RK was treated by PCNL.

SUMMARY AND CONCLUSIONS

Unilateral percutaneous access with serial or balloon dilators resulted in similar acute (hours) declines in porcine renal filtration and perfusion, and tubular transport function, i.e. vasoconstriction in both kidneys with decreased tubular organic anion transport localized to the treated kidney. Both tract dilation procedures showed similar structural changes consistent with blunt trauma and ischemia. Short-term (3-day) recovery from percutaneous access surgery demonstrated that renal hemodynamic function had largely recovered, whereas the kidney's ability to eliminate organic anions, and perhaps organic cations, in the urine remained impaired. This could potentially have important clinical implications as these renal tubular transporters are primarily involved in the elimination of many drugs, toxins and endogenous compounds from the body. Finally, unilateral PCNL in human patients resulted in an acute decline in glomerular function, and initial renal perfusion imaging of a single patient indicated that PCNL was also associated with bilateral renal vasoconstriction. The similarity of human and animal responses to the percutaneous access procedure suggests that the pig may be a good model to study the human renal response to PCNL.

ACKNOWLEDGMENTS

This study was supported by funds from Boston Scientific Co.

REFERENCES

1. J. W. Segura, D. E. Patterson, A. J. LeRoy, H.J. Williams, Jr., D. M. Barrett, R. C. Benson, Jr., G. R. May and C. E. Bender, *J. Urology* **134**, 1077-1081 (1985).
2. J. S. Wolf, Jr. and R. V. Clayman, *Urologic Clinics of North America* **24**, 43-58 (1997).
3. R. Davidoff and G. C. Bellman, *J. Urology* **157**, 1229-1231 (1997).

4. K. M. Al-Kohlany, A. A. Shokeir, A. Mosbah, T. Mohsen, A. M. Shoma, I. Eraky, M. El-Kenawy and H. A. El-Kappany, J. *Urology* **173**, 469-473 (2005).
5. G. M. Preminger, *Urol. Res.* **34**, 108-111 (2006).
6. A. A. Shokeir, K. Z. Sheir, A. R. El-Nahas, A. M. El-Assmy, W. Eassa and H. A. El-Kappany, J. *Urology* **176**, 706-710 (2006).
7. M. E. Mayo, J. N. Krieger and T. G. Rudd, *J. Urology* **133**, 167-169 (1985).
8. M. Eshghi, R. G. Schiff and A. D. Smith, *Urology* **33**, 120-124 (1989).
9. J. R. Chatham, T. E. Dykes, W. G. Kennon and B. F. Schwartz, *Urology* **59**, 522-526 (2002).
10. M.S. Dawaba, A. A. Shokeir, A. T. Hafez, A. M. Shoma, M. T. El-Sherbiny, A. M. I. Eraky, M. El-Kenawy and H. A. El-Kappany, *J. Urology* **172**, 1078-1081 (2004).
11. L. R. Willis, A. P. Evan, B. A. Connors, P. Blomgren, N. Fineberg and J. E. Lingeman, *J. Am. Soc. Neph.* **10**, 1753-1762 (1999).
12. J. E. Lingeman, D. A. Lifshitz and A. P. Evan, "Surgical Management of Urinary Lithiasis," in *Campbell's Urology*, edited by A. B. Retik et al., Saunders, Philadelphia, 2002, pp. 3361-3451.
13. J. B. Pritchard and D. S. Miller, *Physiol. Rev.* **73**, 765-796 (1993).
14. Y. Hagos, A. Bahn, A. R. Asif, W. Krick, M. Sendler and G. Burckhardt, *Biochimie* **84**, 1219-1222 (2002).
15. S. H. Wright and W. H. Dantzler, *Physiol. Rev.* **84**, 987-1049 (2004).
16. B. A. Connors, A. P. Evan, L. R. Willis, J. R. Simon, N. S. Fineberg, D. A. Lifshitz, A. L. Shalhav, R. F. Paterson, R. L. Kuo and J. E. Lingeman, *Nephron Physiol.* **95**, 67-75 (2003).
17. Y. Shao, B. A. Connors, A. P. Evan, L. R. Willis, D. A. Lifshitz and J. E. Lingeman, *Anat Rec Part A.* **275A**, 979-989 (2003).
18. H. R. Brady, B. M. Brenner, M. R. Clarkson and W. Lieberthal, "Acute renal failure," in *The Kidney*, edited by B. M. Brenner, Saunders, Philadelphia, 2004, pp. 1215-1292.
19. V. L. Schuster and D. W. Seldin, "Renal clearance," in *The Kidney: Physiology and Pathophysiology*, edited by D. W. Seldin and G. Giebisch, Raven Press, New York, 1985, pp. 365-395.

VI. URETERAL PHYSIOLOGY AND STENTS

The Role of Ureteral Relaxation in the Promotion of Stone Passage

Kim Davenport, Anthony G. Timoney, and Francis X. Keeley, Jr.

Bristol Urological Institute, Southmead Hospital, Westbury-on-Trym, Bristol, BS10 5NB, UK

Abstract. In order to promote stone passage in renal colic, we must first understand normal ureteral activity and how this is affected by the presence of a stone. Measuring normal ureteral activity in humans is difficult without the use of invasive methods or techniques which in themselves may affect peristalsis. Monitoring the activity during confirmed renal colic is even more difficult and virtually impossible. Both animal and human studies have therefore been used in an attempt to understand the physiology of the ureter and how this is affected by the presence of a stone. Using this knowledge, drugs can be used to alter the behavior of the ureter in an attempt to promote stone passage. Peristalsis has always been thought to be essential to allow stone passage and therefore it has been necessary to determine whether stone passage occurs by promotion of ureteral activity or by smooth muscle relaxation. Research indicates that drugs which allow continued peristalsis whilst preventing the increased uncoordinated activity seen in renal colic would be the most advantageous. The alpha-1A-adrenoceptor antagonists are the most effective drugs to date.

Keywords: alpha antagonists, calcium channel antagonists, peristalsis, renal colic, ureter.
PACS: 87.19.Ff

INTRODUCTION

The use of pharmacological agents to promote stone passage in renal colic is not a new concept. An understanding of ureteral physiology and the pathological changes occurring in the presence of a ureteral stone is essential to determine those agents most likely to have a beneficial effect. Measuring normal ureteral activity in humans is difficult without the use of invasive methods or techniques which in themselves may affect peristalsis. Monitoring the activity during confirmed renal colic is even more difficult and virtually impossible. Both animal and human studies have therefore been performed. Those agents capable of causing ureteral smooth muscle relaxation have the most beneficial effect clinically; however the *in vivo* action on the human ureter remains unclear. Peristalsis has always been thought to be essential to allow stone passage and therefore it has been necessary to determine whether stone passage occurs by modulating ureteral activity or by causing smooth muscle relaxation. This chapter summarizes current research in this area.

CP900, *Renal Stone Disease, 1st Annual International Urolithiasis Research Symposium,*
edited by A. P. Evan, J. E. Lingeman, and J. C. Williams, Jr.

URETERAL PHYSIOLOGY

Ureteral peristalsis may be triggered spontaneously via the pacemaker cells located at the pelvic-calyceal junctions, by external stimuli which may be electrical, mechanical (e.g. stretch) or chemical or conduction from an adjacent excited cell.

In the resting state, the smooth muscle cell membrane potential is approximately -60mV and determined by the movement of potassium along its concentration gradient. If the stimulus is strong enough to decrease the transmembrane potential to the threshold potential, an action potential is generated. This is the primary event in the conduction of a peristaltic impulse and is capable of acting as the stimulus for excitation of adjacent quiescent cells to produce a coordinated ureteral contraction.

Excitation leads to an influx of calcium into the cell which results in the upstroke of the action potential. This is slow as compared to heart or skeletal muscle accounting for the slower conduction velocity seen in the ureter.

The action potential plateaus as a result of persistent calcium influx plus sodium influx via voltage dependent channels. The high intracellular calcium concentration triggers an outward movement of potassium via calcium dependent potassium channels causing repolarization.

In the pacemaker cells, the electrical activity arises spontaneously. The cell resting potential undergoes slow spontaneous depolarization until it reaches the threshold potential at which point an action potential is generated.

The contractile proteins, actin and myosin are located within the sarcoplasm of the ureteral cell. The contractile activity of each ureteral smooth muscle cell is dependent on the free sarcoplasmic calcium concentration in the region of the contractile proteins.

The release of calcium from the sarcoplasmic reticulum during excitation activates a cascade reaction resulting in cross-bridge formation between the myosin heads and the actin filaments producing a contraction. Relaxation occurs following reuptake of calcium into the sarcoplasmic reticulum.

Conduction between adjacent cells occurs via intermediate junctions at a conduction velocity of 2-6 cm/sec [1]. The volume and frequency of contractions can vary in relation to glomerular filtration; for example, both volume and frequency increase during diuresis.

THE ROLE OF THE SYMPATHETIC NERVOUS SYSTEM

Ureteral peristalsis can occur without neuronal stimulation via the pacemaker cells. However the nervous system, predominantly the sympathetic nervous system, appears to play a modulating role. Adrenergic receptors are found along the length of the ureter [2,3] but mainly in the intramural segment. The alpha-adrenergic receptors are most prominent.

Alpha-adrenergic receptors are subdivided into alpha_1 and alpha_2 adrenoceptors [4]. Alpha_1 adrenoceptors predominate in the human ureter and are further subdivided pharmacologically into alpha_{1A}, alpha_{1B} and alpha_{1D} adrenoceptors [5]. The density of

$alpha_1$ adrenoceptors is greatest in the distal ureter (52.5 ± 5.4 fmol/mg protein) as compared with the mid and proximal ureter (25.2 ± 1.7 fmol/mg protein and 23.4 ± 0.4 fmol/mg protein respectively). $Alpha_{1A}$ and $alpha_{1D}$ adrenoceptors predominate over $alpha_{1B}$ at all levels. Activation leads to IP_3 and DAG production resulting in smooth muscle contraction.

THE EFFECT OF STONE ON URETERAL ACTIVITY

The presence of a stone within the ureter initially stimulates peristalsis in an attempt to move the stone. If the stone becomes lodged, then the surrounding smooth muscle goes into spasm, which is presumed to have a negative effect on the probability of stone passage. Accompanying edema and inflammation further narrow the ureter at the level of the stone. Proximal to the stone, ureteral peristalsis increases in an attempt to move the stone resulting in the characteristic pain of renal colic.

There is much debate as to whether peristalsis is necessary to promote stone passage or whether relaxation of ureteral smooth muscle would aid passage. It has been stipulated in the past that ureteral peristalsis is essential to allow spontaneous stone passage. However, irritation and stretch stimulation of the ureter by the stone may result in increased uncoordinated peristalsis [6], which may actually hinder stone passage. In a canine *in vivo* model of acute obstruction, the mean peristaltic rate, baseline pressure and peak pressures above the level of obstruction were all shown to increase significantly [7]. Conversely below the level of obstruction, the mean peristaltic rate remained unchanged but the baseline and peak pressures generated were both significantly reduced.

In an *in vivo* study yet to be published, we recorded human ureteral activity during an episode of pain similar to renal colic using a ureteral pressure transducer catheter [8]. The recording obtained demonstrated increased uncoordinated contractions of higher pressures than those usually recorded in the human ureter using the same catheter (see Figs. 1 and 2). Control of this increased, uncoordinated ureteral activity may promote normal peristalsis allowing stone passage.

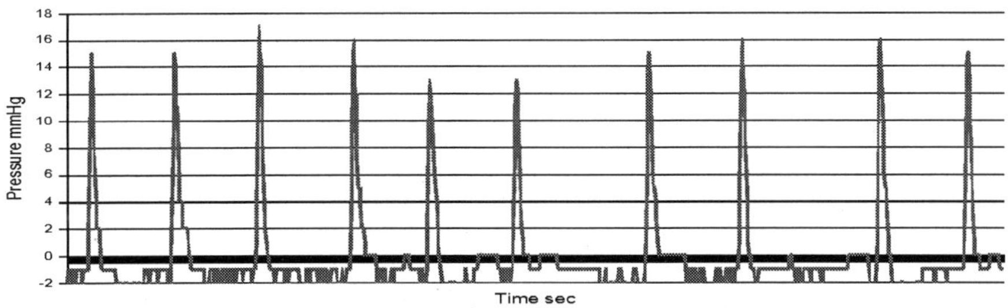

FIGURE 1. 3-minute recording of proximal human ureteral activity obtained 24 hours post-ureteroscopy using the ureteral pressure transducer catheter.

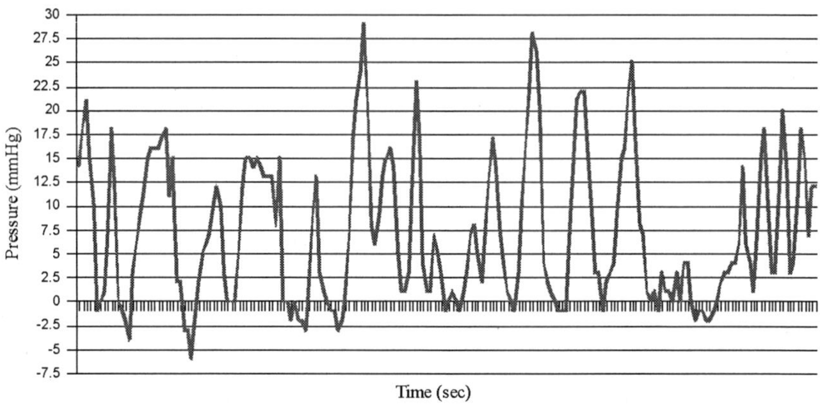

FIGURE 2. 3-minute recording of human ureteral activity during pain typical of acute renal colic using the ureteral pressure transducer catheter.

METHODS FOR MONITORING URETERAL MUSCLE ACTIVITY

In Vitro Methods

Isolated animal and human tissue segments have proven to be useful in the investigation of ureteral physiology. However it is now known that the animal from which the ureter is obtained may affect the results. The most commonly used animal tissues are from pig, dog, guinea pig, rat, rabbit and sheep. Comparative studies have shown pig and sheep ureters to be more histologically similar to human ureter as compared with canine ureter [9]. In view of the differences seen between species, human tissue is now preferred.

Human ureteral tissue can be obtained at the time of open nephrectomy or cystectomy provided the ureter is patent, functional and disease free prior to removal. The tissue must be placed into a physiological buffered solution maintained at 4°C on removal until experimentation to maintain function. Ureteral specimens may be suspended as horizontal rings or longitudinal strips. They require continuous irrigation with a physiological buffered solution aerated with 95% oxygen/5% carbon dioxide mixture and maintained at 37°C. The ureteral strips are prepared, suspended within water baths and attached to a force transducer to allow changes in tension to be recorded. A resting tension is applied to the ureteral segment at the outset and the tissues are allowed to equilibrate within the buffer solution.

Spontaneous contractions are not seen in all human ureteral specimens. When present, the contraction frequency *in vitro* ranges from 1-10 contractions per minute, with the majority of studies reporting rates of 1-2 per minute [10-13].

Two general types of mechanical activity can be distinguished: phasic and tonic contractions. Phasic activity is characterized by regular rhythmic changes in tension, which can be modified both in amplitude and frequency. In its purest form the baseline is always reached between two contractions, for example, spontaneous contractions. In contrast, tonic contractions reach a maximal tension, which is maintained over time under constant conditions.

Drug responses can be measured either by recording the effect on spontaneous contraction rates or by stimulating phasic or tonic contractions and recording the effect the drug has on tension generation. To test the drug response, the drug is added to the physiological solution at various concentrations. These solutions can then be applied to the ureter following equilibration to record the effect on spontaneous contraction frequency and amplitude. Alternatively, electrical field stimulation can be used to stimulate individual contractions.

Chemical stimulation can also be used, predominately carbachol (a muscarinic agonist) or potassium-enriched physiological solutions. The response to a pharmacological agent can then be determined by comparing the increase in tone generated by the stimulant with the response when the drug is used in addition to the stimulant. The drug response is expressed as the percentage change in tone as compared with resting levels.

Spontaneous contractions are preferred to prevent interference by artificial stimulation, however these are inconsistently seen.

In Vivo Methods

The physiology of the upper urinary tract has been studied *in vivo* in both animal and human models since the early 1900's. Many extraluminal and intraluminal methods have been described combining ureteral catheters with strain gauges, strain gauge manometers or electromanometers [14-19], endoluminal ultrasound [20] and laparoscopic ultrasound [21-22]. Ureteral contraction frequency is relatively easy to measure, however contraction pressures are far more difficult as they require intraluminal methods which are far from ideal.

The limitations of the studies to date include:

- Antegrade or retrograde instrumentation of the ureter to site a catheter may disturb normal physiology.
- Extraluminal methods are invasive and require open or laparoscopic surgery to site the sensors; these methods are therefore rarely possible in human subjects.
- Animal studies may not always be representative of human ureteral activity [23].
- The preparation for general anesthesia (nil by mouth) and the anesthetic drugs themselves may affect excretory function [24] and ureteral peristalsis [25].
- Many recordings have been made over short periods of time leading to incorrect assumptions and preventing trends over time to be determined [17-19].

There is a need, therefore, for a method to allow monitoring over longer periods of time in human subjects and, if sited at cystoscopy under general anesthetic, could be left *in situ* for long enough to allow metabolism and excretion of the anesthetic agents and ureteral activity to recover following the instrumentation.

IN VITRO AND IN VIVO STUDIES TO DETERMINE THE ROLE OF SMOOTH MUSCLE RELAXANT DRUGS IN RENAL COLIC

By understanding ureteral physiology, pharmacological agents can be designed to reduce ureteral tone and control peristalsis. Previous research has suggested that there are many drugs in current use capable of influencing normal ureteral physiology and decreasing peristaltic frequency or tone generation *in vitro*. The most promising drugs for use in clinical practice to reduce ureteral activity, which are already in use, appear to be non-steroidal anti-inflammatory drugs, calcium channel antagonists and alpha-$_1$-adrenoceptor antagonists.

Non-steroidal anti-inflammatory drugs

Non-steroidal anti-inflammatory drugs (NSAIDs) inhibit prostaglandin synthesis by non-selective cyclo-oxygenase inhibition, preventing stimulation of smooth muscle contraction by prostanoids (prostaglandins, thromboxanes and prostacyclin). NSAIDs provide excellent analgesia in renal colic. In the laboratory, these drugs appear to reduce ureteral activity and in some cases, ablate all ureteral activity [10,26]. However, despite diclofenac and indomethacin being highly effective in reducing the number of new colic episodes and admissions to hospital, in clinical trials they do not affect the time to stone passage or the stone passage rate in renal colic [27-29].

Calcium Channel Antagonists

Calcium is necessary for the development of action potentials and therefore contraction of the ureter. Calcium channel blockers interfere with the inward displacement of calcium ions through the slow channels of active cell membranes and so would be expected to have an inhibitory effect on ureteral function.

There have been many studies investigating the use of nifedipine in renal colic [30-33]. Unfortunately all four studies have combined the use of nifedipine with a steroid. All four studies have indicated advantages to the use of nifedipine in renal colic. Since all have combined nifedipine with steroid, it is unclear as to the degree of benefit incurred with the use of nifedipine alone. Steroids not only have an anti-inflammatory effect on the ureter and so reduce edema at the level of the stone but they may also cause a degree of ureteral smooth muscle relaxation. All four studies have predominantly involved distal ureteral calculi and so it remains unclear as to whether the beneficial effects apply to stones at all levels or are limited to distal ureteral stones.

Alpha$_{1A}$-adrenoceptor Antagonists

It may be that stone passage is hindered by the overactive ureter but that more controlled contractions, as opposed to complete ablation of all contractions, are necessary to aid stone passage. Within the sympathetic nervous system, alpha$_1$ adrenergic fibers are excitatory; therefore, by blocking the alpha$_1$-adrenergic receptors, smooth muscle relaxation and a reduction in contraction frequency should occur.

Since the sympathetic nervous system only has a modulating role, pacemaker driven peristalsis should continue.

Tamsulosin is an alpha$_1$-adrenoceptor antagonist, which binds selectively and competitively to postsynaptic alpha$_1$-receptors, in particular to the subtype alpha$_{1A}$. There are no published studies in the literature demonstrating the effect of tamsulosin on the human ureter *in vitro* or *in vivo*. However there are many studies demonstrating the relaxant effects of non-selective alpha-adrenoceptor antagonists, namely phentolamine.

Tamsulosin has been used to promote stone passage in renal colic in many trials, but only in the treatment of distal ureteral calculi. All studies have shown a beneficial effect. These are summarized in a meta-analysis by Hollingsworth et al [34]. However many have been non-randomized, performed without blinding or placebo or in conjunction with other drugs making interpretation of results difficult.

Direct Comparison between NSAIDs, Calcium Channel Antagonists and Alpha$_{1A}$-adrenoceptor Antagonists

We have published results from an *in vitro* study comparing the effects diclofenac, nifedipine and tamsulosin had on human ureteral activity to determine the promoting factor for stone passage [35]. Human ureter obtained at the time of open cystectomy or nephrectomy was used to determine the effect these drugs had on activity *in vitro*. Thirty-nine patients took part, providing 201 strips. Brading-Sibley tissue baths were used to perform this experiment. A tonic muscle contraction was first stimulated using potassium enriched physiological Kreb's solution. Each of the three drugs was then applied in solution to each strip in increasing concentrations and the percentage reduction in contraction tone was calculated.

At all drug concentrations, the *in vitro* relaxant effect of nifedipine and 5-methylurapidil (5-MU, representing tamsulosin) was greater than diclofenac (see Fig. 3). At 10^{-5}M concentration, the median reduction in tension generation for proximal and distal ureter seen in response to diclofenac, nifedipine and 5-MU was 18% vs. 5%, 47% vs. 57% and 33% vs. 65% respectively. Nifedipine and 5-MU predominantly affected the distal ureter [35].

In order to determine the effect these drugs had on human ureteral activity *in vivo*, we used a specially designed ureteral pressure transducer catheter. With REC approval and informed consent, the catheter was inserted into the normal contralateral ureter following ureteroscopy for stone and left *in situ* for 24 hours. The patient was randomized to receive oral diclofenac, tamsulosin or nifedipine. Ureteral activity was monitored using an ambulatory recorder for one hour prior to ingestion of the drug (Fig. 1) and continued to the time of maximal drug concentration within the body (Tmax). All *in vivo* studies were performed on the proximal ureter. An example of the results obtained is shown in Table 1 [8].

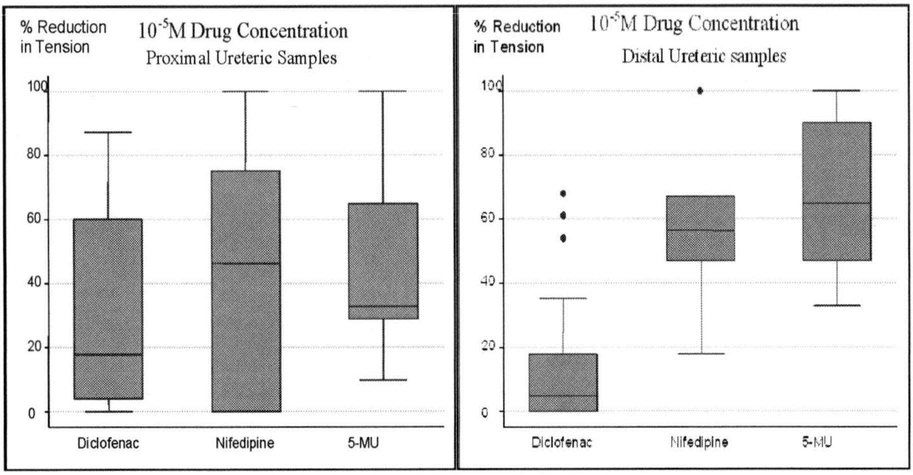

FIGURE 3. Percentage reduction in tension generation at 10^{-5} M drug concentration.

TABLE 1: Typical results obtained pre- and post-drug administration using the ureteral pressure transducer catheter.

	Patient	Contraction Frequency/min			Pressure Generation/mmHg		
		Median	IQR	p	Median	IQR	p
Diclofenac	3: Pre	2	2-2		28	23.2-32	
	Post	2	1-2	0.05	60	58-61	<0.001
Nifedipine	6. Pre	1	0.8-3		35	32-39	
	Post	0	0-2	0.01	22	11.5-25	<0.001
Tamsulosin	8. Pre	4.1	3-5		21	19-23	
	Post	3.1	2-3.8	<0.001	11.9	9-14	<0.001

Diclofenac and nifedipine produced inconsistent ureteral pressure responses but had little effect on contraction frequency. Tamsulosin significantly reduced ureteral contraction pressure but had no effect on contraction frequency.

Nifedipine and 5-MU produced greater ureteral relaxation *in vitro* as compared with diclofenac. Nifedipine and 5-MU predominantly relaxed distal ureter. *In vivo*, varying results were seen for diclofenac and nifedipine; however, even in the proximal ureter, tamsulosin caused a significant reduction in ureteral contraction pressure. Most importantly, peristalsis was maintained despite the use of these drugs.

From this work, promotion of stone passage appears to be directly related to *in vitro* smooth muscle relaxation. *In vivo*, these results suggest that tamsulosin is clinically effective by maintaining ureteral contractions whilst preventing increases in ureteral contraction pressures in response to irritation by a stone. However, it remains extremely difficult to test this theory *in vivo*.

CONCLUSION

Research indicates that drugs which allow continued peristalsis whilst preventing the increased uncoordinated activity seen in renal colic would be the most effective for facilitating spontaneous stone passage. The $alpha_{1A}$-adrenoceptor antagonists are the most effective drugs to date in both *in vitro* and *in vivo* human studies. In order to determine the true clinical effectiveness of $alpha_{1A}$-adrenoceptor antagonists in renal colic, we have commenced a multicenter, randomized, double blind clinical trial using tamsulosin versus placebo for patients with confirmed ureteral stones. This study aims to recruit 250 patients and will determine the beneficial effect of tamsulosin for both proximal and distal ureteral stones.

ACKNOWLEDGMENTS

We thank Mr. Sibley and Mr. Whittlestone for the loan of the Brading-Sibley tissue bath and the MacLab data acquisition software necessary for the *in vitro* ureteral experiments, and the University of Bristol for the loan of the laboratory space.

REFERENCES

1. JA Ross, P Edmond, IS Kirkland. In: Behaviour of the human ureter in health and disease. Edinburgh: Churchill Livingstone, 1972
2. RM Weiss, AL Bassett, BF Hoffman. Adrenergic innervation of the ureter. Invest Urol 16 (2), 123-127 (1978).
3. T Morita, M Ando, K Kihara, H Oshima. Function and distribution of autonomic receptors in canine ureteral smooth muscle. Neurourol and Urodynamics 13, 315-321 (1994).
4. SZ Langer. Presynaptic regulation of catecholamine release. Biochem Pharmacol 23, 1793-1800 (1974).
5. S Sigala, M Dellabella, G Milanese, S Fornali, S Faccoli, F Palazzolo, A Peroni, G Mirabella, SC Cunico, P Spano, G Muzzonigro G. Evidence for the presence of alpha1 adrenoceptor subtypes in the human ureter. Neurourol Urodyn 24 (2), 142-148 (2005).
6. JG Rose, JY Gillenwater. Pathophysiology of ureteral obstruction. Am J Physiol 225, 830-837 (1973).
7. AR Crowley, JC Byrne, E Darracott Vaughan, DN Marion. The effect of acute obstruction on ureteral function. J Urol 143, 596-599 (1990).
8. K Davenport, "The Role of Ureteric Relaxation in the Promotion of Spontaneous Stone Passage in Ureteric Colic", M.D. Thesis, University of Bristol, 2006.
9. JS Wolf Jr, PA Humphrey, HJ Rayala, SM Gardner, RB Mackey, RV Clayman. Comparative ureteral microanatomy. J Endourol 10, 6527-6531 (1996).
10. SY Nakada, TJ Jerde, DE Bjorling, R Saban. Selective cyclooxygenase-2 inhibitors reduce ureteral contraction in vitro: A better alternative for renal colic? J Urol 163, 607-612 (2000).
11. A Sahin, I Erdemli, M Bakkaloglu, A Ergen, I Basar, D Remzi. The effect of nifedipine and verapamil on rhythmic contractions of human isolated ureter. Arch Int Phys, Biochim, Biophys 101, 245-247 (1993).
12. TJ Jerde, R Saban, SY Nakada. Evaluation of ureteric contraction: a comparison among ring, spiral cut and longitudinal segments. BJU Int 83, 95-100 (1999).
13. A Sivrikaya, OF Celik, N Sivrikaya, GK Ozgur. The effect of diclofenac sodium and papaverine on isolated human ureteric smooth muscle. Int Urol and Neph 35, 479-483 (2003).
14. HG Hanley. The electro-ureterogram. Br J Urol 25 (4), 358- (1953).

15. EL Corey, EH Fite Jr, SA Vest. Electropotential changes in the normal human ureter. J Urol 75 (2), 244- (1956).
16. SR Weinberg, TJ Maletta, NY Brooklyn. Measurement of peristalsis of the ureter and its relation to drugs. JAMA 175 (1),109- (1961).
17. JA Ross, P Edmond, J Coull, D Simpson. The 'dynamic function' of the intact human renal pelvis and ureter. Brit J Surg 52 (8), 617- (1965).
18. JA Ross, P Edmond, J Coull, J Griffiths. Observations on the physiology of the human renal pelvis and ureter. J Urol 97: 449- (1967).
19. P Edmond, JA Ross, IS Kirkland. Human ureteral peristalsis. J Urol 104, 670- (1970).
20. H Roshani, NF Dabhoiwala, T Dijkhuis, KH Kurth, WH Lamers. An in vivo endoluminal ultrasonographic study of peristaltic activity in the distal porcine ureter. J Urol 163, 602- (2000).
21. HL Helin, P Kirkinen, S Purhonen, J Penttinen. Ultrasonography of the ureter during laparoscopic, abdominal and radical hysterectomy. Ultrasound Obstet Gynaecol 12 (3), 207- (1998).
22. R Venkatesh, J Landman, SD Minor, DI Lee, J Rehman, R Vanlangendonck, M Ragab, K Morrissey, CP Sundaram, RV Clayman. Impact of a double-pigtail stent on ureteral peristalsis in the porcine model: Initial studies using a novel implantable magnetic sensor. J Endourol 19 (2), 170-176 (2005).
23. MJ Stower, AG Clarke, JW Wright, JD Hardcastle. Effect of glucagons on ureteric peristalsis in man, pig, rabbit and rat. J Urol 131, 822-824 (1984).
24. EM Papper. Renal function during general anesthesia and operation. JAMA 152, 1686-1689 (1953).
25. CJ Young, A Attele, A Toledano, R Nunez, J Moss. Volatile anaesthetics decrease peristalsis in the guinea pig ureter. Anaesthesiology 81, 452-458 (1994).
26. TJ Jerde, JL Calaman-Dixon, DE Bjorling, SY Nakada. Celecoxib inhibits ureteral contractility and prostanoid release. Urol 65, 185-190 (2005).
27. E Laerum, OE Omundsen, JE Gronseth, A Christianson, HE Fagertun. Oral diclofenac in the prophylactic treatment of recurrent renal colic: A double blind comparison with placebo. Eur Urol 28, 108-111 (1995).
28. L Grenabo, D Holmlund. Indomethacin as prophylaxis against recurrent ureteral colic. Scand J Urol Nephrol 18, 325-327 (1984).
29. D Kapoor, S Weitzel, J Mowad, S Melanson, J Gillen. Use of indomethacin suppositories in the prophylaxis of recurrent ureteral colic. J Urol 142, 1428-1430 (1989).
30. L Borghi, T Meschi, F Amato, A Novarini, A Giannini, C Quarantelli, F Mineo. Nifedipine and methylprednisolone in facilitating ureteral stone passage: A randomised, double-blind, placebo-controlled study. J Urol 152, 1095-1098 (1994).
31. F Porpiglia, P Destefanis, C Fiori, D Fontana. Effectiveness of nifedipine and deflazacort in the management of distal ureteric stones. Urology 56 (4): 579-582 (2000).
32. JT Cooper, GM Stack, TP Cooper. Intensive medical management of ureteral calculi. Urology 56(4), 575-578 (2000).
33. A Saita, A Bonaccorsi, F Marchese, SV Condorelli, M Motta. Our experience with nifedipine and prednisolone as expulsive therapy for ureteral stones. Urol Int 72 (1), 43-45 (2004).
34. JM Hollingsworth, MAM Rogers, SR Kaufman, TJ Bradford, S Saint, JT Wei, BK Hollenbeck. Medical therapy to facilitate urinary stone passage: a meta-analysis. Lancet 368, 1171-1179 (2006).
35. K Davenport, AG Timoney, FX Keeley. A comparative in vitro study to determine the beneficial effect of calcium channel and alpha-1-adrenoceptor antagonism on human ureteric activity. BJU Int 98 (3), 651-655 (2006).

Evidence for Alpha Receptors in the Human Ureter

Ralph Madeb, Joy Knopf, Dragan Golijanin, Patricia Bourne, and Erdal Erturk

Department of Urology and Pathology, University of Rochester School of Medicine, 601 Elmwood Avenue, Box 656, Rochester, NY

Abstract. An immunohistochemical and western blot expression analysis of human ureters was performed in order to characterize the alpha-1-adrenergic receptor distribution along the length of the human ureteral wall. Mapping the distribution will assist in understanding the potential role alpha -1-adrenergic receptors and their subtype density might have in the pathophysiology of ureteral colic and stone passage. Patients diagnosed with renal cancer or bladder cancer undergoing nephrectomy, nephroureterectomy, or cystectomy had ureteral specimens taken from the proximal, mid, distal and tunneled ureter. Tissues were processed for fresh frozen examination and fixed in formalin. None of the ureteral specimens were involved with cancer. Serial histologic sections and immunohistochemical studies were performed using antibodies specific for alpha-1-adrenergic receptor subtypes (alpha 1a, alpha 1b, alpha 1d). The sections were examined under a light microscope and scored as positive or negative. In order to validate and quantify the alpha receptor subtypes along the human ureter, Western blotting techniques were applied. Human ureter stained positively for alpha -1-adrenergic receptors. Immunostaining appeared red, with intense reaction in the smooth muscle of the ureter and endothelium of the neighboring blood vessels. There was differential expression between all the receptors with the highest staining for alpha-1D subtype. The highest protein expression for all three subtypes was in the renal pelvis and decreased with advancement along the ureter to the distal ureter. At the distal ureter, there was marked increase in expression as one progressed towards the ureteral orifice. The same pattern of protein expression was exhibited for all three alpha -1-adrenergic receptor subtypes. We provide preliminary evidence for the ability to detect and quantify the alpha-1-receptor subtypes along the human ureter which to the best of our knowledge has never been done with immunohistochemistry and molecular techniques. These findings may lend support to the preliminary studies of the effectiveness of alpha-receptor blockade on ureteral colic and stone passage.

Keywords: Alpha receptor, immunohistochemistry, molecular analysis, human ureter.
PACS: 87.19.Ff

INTRODUCTION

Early physiologic studies revealed alpha-1-adrenergic receptor-like function in the ureter of humans, pigs, dogs and horses[1-4]. Further studies demonstrated that the density of alpha-1-adrenergic receptors in ureteral smooth muscle cells was significantly higher than other adrenergic receptors[1,4-6]. Studies performed with human ureters by Malin et al. noted alpha- and beta-adrenergic receptors in the human

CP900, *Renal Stone Disease, 1st Annual International Urolithiasis Research Symposium,* edited by A. P. Evan, J. E. Lingeman, and J. C. Williams, Jr.

ureter, where alpha-adrenergic receptors appeared to be predominant, as in the animal ureter[1]. Furthermore, alpha-1-adrenergic antagonists have proved to inhibit basal tone, peristaltic frequency, and ureteral contractions[1,2,4,5,7-12]. Despite these studies, adequate mapping of these receptors in the human ureter has not been performed.

Several studies have focused on the role of the adrenergic system in ureteral physiology [1,2,4,5,7-12]. In general, the main alpha-adrenergic agonist, noradrenaline, induces a positive chronotropic effect, increasing ureteral peristaltic frequency, and a positive inotropic effect, increasing muscle tone until ureteral obstruction (spasm) occurs at high doses. The blockade of alpha-adrenergic receptors by specific antagonists results in decreased ureteral peristaltic amplitude and frequency with consequent reduction of intraureteral pressure. The resulting ureteral spasm causes an increase in fluid transport ability [1,2,4,5,7-12]. Morita et al.[3] reported a significantly higher density of alpha-1-adrenoceptors than alpha -2-and beta-adrenoceptors in the canine ureter. These earlier studies elucidated the sympathetic response of the human ureter. With these established physiologic principles, small clinical studies have been performed to see if alpha-blockade with alpha-1- adrenergic receptor inhibitors could be beneficial. Although preliminary data have been encouraging [13-17], scientific basis for the use of alpha-adrenergic receptor blockers is lacking. Our goal was to map the distribution of the alpha-1-receptors along the human ureter. Subsequently, this will assist in understanding the potential role alpha-1-adrenergic receptors and their subtype density might have in the pathophysiology of ureteral colic and stone passage.

MATERIALS AND METHODS

Patient Selection and Tissue

Patients diagnosed with either renal cancer or bladder cancer and who underwent nephrectomy or cystectomy were counseled about urologic tissue banking. Any ureter that had a primary disease, such as cancer or any other ureteral pathology, was excluded from the study. Intramural (tunneled) ureter and ureteral orifice specimens were retrieved from the side opposite of the bladder pathology. After written informed consent for urologic tissue banking—per our institutional review board approval protocol—was obtained, specimens from renal pelvis, proximal, mid, distal and tunneled ureter were collected. After harvesting the necessary specimens, all tissues were saved in the urologic tissue bank at the University of Rochester Medical Center. Tissues were processed for fresh frozen examination and/or fixed in formalin and embedded in paraffin. Immunohistochemical studies were performed on serial sections of paraffin-embedded tissues using antibodies specific for alpha-1-adrenergic receptor (AR) subtypes (alpha-1A, alpha-1B, alpha-1D-AR). The sections were then examined under a light microscope and scored as positive or negative for expression of alpha-1-adrenergic receptor subtypes. In order to validate and quantify the presence of alpha receptor subtypes along the human ureter, reverse transcriptase polymerase chain reaction (RT-PCR) and Western blotting techniques were performed on the same section of frozen ureter.

Immunohistochemical Analysis

Immunohistochemistry was performed on tissue snap-frozen with liquid nitrogen and on formalin-fixed, alpha paraffin-embedded tissue sections using rabbit polyclonal antibodies (Novus Biologicals Inc; Littletone, CO 80160) to alpha-1B AR (Cat. No. NLS697, used at 1:200), alpha-1A AR (Cat. No. SP4061P, used at 1:400) and alpha-lD AR (Cat. No. SP4062P, used 1:400). Cryostat sections were stored at -25°C until ready for staining then fixed in ice cold acetone for 6 minutes, air dried, and placed into fresh Tris buffer for 5 minutes before staining. Staining was completed on the Dako autostainer as described below for paraffin embedded tissues without heat retrieval. Paraffin embedded tissues were sectioned at 5 mm thickness and floated on distilled water at 45°C. Sections were mounted on chemically charged slides, dried at room temperature until opaque, and then placed in the oven at 57°C overnight. Sections were deparaffinized and quenched with 3% hydrogen peroxide for 6 minutes. They were then cleared in running water followed by TBS (50mM Tris-hydrogen chloride, 150mM sodium chloride, and 0.05% Tween 20 at pH 7.6). Pretreatment: Antigen unmasking was performed on all three antibodies by the following method. Pre-heated (95°C-99°C) Dako antigen retrieval solution (Citrate Buffer pH 6.1) in a Black and Decker steamer [Shelton, Ct. 06484 Model HS800] for 30 minutes followed by a 15 minute cool-down period. Slides were rinsed with Tris Buffered Saline (TBS) for 5 minutes and mounted in the Dako autostainer. Slides were covered with fresh TBS to prevent drying during mounting. The sections were incubated with the primary antibodies at the specified dilution at room temperature for 60 minutes followed by separate 30-minute incubation in both goat anti-rabbit IgG-Biotin (Vector Laboratories, Inc. Burlingame, Ca) and Streptavidin-HRP (Jackson Labs). Slides were developed with AEC+ (Dako, Carpinteria, CA) for 10 minutes, rinsed in running distilled water, counterstained in Modified Mayer's Hematoxylin, blued in 0.3% ammonia water followed by a tap water rinse. Slides were mounted using an aqueous media and viewed under light microscopy. Adrenal gland was used as a positive control and vascular smooth muscle as an internal positive control.

Western Blotting

Biopsy tissue was received and stored at -85°C prior to analysis. Protein was extracted from umbilical cord, ureter, and kidney (normal and tumor biopsy) for western analysis. Tissue was cut into small pieces then mechanically homogenized in RIPA Lysis Buffer (Upstate Biotechnology) with 1:100 Protease Inhibitor Cocktail (Sigma) and frozen at -85°C. Tissue slurry was thawed on ice and vortexed vigorously; solids were removed by centrifugation. Protein concentration was quantified using a Bradford assay (BioRad Protein Assay reagent), and 50 μg protein was loaded on a 7.5% acrylamide gel then transferred to 0.45 um nitrocellulose membrane. The membrane was blocked overnight at 4°C in 5% milk in Tris-HCl buffer with Tween 20 then reacted with primary antibodies alpha 1A-AR, alpha 1B-AR, or alpha 1D-AR obtained from Santa Cruz. Antibody incubation (1:500) was performed for 1.5 hours at room temperature, followed by horseradish peroxidase-conjugated secondary antibody treatment. Detection with ECL reagents (Amersham) on X-omat film (Kodak) revealed bands at 51 kD for alpha-1A-AR, 57 kD for alpha 1B-AR and 60 kD for alpha-1D-AR antibodies. Sections of renal pelvis, proximal ureter, and mid ureter were obtained from a single patient undergoing nephrectomy; tissue from distal ureter, tunnel ureter and ureteral orifice were obtained from patients undergoing cystectomy.

RT-PCR Analysis

Tissue sections from lung, placenta, umbilical cord, and ureter were flash frozen in liquid nitrogen and stored at -85°C prior to analysis. Tissue was mechanically homogenized and RNA extracted using RNAqueous 4-PCR kit (Ambion) protocol. One microgram of total RNA was reverse transcribed with Roche Transcriptor Reverse Transcriptase reagents utilizing an oligo dT primer; a control reaction for genomic DNA contamination omitting the reverse transcriptase was performed in parallel. PCR amplification of cDNA was performed using High Fidelity Taq Polymerase (Promega), with primers and conditions specific for alpha-1A, alpha-1B, and alpha-1D-AR as described by Fauer[18].

RESULTS

Thirty ureteral segments were harvested from nephrectomy and cystectomy specimens for immunohistochemical and molecular analysis. Because the lung, adrenal, placenta, and aorta are known to possess alpha1-ARs, these tissues were obtained from the pathology tissue bank and used as positive controls [19-21]. Immunohistochemical stains for alpha-1A, alpha-1B, and alpha-1D adrenergic receptors demonstrated the presence of receptors in the smooth muscle of the wall of the ureter. The reaction was demonstrated by a reddish brown deposit within the tunica media of the smooth muscle of the ureter with the collagen/connective and urothelial tissue showing no signal (staining blue, see Fig. 1). Interestingly, the intensity of staining of the adrenergic receptors decreased in each class (alpha -1A, alpha -1B and alpha -1D) from the renal pelvis to the distal ureter, with a marked increase in staining from the distal to the tunneled ureter (Fig. 1).

This pattern was repeated among all the samples examined and was consistent in each subclass in both the frozen and paraffin embedded specimens. Immunoreactivity for the alpha-1D-adrenergic receptor was detected more intensely than the other subtypes (Fig. 2; right panel).

Appropriately sized RT-PCR cDNA products for alpha-1A, alpha-1B and alpha-1D were obtained from lung, placenta, umbilical cord and all ureter specimens, thereby confirming the transcription of all three receptors in human ureter (Fig. 3).

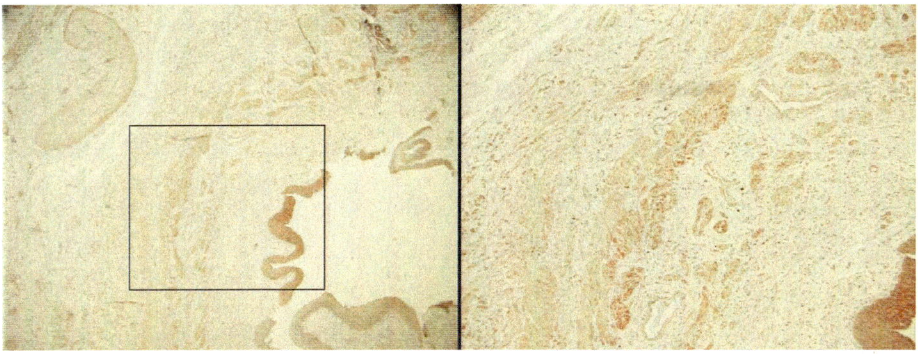

FIGURE 1. Immunohistochemical staining of human ureter for α-1-adrenorecptors. Immunostaining appears red, with intense membrane reaction in the smooth muscle of the ureter and endothelium of the neighboring blood vessels, while surrounding connective and urothelial tissue has no signal and appears blue.

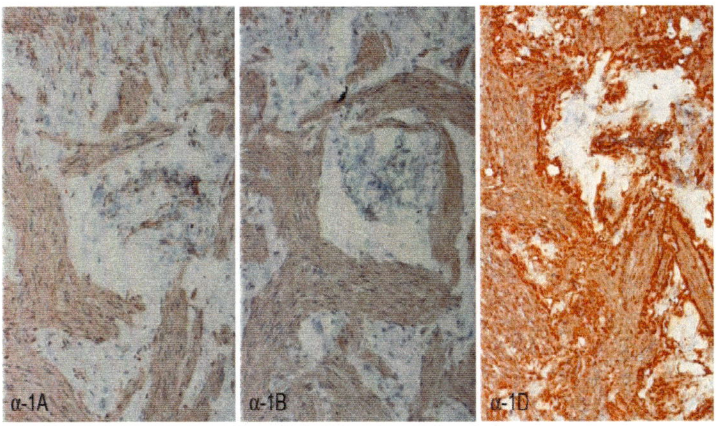

FIGURE 2. Immunohistochemical staining of serial sections through the renal pelvis of all three alpha-receptor subtypes. Alpha-1D appears to exhibit the highest degree of staining.

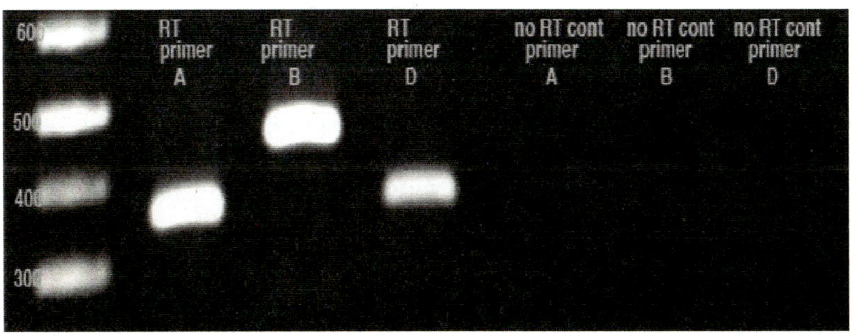

FIGURE 3. Appropriate sized cDNA products confirming ureteral RNA expression of the three alpha-receptor subtypes by RT-PCR.

In the Western blotting of extracts prepared from adult human ureters, the antibody against alpha-1-ARs recognized a major protein with molecular weights of 55, 65, 80 kDa respectively (not shown). Appropriate sized bands were obtained for all three receptors in protein extracts from lung, kidney, and umbilical cord (positive controls) and all ureter specimens (not shown). Protein expression of adrenergic receptors varied along the length of the ureter. As was seen with the immunohistochemical analysis along the ureter, the degree of expression of the alpha-receptors was highest at the renal pelvis and decreased toward the distal ureter. From the distal ureter onward, there was a marked re-increase in expression towards the ureteral orifice. The relative expression as measured by optical densitometry is shown in Fig. 4.

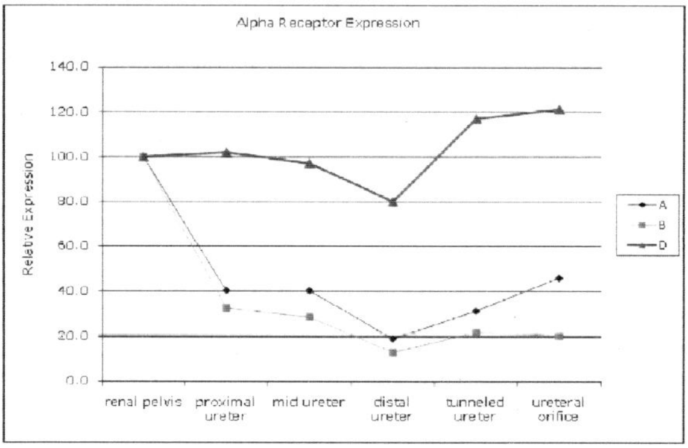

FIGURE 4. Alpha receptor protein expression along the length of the entire human ureter.

DISCUSSION

Prior pharmacologic studies have demonstrated the functional significance of adrenergic receptors in the human ureter [1-6,8,10]. Through use of immunohistochemistry, western blotting, and RT-PCR, this research demonstrates the presence and distribution of the alpha adrenergic receptor system in the tunica media of the ureteral smooth muscle along the human ureter. As Figs. 1 and 2 demonstrate, there is an intense reddish brown deposit within the tunica media of the smooth muscle of the ureter representing the alpha-adrenergic receptors; the collagen/connective tissue shows no signal. This staining pattern was consistent for all alpha-receptor subtypes with the degree of intensity strongest for the alpha-1D subtype and weakest for the alpha-1B subtype.

When using immunohistochemistry for validation, polyclonal antibodies, such as those used here, may display different degrees of reactivity. This can cause each antibody to stain and appear differently under the light microscope leading to a possible misrepresentation of the relative receptor densities. Thus, we used molecular techniques to validate our findings, which confirmed a greater degree of expression of the alpha-1D subtypes (Figs. 3 and 4). This same finding has been reported in a recent study using only RT-PCR with competitive radioligand binding assays [22,23]. The characterization of the different receptor subtypes along the ureter is needed to predict the existence of a pharmacological 'uroselectivity' in the ureter that would provide a rationale for selective pharmacologic therapy [24-26].

Also interesting in this study is the demonstration that the degree of expression of each receptor subtype varied along the length of the ureter. Both immunohisto-chemical and molecular analyses display the highest density of each receptor subtype at the renal pelvis with decrement along the ureter until the most distal section where there was again an increase in expression and density toward the tunneled ureter and ureteral orifice. We have postulated a possible physiologic role for such a distribution. When a bolus of urine enters the large surface area of the renal pelvis, a great degree of force is needed to organize and propel the urine down the narrow ureteral lumen. Therefore, the renal pelvis exhibits a random but high density distribution of all three receptor subtypes. Greater expression of the alpha-1-receptors in the proximal ureter allows muscular compression of the smooth muscle wall to propel the urine distally. Since mid-ureteral luminal diameter is less than in the pelvis and proximal ureter, less muscle tone is necessary to achieve a similar degree of coaptation to propel the urine bolus. If the mid ureter had a greater degree of expression of alpha innervation, it seems plausible that ureteral spasm could be precipitated, resulting in reflux of urine to the renal pelvis or the need for increased renal pelvic pressure to continue the antegrade transport of urine. Once the urine has passed the crossing iliac vessels however, an anatomical barrier is formed, which functionally closes off the ureter against anti-peristaltic waves. The distal increase in expression of alpha-receptors may then serve physiologically to assist in propulsion of urine toward the urinary bladder and prevent vesicoureteral reflux (by negating ureteral tone in this region) without initiating retrograde flow. It would also then be plausible to assume that beta-receptor expression (which usually mediates relaxation in the digestive and urinary system) would demonstrate inverse expression.

Recently, there has been great interest in using alpha receptor blockade for patients with urinary lithiasis, an approach referred to as 'medical expulsive therapy' [13-17]. Several pioneering studies have already addressed the presence and function of the autonomic nervous system in the ureter [1-10,19,27]. Both animal and human studies have confirmed opposing effects of the alpha and beta adrenergic systems on ureteral physiology. This is similar to the effects that the autonomic system has on other parts of the body including the eye, heart, and gastrointestinal tract. Early on, Weiss and Morita et al. demonstrated that the alpha adrenergic contractile activity dominates the relaxing effects of beta-stimulation [4-6,10]. It was then demonstrated that alpha-adrenergic receptors modulate both ureteral tone and the volume of urine passing through the ureter. Based chiefly on these pharmacologic findings, several studies have shown that the alpha-1D-blocker tamsulosin could aid and induce rapid expulsion of juxtavesical urinary calculi [13,14,16,17]. Our findings lend support to these studies, as our results indicate that there is expression of alpha-1D receptors in the uretero-vesical junction. By blocking ureteral contraction, the distal ureter may dilate allowing for expulsion of distal ureteral stones.

Although these reports suggest encouraging efficacy for alpha-blockade on stone passage, the data is preliminary and derived only from a select group of patients. Moreover, the alpha receptor adrenergic system is only one system of many affecting ureteral function and physiology. Presence of beta 'relaxation' adrenergic receptors, as well as histaminic, prostaglandin, and dopaminergic systems have all been demonstrated in the human ureter. Their exact roles in ureteral physiology and function have yet to be determined. Further investigational research with newer immunohistochemical and molecular techniques is needed in order to elucidate the intricate and complex interactions of these receptor families on ureteral physiology. Then, hopefully, a rational approach can be developed for predicting which calculi can be treated with medical therapy.

CONCLUSION

We provide evidence for the ability to detect and quantify alpha-1-receptor subtypes along the human ureter, which, to the best of our knowledge, has not been done with immunohistochemistry and molecular techniques. These findings lend support to the preliminary studies of the effectiveness of alpha-receptor blockade in ureteral colic and stone passage. Further research is warranted to determine the precise role of other receptor families in ureteral physiology and function.

REFERENCES

1. Malin JM, Jr., Deane RF, Boyarsky S. Characterisation of adrenergic receptors in human ureter. Br J Urol 1970: 42(2):171-174.
2. Morita T, Wada I, Suzuki T, Tsuchida S. Characterization of alpha-adrenoceptor subtypes involved in regulation of ureteral fluid transport. Tohoku J Exp Med 1987: 152(2):111-118.
3. Morita T, Ando M, Kihara K, Oshima H. Function and distribution of autonomic receptors in canine ureteral smooth muscle. Neurourol Urodyn 1994: 13(3):315-321.
4. Weiss RM, Bassett AL, Hoffman BF. Adrenergic innervation of the ureter. Invest Urol 1978: 16(2):123-127.
5. Weiss RM. Ureteral function. Urology 1978: 12(2):114-133.
6. Weiss RM. Effects of obstruction and age on the mechanical properties of the ureter. Nippon Heikatsukin Gakkai Zasshi 1978: 14 Suppl:47-49.
7. Caine M, Raz S. Some clinical implications of adrenergic receptors in the urinary tract. Arch Surg 1975: 110(3):247-250.
8. Caine M. Pharmacologic receptors in the urinary tract. Compr Ther 1983: 9(8):9-14.
9. Caine M. Alpha-adrenergic mechanisms in dynamics of benign prostatic hypertrophy. Urology 1988: 32(6 Suppl):16-20.
10. Morita T, Wada I, Saeki H, Tsuchida S, Weiss RM. Ureteral urine transport: changes in bolus volume, peristaltic frequency, intraluminal pressure and volume of flow resulting from autonomic drugs. J Urol 1987: 137(1):132-135.

11. Raz S, Zeigler M, Caine M. Hormonal influence on the adrenergic receptors of the ureter. Br J Urol 1972: 44(4):405-410.
12. Testa R, Guarneri L, Taddei C, Poggesi E, Angelico P, Sartani A et al. Functional antagonistic activity of Rec 15/2739, a novel alpha-1 antagonist selective for the lower urinary tract, on noradrenaline-induced contraction of human prostate and mesenteric artery. J Pharmacol Exp Ther 1996: 277(3):1237-1246.
13. Dellabella M, Milanese G, Muzzonigro G. Efficacy of tamsulosin in the medical management of juxtavesical ureteral stones. J Urol 2003: 170(6 Pt 1):2202-2205.
14. Porpiglia F, Ghignone G, Fiori C, Fontana D, Scarpa RM. Nifedipine versus tamsulosin for the management of lower ureteral stones. J Urol 2004: 172(2):568-571.
15. Resim S, Ekerbicer HC, Ciftci A. Role of tamsulosin in treatment of patients with steinstrasse developing after extracorporeal shock wave lithotripsy. Urology 2005: 66(5):945-948.
16. Resim S, Ekerbicer H, Ciftci A. Effect of tamsulosin on the number and intensity of ureteral colic in patients with lower ureteral calculus. Int J Urol 2005: 12(7):615-620.
17. Yilmaz E, Batislam E, Basar MM, Tuglu D, Ferhat M, Basar H. The comparison and efficacy of 3 different alpha1-adrenergic blockers for distal ureteral stones. J Urol 2005: 173(6):2010-2012.
18. Faure C, Gouhier C, Langer SZ, Graham D. Quantification of alpha 1-adrenoceptor subtypes in human tissues by competitive RT-PCR analysis. Biochem Biophys Res Commun 1995: 213(3):935-943.
19. Guimaraes S, Moura D. Vascular adrenoceptors: an update. Pharmacol Rev 2001: 53(2):319-356.
20. Novakova M, Myslivecek J. Identification of all alpha1-adrenoceptor subtypes in rat lung. Gen Physiol Biophys 2005: 24(3):349-353.
21. Resch BE, Ducza E, Gaspar R, Falkay G. Role of adrenergic receptor subtypes in the control of human placental blood vessels. Mol Reprod Dev 2003: 66(2):166-171.
22. Sigala S, Peroni A, Mirabella G, Fornari S, Palazzolo F, Pezzotti G et al. Alpha1 adrenoceptor subtypes in human urinary bladder: sex and regional comparison. Life Sci 2004: 76(4):417-427.
23. Sigala S, Dellabella M, Milanese G, Fornari S, Faccoli S, Palazzolo F et al. Evidence for the presence of alpha1 adrenoceptor subtypes in the human ureter. Neurourol Urodyn 2005: 24(2):142-148.
24. Andersson KE. Alpha-adrenoceptors and benign prostatic hyperplasia: basic principles for treatment with alpha-adrenoceptor antagonists. World J Urol 2002: 19(6):390-396.
25. Chapple C, Andersson KE. Tamsulosin: an overview. World J Urol 2002: 19(6):397-404.
26. Kirby R, Andersson KE, Lepor H, Steers WD. alpha(1)-Adrenoceptor selectivity and the treatment of benign prostatic hyperplasia and lower urinary tract symptoms. Prostate Cancer Prostatic Dis 2000: 3(2):76-83.
27. Caine M. Alpha-adrenergic blockers for the treatment of benign prostatic hyperplasia. Urol Clin North Am 1990: 17(3):641-649.Brown and K. Austin, *The New Physique*, Publisher City: Publisher Name, 2005, pp. 25-30.

The Role of Pharmacology in Ureteral Physiology and Expulsive Therapy

Travis J. Jerde and Stephen Y. Nakada

University of Wisconsin School of Medicine and Public Health; Department of Surgery/ Division of Urology; Madison, WI 53792, USA

Abstract. Research in the field of ureteral physiology and pharmacology has traditionally been directed toward relaxation of ureteral spasm as a mechanism of analgesia during painful ureteral obstruction, most often stone-induced episodes. However, interest in this field has expanded greatly in recent years with the expanded use of alpha-blocker therapy for inducing stone passage, a usage now termed "medical expulsive therapy". While most clinical reports involving expulsive therapy have focused on alpha receptor or calcium channel blockade, there are diverse studies investigating pharmacological ureteral relaxation with novel agents including cyclooxygenase inhibitors, small molecule beta receptor agonists, neurokinin antagonists, and phosphodiesterase inhibitors. In addition, cutting edge molecular biology research is revealing promising potential therapeutic targets aimed at specific molecular changes that occur during the acute obstruction that accompanies stone disease. The purpose of this report is to review the use of pharmacological agents as ureteral smooth muscle relaxants clinically, and to look into the future of expulsive therapy by reviewing the available literature of ureteral physiology and pharmacology research.

Keywords: ureter, expulsive therapy, pharmacology, smooth muscle, relaxation.
PACS: 87.19.Ff; 87.54.Hk

INTRODUCTION

The mechanistic effects of pharmacologic agents on ureteral physiology have been studied for nearly four decades. The focus of this field of research has traditionally been toward identifying pharmacological agents useful in treating the painful symptomology associated with acute ureteral obstructions, most notably urinary stone disease. Many studies have evaluated compounds that have relaxed ureteral smooth muscle tone or spasm, a process that is known to potentiate the pain associated with acute obstructions. In 2003, Dellabella and associates found that stone passage rate improved significantly in response to tamsulosin, a selective alpha receptor antagonist usually prescribed for the treatment of benign prostatic hypertrophy [1]. This observation has now been repeated by several investigators. These findings have added substantial relevance to research in ureteral physiology and pharmacology, and dramatically shifted the focus of this research from pain management to expulsive therapy.

CP900, *Renal Stone Disease, 1st Annual International Urolithiasis Research Symposium,*
edited by A. P. Evan, J. E. Lingeman, and J. C. Williams, Jr.

While alpha receptor blockers remain the focus of clinical studies in ureteral pharmacology and expulsive therapy, numerous compounds have been investigated in basic ureteral pharmacology studies including cyclooxygenase inhibitors, neurokinin antagonists, beta receptor agonists, and phosphodiesterase inhibitors [2-8]. Given the efficacy of these novel compounds in vitro, they may ultimately prove to be particularly effective in expulsive therapy when translated to clinical studies. This report focuses on the current knowledge of ureteral pharmacology as it relates to ureteral smooth muscle relaxation, the proposed mechanism of expulsive therapy, with the hope of generating ideas for future clinical studies using these therapeutics toward improved outcomes in inducing ureteral stone passage and treating pain.

In order to put this discussion in proper context, this report begins with a discussion on basic ureteral physiology and a review of ureteral coordinated ureteral contraction (peristalsis) and hypercontractility during the obstructive condition. Next, literature on clinical studies of expulsive therapy will be reviewed, followed by a discussion of basic science in vitro and animal studies of ureteral pharmacology. It is likely that the future of expulsive therapy will arise from these studies.

BASIC URETERAL PHYSIOLOGY

Visceral urinary tissues, including the urethra, bladder, and ureter, are luminal structures consisting of an epithelial layer (urothelium), a mucosal layer containing capillaries and sensory and motor nerve terminals, the functional smooth muscle layer, and a surrounding layer of adventitia and serosa [9]. The urothelium is comprised of seven layers of urothelial cells that are oriented to basal-lateral and apical surfaces similar to other epithelial layers. While the urothelium has long been thought of as functioning as a protective surface of the urinary tract, it is now known that urothelial cells are critical to ureteral function [10]. Urothelial cells sense chemical signals in the urinary lumen, perceive pressure and distension-related events, and are critical in maintaining the gnotobiotic condition of intraluminal urinary organs. In response to changes in the luminal environment, urothelial cells signal to the smooth muscle, neurons, and capillaries via release of prostanoids, catecholamines, and cytokines, causing alterations in the function of the organ [10]. While the study of this cross-layer interactive environment is novel in the ureter and bladder, it is well established in epithelial-stromal interactions of the prostate and many analogous relationships are present throughout the urinary tract [11].

The mucosal layer of urinary tissues contains microvasculature and neuronal tissue. As such, it is a major communication point between the ureter or bladder and the rest of the body, particularly the cardiovascular and nervous systems. Pain mediators released from the urothelium act on sensory nerve terminals in this layer sending pain signals to the brain, and motor nerve axons extending from their dorsal root cell bodies communicate with the smooth muscle from this layer [10]. While they are extremely uncommon during stretch and distension, edema, hemorrhage, and inflammatory cell infiltrate present in this layer in response to infection or chemical stimuli, and are commonly present during urinary tract infections and interstitial cystitis [12].

The smooth muscle layer of the urinary tract is responsible for contraction, peristalsis (in the ureter), and structural support [13]. The smooth muscle is divided into two sub-layers: an inner layer of helical cellular arrangement and an outer layer of mesh-like cellular arrangement [13]. In the ureter, the inner helical layer is responsible for contractile function of the tissue, while the outer mesh-like layer provides structural support. Normal contraction of smooth muscle is the result of electrical activity of the smooth muscle cell membrane. In a resting smooth muscle cell, the membrane potential is approximately 80 mV [9]. When stimulated by chemical signal or cell-to-cell electrical conduction, Na^+ and K^+ ion conductance increases the membrane potential to 50 mV, at which point an action potential is generated. At this point, smooth muscle cells lose their preferential permeability to K^+ and become more permeable to Ca^{++} ions moving into the cell, primarily via L-type Ca^{++} channels [9]. This increase in intracytosolic calcium concentration ($[Ca^{++}]_i$) results in activation of calcium-dependent calmodulin (CaM). CaM activates myosin light chain kinase, which phosphorylates myosin, activating it as a motor protein to migrate up actin filaments thereby contracting the cell. In the case of normally functioning tissue, the increase in $[Ca^{++}]_i$ during upstroke of the action potential eventually activates outward Ca^{++}-dependent K^+ currents such that repolarization occurs and membrane potential is returned to its resting level [9].

In the ureter, this depolarization-repolarization cycle is coordinated in a peristaltic wave, where electrical potentials are generated in pacemaker tissue within the renal pelvis and propagated distally from cell to cell membrane conduction at intermediate junctions [9]. Smooth muscle cells possess resistive and capacitative membrane properties conducive to propagation of electrical currents. Such currents are generated in interstitial cells of Cajal in a rhythmic fashion [9]. Urine propulsion is performed in a bolus fashion, where small local distensions induce mediator release in concert with electrical wave potentials [9]. The result is coordinated peristalsis of urine from the renal pelvis to the bladder.

Hormones that elevate $[Ca^{++}]_i$ including prostanoids, neuropeptides, and cytokines, as well as integrin signaling, can induce smooth muscle cell contractility and increase ureteral contractility [14]. In the case of kidney-stone-induced obstruction, the activation of these cascades occurs, potentiating contraction. Contractility of urinary tract smooth muscle increases luminal pressure and contact (in the case of calculi) with the noxious stimulus, intensifying the pain cascade. Prostanoids, neuropeptides, and catecholamines activate $G_{\alpha}q$-protein coupled receptors (GPCRs) of the seven-transmembrane domain superfamily [15]. These ligand-receptor interactions lead to the activation of phospholipase C-β (PLCβ), which catalyzes the synthesis of inositol triphosphate (IP_3) and diacylglycerol (DAG) from phosphoinositol bisphosphate (PIP_2). IP_3 opens IP_3-sensitive calcium channels on the sarcoplasmic reticulum and mitochondria, causing Ca^{++} flux into the cytosol where it can interact with CaM and induce the actin-myosin contractile cascade [15]. It is likely that pharmacologic inhibition of prostanoid synthesis, neuropeptide receptors, alpha-adrenergic receptors, or phosphodiesterases ultimately works by preventing the activation of the above-mentioned signal transduction mechanisms, leading to smooth muscle relaxation, spasm-induced pain relief, and stone passage.

CLINICAL STUDIES OF EXPULSIVE THERAPY

Tamsulosin

Prior to 2003, most ureteral physiology studies were conducted seeking novel ureteral smooth muscle relaxants to relieve the pain associated with ureteral spasm. In 2003, Dellabella and associates showed that the selective alpha adrenoreceptor antagonist tamsulosin increases stone passage rate from 70% to 100%, and decreased passage time from 111 hrs to 66 hrs, with 30 patients in each arm [1]. This same research group reported two years later that tamsulosin given alone produced a 90% stone free rate at a median time of 120 hours. Cervenakov and associates reported similar efficacy increases by tamsulosin [16]. In similar studies, DeSio et al reported that tamsulosin increased stone passage rate from 58% with diclofinac and aescin (anti-inflammatory drugs) alone to 90% with tamsulosin treatment [17]. Median passage time improved from 180 hours with anti-inflammatories alone to 116 hours with tamsulosin [17].

Non-selective Alpha Antagonists

Tamsulosin is considered a selective alpha-receptor antagonist [18], meaning it is selective for alpha-1A and 1D receptors (for review, please see Michelotti et al, 2000 [19]). However, non-selective alpha blockers have been shown to produce similar stone passage success rates as tamsulosin [20]. Yilmaz and associates report that tamsulosin, terazosin, and doxazosin all similarly increased stone passage rate from controls, from 52% to 79%, 78%, 75%, respectively [20]. In addition, Mohseni and associates have confirmed these findings with terazosin [21]. While it is clear that more studies need to be conducted to carefully compare the efficacy and safety of various alpha-receptor antagonists in stone passage, these early reports suggest that non-selective alpha blockade might be a viable treatment option in patients in which non-selective alpha-blockers are not contraindicated for other health concerns.

Calcium Channel Blockers

While alpha receptor antagonists have received the most attention as pharmacologic agents inducing stone passage, calcium channel blockers have performed equally well in clinical studies to date. Borghi and associates found that nifedipine increased stone passage rate from 65% to 87% [22]. Similar efficacy was reported by Saita and associates [23], while Porpiglia and associates report that nifedipine increased stone passage from 33% to 71%, and median passage time from 20 days to 7 [24]. Though no conclusive, large randomized study comparing alpha blockers to calcium channel blockers has been reported, an extensive meta-analysis by Hollingsworth et al.

calculates that calcium channel blockers' expulsive rate relative to control is 1.90 compared to 1.54 for tamsulosin [25]. The authors of this article conclude that both therapies are significantly improved over non-treated subjects, but there is no significant difference to date between alpha receptor antagonism and calcium channel blockade. This conclusion is supported by small comparison studies [26-27]. It is important to note that the large range of values and inconsistencies in the literature reports (inclusion criteria, stone size, location, etc.) make concrete comparisons difficult.

Corticosteroids

Numerous studies have looked at corticosteroids in combination with either alpha antagonists or channel blockers, but few have compared these compounds to other drug classes. To date, steroids appear to have additive effect with other drugs, but little efficacy alone [28]. When administered with deflazacort (a corticosteroid) tamsulosin increased stone passage rate increased to 97% (from 90%) with a median time of 72 hours [29]. At present, it appears corticosteroids may provide a modest improvement in stone passage when used in combination with either alpha antagonist or calcium blocker, but appear to have no significant effect alone.

Expulsive Therapy with SWL

Pharmacologic expulsive therapy also appears to have efficacy when used in combination with lithotripsy. Three studies to date have evaluated shockwave lithotripsy in combination with tamsulosin treatment, and all three report significant improvements in pain scores and number of renal/ureteral colic episodes [30-32]. In addition, studies by Gravina et al. and Kupeli et al. demonstrate that stone-free rates were significantly higher in patients on tamsulosin therapy relative to controls [31-32]. While further study is needed to fully characterize pharmacologic intervention in combination with SWL and comparisons between drug classes in this indication have yet to be performed, early studies in this area suggest that ureteral relaxant therapy may improve the efficacy of conventional stone treatments.

Summary

While the clinical treatment of pharmacologic expulsive therapy for kidney stones continues to evolve, several important concepts arise from clinical studies to date. Alpha adrenergic antagonism and calcium channel blockade significantly enhance stone passage rate relative to controls. At present, there appears to be no significant difference between these two drug classes with regard to clinical efficacy. In addition, most evidence suggests that non-selective alpha receptor antagonists, including doxazosin, have similar efficacy to tamsulosin at improving stone passage rates and median passage time. Corticosteroids may slightly enhance the expulsive efficacy of other therapeutics, but appear to have limited or no effect alone. Finally, early reports suggest that expulsive therapy enhances the effectiveness of conventional stone therapy.

IN VITRO STUDIES OF URETERAL RELAXATION

In depth pharmacological analysis of the ureter began in the early 1970's. The goal of this research was to further the basic knowledge of this understudied organ with the hope that ureteral smooth muscle relaxation might benefit renal hydronephrosis proximal to obstruction and pain associated with urinary obstructions, including stones. Stone expulsion was not an objective. While anecdotal evidence suggested ureteral smooth muscle relaxation would relieve pain associated with acute ureteral obstruction, Laird and associates provided direct evidence that spasm and hypercontractility significantly potentiate the pain response in 1997 [33]. Many antagonists/enzyme inhibitors were studied for pharmacological activity, working toward developing non-narcotic therapeutics for analgesia using ureteral smooth muscle relaxation as a model. Regardless, the belief was that inhibiting contraction of the ureter, and therefore peristalsis, would prevent stone passage rather than promote it. Today, there is substantial evidence that pharmacologic relaxation of the ureter enhances stone passage rate. As such, the clinical studies previously reviewed have added substantial gravity and energy to the field of ureteral physiology and pharmacology, with the hope that drugs originally investigated to relieve pain might be candidates for expulsive therapy. Because alpha receptor antagonists and calcium channel blockers may not be suitable for all patients, it is critical to look to the currently available knowledge of pharmacologic agents in vitro as a source of therapeutic candidates in the future expulsive therapy.

Cyclooxygenase Inhibitors

Cyclooxygenase (COX) inhibitors have been studied in ureter since 1986, and have proven successful at inhibiting ureteral contractility in numerous studies [2-4,34-36]. COX catalyzes the synthesis of prostanoids from arachidonic acid and exists in two isoforms: COX-1 and COX-2 [37]. Though COX-1 can be regulated, it is usually considered to be expressed constitutively. In contrast, COX-2 is highly inducible by inflammatory and mechanical stimuli, and is highly induced during ureteral obstruction [38-40]. Because prostanoids are highly potent smooth muscle contractants, inhibition of their synthesis expectedly causes smooth muscle relaxation. Nonselective COX inhibitors have been successful in treating the pain associated with urinary calculi [41-43], and these compounds produce complete ureteral relaxation overtime, unlike other compounds. Interestingly, ureteral contractility is inhibited by nonselective and COX-2 selective inhibitors (including celecoxib) equally well, suggesting a primary role for COX-2-derived prostanoids in this system [4,34,36].

Despite promising in vitro data, use of COX inhibitors in expulsive therapy may be limited. Prostacyclin-driven contralateral renal vasodilation is COX-2 dependent, explaining the high rate of renal insufficiency with these compounds, particularly in the face of obstruction [44]. In addition, there are conflicting reports on the effect of COX inhibitors on stone passage rates, with most reporting minimal or no effect despite clear efficacy in ureteral relaxation relative to alpha receptor antagonists [45-47]. It has been proposed that this may be due to a complete inhibition of contraction of the ureter by COX inhibitors, whereas alpha antagonists may block spasm but not coordinated peristalsis [48]. However, this assertion is yet to be supported by clear scientific evidence. Future related research might be directed toward specific prostanoid receptor antagonism, as it has been shown that the EP-3 prostanoid receptor plays a role ureteral contractility [49-50]. However, studies in this area are limited by lack of quality specific antagonists at present.

Phosphodiesterase Inhibitors

Phosphodiesterase (PDE) inhibitors have been studied in the ureter since the late 1980's. PDE inhibitors produce substantial effects on ureteral contractility, and appear to be nearly as efficacious as COX inhibitors [51-53]. PDE enzymes degrade the cyclic nucleotides, cAMP and cGMP, and the mechanism of these compounds is inhibition of this process. The resulting elevation of cyclic nucleotide concentrations leads to smooth muscle relaxation via activation of protein kinase A and subsequent phosphorylation and inhibition of myosin light chain kinase. PDE exist in seven isoforms, each with varying specificities for cAMP and cGMP [37]. Specific inhibition of the PDE-IV isoform has repeatedly shown greater efficacy than inhibition of the other isoforms [51], though it appears that PDE-V isoform inhibition does cause ureteral relaxation [53]. Of the clinically available drugs studied to date, rolipram, a selective PDE-IV inhibitor, has been shown to be the most potent PDE inhibitor in vitro at inhibiting ureteral contractility [52]. However, PDE-IV inhibitors are notoriously high in systemic effects, and this would likely limit their clinical utility particularly in a market pre-possessing alpha receptor and calcium channel inhibitors [54].

Neurokinin Receptor Antagonists

Among the most efficacious ureteral contractility inhibitors are the neurokinin receptor antagonists. There are three known neurokinin receptors in mammals: NK-1, NK-2, and NK-3; each receptor has preferential affinity for the ligands substance P, neurokinin A, and neurokinin B, respectively [55]. Antagonism of these receptors prevents activation of G-protein coupled receptor signaling cascades, phospholipase C synthesis and ultimately, calcium flux, thereby causing relaxation [55]. The NK-2 receptor is clearly the most dominant NK receptor in the ureter, and inhibition of this receptor inhibits both spontaneous and inducible contractility [5-6]. Though these compounds have not been evaluated clinically, NK-2 antagonism would likely offer analgesia and possibly, enhanced stone passage via ureteral relaxation. Systemic effects of these compounds have not been evaluated to date, as none of these compounds are as of yet clinically available. Future research in this field should include development of clinically-available NK antagonists.

Adrenergic Receptor Agonists/Antagonists

While the presence and activity of adrenergic receptors in the ureter has long been described, the use of specific receptor modulators in ureteral physiology studies has been recently buoyed by clinical reports of stone passage induced by these compounds. There are three groups of adrenergic receptors: alpha-1 receptors that induce contractility by phospholipase-C and calcium-dependent signaling; alpha-2 receptors that induce contractility by inhibition of cyclic nucleotide signaling; and beta receptors that inhibit contractility by induction of cyclic nucleotide signaling [19]. Despite the clinical efficacy of alpha-receptor antagonists at inducing stone passage, these compounds appear to have less efficacy in vitro than the above mentioned classes of inhibitors. However, Nakada and associates have recently reported that alpha receptor antagonism causes complete ureteral relaxation only in the presence of epinephrine, the endogenous ligand of both alpha and beta receptors [56]. This suggests a key role for beta receptors in alpha antagonist efficacy, such that beta activation by epinephrine is unopposed during alpha receptor antagonism. While this has yet to be proven experimentally, studies using selective beta agonists have shown remarkable relaxation of ureteral smooth muscle [7], further supporting a role for beta receptors in this system. Selective beta agonists are available clinically for the treatment of asthma, and future studies of expulsive therapy will likely include these compounds.

Future Studies in Ureteral Physiology and Pharmacology

Several other interesting pharmacologic compounds have been evaluated in ureteral smooth muscle relaxation. 5-hydroxytryptamine (5-HT, serotonin) receptor antagonists have shown efficacy in relaxing the ureter [57], and these compounds may become of greater interest upon further receptor characterization in the ureter. Similarly, many adenosine receptor subtypes exist in the ureter, and Hernandez and associates have reported that A2B adenosine receptors mediate ureteral relaxation [58]. Selective agonists of this receptor may ultimately prove useful in relaxing the ureter and promoting stone passage. Finally, the tricyclic antidepressant amitriptyline has been shown to relax ureteral smooth muscle, though a mechanism for this action has not been defined [59].

Novel experimental models hold the potential to dynamically shift the experimental direction of ureteral research in the future. An in vivo animal model developed by Venkatesh and associates is able to measure ureteral contractility rates in vivo [60]. Using this model, this group has evaluated the in vivo relaxation effects of calcium channel blockers, neurokinin receptor antagonists, and theophyline. Future studies with this model would likely include characterizing the effects of known relaxants in vivo, in vitro, and in clinical studies.

Novel molecular and cellular biology techniques will allow the systematic determination of new therapeutic targets using genetic and biochemical knockdown of specific molecules within ureteral cells. A model developed by Jerde et al has been used to characterize COX-2 induction in ureteral-derived primary epithelial cells in culture [40]. Using this model, our group has found that mechanically-induced COX-2 expression in cell culture mimics that of the in vivo condition. Distension-induced COX-2 expression is regulated at transcriptional and post-transcriptional levels (via mRNA stability), and is dependent upon calcium and protein kinase C-zeta signaling [61]. Future studies springing from this work would be directed toward development of a novel protein kinase C zeta inhibitor and evaluation of this compound in vitro, in animals, and ultimately, in expulsive therapy.

Summary

Relaxation of the ureter in the lab has been studied for many years, primarily for developing improved analgesia. Experimental studies show the most effective compounds have been the NSAIDs, PDE-IV inhibitors, and NK antagonists. COX inhibitors are very successful at reducing ureteral contractility, but produce systemic effects that are pronounced during acute obstruction, limiting their clinical utility. Although alpha receptor antagonism had modest effects on ureteral contractility in vitro, the presence of epinephrine significantly enhances the effect, suggesting a likely role for the beta receptors. This hypothesis is supported by studies using selective beta receptor agonists. Cellular and molecular studies are identifying new therapeutic targets (such as PKCζ) that may minimize systemic effects while optimizing therapeutic effect. Future work in ureteral physiology and pharmacology will likely include translating in vitro and molecular studies to the clinics and improving drug development of novel therapeutic agents identified in vitro or in cell assays.

ACKNOWLEDGMENTS

The authors extend their sincere appreciation to Drs. William Mellon, Dale Bjorling, Ricardo Saban, and Debra Hullett for expert input in pharmacological and molecular biological studies conducted by our laboratory, and Tawnya Cary-Coyle, Kwadwo Owusu-Ofori, Jamie Calamon-Dixon, Dr. Patrick Lowry, and Dr. Murali Ankem for conducting research in our laboratory which is referenced in this report.

REFERENCES

1. Dellabella M, Milanese G, Muzzonigro G. *J. Urol.* **170,** 2202-2205 (2003).
2. Thulesius O, Ugaily-Thulesius L, Angelo-Khattar M. *Acta. Physiol. Scand.* **127,** 485-490 (1986).
3. Cole RS, Fry CH, Shuttleworth KE. *Br J Urol.* **61,** 19-26 (1988).
4. Jerde TJ, Calamon-Dixon JL, Bjorling DE, Nakada SY. *Urology.* **65,** 185-190 (2005).
5. Patacchini R, et al. *Br J Pharmacol.* **125,** 987-996 (1998).
6. Nakada SY, Jerde TJ, Bjorling DE, Saban R. *J. Urol.* **166,** 1534-1538 (2001).
7. Tomiyama et al. *J. Pharmacol. Sci.* 92: 411-419 (2003).
8. Kuhn et al, *Urol Res.* **28,** 110-115 (2000).
9. Weiss RM. "Physiology and Pharmacology of the Renal Pelvis and Ureter." In *Campbell's Urology*. Edited by Walsh PC, Retik AB, Vaughan ED, Wein A. Philadelphia, PA, WB Saunders, 1998, pp.839-869.
10. Birder L. *Scand. J. Urol. Nephrol.* **215,** 48-53 (2004).
11. Wong YC, Wang YZ. *Int Rev Cytol.* **199,** 65-116 (2000).
12. Itano NM, Malek RS. *J Urol.* **165,** 805-807 (2001).

13. Morita T, Ando M, Kihara K, Oshima H. *Urol Int.* **55,** 123-127 (1995).
14. Young LS, Hegarty NJ, Fitzpatrick JM. "Upper urinary tract obstruction" in *The Scientific Basis of Urology*. Edited by Mundy AR, Fitzpatrick JM, Neal DE, and George NJR. Oxford, UK, Isis Medical Media, 1999.
15. Kiselyov K, Shin DM, Muallem S. *Cell Signal.* **15,** 243-253 (2003).
16. Cervenakov I, et. al. *Int. Urol. Nephrol.* **34,** 25-29 (2002).
17. DeSio et al. *J. Endourol.* **20,** 12-16, (2006).
18. Wilde MI, McTavish D. *Drugs* **52,** 883-898 (1996).
19. Michelotti GA, Price DT, Schwinn DA. *Pharmacol. Ther.* **88,** 281-309 (2000).
20. Yilmaz E, et al. *J Urol.* **173,** 2010-2012 (2005).
21. Mohseni MG, Hosseini SR, Alizadeh F. *Saudi Med. J.* **27,** 838-840 (2006).
22 Borghi J. et al. *J.Urol.* **152,** 1095-1098 (1994).
23. Saita A. et al. *Urol. Int.* **72,** 43-45 (2004).
24. Porpiglia F. et al. *Urology* **56,** 579-582 (2000).
25. Hollingsworth et al. *The Lancet* **368,** 1171-1179 (2006)
26. Porpiglia F. et al. *J Urol.* **172:** 568-571 (2004).
27. Dellabella M, Milanese G, Muzzonigro G. *J Urol.* **174,** 167-172 (2005).
28. Porpiglia et al, *Eur. Urol.* **50,** 339-344 (2006).
29. Dellabella et al. *UROLOGY* **66,** 712-715 (2005).
30. Resim S, Ekerbicer HC, Ciftci A. *Urology* **66,** 945-948 (2005).
31. Gravina GL, et. al. *Urology* **66,** 24-28 (2005).
32. Kupeli B, et. al. *Urology* **64,** 1111-1115 (2004).
33. Laird et al. *Am. J. Physiol.* **272,** R1409-R1414 (1997).
34. Nakada SY, Jerde TJ, Bjorling DE, Saban R. *J. Urol.* **163,** 607-612 (2000)
35. Mastrangelo D. et al. *Urol. Res.* **28,** 376-382 (2000).
36. Davidson ME, Lang RJ. *Br. J. Pharmacol.* **129,** 661-670 (2000).
37. Bushnik T, Conti M. *Biochem. Soc. Trans.* **24,** 1014-1019 (1996).
38. Nakada SY, et al. *J. Urol.* **168,** 1226-1229 (2002).
39. Norregaard R. et al. *Kidney Int.* **70,** 872-881 (2006).
40. Jerde TJ, Mellon WS, Bjorling DE, Nakada SY. *J. Pharmacol. Exp. Ther.* **317:** 965-972 (2006).
41. Basar I. et. al. *Int. Urol. Nephrol.* **23,** 227-230, (1991).
42. Ahmad M, Chaughtai MN, Khan FA. *J. Pak. Med. Assoc.* **41,** 268-270 (1991).
43. al-Sahlawi KS, Tawfik, OM: *Eur. J. Emerg. Med.* **3,** 183. (1996)
44. Hernandez J, Astudillo H, Escalante B. *Am. J. Physiol. Renal Physiol.* **282,** F592-598 (2002).
45. Laerum E. et. al. *Eur. Urol.* **28,** 108–111 (1995).
46. Grenabo L, Holmlund D. *Scand. J. Urol. Nephrol.* **18,** 325–327 (1984).
47. Kapoor DA, Weitzel S, Mowad JJ, Melanson S, Gillen J. *J Urol.* **142,** 1428–30 (1989)
48. Davenport K, Timoney AG, Keeley FX. *BJU Int.* **98,** 651-655 (2006).
49. Ankem M, Jerde TJ, Wilkinson ER, Nakada SY: *J. Endourol.* **19,** 1088-1091 (2006).
50. Lowry PS, Jerde TJ, Bjorling DE, Maskel JL, Nakada SY. *J. Endourol.* **19,** 183-187 (2004).
51. Stief CG. et. al. *Urol. Int.* **55,** 183-189 (1995).
52. Becker AJ. et al. *J. Urol.* 160, 920-925 (1998).
53. Uckert S, et. al. *Eur. Urol.* **50,** 1194-1207 (2006).
54. Lehnart SE, Marks AR. *Expert Opin. Ther. Targets.* **10,** 677-688 (2006).
55. Regoli D, Nguyen K, Calo G. *Ann N Y Acad Sci.* **812,** 144-146. (1997).
56. Nakada SY, Moon TD, Hedican SP, Jerde TJ: *J. Urol.***173,** A1104 (2005).
57. Hernandez M. et al. *Br. J. Pharmacol.* **138,** 137-144, (2003).
58. Hernandez M, et al. *Br. J. Pharmacol.* **126,** 969-978 (1999).
59. Archar et al. *Kidney Int.* **64,** 1356-1364 (2003).
60. Venkatesh R. et. al. *J. Endourol.* **19,** 170-176 (2005).
61. Jerde TJ, Mellon WS, Bjorling DE, Nakada SY. *J.Urol.* **175,** A542 (2006).

Advances in Ureteral Stent Design

John D. Denstedt

Division of Urology, Department of Surgery, Schulich School of Medicine and Dentistry, The University of Western Ontario, London, Ontario, CANADA

Abstract. Ureteral stents are commonly used in urolithiasis patients for relief of obstruction or in association with stone treatments such as ureteroscopy and extracorporeal shock wave lithotripsy. There are currently many different bulk materials and coatings available for the manufacture of ureteral stents, however the ideal material has yet to be discovered. All potential biomaterials must undergo rigorous physical and biocompatibility testing before commercialization and use in humans. Despite significant advances in basic science research involving biocompatibility issues and biofilm formation, infection and encrustation remain associated with the use of biomaterials in the urinary tract. There have been many significant advances in the design of ureteral stents in recent years and these will be highlighted along with a discussion of future aspects of biomaterials and use of stents in association with urolithiasis.

Keywords: ureteral stents, biocompatible materials
PACS: 01.30.Cc; 81.05.Zx

INTRODUCTION

Ureteral stents have become an important part of contemporary urologic practice since Finney [1] and Hepperlen [2] and colleagues first described the double-J stent and single-pigtail stent [3], respectively. Since that time, there have been many advances in design that have been directed at improving biocompatibility and reducing stent related morbidity. Ureteral stents are very commonly placed in patients with urolithiasis, either to relieve obstruction or in association with interventions, such as extracorporeal shock wave lithotripsy, ureteroscopy or percutaneous surgery. Although significant advances in basic science research involving biocompatibility issues and biofilm formation have been achieved, infection and encrustation remain problems associated with stents in the urinary tract and therefore limit their long-term use. In recent years, different raw biomaterials have made the transition from laboratory research to widespread use in the clinical realm. However, despite ongoing intensive basic science and clinical research, the ideal biomaterial is yet to be discovered. Nonetheless, there have been many significant advances in the design of ureteral stents, and these will be highlighted along with a discussion of the future of biomaterials in the urinary tract.

CP900, *Renal Stone Disease, 1st Annual International Urolithiasis Research Symposium,*
edited by A. P. Evan, J. E. Lingeman, and J. C. Williams, Jr.

STENT BIOMATERIALS AND COATINGS: WHAT IS AVAILABLE?

The biomaterials currently placed in the urinary tract are most commonly composed of synthetic polymeric compounds including polyurethane, silicone and other proprietary combinations of "plastic" materials. Silicone, composed of alternating silicone and oxygen atoms, is the current gold standard with respect to tissue compatibility owing to its nontoxic and inert nature [4]. Silitek is a proprietary silicone-based block copolymer. C-Flex is a proprietary silicone-modified styrene/ethylene/butylenes block copolymer and percuflex is a proprietary olefinic block copolymer. Each of these biomaterials has been used widely and successfully in the urinary tract whether it be in the form of urethral catheters or ureteral stents. Hydrogels are the coating most commonly used for urinary tract devices at present. Hydrogels are composed of a hydrophilic polymer that allows water to be trapped in the chemical structure. This reduces the coefficient of friction of the material, which improves biocompatibility by reducing frictional irritation and cell adhesion at the biomaterial— tissue interface. Furthermore there is some evidence that hydrogel coatings result in a reduction of encrustation [5].

STENT BIOMATERIALS: WHAT IS NEW?

Recently, there have been a number of interesting publications assessing new urinary tract biomaterials and coatings. One material that was tested in an study by Laaksovirta and associates [6] is a self-reinforced L-lactide-glycolic acid copolymer, molar ratio 80:20 (80% L-lactide and 20% glycolic acid). In a chronic rabbit implantation model, the authors tested the biocompatibility of this material both in muscle tissue and in the urinary tract. Urethral stents of self-reinforced L-lactide-glycolic acid copolymer or steel were inserted via cystoscopy into the rabbit prostatic urethra and removed as much as 3 months later. The copolymer stents were soft and had been almost completely degraded at 3 months. The material did not encroach into the urethral wall and there was no encrustation.

In another recent study, Nitinol was evaluated as a urinary stent material in an animal model [7]. Nitinol is a nickel-titanium allow that has gained widespread use for many disposable devices for urology, including guidewires, stone graspers, and stone baskets. In an in vivo canine model, a novel application was evaluated in the form of a polyurethane-covered retrievable, expandable urethral Nitinol stent. Unfortunately, the study was complicated by stent migration, failed stent removal, and accumulation of granulation tissue at both ends of the stent, leading the authors to conclude that some design modifications were necessary.

Bioabsorbable or dissolvable biomaterials have recently been developed for ureteral drainage stents to eliminate the need for cystoscopic removal. Moreover, such a biodegradable stent would shorten the period of suffering for the patient and possibly eliminate the problem of forgotten or neglected stents. To this end, Olweny and colleagues [8] evaluated the use of poly-L-lactide-co-glycolide (PLGA) bioabsorbable ureteral stent following Acucise (Applied Medical Resources, Rancho Santa Margarita, CA) balloon incision endopyelotomy in a porcine model. This self-reinforced stent was similar to a standard ureteral stent with respect to fluid flow results and postoperative appearance on retrograde pyelography. However, the PLGA stent was found to have less favorable biocompatibility than a standard stent, as indicated by inferior healing of the ureteral musculature.

The development of tissue-engineered stents is in its infancy, but this area has the potential to revolutionize biomaterial science and clinical applications of biomaterials. The use of autologous tissue would be advantageous because of its inherent biocompatibility. Using a novel approach in a very interesting study, Amiel and colleagues [9] investigated the feasibility of stents created from chondrocytes using *in vitro* and *in vivo* models. Remarkably, they were successful in creating cartilaginous stents *in vitro* and *in vivo* using chondrocyte-seeded polymer matrices. They proposed that this technology might one day become clinically useful in the treatment of urethral or ureteral strictures.

STENT COATINGS: WHAT IS NEW?

The goals of coating ureteral stents are to facilitate passage over a guidewire beyond an obstruction (i.e., to decrease friction) and to reduce, or eliminate biofilm formation and encrustation. To this end, Tunney and colleagues [10] reported on a new hydrophilic coating, polyvinylpyrrolidone, applied to polyurethane. In an *in vitro* model, the coating resulted in a decrease in both hydroxyapatite encrustation and adherence of a hydrophobic *Entercoccus faecalis* isolate. On the basis of these results, the authors concluded that coatings of polyvinylpyrrolidone might prevent bacterial biofilm formation and encrustation on biomaterials in the urinary tract and therefore warrant further evaluation.

Another coating that has potential for reducing encrustation is the phosphorylcholine group of compounds. In a recent human clinical trial, uncoated and phosphorylcholine-coated ureteral stents were examined by scanning electron microscopy 12 weeks after implantation. The phosphorylcholine-coated stents were less vulnerable to encrustation and colonization by bacterial biofilm than were the uncoated stents [11].

A novel approach to reducing biomaterial-related urinary tract encrustation involves coating biomaterials with oxalate-degrading enzymes derived from *Oxalobacter formigenes*. This anaerobic bacterium is capable of degrading oxalate through its production of several enzymes including oxalyl coenzyme A decarboxylase (OXC) and formyl coenzyme A transferase (FRC). Watterson and coworkers demonstrated incubation-based coating of OXY and FRC on silicone disks. In an *in vivo* rabbit bladder implantation model, they found a reduction in the amount of encrustation on the enzyme-coated disks versus control disks after a 30-day implantation [12].

In another recent publication, Multanen and associates, [13] assessed the biocompatibility, encrustation and biodegradation properties of silver nitrate and ofloxacin-blended caprolactone-L-lactide copolymer-coated self-reinforced poly-L-lactic acid (SR-PLLA) urospiral urethral stents in a rabbit model. The silver nitrate and ofloxacin-blended copolymer-coated urospiral stents had good biocompatibility properties and caused less tissue reaction than stents with a pure copolymer coating. Furthermore, the silver nitrate coating was effective in preventing biofilm formation and stent encrustation.

RECENT ADVANCES IN STENT DESIGN

Changes in ureteral stent design have been aimed at reducing the morbidity, namely discomfort, bladder irritability, migration, infection, encrustation, and the need for an additional cystoscopic procedure to remove the stent. There are many novel stent designs that have been introduced over the past few years, each of which is discussed below.

Mesh Stents

One effort to preserve drainage while minimizing irritative symptoms was the development of a lightweight, self-expanding mesh stent. In an established porcine animal model, Olweny and coworkers [14] compared tissue reaction and flow characteristics of a mesh stent with those of a standard 7F double-pigtail polyurethane stent. Although the difference was not statistically significant, the mesh stent tended to result in less inflammation along the urinary tract at 1 week. Furthermore, the flow rate through the mesh stent tended to be greater than that through the standard stent at both 1 and 6 weeks.

The flow characteristics of the mesh stent were compared with those of other stents in a separate porcine animal study. The greatest flow was seen with the mesh stent.

Tail Stents

Attempts to decrease ureteral stent-related bladder irritability have led to the development of a specialty device known as the Tail Stent (Microvasive Urology/Boston Scientific). This stent has a 7F proximal pigtail and a shaft that tapers to a lumenless straight 3F distal tail that resides in the bladder. To date, this stent has been assessed in two randomized clinical studies. The first was a single-blind trial in 60 patients, in which Tail Stents produced significantly fewer irritative voiding symptoms than standard 7F double-pigtail stents [15]. The second study assessed outcomes following percutaneous nephrolithotomy in 40 patients, comparing a Tail Stent with a 18F Councill nephrostomy tube for postoperative drainage versus a 24F re-entry Malecot nephrostomy tube [16]. The results were favorable for the group with the Tail Stents, as marked by a statistically significant reduction in postoperative flank pain.

Dual-durometer Stents

There is some evidence that ureteral stents that are composed of softer biomaterials are better tolerated than harder stents [17]. However, softer stents have a weaker renal coil strength and are therefore more likely to migrate and also are more difficult to push past an obstructing stone. Attempts at addressing these issues, namely, to facilitate stent placement, reduce migration, and minimize patient discomfort, have led to the development of dual-durometer stents. These stents incorporate a smooth transition from a firm biomaterial at the renal end to a soft biomaterial at the bladder end. Two such devices are the Sof-Curl (ACMI) and the Polaris (Microvasive Urology/Boston Scientific) stents, which have long tapered tips at the renal end and are coated with a hydrophilic-bonded hydrogel that decreases their coefficients of friction [18]. Their firm proximal end and hydrophilic coating allow for ease of access through the ureteral orifice and facilitate negotiation past obstruction, and the soft distal end results in decreased patient discomfort. In a study comparing six ureteral stents, the Polaris was shown to have superior lubricity (which eases stent passage) and lower flexural strength (which minimizes bladder discomfort). Unfortunately, not all contemporary hydrophilic-coated stents were assessed in this study.

FUTURE OF URETERAL STENTING

Drug-coated and drug-eluting stents

It is very likely that a variety of pharmacologically active agents will be incorporated into ureteral stents, similar to the stents in final testing stages for treating diseased coronary arteries [19]. These drugs could be applied directly to the polymeric surface of the biomaterial (surface coating) and be pharmacologically active at the surface, preventing infection or encrustation. Alternatively, drugs could be incorporated into the core of the polymeric structure of the biomaterial, being delivered into the local environment in a sustained-release fashion (drug-eluting) and consequently have potential activity at the level of the urothelium.

An interesting approach to achieving controlled release of a drug in the ureter has been reported recently [20]. In this study, large multilamellar liposomes that entrapped dexamethasone were prepared, and in an *in vitro* setting, 51% of the drug was released from the biomaterial in artificial urine over a 48-hour period. Although early in their development, techniques such as this one hold promise for controlled release of drugs from ureteral stents into the local urinary environment.

CONCLUSION

Ureteral stents will continue to be an essential tool in the practicing urologist's armamentarium. Ongoing research is essential to optimize biocompatibility and decrease stent-related complications such as pain, bladder irritability, infection, and encrustation within the urinary tract. There has been great interest in this field of research, as marked by the introduction of new biomaterials, coatings and ureteral stent designs. The future of biomaterial research is promising with continued insights into biomaterial science, further improvements in clinically available ureteral stents and a significant reduction in stent-related morbidity.

REFERENCES

1. Finney RP. Experience with new double-J ureteral catheter stent. *J Urol* 1978;120-678
2. Hepperlen TK, Mardis HK. Pigtail stent termed means of lessening ureteral surgery. *Trends Clin Urol* 1978;1-405
3. Watterson JD, Cadieux P, Denstedt JD. Ureteral stents: Which, when, and why? *AUA Update Series* 2002;21(16):122
4. Denstedt JD, Wollin TA, Reid G. Biomaterials used in urology: Current issues of biocompatibility, infection, and encrustation. *J Endourol* 1998;12-493
5. Mardis HK, Kroeger RM. Ureteral stents: Materials. *Urol Clin North Am* 1988;15-471
6. Laaksovirta S, Laurila M, Isotalo T, et al. Rabbit muscle and urethral in situ biocompatibility properties of the self-reinforced L-lactide-glycolic acid copolymer 80:20 spiral stent. *J Urol* 2002;167:1527
7. Ko GY, Kim GC, Seo TS, et al. Covered, retrievable, expandable urethral Nitinol stent: Feasibility study in dogs. *Radiology* 2002;223:83
8. Olweny EO, Landman J, Andreoni C, et al. Evaluation of the use of a biodegradable ureteral stent after retrograde endopyelotomy in a porcine model. *J Urol* 2002;167:2198
9. Amiel GE, Yoo JJ, Kim BS, Atala A. Tissue engineered stents created from chondrocytes. *J Urol* 2001;165:2091
10. Tummey MM, Gorman SP. Evaluation of a poly (vinyl pyrrolidone) coated biomaterial for urological use. *Biomaterials* 2002;23:4601
11. Stickler DJ, Evans A, Morris N, Hughes G. Strategies for the control of catheter encrustation. *Int J Antimicrob Agents* 2002;19:499
12. Watterson JD, Cadieux PA, Beiko DT, et al. Oxalate-degrading enzymes from Oxalobacter formigenes: A novel device coating to reduce urinary tract biomaterial-related encrustation. *J Endourol* 2003;17(5):269
13. Multanen M, Tammela TL, Laurila M, et al. Biocompatibility, encrustation and biodegradation of ofoxacine and silver nitrate coated poly-L-lactic acid stents in rabbit urethra. *Urol Res* 2002;30:227
14. Olweny EO, Portis AJ, Sundaram CP et al. Evaluation of a chronic indwelling prototype mesh ureteral stent in a porcine model. *Urology* 2000;56:857
15. Dunn MD, Portis AJ, Kahn SA, et al. Clinical effectiveness of new stent design: randomized single and double-pigtail stents. *J Endourol* 2000;14:195
16. Liatsikos EN, Hom D, Dinlenc CZ, et al. Tail Stent versus re-entry tube: a randomized comparison after percutaneous stone extraction. *Urology* 2002;59:15

An Everting Ureteral Access Sheath: Concepts and *In Vitro* Testing

Keith L. Lee and Marshall L. Stoller

Department of Urology, University of California San Francisco

Abstract. Ureteral access sheaths have been a recent innovation in facilitating ureteral stone surgery. Once properly placed, access sheaths allow the movement of ureteroscopes and other instruments through the ureter with minimal injury to the urothelium. However, there are shortcomings of the current device designs. Initial sheath placement requires significant force, and shear stress can injure the ureter. In addition, inadvertent advancement of the outer sheath without the inner introducer stylet can tear and avulse the ureter. A novel eversion design incorporating a lubricous film provides marked improvement over current access sheaths. In bench top and animal models, the eversion shealths require less force during advancement, cause less injury to the urothelial tissue, and have a lower potential of introducing extraneous materials (*e.g.*, microbes) into a simulated urinary tract. While, the everting design provides important advantages over traditional non-everting designs, further preclinical and clinical trials are required.

Keywords: urolithiasis, ureteral access sheath, ureteroscopy
PACS: 81.05.Zx

CLINICAL UTILITY OF URETERAL ACCESS SHEATHS

Ureteral access sheaths are a relatively recent innovation in urological surgery as a tool in facilitating repeated insertions of ureteroscopes during lithotripsy. The use of ureteral access sheaths have been shown to shorten operative times, lower operative costs, reduce the risk of ureteral trauma, and dilate a restrictive ureteral orifice [1-4]. These access sheaths currently are available with outer diameters ranging from 12 to 16 French and internal diameters of 10 to 14 French.

While access sheaths provide a pathway for multiple passes of ureteroscopes and other tools, the use of these devices is not without incident. Advancement of these devices can produce substantial shear forces to the ureter wall, and the tip can injure the underlying urothelium as the sheath is advanced. Forceful dilation of the ureteral orifice (UO) also can result in edema, necessitating placement of a stent at the end of the procedure. Pressure of the cannula against the intubated ureter has been shown to reduce blood flow in the compressed tissue, increasing risks for ischemic injury [5,6]. Many of these deleterious effects can be attributed to the sheath advancement method. An alternative design minimizing shear forces can be safer and more effective.

CP900, *Renal Stone Disease, 1st Annual International Urolithiasis Research Symposium,*
edited by A. P. Evan, J. E. Lingeman, and J. C. Williams, Jr.

Novel Device Design Incorporating an Everting Film

As instruments advance through the urethra or ureter, they exert shear forces against the urothelium, which can cause injury and may contribute to post-operative dysuria and hematuria. In order to minimize the shear or axial forces exerted against the urothelium during advancements, a novel device design has emerged based upon the concept of an everting catheter. The lumen of the device contains a film which is dispensed from the tip of the device as the cannula is advanced (Fig. 1). In this manner, the device produces radial force during its advancement but minimal axial force. Minimizing axial movement also will reduce the likelihood of moving exogenous material up into the urinary tract.

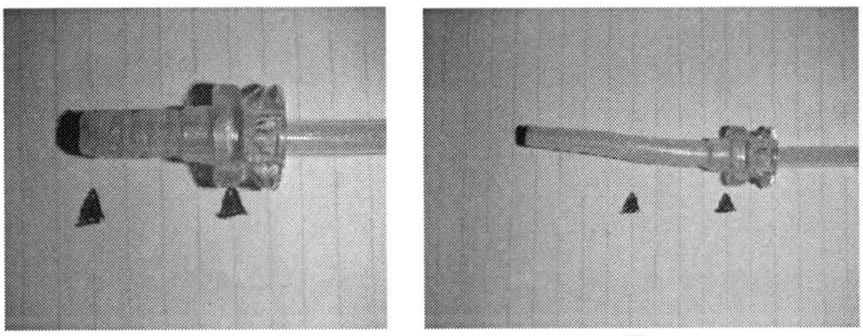

A. B.

FIGURE 1. Representative of the mechanism of the everting design. A. The film is attached to a ring on the outside of the cannula, with the majority of the film loaded into the lumen of the cannula. B. During eversion, the ring remains static while the film everts from the lumen of the device at its tip as the cannula advances.

Force Reduction During Advancement through a Lumen

Initial work with an everting urethral introducer sheath that had an outer diameter of 21 French attempted to quantify differences in forces generated as everting and non-everting devices were advanced in an artificial urethral model [7]. A urethral model of silicone was molded with a lumen of 5 mm (approximately 15 Fr) and loaded into a motorized test stand attached to a digital force meter. Advancing a 21 Fr everting device required significantly less force than for a simulated 18 Fr cystoscope or a lubricated 21 Fr non-everting dilator (Fig. 2).

Working in a similar set-up, measurements were made of the forces generated in order to dilate simulated urethra strictures with orifices of 15 Fr and 20 Fr using an everting 23 Fr introducer sheath, or 16 Fr and 22 Fr non-everting followers. The mean force generated with the everting 23 Fr everting device during advancement through the 15 Fr simulated stricture was comparable to that generated by the 16 Fr follower, even though the everting device was significantly larger in diameter. In comparison to the forces generated with the non-everting 22 Fr follower, those generated by the everting 23 Fr design moving through a 20 Fr stricture were significantly less (Fig. 3) [8,9].

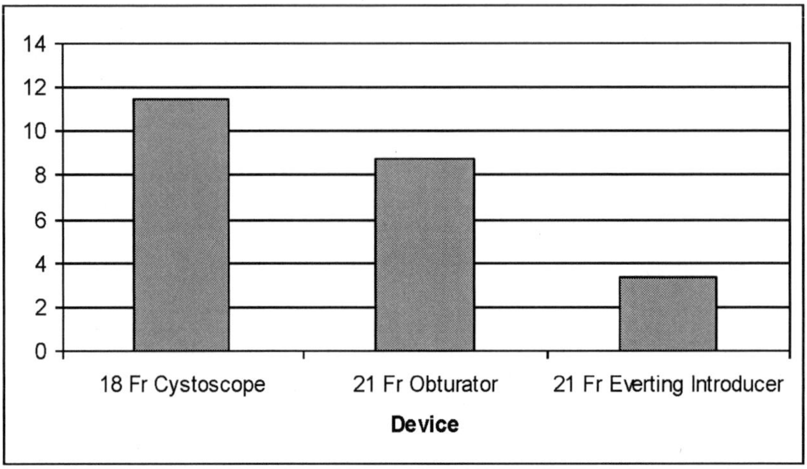

FIGURE 2. Mean peak forces (in pounds) generated while advancing three urological devices up a simulated urinary lumen that was 15 Fr (5 mm) in diameter.

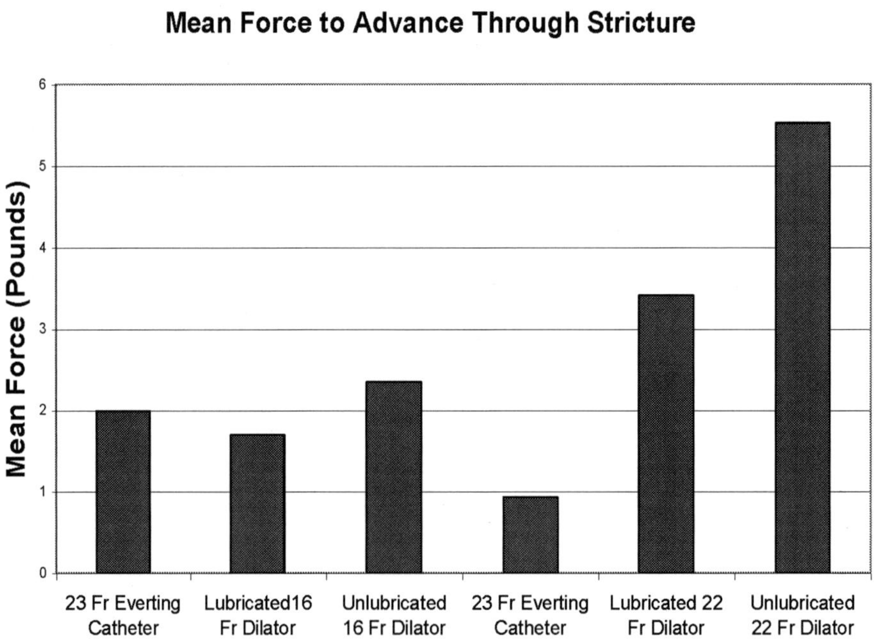

FIGURE 3. Mean peak forces generated while advancing a 23 Fr everting introducer sheath through either a 15 Fr or 20 Fr simulated stricture in comparison to the peak forces generated while advancing lubricated and unlubricated 16 Fr and 22 Fr followers through stricture orifices 15 Fr and 20 Fr in diameter, respectively.

To simulate dilation of the UO, we developed a bench top model that mimicked the UO in a silicone disc. A noneverting 14 Fr outer diameter ureteral access device, the Navigator (Boston Scientific Corporation), was advanced through the opening. The mean force necessary was 7.2 Newtons. We then loaded a length of film into the lumen of the Navigator sheath and attached the film to a small ring on the outer cannula of the device. This produced a Navigator sheath that would make use of the everting film design. With the mechanics of an everting film, the mean force for the 14 Fr Navigator sheath to advance through the 3 mm opening in the silicone disc was 1.4 Newtons (Figure 4). Clearly, the reduction in axial movement of the everting device as it is advanced through a restrictive lumen resulted in significant mechanical advantages.

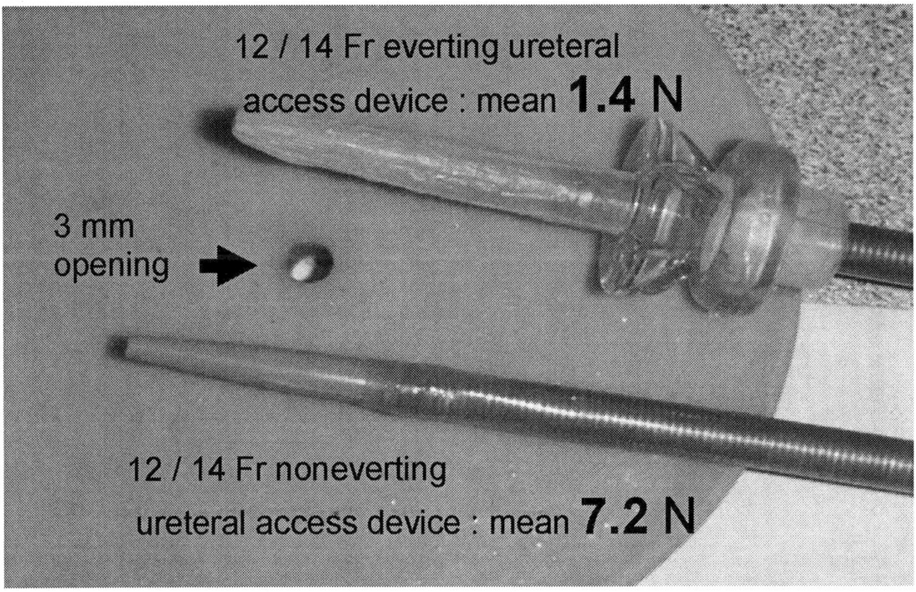

FIGURE 4. Simulated ureteral orifice and mean force required to advance the traditional 12/14 F ureteral access sheath with and without the everting sheath.

Force Reduction During Simulated Ureter Advancement

Using an automated test stand, researchers at Johns Hopkins measured the maximum force generated when advancing 0.035 inch diameter guide wires, 6 Fr ureteral catheters over guide wires, and 6.5 Fr everting catheters [10]. The test model simulated passage of wires and catheters pass embedded stones. Despite the large discrepancy in size, the 6.5 Fr everting catheter generated peak forces that were comparable to those generated by the guide wires alone in both advancement up the simulated ureter and then pass the embedded stone (Figs. 5 and 6).

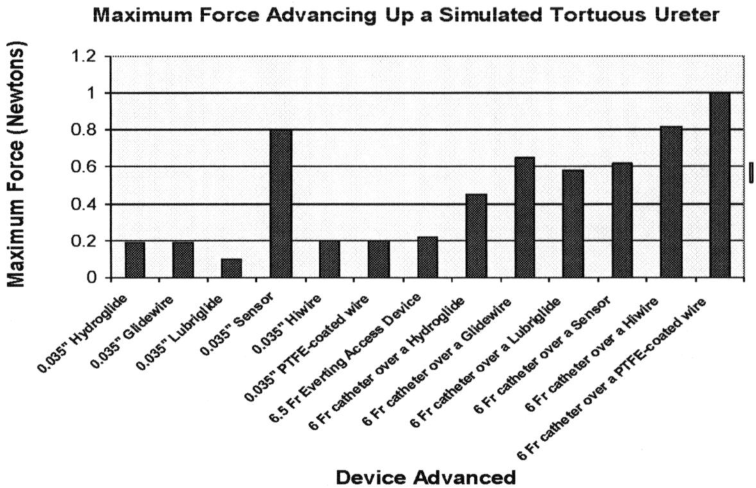

FIGURE 5. Mean peak force (in Newtons) generated during the advancement of 0.035 inch guide wires, 6 Fr non-everting catheters, and a 6.5 F everting catheter in a torturous ureter model.

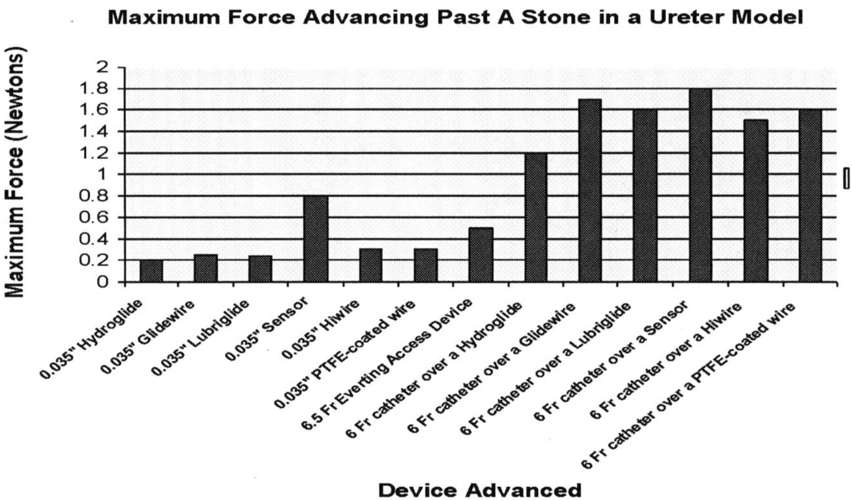

FIGURE 6. Mean peak force (in Newtons) generated during the advancement of 0.035 inch guide wires, 6 Fr non-everting catheters, and a 6.5 F everting catheter past an embedded stone.

Reduction in Injury to Ureteral Urothelium

The reduction in force with the everting sheath should result in decreased potential of mucosal injury during device advancement. This was evaluated *in vitro* with porcine ureteral systems. Twelve ureters were first excised *en bloc*. In five of the systems (i.e., 10 ureters) a 6.5 Fr everting ureteral access sheath was advanced up one ureter, and a 5 Fr open-ended ureteral catheter over a guide wire was advanced up the contralateral ureter. One system served as the control. After removal of the devices 10 mL of a 30% fluorescein solution were injected into the renal pelvis and allowed to drain distally. Injured urothelium will stain with fluorescein. Each ureter was then bivalved, washed with 10 mL of saline and observed for trauma under the illumination of a Wood's lamp. As a group, there was less ureteral fluorescein staining seen when the everting sheath was used. This difference was dramatic when compared to that seen with conventional ureteral access methods. In fact, the levels of fluorescein staining noted in 3 ureteral units were comparable to that of the non-manipulated control. In the remaining 2 systems, the trauma noted with staining was similar between the conventional and the everting devices [11]. Additional studies are of course needed to assess the clinical impact of these findings.

Minimizing Retro-Propulsion of Extraneous Material

Inadvertent introduction of microbes and extraneous material into the urethra and ureter can occur during placement of access sheaths. The libricous coating combined with the everting design can reduce seeding of the urinary tract compared to traditional designs. In an *in vitro* model, the tips of everting and non-everting catheters were dipped in solution of ampicillin-resistant Escherichia coli, then advanced 2.7, 5.5 and 11 cm in a urinary tract models until they reached a well containing Luria-Bertani broth. Following this exposure, 4 mL of the broth was cultured. The optical density of the solution was then measured to give an estimation of the bacterial load. The mean bacterial load was significantly lower with the everting device compared to the non-everting catheter for all advancement groups [12]. The everting design can reduce retro-propulsion of extraneous bacteria into the urinary tract. This could lower the incidence of infectious complications during ureteral manipulation.

SUMMARY

Ureteral access sheaths can facilitate ureteroscopic procedures but improper or forceful use can be associated with dire complications. The novel everting ureteral sheath provides advantages over traditional non-everting designs because less force is required for their placement. This should minimize complications such as ureteral perforations, tears, or avulsions. Nevertheless, clinical trials are required to determine the true efficacy and safety of these "second generation" ureteral access sheaths.

REFERENCES

1. Monga M. Accessory instrumentation for ureteroscopy. *Curr Opin Urol* 2004; 14: 107-109.
2. Vanlangendonck R, J Landman. Ureteral access strategies: pro-access sheath. *Urol Clin N Am* 2004; 31: 71-81.
3. Kourambas J, RR Byrne, GM Preminger. Does a ureteral access sheath facilitate ureteroscopy? *J Urol* 2001; 165: 789-793.

4. Monga M, *et al.* Prospective randomized comparison of 2 ureteral access sheaths during flexible retrograde ureteroscopy. *J Urol* 2004; 172: 572-573.
5. Abrahams HM, ML Stoller. The argument against the routine use of ureteral access sheaths. *Urol Clin N Am* 2004; 31: 83-87.
6. Lallas CD, *et al.* Laser Doppler flowmetric determination of ureteral blood flow after ureteral access sheath placement. *J Endourol* 2002; 16(8): 583-590.
7. Rubenstein JN, *et al.* Novel everting urologic access sheath: decreased axial forces during insertion. *J Endourol* 2005; 19(10): 1216-1220.
8. Heine JP. Utility of an everting catheter to dilate urethral strictures: ex vivo and one case study results. Poster presentation at the Western Section American Urological Society Annual Meeting, August 2005.
9. Adam C, *et al.* Utility of an everting sheath to dilate urethral strictures. Oral presentation at the European Association of Urology Annual Meeting, March 2006.
10. Patriciv A, *et al.* An automatic method for guide-wire and catheter evaluation. Poster presentation at the Engineering and Urology Society Annual Meeting, May 2005.
11. Stoller ML, *et al.* An *in vitro* assessment of urothelial trauma with a novel everting access sheath. *J Endourol* 2005; 19(6, Supl): A11.
12. Camargo AHLA, *et al.* Novel everting urologic access sheath: potential advantages of decreased cellular advancement. *J Endourol* 2006; 20(2): 153-156.

VII. SHOCK WAVE LITHOTRIPSY: MECHANISMS OF SHOCK WAVE ACTION AND STRATEGIES FOR IMPROVED SWL

Shock Wave Injury to the Kidney in SWL: Review and Perspective

James A. McAteer[*], Andrew P. Evan[*], Lynn R. Willis[†], Bret A. Connors[*], James C. Williams, Jr. [*], Yuri A. Pishchalnikov[*], and James E. Lingeman[‡]

Departments of [*]Anatomy and Cell Biology, and [†]Pharmacology and Toxicology, Indiana University School of Medicine, Indianapolis, IN 46202-5120, USA;
[‡]Methodist Hospital Institute for Kidney Stone Disease, Indianapolis, IN 46202, USA

Abstract. Shock wave lithotripsy (SWL) is a first-line option for treatment for urinary calculi—particularly effective for the removal of uncomplicated stones from the upper urinary tract. The success of lithotripsy is tempered, however, by the occurrence of acute injury that has been reported to progress to long-term complications. SW trauma to the kidney is a vascular lesion characterized by parenchymal and subcapsular bleeding. The acute lesion is dose-dependent, and typically localized to the focal volume of the lithotripter. Cavitation has been implicated in vessel rupture, but SW-shear has the potential to be a primary mechanism for damage as well. Possible chronic adverse effects of SWL may include new-onset hypertension, development of diabetes, and exacerbation of stone disease. If acute trauma could be reduced, it seems likely that serious long-term effects could be minimized, or even eliminated. Reducing the dose of SW's needed for stone breakage is one option. Improved coupling improves stone breakage, and slowing SW rate significantly improves stone-free outcomes. Experiments with animals now show that treatment protocols can be designed to protect against tissue injury. Initiating treatment with low energy SW's dramatically reduces lesion size, and reducing the rate of SW delivery virtually eliminates SW trauma altogether. SWL stands to gain from new advances in technology, as lithotripters become safer and more effective. Perhaps the greatest progress will be made when we have determined the physical mechanisms of SW action both for stone breakage and tissue damage, and have better characterized the biological response to SW's—as this will provide the principles needed to achieve the best combination of safety and efficiency with whatever lithotripter is at hand.

Keywords: shock wave lithotripsy, kidney, trauma, kidney stones, animal models
PACS: *43.25.Cb, *43.40.Jc, 87.53.Tf, 87.19.Rr; 87.54.Hk

INTRODUCTION

It is well documented that renal injury occurs as a side effect of SWL, and considerable progress has been made in characterizing the acute effects of SW trauma, particularly in experimental animals. Still, we are just beginning to appreciate the causes of SW injury, the acoustic mechanisms involved, and the physiologic risk factors that appear to potentiate adverse effects. It is also clear that we have a fairly limited understanding of the long-term consequences of SW treatment. With this in mind, it seems reasonable to take stock of the field, redefine the problem of adverse

CP900, *Renal Stone Disease, 1st Annual International Urolithiasis Research Symposium*, edited by A. P. Evan, J. E. Lingeman, and J. C. Williams, Jr.

effects, and assess what can be done to help make shock wave lithotripsy safer and more effective.

THE CHARACTERISTICS OF ACUTE SWL INJURY TO THE KIDNEY

Shock Waves Rupture Blood Vessels

Animal studies leave no doubt that SW's can cause hemorrhage to the kidney vasculature [1-5]. The pig is the accepted model of renal injury in SWL [4-6]. Detailed morphological analysis of pig kidneys treated with a clinical dose of SW's has shown that veins are particularly susceptible to SW injury, and a broad range of vessels—from vasa recta and cortical capillaries, to arcuate and intralobular vessels—are damaged by SW's [2,3,7,8]. The vast majority of research in SWL injury has been conducted using the Dornier HM3 lithotripter, a water bath-style, spark-gap machine, but all lithotripters that have been studied create a vascular lesion [9].

Vascular Trauma in SWL Can Cause Parenchymal Hemorrhage and Subcapsular Hematomas

The occurrence of hematomas is a potentially significant finding. Certainly, mild subcapsular hematomas can be uncomplicating, but big bleeds can seriously compromise renal function, and can lead to acute renal failure [10-21]. Hematoma rates may depend on the type of lithotripter, and values between about 1 and ~12% can be found in the literature [reviewed in 7]. Even higher rates have been reported using CT or MR imaging [22,23]. There are also data suggesting that age is a risk factor for the development of perinephric hematomas in SWL, with the incidence of hematomas increasing about 2-fold per decade [13].

The Hemorrhagic Lesion in SWL Is Dose-dependent, and Proper Detection and Quantitation of Injury Requires a Rigorous Methodology

Lesion size, the volume of hemorrhagic tissue in the kidney, increases with SW number and with the power setting of the lithotripter [24-27]. It is often possible to see such trends by gross visual inspection alone, but quantitation of the histologic lesion gives a much better means to localize sites of hemorrhage, and determine the extent of damage. A method that has proven to be both sensitive and objective is to perform *in situ* perfusion fixation, followed by instillation of the vasculature with pigmented microfil to mark the patent vasculature [28]. The kidney is then embedded whole in paraffin, and serially sectioned at 40 μm. The cut face of the kidney is photographed—systematically selected representative sections—and areas of parenchymal hemorrhage are outlined and measured (morphometric segmentation) to determine lesion size. By this method the entire kidney is serially sectioned, areas of hemorrhage exclusively within the parenchyma are segmented to exclude the renal pelvis and calyceal system, and the lesion is expressed as percent of functional renal volume (%FRV) [7].

Research on Renal Injury in SWL Requires an Intact, Physiologically Competent, Viable Animal Model

Patient studies have shown that SW's trigger a rapid reduction in renal blood flow in both the treated and the contralateral kidney, and data suggest that the effect can be long-lasting [29,30]. The overall importance of this hemodynamic response has yet to be fully worked out, but vasoconstriction may be a critical event in the protective effect of initiating SWL treatment with low energy SW's, as has been observed in pigs [31]. Observation of the responsiveness of the kidney to SW's is also a reminder of the importance of using the appropriate animal model to assess SWL trauma. Some laboratories have reported using cadaver and slaughterhouse kidneys to assess for SW injury [32]. Unfortunately, no matter how freshly excised the kidney may be, it will not show a normal physiologic response. SW injury to the kidney is dominated by vascular trauma. If the vasculature of the model is not anatomically intact and physiologically competent, the damage that occurs upon treatment with SW's cannot be expected to represent what occurs in SWL, and such a model has limited-to-no practical value.

EVIDENCE FOR LONG-TERM ADVERSE EFFECTS IN SWL, AND WHY CHRONIC INJURY IS A CONCERN

Acute Vascular Trauma to the Kidney in SWL Leads To Scarring and Loss of Functional Renal Mass

The acute vascular lesion caused by SW's can progress to scar formation. Thus, parenchymal hemorrhage can result in a chronic loss of nephrons—a loss of functional renal mass. Chronic damage of this sort was first reported in a study with experimental animals, in which dogs that were treated using the Dornier HM3 lithotripter showed fibrosis after one month, with the severity of scarring dependent on the dose of SW's applied [1]. A study in rabbits likewise showed a dose-dependent increase in scar formation one month after treatment, with a significant rise (nearly 10 fold higher) in scar volume with treatment at 2000 SW's compared to 1000 SW's [33]. The renal medulla may be particularly susceptible to SW damage, and a study in pigs has shown that treatment with a clinical dose of SW's can lead to complete atrophy of renal papillae within the target site, observed at 3 months post-SWL [16]. Scar formation has also been reported in patients, in which Single Photon Emission CT was used to measure exclusion of Technicium-99 label from areas of poor vascular perfusion [34]. Patients were scanned before and 30 days following SWL, with a loss of marker uptake observed in half the subjects. The scars that developed in these patients measured larger (mean 19x15 mm) than the focal zone of the lithotripter (EDAP-PEL) that was used. These reports all suggest that lasting damage can occur as a consequence of SWL but, clearly, more work is needed to characterize the long-term consequences of treatment, and to determine the relationship between acute injury and lasting damage.

New-onset Hypertension Has Been Reported, with Increased Risk for Older Patients

Hypertension is a potential consequence of SWL and there is evidence to suggest that the occurrence of new-onset hypertension in lithotripsy patients is related to the dose of SW's they received [9]. Clearly this topic has stimulated spirited debate, but the implications posed by reports showing a link between SWL and hypertension cannot help but be cause for concern [2,7,9,35-42]. A prospective study by Janetscheck and colleagues shows an alarming increase in intrarenal resistive index in patients 60 years of age and older [36]. This finding implies that SW treatment for stone disease can have serious long-term effects, and that age may be a critical risk factor for significant adverse effects in SWL [41]. It is not clear precisely what mechanisms might be at play in the cellular response to SW's that could lead to hypertension. However, the observation that SW's can stimulate glomerular mesangial cell proliferation in pigs, still evident one month after treatment, suggests a condition that if unresolved could be a potential causative factor in the development of hypertension [43].

A Potential Link Has Been Proposed Between SWL and the Development of Diabetes

In a patient follow-up study, Krambeck and colleagues report an association between SW dose for treatment of upper urinary tract stones, and the development of diabetes mellitus [35, also see Dr. Krambeck's paper in this volume]. Here, again, the potential cellular mechanisms at play leading to such a response are not known, but one would expect this involves direct SW damage to the pancreas. Patient studies have reported SW trauma to the pancreas, and detected increased serum and urinary amylase levels following SWL [44-47]. Clearly the pancreas lies along the acoustic axis during treatment of either kidney, but it is also true, although not widely appreciated, that SW's targeted at urinary stones have the potential to cause significant trauma outside the SW-axis. A recent study in which gas-laden microspheres were injected into the circulation of pigs during SW administration has shown that SW pressures exceeding the threshold for vessel-damaging cavitation can occur a considerable distance off the geometric SW axis of the lithotripter [48]. That is, with abundant cavitation nuclei present in the vasculature, SW's targeted at the lower pole of the left kidney caused extensive hemorrhage throughout the abdominal viscera, even the contralateral kidney. Thus, it should be recognized that SWL treatment of stones in the kidney and upper ureter carries the potential to deliver a damaging dose of SW's to the pancreas.

Multiple Lithotripsies May Exacerbate Stone Disease

Epidemiological studies indicate that over the past three decades the percentage of calcium phosphate (CaP) in stones has been on the rise and, indeed, the data suggest a transition from calcium oxalate (CaOx) stones to CaP stones [49]. In looking for factors that might explain this, Parks and colleagues observed a striking positive correlation between the percent CaP in stones and the number of lithotripsy sessions per patient [50]. The number of SWL sessions was higher for CaP stone formers than for CaOx stone formers, and highest for patients whose stones contained brushite, even when corrected for number of stones and duration of stone disease. Brushite stones typically present a more complicated pathology than CaOx stones. Unlike CaOx stones, which appear to develop in association with papillary interstitial mineral, brushite stones develop from crystalline deposits that plug the papillary collecting ducts—causing further cell damage that can lead to advanced tissue alterations, such as tubular atrophy and papillary fibrosis [51]. The correlation between SWL and the occurrence of brushite stones is concerning, as this implies that for some patients, multiple sessions of SWL may lead to the development of a more advanced pathology involving stones (brushite) that generally do not respond well to subsequent SW treatment.

WHAT PHYSICAL MECHANISMS CAUSE SHOCK WAVE INJURY?

Cavitation Is Strongly Implicated in SW Trauma, But May Not Be the Only Cause of injury

Cavitation within blood vessels is believed to play an important role in the vascular trauma that characterizes tissue injury in SWL [9,52]. This is shown by studies in which cavitation is enhanced by injecting micro-bubbles or gas-laden micro-carrier beads into the circulation during SWL, resulting in increased hemorrhage [48,53]. Also, strategies to suppress cavitation, such as using tandem SW's or a phase-reversed waveform to interrupt bubble growth, dramatically reduce tissue damage [54,55].

The search to determine just how bubbles go about rupturing vessels has proven to be an interesting problem. Decades of research in physics and engineering on the disruptive force of inertial cavitation, has shown that when a cavitation bubble collapses it can generate a fluid micro-jet that delivers great force to a very small area [56]. This is the mechanism by which cavitation bubbles chip away at metal surfaces, such as the erosion that often occurs to ship's propeller blades. If a cavitation bubble were to grow and collapse within a blood vessel, the force of its micro-jet would surely break the vessel wall. At question, however, is whether a cavitation bubble within a vessel can grow large enough to undergo such forceful collapse. Inertial cavitation typically involves bubbles that grow to a size of one to several millimeters in diameter before collapse. This is too large to occur within the micro-vessels of the kidney that are damaged during SWL. Zhong and colleagues tested the idea that vessel rupture could be caused by bubble expansion [52,57]. They set up an *in vitro* system in which a laser fiber was used to excite bubble expansion within the lumen of a segment of micro-dialysis tubing, and were able to photograph the rupture of this vessel phantom.

Whether it is bubble expansion, or bubble micro-jets, or possibly the secondary SW's generated when bubbles collapse symmetrically that is responsible for vessel rupture, it is important to note that cavitation does not occur readily in circulating blood [53]. Also, studies using sensitive methods of cavitation detection have shown that it takes hundreds of SW's to generate bubble activity in tissue within the living kidney [58]. This suggests that the occurrence of cavitation may be highly dependent on the intravascular micro-environment, and possibly the presence of minute particles that may serve as nuclei for cavitation bubble formation. It is not known what constitutes a natural cavitation nucleus in the circulatory system, but the fact that cavitation does not initiate readily suggests that the circulation is relatively free of such particles [53]. Thus, cavitation appears to be an important player in SW damage, but one wonders if other factors may be involved as well.

Shear Has the Potential to Damage Tissue, Particularly at Fast SW Rate

Cavitation may not be the driving force for SW injury. That is, bubble expansion (or collapse) may not be the primary mechanism responsible for tissue damage. *In vitro* studies have shown that when isolated cells are placed under static pressure in excess of the threshold for cavitation, SW's induce cell lysis significantly higher than in untreated controls [59]. That is, in the absence of cavitation, SW's still caused cell injury. Pigs treated with SW's from an HM3 lithotripter fitted with a reflector insert that suppressed cavitation without significantly affecting pulse amplitude, exhibited dramatically reduced vessel damage compared to animals treated with the standard reflector, but still showed some bleeding involving vessels of the renal papillae [55]. That is, the region of the kidney that is the most sensitive to SW's showed injury in the absence of cavitation. A study involving numerical modeling of tissue compartments in the kidney, presented in these proceedings [See Dr. Freund's paper in this volume, pp. 356-359], suggests that stress can accumulate within the kidney parenchyma if the rate of SW delivery is faster than the displacement relaxation time of the tissue. The Freund model predicts that the magnitude of shear deformation of tissue will be different for different regions of the renal papilla, and that the region closest to the tip of the papilla, where the kidney is most sensitive to SW's, will exhibit the greatest strain. The study suggests that vessel failure could be induced by shear, and that subsequent hemorrhage and pooling of blood could then create an environment conducive to cavitation, and further SW damage.

INJURY IS DOSE-DEPENDENT, AND THERE APPEARS TO BE A THRESHOLD FOR SIGNIFICANT SW TRAUMA

SW Damage Jumps Dramatically after ~1000 SW's

SW injury to the kidney is dose-dependent [2,7,24-26]. Damage increases as more SW's are delivered, and injury is greater at higher SW energy levels, but it is clear that whereas renal injury is cumulative, it is not linear. Studies in the pig in which the volume of hemorrhagic tissue was quantified, showed that a dose of 2000 SW's at 24kV from the HM3 lithotripter produced a lesion measuring ~6% of functional renal volume [31]. Treatment with half that dose (1000 SW's) at the same energy setting gave a lesion of only 0.2%FRV [7]. That is, the injury produced by 1000 SW's was barely detectable, and doubling the dose increased the lesion about 30 fold. These data in the pig strongly suggest that there is a threshold for the initiation of injury that, if exceeded, can result in significant trauma. This level of acute injury is in agreement with data for evidence of long-term damage in rabbits, where the size of parenchymal scars measured one month following treatment increased from ~1.4% at 1000 SW's to over 12% at 2000 SW's [33].

An important challenge is that we do not know where the threshold for significant SW injury truly lies. Data for the HM3 localize the threshold only vaguely, and begin to define it for just one lithotripter, and for only one energy setting, at that. One would expect that the threshold for measurable injury would depend not only on the number of SW's, and the power or kV of the pulses, but also on the acoustic signature of the particular lithotripter—the dimensions and energy density of the focal volume, and possibly even the rate of SW delivery. That is, since acoustic output is different for different lithotripters, the threshold for injury should be different, and should depend on treatment parameters. Further, just as kidney size and the health of experimental animals have been shown to affect the renal response to SW's, the health status of the subject should also affect the threshold for injury [4,13,36,42,60].

Thresholds for SW Injury Could Be Determined in an Appropriate Animal Model

Clearly it would be valuable to know the number of SW's that can be delivered safely at typical treatment settings, and this is a reasonable problem to address with a relevant animal model such as the pig. At the present time, the most clear-cut metric of SWL injury is lesion size, and the method to determine lesion volume is well defined [28]. Such data collected for popular lithotripters could give a reasonable approximation of the damage expected with a given dose. That is, it may be possible to determine the maximum dose that is safe for a particular lithotripter, and this information could be a useful guideline.

Cavitation Detection Could Be a Means to Monitor SW Damage in Real Time

As so many factors have the potential to affect the injury threshold for an individual patient, it would also be valuable to have a means to detect injury in the making. This is not out-of-the-question and, indeed, cavitation detection has been proposed as a means to do this [61]. The approach is to use acoustic monitoring such as focused directional transducers to listen for bubble noise, or B-mode ultrasound to visualize cavitation echogenicity during treatment. In concept, a robust cavitation signal originating within the kidney parenchyma would indicate that conditions are right for vessel damage, signaling the need to stop treatment. This makes good sense, but a problem encountered in early attempts was difficulty in localizing cavitation to the renal parenchyma. A recent study shows that using US simultaneously with passive cavitation detection gives precise localization, and suggests that with proper characterization of the signal, cavitation can be detected in the kidney parenchyma using diagnostic ultrasound alone [58]. Thus, it now seems feasible that ultrasound monitoring during SWL could be used to detect the occurrence of cavitation in tissue, and this information could help decision making during treatment.

TREATMENT STRATEGIES TO MAKE SWL SAFER AND MORE EFFECTIVE

New lithotripter technologies may eventually be developed to make SWL safer and more effective, but what can be done now to improve how lithotripsy is performed using the lithotripters we currently have at hand? The answer may be fairly simple—slow down, and treat at lower energy.

Stone Clearance Is Improved at 60 SW/min Compared to 120 SW/min

Several clinical studies have now reported that slowing the rate of SW delivery to 60 SW/min breaks stones more effectively, giving better outcomes than treatment at the typical rate of 120 SW/min [62-67]. This positive effect of slowing SW rate is seen with both electrohydraulic and electromagnetic lithotripters. The obvious advantage of improving the efficiency of SW action is that fewer SW's should be needed for treatment [62]. A potential disadvantage is that slower rate can increase overall treatment time. How much an increase in treatment time may depend on how the treatment end point is determined (i.e. the quality of imaging used to assess breakage).

The idea that simply slowing SW rate can break stones better may be difficult at first to appreciate, but recent studies give clues to the physical mechanisms involved. Cavitation bubble collapse at the stone surface contributes to stone comminution, but bubble growth along the acoustic axis can interfere with delivery of shock wave energy to the stone. Cavitation is enhanced at fast SW rate because as bubbles collapse they spawn micron sized micro-bubbles that can persist between pulses. Such micro-bubbles act as cavitation nuclei, seeding new cavitation initiated by subsequent SW's [68]. The shorter the interval between SW's, the more cavitation nuclei survive, and the greater the number of new cavitation bubbles that form. Bubble interference at fast rate does not appear to be a matter of blockage or deflection of the pulse, but instead involves transfer of energy from the tensile phase of the SW into bubble growth. That is, cavitation increases as SW's are delivered at faster rate, but the leading positive pressure phase of the SW is virtually unaffected, and it is the trailing negative wave that is reduced [69]. It is as yet not entirely clear how the reduction of negative pressure in the SW impacts stone breakage, but it has been predicted that this should reduce the amplitude of shear waves within the stone, as well as affect the dynamics of bubble cluster collapse at the stone surface [70,71].

Step-wise SWL Protects against SW Injury

One of the most exciting findings in lithotripsy research is the observation that treatment with a priming dose of low amplitude SW's can have a dramatic tissue-protective effect. That is, initiating treatment at a low power setting before shifting to higher amplitude pulses results in a significant reduction in lesion size [31]. This observation comes from work using the pig model. The findings are significant because they suggest a potential treatment strategy to reduce adverse effects. How the observation came to light is also instructive, as the experimental design behind the study validates the importance of using an appropriate animal model for this sort of work. In studies to characterize SWL injury to the kidney using a clinical dose of SW's from the Dornier HM3, one group of animals was treated with 2000 SW's at 24 kV (120 SW/min) targeted to the lower renal pole. This dose created a lesion measuring ~6% functional renal volume (FRV). A pilot group of pigs received the same dose of SW's to both renal poles. That is, a dose of 2000 SW's at 24 kV was delivered first to the lower pole, then 2000 SW's were targeted to the upper pole of the same kidney. The lesion in the lower pole was as expected, but there was virtually no damage to the upper pole. Treatment of the lower pole had protected the upper pole from injury. Subsequent experiments determined that as few as 100 SW's delivered to one pole at 12 kV (28.8±10.8 MPa) prior to treatment of the same site with 2000 SW's at 24 kV (41.4±5.3 MPa), reduced lesion size to only 0.3% FRV. Thus, "pre-treatment" with low energy SW's protected the kidney from subsequent injury. The physiologic mechanism responsible for this protective effect has yet to be fully characterized, but assessment of renal hemodynamics shows that SW's induce transient vasoconstriction in the treated kidney (and in the contralateral kidney as well). Increased vascular tone may make vessels less susceptible to damage due to cavitation or shear stress. The responsiveness of the living, intact kidney is, thus, an important feature of this animal model. The main result observed using the "protection protocol" in experimental animals—significantly reduced tissue damage—suggests that a similar, step-wise treatment protocol might reduce kidney injury in clinical SWL.

Treatment at Reduced SW Rate Minimizes SW Trauma while Improving Stone Breakage

Results from a study in pigs suggest that slowing the rate of SW delivery to 30 SW/min reduces lesion size to less than 0.1% FRV [72,73]. That is, slowing SW rate affords protection against kidney injury equivalent to that observed using the step-wise, "protection protocol". Since stone breakage is also improved at slow SW rate, this finding opens the possibility that reducing the rate of SW delivery could be a means to improve both the safety and efficacy of SWL.

Improved Coupling Reduces the Number of SW's Needed for Stone Comminution

Most modern lithotripters employ a dry treatment head that is coupled to the patient with a medium of high acoustic transmission such as gel or oil. Development of the dry head was an important advance in the evolution of the lithotripter, making it possible for lithotripters to be transportable, and substantially improving access to SWL. Unfortunately, it is difficult to achieve good coupling with a dry-head device. Typical protocols used to prepare a patient for treatment create air pockets at the coupling interface, and these defects can be a significant barrier to SW transmission. *In vitro* studies have shown that coverage by air pockets of just 2% of the coupling interface reduced stone breakage by 20-40% [74]. The quality of coupling is also highly variable, and it is conceivable that variability in coupling may contribute to variability in clinical outcomes.

Poor coupling may be a factor in adverse effects. When coupling is poor more SW's are needed to break the stone. Though the pressure amplitude of the pulses is reduced, they still generate negative pressure that is well above the threshold for cavitation, thus they still have the capacity to injure blood vessels. Because poor coupling is less efficient, it takes more SW's to break the stone, and delivery of more SW's has the potential to cause more injury. A further difficulty concerning coupling is that the interface between the treatment head and the skin is not readily visible. One does not know when defects are present. However, recent *in vitro* tests [see Pishchalnikov *et al.* in these proceedings, pp. 368-371] show that it is possible to improve on the quality of coupling—that how the gel is applied, matters. Taken together, these observations suggest that coupling, an aspect of lithotripsy that is generally taken for granted, is problematic, but that with attention to detail, this aspect of treatment can be improved.

CONCLUSIONS

Basic research has done a great deal to characterize the acute effects of SW's, and there has been considerable progress in understanding the physical mechanisms of SW action in stone breakage and tissue damage. Although we know that the vascular lesion in SWL can progress to scarring and loss of functional renal mass, we know very little about the long-term consequences of acute SW trauma. Clinical findings such as the suggestion of new-onset hypertension in older patients, the apparent link between multiple lithotripsies and a transition to brushite stone disease, and the possibility that some patients may even develop diabetes as a result of treatment for their stones, seem reason enough to invest more effort in determining the causes and consequences of long-term adverse effects in SWL, and encourage us to find practical strategies to make lithotripsy truly safe.

ACKNOWLEDGMENTS

This work was funded by NIH grant DK-43881

REFERENCES

1. R. Newman, R. Hackett, D. Senior, K. Brock, J. Feldman, J. Sosnowski, and B. Finlayson. Pathological effects of ESWL on canine renal tissue, *Urology* 29, 194-200 (1987).
2. A.P. Evan and J.A. McAteer. Q-Effects of shock wave lithotripsy. In: *Kidney Stones: Medical and Surgical Management*, FL Coe, MJ Favus, CYC Pak, JH Parks, GM Preminger (eds), Lippincott-Raven, Philadelphia, pp. 549-570 (1996).
3. Y. Shao, B.A. Connors, A.P. Evan, L.R. Willis, D.A. Lifshitz, and J.E. Lingeman. Morphological changes induced in the pig kidney by extracorporeal shock wave lithotripsy: nephron injury, *Anat Rec* 275, 979-989 (2003).
4. A.P. Evan, L.R. Willis, J.E. Lingeman, and J.A. McAteer. Renal trauma and the risk of long-term complications in shock wave lithotripsy, *Nephron* 78,1-8 (1998).
5. A.P. Evan, L.R. Willis, B. Connors, G. Reed, J.A. McAteer, and J.E. Lingeman. Shock wave lithotripsy-induced renal injury, *Am J Kidney Disease* 17, 445-450 (1991).
6. A.P. Evan, J.A. McAteer, C.P. Steidle, L.R. Willis, N. Hockley, R. Saint, A. Hawk, B.A. Connors, S.A. Kempson, J.E. Lingeman. The mini-pig: an ideal large animal model for studies of renal injury in ESWL research. In: *Shock Wave Lithotripsy 2,* JE Lingeman & DM Newman (Ed), Plenum Press, New York, pp.35-40, (1989).
7. A.P. Evan and L.R. Willis. Extracorporeal shock wave lithotripsy: complications. In: *Smith's Textbook on Endourology*. Smith AD, Badlani GH, Bagley DH, Clayman RV, Docimo SG, Jordan GH, Kavoussi LR, Lee BR, Lingeman JE, Preminger GM, Segura JW (eds), Hamilton, Ontario, Canada, BC Decker, Inc, pp: 353-365 (2007).
8. L.R. Willis, A.P. Evan, B.A. Connors, P. Blomgren, N.S. Fineberg, and J.E. Lingeman. Relationship between kidney size, renal injury, and renal impairment induced by shock wave lithotripsy, *J Am Soc Nephrol* 10, 1753-1762 (1999).
9. J. Lingeman, M. Delius, A. Evan, M. Gupta, K. Sarica, W. Strohmaier, J. McAteer, and J. Williams. Bioeffects and physical mechanisms of SW effects in SWL. In: *Stone Disease: First International Consultation on Stone Disease*. J Segura, P Conort, S Khoury, C Pak, GM Preminger, D Tolley (eds.), Heath Publications, Paris, pp. 251-286 (2003).
10. J.V. Kaude, C.M. Williams, M.R. Millner, K.N. Scott, and B. Finlayson. Renal morphology and function immediately after extracorporeal shock wave lithotripsy, *Am J Roentgenol* 145, 305-313 (1985).
11. R.C. Newman, L. Bezirdjian, G. Steinbock, and B. Finlayson. Complications of extracorporeal shock wave lithotripsy: prevention and treatment, *Seminars Urol* 4, 170-174 (1986).
12. P.M. Knapp, T.B. Kulb, J.E. Lingeman, D.M. Newman, J.H.O. Mertz, P.G. Mosbaugh, and R.E. Steele. Extracorporeal shock-wave lithotripsy-induced perirenal hematomas, *J Urol* 139, 700-703 (1988).

13. N.B. Dhar, J. Thornton, M.T. Karafa, and S.B. Streem. A multivariate analysis of risk factors associated with subcapsular hematoma formation following electromagnetic shock wave lithotripsy, *J Urol* 172, 2271-2274 (2004).
14. A. Treglia and M. Moscoloni. Irreversible acute renal failure after bilateral extracorporeal shock wave lithotripsy, *J Nephrol* 12,190-192 (1999).
15. S.C. Sherman and A. Dogon. Subcapsular renal hematoma after shock wave lithotripsy, *J Emergency Med* 30, 437-439 (2006).
16. J.E. Lingeman, B. Matlaga, and A.P. Evan. Surgical management of urinary lithiasis. In: Walsh, P.C., Retik, A.B., Vaughan, E.D. Wein, A.J. eds., *Campbell's Urology*, Philadelphia, W.B Saunders Company, Chapter 44, pp: 1431-1507 (2006).
17. G. Liguori, C. Trombetta, S. Bucci, L. Salame, S. Savoldi, and E. Belgrano. Reversible acute renal failure after unilateral extracorporeal shock-wave lithotripsy, *Urol Res* 32, 25-27 (2004).
18. A.K. Tuteja, J.P. Pulliam , T.H. Lehman, and L.W. Elzinga. Anuric renal failure from massive bilateral renal hematoma following extracorporeal shock wave lithotripsy, *Urology* 50, 606-608 (1997).
19. L.S. Baskin, and M.L. Stoller. Severe haemorrhage after extracorporeal shock wave lithotripsy: radiological evaluation, *Brit J Urol* 69, 214-215 (1992).
20. D.E. Maziak, A. Ralph-Edwards, M. Deitel, J. Wait, H.J. Watt, and A. Marcuzzi. Massive perirenal and intra-abdominal bleeding after shock-wave lithotripsy: case report, *Can J Surg* 37, 329-332 (1994).
21. J.V. Kaude, C.M. Williams, M.R. Millner, K.N. Scott, and B. Finlayson. Renal morphology and function immediately after extracorporeal shock-wave lithotripsy, *Am J Roentgenol* 145, 305-313 (1985).
22. J.I. Rubin, P.H. Arger, H.M. Pollack, M.P. Banner, B.G. Coleman, M.C. Mintz, and K.N. VanArsdalen. Kidney changes after extracorporeal shock wave lithotripsy: CT evaluation, *Radiology* 162, 21-24 (1987).
23. B. R. Baumgartner, K.W. Dickey, S.S. Ambrose, K.N. Walton, R.C. Nelson, and M.E. Bernardino. Kidney changes after extracorporeal shock wave lithotripsy: appearance on MR imaging, *Radiology* 163, 531-534 (1987).
24. L.R. Willis, A.P. A.P. Evan, B.A. Connors, Y. Shao, P.M. Blomgren, J.H. Pratt, N.S. Fineberg, and J.E. Lingeman. Shockwave lithotripsy: dose-related effects on renal structure, hemodynamics, and tubular function, *J Endourology* 19, 90-101 (2005).
25. B.A. Connors, A.P. Evan, P.M. Blomgren, L.R. Willis, R.K. Handa, D.A. Lifshitz, J.E. Lingeman, and J. Ying. Reducing shock number dramatically decreases lesion size in a juvenile kidney model, *J Endourology* 20, 607-611, (2006).
26. B.A. Connors, A.P. Evan, L.R. Willis, P.M. Blomgren, J.E. Lingeman, and N.S. Fineberg. The effect of discharge voltage on renal injury and impairment caused by lithotripsy in the pig, *J Am Soc Nephrol* 11, 310-318 (2000).
27. L.R. Willis, A.P. Evan, B.A. Connors, Y. Shao, P.M. Blomgren, J.H. Pratt, N.S. Fineberg, and J.E. Lingeman. Shockwave lithotripsy: dose-related effects on renal structure, hemodynamics, and tubular function, *J Endourol* 19, 90-101 (2005).
28. P.M. Blomgren, B.A. Connors, J.E. Lingeman, L.R. Willis, and A.P. Evan. Quantitation of shock wave lithotripsy-induced lesion in small and large pig kidneys, *Anat Rec* 249, 341-348 (1997).
29. M.R. Mostafavi, Chavez D.R., J. Cannillo, B. Saltzman, and P.V. Prasad. Redistribution of renal blood flow after SWL evaluated by Gd-DTPA-Enhanced magnetic resonance imaging, *J Endourol* 12, 9-12 (1998).
30. D. Eterovic, L. Juretic-Kuscic, V. Capkun and Z. Dujic. Pyelolithotomy improves while extracorporeal lithotripsy impairs kidney function, *J Urol* 161, 39-44 (1999).
31. L.R. Willis, A.P. Evan, B.A. Connors, R.K. Handa, P.M. Blomgren, and J.E. Lingeman. Prevention of lithotripsy-induced renal injury by pretreating kidneys with low-energy shock waves, *J Am Soc Nephrol* 17, 663-673, (2006).

32. TH. Bergsdorf, S. Thuroff, and CH. Chaussy. The isolated perfused kidney: an in vitro test system for evaluation of renal tissue damage induced by high-energy shockwaves sources, *J Endourol* 19, 883-888 (2005).
33. J.S. Morris, D.A. Husmann, W.T. Wilson, and G.M. Preminger. Temporal effects of shock wave lithotripsy, *J Urol* 145, 881-883 (1991).
34. E. Lechevallier, S. Siles, J.C. Ortega, and C. Coulange. Comparison by SPECT of renal scars after extracorporeal shock wave lithotripsy and percutaneous nephrolithotomy, *J Endourol* 7, 465-467 (1993).
35. A.E. Krambeck, M.T. Gettman, A.L. Rohlinger, C.M. Lohse, D.E. Patterson, and J.W Segura. Diabetes mellitus and hypertension associated with shock wave lithotripsy of renal and proximal ureteral stones at 19 years of followup, *J Urol* 175, 1742-1747 (2006).
36. G. Janetschek, F. Frauscher, R. Knapp, G. Höfle, R. Peschel, and G. Bartsch. New onset hypertension after extracorporeal shock wave lithotripsy: age related incidence and prediction by intrarenal resistive index, *J Urol* 158, 346-351 (1997).
37. R. Knapp, F. Frauscher, G. Helweg, W. Judmaier, H. Strasser, G. Bartsch, and D. zur Nedden. Blood pressure changes after extracorporeal shock wave nephrolithotripsy: prediction by intrarenal resistive index, *Eur Radiology* 6, 665-669 (1996).
38. J. Lemann Jr., A.J. Taylor, B.D. Collier, and E.O. Lipchik. Kidney hematoma due to extracorporeal shock wave lithotripsy causing transient renin mediated hypertension, *J Urol* 145, 1238-1241 (1991).
39. C.M. Williams, J.V. Kaude, R.C. Newman, J.C. Peterson, and W.C. Thomas. Extracorporeal shock-wave lithotripsy: long-term complications, *Am J Roentgenol* 150, 311-315 (1988).
40. F. Frauscher, G. Hofle, and G. Janetschek. A randomized controlled trial to assess the incidence of new onset hypertension in patients after shock wave lithotripsy for asymptomatic renal calculi [comment], *J Urol* 162, 806 (1999).
41. R. Knapp, F. Frauscher, G. Helweg, D. zur Nedden, H. Strasser, G. Janetschek , and G. Bartsch. Age-related changes in resistive index following extracorporeal shock wave lithotripsy, *J Urol* 154, 955-958 (1995).
42. P. Bataille, G. Cardon, M. Bouzernidji, N. El Esper, A. Pruna, A. Ghazali, P.F. Westeel, J.M. Achard, and A. Fournier. Renal and hypertensive complications of extracorporeal shock wave lithotripsy: who is at risk?, *Urol Int* 62, 195-200 (1999).
43. B. Banner, D. Ziiesmer, and L.A. Collins. Proliferative glomerulopathy following shock wave lithotripsy in the pig, *J Urol* 146, 1425-1428 (1991).
44. J.E. Lingeman, D. Newman, J.H.O. Mertz, P.G. Mosbaugh, R.E. Steele, R.J. Kahnoski, T.A. Coury, and J.R. Woods. Extracorporeal shock wave lithotripsy: the Methodist Hospital of Indiana experience, *J Urol* 135, 1134-1137 (1986).
45. G.W. Drach, S. Dretler, W. Fair, B. Finlayson, J. Gillenwater, D. Griffith, J. Lingeman, and D. Newman. Report of the United States cooperative study of extracorporeal shock wave lithotripsy, *J Urol*, 135, 1127-1133 (1986).
46. K.D. Mullen, J.H. Hoofnagle, and E.A. Jones. Shock wave-induced pancreatic trauma, *Am J Gastroenterol* 86, 630-632 (1991).
47. I. Hassan and S.P. Zietlow. Acute pancreatitis after extracorporeal shock wave lithotripsy for a renal calculus, *Urology* 60, 1111 (2002).
48. B.R. Matlaga, J.A. McAteer, B.A. Connors, R.K. Handa, A.P. Evan, J.C. Williams, J.E. Lingeman, and L.R. Willis. The potential for cavitation-mediated tissue damage in shock wave lithotripsy, (In Press: *J Endourology*)
49. N. Mandel, I. Mandel, K. Fryjoff, T. Rejniak, and G. Mandel. Conversion of calcium oxalate to calcium phosphate with recurrent stone episodes, *J Urol* 169, 2026-2029 (2003).
50. J.H. Parks, E.M. Worcester, F.L. Coe, A.P. Evan and J.E. Lingeman. Clinical implications of abundant calcium phosphate in routinely analyzed kidney stones, *Kidney Int* 66, 777-785 (2004).
51. A.P. Evan, J.E. Lingeman, F.L. Coe, Y. Shao, J.H. Parks, S.B. Bledsoe, C.L. Phillips, S. Bonsib, E.M. Worcester, A.J. Sommer, S.C. Kim, W.W. Tinmouth, and M. Grynpas. Crystal-associated nephropathy in patients with brushite nephrolithiasis, *Kidney Int* 67, 576-591 (2005).

52. Zhong P, Cioanta J, Zhu S, Cocks FH, Preminger GM. Effects of tissue constraint on shock wave-induced bubble expansion in vivo, *J Acoust Soc Am* 104, 3126-3129 (1998).
53. E.L. Carstensen, S. Gracewski, and D. Dalecki. The search for cavitation in vivo, *Ultrasound Med Biol* 26, 1377-1385 (2000).
54. P. Zhong and Y. Zhou. Suppression of large intraluminal bubble expansion in shock wave lithotripsy without compromising stone comminution: Methodology and *in vitro* experiments, *J Acoust Soc Am* 110, 3283-3291 (2001).
55. A.P. Evan, L.R. Willis, J.A. McAteer, M.R. Bailey, B.A. Connors, Y. Shao, J.E. Lingeman, J.C. Jr. Williams, N.S. Fineberg, and L.A. Crum. Kidney damage and renal functional changes are minimized by waveform control that suppresses cavitation in SWL, *J Urol* 168,1556-1562 (2002).
56. L.A. Crum. Cavitation microjets as a contributory mechanism for renal calculi disintegration in ESWL, *J Urol* 140, 1587-1590, (1988).
57. P. Zhong, Y. Zhou, and S. Zhu. Dynamics of bubble oscillation in constrained media and mechanisms of vessel rupture in SWL, *Ultrasound Med Biol* 27, 119-134 (2001).
58. M.R. Bailey, Y.A. Pishchalnikov, O.A. Sapozhnikov, R.O. Cleveland, J.A. McAteer, N.A. Miller, I.V. Pishchalnikova, B.A. Connors, L.A. Crum, and A.P. Evan. Cavitation detection during shock wave lithotripsy, *Ultrasound Med Biol* 31, 1245-1256 (2005).
59. J.C. Williams, J.F. Woodward, M.A. Stonehill, A.P. Evan, and J.A. McAteer. Cell damage by lithotripter shock waves at high pressure to preclude cavitation, *Ultrasound Med Biol* 25, 1445-1449 (1999).
60. L.H. Newman and B. Saltzman. Identifying risk factors in development of clinically significant post-shock-wave lithotripsy subcapsular hematomas, *Urology* 38, 35-38 (1991).
61. R.O. Cleveland, O.A. Sapozhnikov, M.R. Bailey, and L.A. Crum. A dual passive cavitation detector for localized detection of lithotripsy-induced cavitation in vitro, *J Acoust Soc Am* 107, 1745-1758 (2000).
62. K.T. Pace, D. Ghiculete, M. Harju, and R.J.D'A. Honey. Shock wave lithotripsy at 60 or 120 shocks per minute: a randomized, double-blind trial, *J Urol* 174, 595-599 (2005).
63. E. Yilmaz, E. Batislam, M. Basar, D. Tuglu, C. Mert, and H. Basar. Optimal frequency in extracorporeal shock wave lithotripsy: prospective randomized study, *J Urol* 66, 1160-1164 (2005).
64. K. Madbouly, A.M. El-Tiraifi, M. Seida, S.R. El-Faqih, R. Atassi, and R.F. Talic. Slow versus fast shock wave lithotripsy rate for urolithiasis: a prospective randomized study, *J Urol* 173, 127-130 (2005).
65. J. Chacko, M. Moore, N. Sankey, and P.S. Chandhoke. Does a slower treatment rate impact the efficacy of extracorporeal shock wave lithotripsy for solitary kidney or ureteral stones?, *J Urol* 175, 1370-1373 (2006).
66. K. Davenport, A. Minervini, S. Keoghane, J. Parkin, F.X. Keeley, and A.G. Timoney. Does rate matter? The results of a randomized controlled trial of 60 versus 120 shocks per minute for shock wave lithotripsy of renal calculi, *J Urol* 176, 2055-2058 (2006).
67. Y. Kato, S. Yamaguchi, J. Hori, M. Okuyama, and H. Kakizaki. Improvement of stone comminution by slow delivery rate of shock waves in extracorporeal lithotripsy, *Intl J Urol* 13, 1461-1465 (2006).
68. Y.A. Pishchalnikov, J.A. McAteer, J.C. Williams Jr,, I. Pishchalnikova, and R.J. VonDerHaar. Why stones break better at slow shock wave rate than at fast rate: In vitro study with a research electrohydraulic lithotripter, *J Endourology* 20, 537-541 (2006).
69. Y.A. Pishchalnikov, O.A. Sapozhnikov, M.R. Bailey, I.V. Pishchalnikova, J.C. Williams, and J.A. McAteer. Cavitation selectively reduces the negative-pressure phase of lithotripter shock waves, *Acoust Res Let Online* 6, 280-286 (2005).
70. O. A. Sapozhnikov, A. D. Maxwell, B. MacConaghy, and M. R. Bailey. A mechanistic analysis of stone fracture in lithotripsy, *J Acoust Soc Am* 112, 1190-1202 (2007).
71. T. Ikeda, M.R. Bailey, B. MacConaghy, and L. Crum. Measurement of reduced stress in model kidney stones with increased rate of shock wave delivery in lithotripsy, *J Acoust Soc Am* 120, 3065 (abstr) (2006).

72. A.P. Evan, J.A. McAteer, B.A. Connors, P.M. Blomgren, and J.E. Lingeman. Renal injury in SWL is significantly reduced by slowing the rate of shock wave delivery, (Submitted)
73. B. A. Connors, A.P. Evan, L.R. Willis, R.K. Handa, J.A. McAteer, and J.E. Lingeman. Reducing shock wave rate decreases renal lesion size and acute functional decline in a SWL model, AUA 2007 Annual Meeting (abstr).
74. Y.A, Pishchalnikov, J.S. Neucks, R.J. VonDerHaar, I.V. Pishchalnikova, J.C. Williams, and J.A. McAteer. Air pockets trapped during routine coupling in dry-head lithotripsy can significantly reduce the delivery of shock wave energy, *J Urol* 176, 2706-2710 (2006).

Shock Wave Lithotripsy: Effects on the Pancreas and Recurrent Stone Disease

Amy E. Krambeck[*], Audrey L. Rohlinger[†], Christine M. Lohse[†], David E. Patterson[*], and Matthew T. Gettman[*]

Departments of Urology[*] and Division of Biostatistics[†] Mayo Clinic College of Medicine 200 1st SW; Rochester, Minnesota, USA

Abstract. Long-term effects of shockwave lithotripsy (SWL) are unknown; however, we recently found an association between SWL and diabetes mellitus in a population based case control cohort. To further study the association between SWL and diabetes mellitus, we determined the immediate impact of SWL on the pancreas as well as the long-term natural history of stone disease following treatment. Chart review identified 630 patients treated with SWL at our institution in 1985. Questionnaires focusing on recurrent stone episodes after SWL were sent to 578 patients alive in 2004. To further assess impact of SWL on the pancreas, pancreatic enzyme measurements were performed on 24 symptomatic stone patients treated in 2006 with ureteroscopy (n=12) and SWL (n=12). Serum amylase and lipase were evaluated pre and post SWL. A $\geq$5 U/L increase in either lab value was considered significant. Among patients in the long-term SWL treatment group, the questionnaire response rate was 58.9% (288/489). Recurrent stone events were noted in 154 (53.5%) of the survey respondents. Characteristics associated with stone recurrences were: gender (p=0.004), age at SWL (p=0.022), BMI (p=0.007), SWL complications (p=0.009), and lower pole SWL (p=0.025). Recurrent stone disease was also associated with the development of diabetes mellitus (p=0.020). In the contemporary group of treated stone patients, pancreatic enzyme analysis demonstrated an increase in serum amylase and lipase in 3 (25.0%) SWL patients and 1 (8.3%) ureteroscopy patient (p=0.273). In conclusion, over half of the patients treated with SWL will develop recurrent stone events. We found a strong association between recurrent stone disease and the development of diabetes mellitus at long-term follow-up. Although not statistically significant due to small number, data in a contemporary treatment cohort suggest the possibility that the pancreas can be adversely affected by SWL.

Keywords: lithotripsy, diabetes mellitus, pancreatic enzymes, kidney calculi, ureteral calculi
PACS: 87.19.Xx; 87.54.Hk

INTRODUCTION

The introduction of shock wave lithotripsy (SWL) by Chaussy and colleagues revolutionized the treatment of stone disease, ushering in the era of minimally invasive management of urinary calculi [1,2]. Today SWL is the preferred treatment by many urologists for symptomatic urinary calculi such that 80-90% of calculi are currently considered to be amenable to SWL [3]. Although this treatment method is considered safe overall, many early deleterious effects to the kidney and surrounding organs have been identified [3-6].

CP900, *Renal Stone Disease, 1st Annual International Urolithiasis Research Symposium,* edited by A. P. Evan, J. E. Lingeman, and J. C. Williams, Jr.

Recently, a study from our institution evaluated the long-term effects of SWL after 19 years of follow-up [7]. In this study, patients were asked to report on new conditions related to organs thought to be in the SWL blast path that developed since their original SWL (Fig. 1). Survey response rate was 59%. Responders were matched 1:1 with regards to age, gender, and year of presentation to a group of urolithiasis patients treated conservatively (i.e. no surgical intervention). We found an increased risk (Odds Ratio, OR=1.47) of developing hypertension at long-term follow-up after SWL compared to the control group. We also found that patients treated with SWL were more likely to develop diabetes mellitus than controls (OR=3.23). This risk persisted in multivariate analysis controlling for presence of obesity on follow-up and change in BMI (OR's of 3.28 and 3.75, respectively). In addition, the development of diabetes mellitus in the SWL group was associated with the number of shocks administered and the total intensity of the treatment (p=0.005 and p=0.007, respectively).

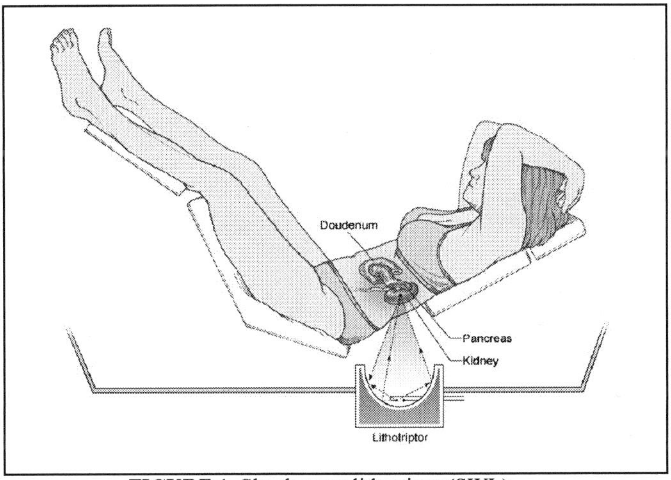

FIGURE 1. Shock wave lithotripsy (SWL).

It is known that the incidence of diabetes mellitus is increased in patients with urolithiasis regardless of age, BMI, or diet [8], but an association between a specific stone treatment and such adverse effects has not previously been published. Although prior studies have demonstrated acute pancreatitis, changes in pancreatic enzymes [4,9-11], and pancreatic hematomas after SWL [12], skepticism still exists as to whether the pancreas is damaged enough to produce structural changes resulting in functional deficits.

Multiple theories may explain the observed association between SWL and diabetes. Shear and cavitational forces, for example, are known to cause soft tissue injury after SWL [11,13]. These forces may alter the islet cell cycle as they pass through the pancreas, leading to an increased rate of cellular apoptosis and eventual diabetes mellitus. Neural tissue studies have demonstrated increased rates of cellular apoptosis when nerve cells are exposed to intense noise shock waves. This effect is accentuated by coexisting surgical lesions [14]. Another theory is that damage to the pancreas results in pancreatic antigen release and eventual pancreatic autoimmune destruction. Pancreatic antigen exposure to the immune system is known to cause diabetes mellitus in certain individuals [15]. Or, simply, SWL may damage limited pancreatic reserves in patients already at increased risk of developing diabetes mellitus.

Other long-term treatment concerns with SWL may be contributing to this association. Since this treatment method relies on passage of stone fragments, the rate of stone recurrence for SWL if fragments persist may be higher than other treatment modalities. Multiple stone recurrences could result in further surgical interventions and increased rates of long-term adverse events. The goal of our current work was to determine the long-term natural history of stone disease after SWL as well as the immediate impact of SWL on pancreatic function in a contemporary SWL treatment cohort.

METHODS

Stone Recurrences after Shock Wave Lithotripsy

After approval from the Mayo Clinic Institutional Review Board a retrospective review identified 630 consecutive patients with renal and ureteral calculi who underwent SWL using an HM-3 lithotripter in 1985. This year marked the first year of SWL at our institution. Preoperative patient demographics, preexisting medical conditions, stone demographics, and treatment characteristics were collected. Preexisting renal insufficiency was defined as serum creatinine greater than 1.4 mg/dL in males and greater than 1.2 mg/dL in females. Preexisting obesity was defined as BMI of 30 or greater. Preexisting hypertension was defined as a diagnosis of hypertension requiring antihypertensive medications. Stone analysis was performed on gravel passed via the urethra after treatment to determine composition. Hematuria with clot retention was considered a postoperative complication.

Survey of Cases

A structured questionnaire was sent to 578 SWL patients listed in our clinic records as being alive in 2004. The questionnaire, which was developed and distributed with the Mayo Clinic Survey Research Center, focused on the development of subsequent stone recurrences after the initial SWL treatment in 1985. The survey inquired about the number of recurrences, date of recurrences, location (right versus left), and method of treatment.

Pancreatic Enzyme Measurements

After approval from the Mayo Clinic Institutional Review Board 24 patients with symptomatic renal or ureteral calculi were enrolled in this prospective study. Stone burden was treated ureteroscopically in 12 patients or with SWL in the remaining 12 patients. Ureteroscopic treatment consisted of laser lithotripsy or basket extraction. The electrohydraulic HM-3 lithotripter was used for SWL. Serum amylase and lipase were evaluated the day prior to the surgical procedure and 2 hours post procedure, prior to dismissal from the outpatient surgical setting. A ≥5 U/L increase in either lab value from preoperative to postoperative was considered a clinical meaningful change. Normal reference ranges at our laboratory for serum amylase and lipase are 26-102 U/L and 10-73 U/L, respectively. All interventions were performed under general anesthesia with paralysis.

Statistical Analysis

Comparisons of age and sex between questionnaire responders and nonresponders were evaluated using the Wilcoxon rank sum and chi-square tests. Associations with SWL features with long-term stone recurrences were evaluated using chi-square and two-sample t tests. Conditional logistic regression models were used to evaluate the risk of long-term stone recurrent events for SWL patients compared with controls. Comparisons of pancreatic enzyme changes between the SWL and ureteroscopy groups were evaluated using a two-sample t-test. Statistical analyses were performed using the SAS software package (SAS Institute, Cary, North Carolina) with $p<0.05$ considered statistically significant.

RESULTS

Stone Recurrence after Shock Wave Lithotripsy

Retrospective Review of All Patients Treated with SWL

Retrospective chart review revealed a total of 687 SWL treatments in 630 patients from January 1, 1985 to December 31, 1985. Eight patients were excluded: 7 due to age and 1 who declined to participate in medical research. Median patient age was 52 years (range 18 to 90). There were 218 females and 404 males. Stone location was left sided in 384 cases, right sided in 295 and bilateral in 57. There were 541 solitary renal stones, 27 multiple renal stones and 114 proximal ureteral stones. According to available stone sizes, 34.9% of the stones were less than 1 cm, 58.4% were 1 cm or greater and 6.6% were partial staghorn calculi. Greater than 50% of the stones were composed of the following: calcium oxalate monohydrate in 292 (43%), calcium oxalate dihydrate in 115 (16.9%), calcium phosphate in 123 (18.1%), uric acid in 28 (4.1%), magnesium ammonium phosphate in 17 (2.5%), cystine in 4 (0.6%), and unknown for 72 (24.8%).

Comparison of Questionnaire Responders and Nonresponders

Of the 578 questionnaires mailed, 89 were returned uncompleted because the patient was deceased. The completed survey response rate was 58.9%. There were no significant differences in age and sex between the 288 responders and 201 nonresponders. Of the questionnaire responders 228 (81.4%) had been referred for SWL and did not return to our institution for postoperative follow-up.

Questionnaire Respondents

Table 1 lists demographics, comorbidities, stone location, and treatment characteristics for the survey respondents. Median patient weight at treatment was 79.0 kg (range 42.0 to 134.5). Stone location in this group was renal in 236 (81.9%) and proximal ureteral in 52 (18.1%). Overall 3 patients received greater than 2,000 shocks in a single setting and 10 received greater than 2,000 shocks as a cumulative amount during multiple SWL's. Of the survey respondents 222 (78.5%) were referred to a nephrology stone clinic in 1985 for metabolic evaluation and treatment. An immediate postoperative complication was noted in 40 of the 288 responders (13.9%), as summarized in Table 2. No clinically significant perinephric hematomas were noted.

TABLE 1. Questionnaire respondents demographics and SWL interventions

Characteristic	No. Pts (%)	Median (range)
Overall	288	
Sex:		
Male	182 (63.2)	
Female	106 (36.8)	
Preoperative Obesity (BMI ≥30)		
Yes	74 (25.7)	
No	212 (73.6)	
Unknown	2 (0.7)	
Preoperative Renal Insufficiency	16 (5.6)	
Preoperative Hypertension	28 (9.7)	
Preoperative Diabetes Mellitus	8 (2.8)	
Stone Side:		
Left	151 (52.4)	
Right	137 (47.6)	
# SWL Treatments		
1	270 (93.8)	
>1	18 (6.2)	
Voltage (kV)	288	20 (19-24)
# Shocks	288	1,100 (300-4,500)
Intensity*	288	22,000 (5,700-55,200)
Total Intensity	288	24,000 (5,700-93,600)

*Patients receiving more than 1 SWL treatment had an average intensity based on the average of their total treatments.

Of the 288 survey respondents, recurrent stone events after original SWL were noted in 154 (53.5%), as summarized in Table 3. Analysis of patient demographics, stone characteristics, and treatment characteristics with stone recurrences was performed (Table 4). Certain patient and treatment characteristics were associated with recurrent stone disease including: gender (p=0.004), age at original SWL (p=0.022), BMI (p=0.007), any complication at original SWL (p=0.009), and SWL of a lower pole stone (p=0.025). Referral to nephrologist in the year 1985 did not predict stone recurrence (p=0.167). Recurrent stone disease was not associated with the subsequent development of new onset hypertension (p=0.088) or renal insufficiency (p=0.167).

Stone recurrence was significantly associated with the subsequent development of new onset diabetes mellitus (p=0.020).

TABLE 2. Postoperative complications

Postoperative Complications	No. Pts (%)
Pain	8 (2.8)
Ureteral Edema/Obstruction	7 (2.4)
Cardiac Event	7 (2.4)
Sepsis	6 (2.1)
Steinstrasse	6 (2.1)
Fever	2 (0.7)
Clot Retention	2 (0.7)
Abscess	1 (0.4)
Venous Thrombosis	1 (0.4)
Hypotension	1 (0.4)
Ureteral Perforation	1 (0.4)

TABLE 3. Recurrent stone events after original SWL

	No. Pts (%)
Any Recurrence	154 (53.5)
Number of Recurrences:	
1	50 (32.5)
2-5	78 (50.6)
6-9	18 (11.7)
$\geq$ 10	8 (5.2)
Management of Recurrence:	
Conservative	88 (57.1)
SWL	90 (58.4)
Ureteroscopy	34 (22.1)
Percutaneous Nephrolithotomy	11 (7.1)
Open Nephrolithotomy	4 (2.6)

Pancreatic Enzyme Measurements

There was no statistically significant difference between the ureteroscopy and SWL groups with regards to patient demographics (Table 5) or stone size. Mean SWL voltage was 20 kV (18-22) and all SWL patients received 2000 shocks. An increase in serum amylase was noted in 3 (25.0%) SWL patients and 1 (8.3%) ureteroscopy patient (p=0.273). An increase in serum lipase was also noted in 3 (25.0%) SWL patients and 1 (8.3%) ureteroscopy patient (p=0.273). All pancreatic enzyme elevations were within the normal laboratory value limits. Only those patients with left sided SWL's demonstrated increases in serum amylase and lipase.

DISCUSSION

Recently a link between diabetes mellitus and patients with urolithiasis has been identified, with urolithiasis patients having a higher rate of diabetes mellitus compared to non-stone formers [8]. Further evidence has demonstrated a link between specific treatments for urolithiasis and the development of adverse medical conditions [7]. Since its introduction, strong evidence has implicated SWL as a cause of transient acute damage to the kidney and surrounding tissues [16]. However, it was not until recently that long-term studies associated SWL with the development of adverse medical conditions such as diabetes mellitus and hypertension [7]. The current study further evaluates this association by analyzing long-term stone recurrence rates after SWL and by evaluating the acute effects of SWL on the pancreas.

TABLE 4. Comparison of patient, stone, and treatment characteristics with recurrent stone events.

Characteristic	P-value
Preexisting Conditions	
Diabetes Mellitus	1.000
Hypertension	0.113
Renal Insufficiency	0.076
Male Gender	0.004
Age	0.022
BMI in 1985	0.007
Nephrology Referral	0.167
Stone Composition	
Calcium Oxalate Monohydrate	0.841
Calcium Oxalate Dihydrate	0.249
Calcium Phosphate	0.319
Uric Acid	0.738
Struvite	1.000
Cystine	1.000
Stone Size	0.875
Stone Location	
Upper	0.240
Mid	0.841
Lower	0.025
UPJ	0.542
SWL Intensity	0.346
Postoperative Complication	0.009
New Onset Conditions	
Diabetes Mellitus	0.020
Hypertension	0.088
Renal Insufficiency	0.167

TABLE 5. Pancreatic enzyme measurement patient demographics

Characteristic	Ureteroscopy	SWL	P-value
Gender			0.681
Male	7	8	
Female	5	4	
Age in years	50	54	0.664
(range)	(22-72)	(33-87)	
Stone Size in cm	0.9	0.7	0.211
(range)	(0.5-1.5)	(0.4-1.5)	

With long-term follow-up approximately 54% of patients will experience a recurrent stone event and many will experience multiple stone events after SWL. These results are similar to the accepted 10-year recurrence rates for calcium oxalate stones treated conservatively 50% [17]. Other intermediate studies (<5 years) following children treated with SWL have demonstrated significant stone recurrences rates, but none as high as 50% [18,19]. We also noted certain preoperative and operative characteristics were associated with stone recurrence such as: age at SWL, obesity, gender, any complication at original SWL, and SWL of lower pole calculi. We did not find an association with preexisting diabetes mellitus, hypertension, or renal insufficiency and recurrent stone disease. However, those patients who developed multiple stone recurrences after their original SWL were more likely to develop new onset diabetes mellitus than those patients who did not experience a recurrence. These findings suggest that recurrent symptomatic stone disease may somehow provoke the development of diabetes mellitus, however the mechanism is unknown. There was no association between recurrent stone disease and the development of new onset hypertension or renal insufficiency. We also found no association between referral to nephrology stone clinic at time of original stone treatment and the development of recurrent stone disease.

Pancreatic enzyme findings in this study provide further evidence that the pancreas is affected by SWL and presents a possible initial mechanistic link between SWL and diabetes mellitus. Although not statistically significant, we did find that more patients in the SWL group (25%) developed subclinical elevations in pancreatic enzymes post procedure compared to the ureteroscopy group (8%). Of note, only those patients with left sided SWL experienced elevation of pancreatic enzymes, which is most likely the result of the anatomic proximity of the pancreas to the left kidney. It also bears mentioning that the one patient in the ureteroscopy group who demonstrated elevations in pancreatic enzymes post procedure was known to have significant peripheral vascular disease and experienced an acute hypotensive episode during the procedure, which may have contributed to the pancreatic enzyme elevations. These findings of pancreatic enzyme elevations after SWL are supported by previous case reports of acute pancreatitis [10-12,16] and those demonstrating pancreatic enzyme elevations after SWL [4,9]. Kirkali et al demonstrated that serum amylase, lipase and urinary amylase were all elevated after SWL of proximal ureteral and renal stones using an electromagnetic lithotripter up to one week post SWL [9]. Pancreatic enzyme elevations did not occur when low ureteral stones were treated implicating direct damage to the pancreas by shock waves.

We do recognize certain limitations of the long-term follow-up study. Patients who died before 2004 were not studied and therefore adverse long-term outcomes in these patients are not available. The response rate to the survey is altered by the proportion of deceased patients. Only 18.6% of the patients were followed at our institution. Therefore, the 58.9% response rate may be falsely low due to surveys sent to unrecognized deceased patients. Due to the multiple different treatments received for stone recurrences, we are unable to accurately determine if subsequent treatment modalities are specifically associated with the development of adverse medical conditions.

CONCLUSION

Among a group of patients treated with SWL at 19 years follow-up 53.5% developed recurrent stone events. Obesity, age, gender, complicated SWL, and treatment of lower pole stones predisposed patients to recurrent stone events. In addition, recurrent stone disease was noted to be associated with the development of new onset diabetes mellitus at long-term follow-up. In 25.0% of patients treated with HM3 SWL, pancreatic enzymes were elevated, yet the increase was not significant when compared to a ureteroscopy control group in this small trial.

ACKNOWLEDGMENTS

We would like to recognize the substantial contributions of Joseph W. Segura, M.D. to the original manuscript.

REFERENCES

1. C. Chaussy, E. Schmiedt, D. Jocham, W. Brendel, B. Forssmann, and V. Walther, *J Urol* 172, 417-20 (1982).
2. C. Chaussy, J. Schuller, E. Schmiedt, H. Brandl, D. Jocham, and B. Liedl. *Urology* 23, 59-66 (1984).
3. J. E. Lingeman, J. R. Woods, and P. D. Toth. *JAMA* 263, 1789-94 (1990).
4. J. E. Lingeman, D. M. Newman, J. H. O. Mertz, P. G. Mosbaugh, R. E. Steele, R. J. Kahnoski, T. A. Coury, and J. R. Woods *J Urol* 135, 1134-7 (1986).
5. K. H. Andreassen, C. Dahl, J. T. Andersen, M. S. Rasmussen, J. D. Jacobsen, and P. Mogensen. *Scand J Urol Nephrol* 31, 245-8 (1997).
6. S. Krysiewicz. *Urol Radiol* 13, 139-45 (1992).
7. A. E. Krambeck, M. T. Gettman, A. L. Rohlinger, C. M. Lohse, D. E. Patterson, and J. W. Segura. *J Urol* 175, 1742-1747 (2006).
8. E. N. Taylor, M. J. Stampfer, and G. C. Curhan. *Kidney Int* 68, 1230-1235 (2005).
9. Z. Kirkali, G. Kirkali, S. Tanci, and Y. Tahiri. *Int Urol Nephrol* 26, 405-408 (1994).
10. I. Hassan, and S. P. Zietlow. *Urology* 60, 1111 (2002).
11. H. Abe, T. Nisimura, S. Osawa, T. Miura, and F. Oka. *Int J Urol* 6, 65-8 (2000).
12. S. Y. Hung, H. M. Chen, Y.Y. Jan, and M. F. Chen. *Hepatogastroenterology* 47, 1162-3 (2000).
13. K. Afshar, G. McLorie, F. Papanikolaou, R. Malek, E. Harvey, J. L. Pippi-Salle, D. J. Bagli, A. E. Khoury, and W. Farhat. *J Urol* 172, 1600-1603.
14. P. Zhong, and G. Preminger, Physics of shock wave lithotripsy, in *Kidney Stones: Medical and Surgical Management*, edited by F. L. Coe, M. J. Favus, C. Y. C. Pak, J. H. Parks, and G. M. Preminger, Lippincott-Raven, Philadelphia, 1996, pp. 529-548.
15. R. Gianani and G. S. Eisenbarth. *Immunol Rev* 204, 232-249 (2005).
16. A. Saljo, Y. L. Huang, and H. A. Hansson. *J Neurotrauma* 20, 787-794 (2003).
17. M. Conlin, Complications of extracorporeal shock wave lithotripsy, in *Complications of Urologic Surgery*, edited by S. S. Tanefa, R. B. Smith and R. M. Ehrlich, W. B. Saunders Co., Philadelphia, 2001, pp. 155-164.
18. A. A. Shokeir, K. Z. Sheir, A. R. El-Nahas, A. M. El-Assmy, W. Eassa, and H. A. El-Kappany. *J Urol* 176, 706-710.
19. J. Uribarri, M. S. Oh, and H. J. Carroll. *Ann Intern Med* 111, 1006-1009 (1989).

The Acoustics of Shock Wave Lithotripsy

Robin O. Cleveland

Dept. of Aerospace and Mechanical Engineering, Boston University, Boston, USA

Abstract. The shock waves employed in lithotripsy are high amplitude acoustics waves. As they propagate through the body to the stone that are affected by coupling to the body and the presence of tissue through which they must pass. Once the shock wave arrives at the stone there is a complex transmission of energy into the stone as the shock wave can couple into compression and shear waves in the stone and produce cavitation in the surrounding fluid. The surrounding tissue is also subject to large physical forces that can result in damage. Physical phenomena that play a role include: generation of sound, nonlinear distortion, attenuation, diffraction, coupling into the body, transmission and mode conversion into the stone. This paper gives a synopsis of some of the relevant physics that applies to shock wave lithotripsy.

Keywords: lithotripsy, shock waves, kidney stones, acoustic propagation
PACS: 43.25.-x; 43.80.-n

INTRODUCTION

Almost a quarter century after the introduction of shock wave lithotripsy there is still no agreement on the physical process by which shock waves fragment kidney stones. It is also accepted that a clinical dose of shock waves results in trauma to kidney tissue. The side-effects provide motivation to develop lithotripters which effectively fragment stones but with reduced trauma to the tissue. Improvements in the performance of lithotripters can only be achieved by understanding how shock waves interact with tissue and kidney stones. An understanding of the physics of shock waves can also provide insight into the optimal use of current lithotripters. The goal here is to provide a brief overview of the physics involved in lithotripsy [1].

RESULTS

Shock wave lithotripters generate shock waves by one of three mechanisms. In an electrohydraulic lithotripter (EHL) an underwater spark generates a spherically diverging shock wave placed at one focus of an ellipsoidal reflector. The spherical wave reflects from the ellipsoid and focuses to the second focus of the ellipse. An electromagnetic lithotripter (EML) uses an electrical coil and a metallic plate. When the coil is excited by a short electrical pulse the plate experiences a repulsive force and this can be used to generate an acoustic wave. If the metallic plate is flat the resulting plane wave can be focused by a lens. If the plate is in the shape of a tube the resulting cylindrical wave can be focused by a parabolic reflector. The piezoelectric lithotripter

CP900, *Renal Stone Disease, 1st Annual International Urolithiasis Research Symposium,*
edited by A. P. Evan, J. E. Lingeman, and J. C. Williams, Jr.

(PEL) uses piezoelectric crystals to form an ultrasonic wave. When a voltage is applied to a piezoelectric crystal it deforms and creates an acoustic wave. The crystals are placed on a spherical cap and geometrical effects allow for the focusing.

The measurement of the acoustic output of a lithotripter is governed by an IEC (International Electrotechnical Commission) standard [2]. A representative shock wave (SW) measured at the focus of an electrohydraulic lithotripter is shown in Fig. 1. The SW consists of a leading compressive pulse, with about 40 MPa peak pressure and duration of 1 μs. It is followed by a rarefractional tail with a peak pressure of about –10 MPa and duration of 4 μs. The aspect of the waveform that makes it a "shock wave" is the shock front rise time which results from the phenomenon of nonlinear distortion. Nonlinear distortion occurs when the amplitude of a sound wave is intense enough that speed varies with the pressure and is described by the following equation: $c=c_0+\beta p/\rho_0 c_0$. Here c is the phase speed for a local acoustic pressure p, c_0 is the small-signal sound speed, β the coefficient of nonlinearity, and ρ_0 the density of the fluid. For the SW shown in Fig. 1 the peak of the wave travels about 120 m/s faster than the usual sound speed. This makes the wave distort and steepen until attenuation becomes strong enough to counteract the nonlinear distortion. When nonlinearity and attenuation are in balance the resulting transition is called a shock. For an EHL the spark source generates a SW from the source. For the EML and PEL the source waveform is not shocked but will distort as it propagates to the focus. For most clinically relevant power settings a shock is produced before the wave reaches the focus. The rise time of the shock front is less than 5 ns in water and around 70 ns in the body [3].

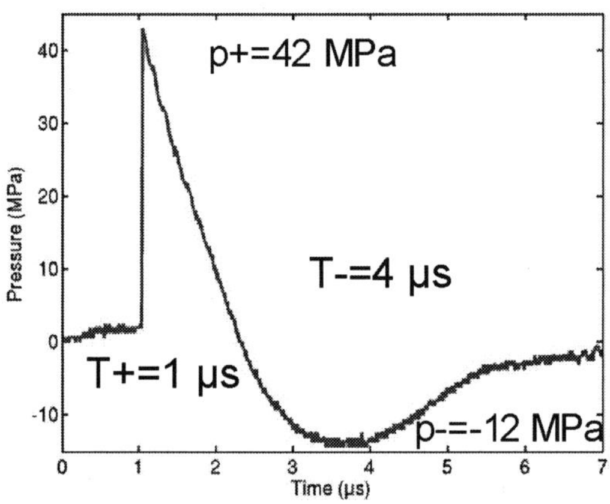

FIGURE 1. Waveform measured at the focus of an EHL: p+ is peak positive pressure, T+ duration of positive phase, p- peak negative pressure and p- duration of negative phase.

The focus of a lithotripter is a geometrical point in space. However, the region of high pressure is limited by a process referred to as diffraction which provides a fundamental limit on the region of space to which a wave can be localized. For a typical EHL the focal spot is a cigar-shaped focal volume about 60 mm long and 12 mm in diameter. In contrast the typical EML has a maximum pressure of around 100 MPa and a focal volume that is 35 mm long and 4 mm in diameter. Reported values for PELs indicate a peak focal pressure of 80 MPa and a focal spot 20 mm long and 3 mm in diameter [4,5].

The smaller, tighter focal spot of an EML or PEL would at first glance appear to be advantageous as it should allow for more accurate targeting and less damage to the tissue. However, *in vitro* experiments (where stones are stationary) indicate that the EM and PE lithotripters, with their very high pressures, are no better at breaking stones that an EHL and often have greater side-effects [6]. The smaller focal spot lithotripters may not be as effective for two reasons. First, if the focal spot is smaller than the size of the stone then only a small volume of the stone will experience the full stress of the wave. This will affect the comminution efficiency of even a perfectly targeted stone. Second, stone motion due to respiration means that many shock waves will miss the stone [7]. This second point may partially explain the higher side-effects reported with the newer lithotripters.

The waveform shown in Fig. 1 was measured in a water path. However in clinical operation the shock wave has a more complex path (Fig 2). The path starts in a coupling liquid, normally water, passes through a membrane into the body, and then propagates through the tissue to the kidney. The presence of the path can dramatically affect the pressure at the focus. For example, where the membrane contacts the skin the presence of bubbles that cover just 8% of the surface area can reduce the peak pressure by 50% [8].

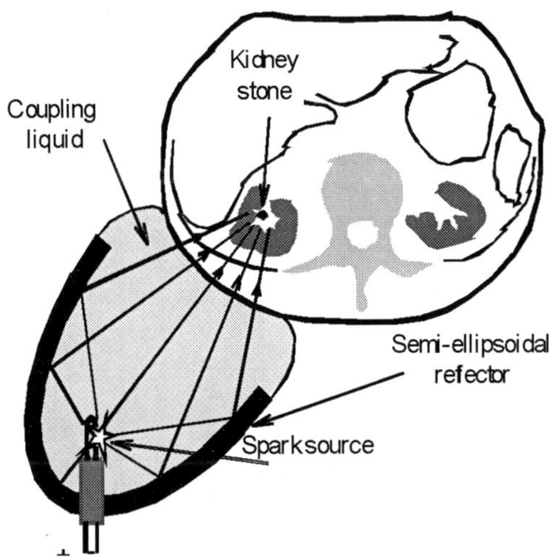

FIGURE 2. Schematic showing shock wave source coupling to the body. Graphic courtesy of Dr. O.A. Sapozhnikov.

Once the shock wave arrives at the stone there are a number of mechanisms by which it may act. Each mechanism has a particular physical process associated with it and there should be accompanying characteristic traits in the development of the failure. The mechanisms considered here, and the anticipated region of action (also indicated in Fig. 1), are as follows:

Spallation occurs after the shock wave enters the stone and subsequently reflects from the rear of the stone. The stone/urine interface inverts the large positive pressure pulse resulting in a large tensile stress near the back wall. Most solids are much weaker in tension than in compression and so the large tensile stress can be expected to make the material fail.

Shear waves occur because kidney stones are elastic solids and can support shear waves as well as compressional waves. The shear waves are most efficiently generated at interfaces that are not normal to the incident shock wave, that is, on the edges of the stone [9] in a squeezing-like mode [10]. Many materials are weak in shear. The interaction of shear waves can also result in regions of high tensile stress [9,11,12].

Cavitation refers to small bubbles/cavities that grow in the urine surrounding the stone due to the large negative pressure tail of the acoustic pulse. The bubbles can collapse with great violence and generate intense shock waves or very powerful microjets of fluid [13] [14]. Cavitation is principally a surface acting mechanism, and experiments indicate that it acts most strongly on the proximal (shock wave incident) surface of the stone [15]. Cavitation bubbles can also exist for seconds after the passage of a shock wave and can result in a barrier to subsequent shock waves and less effective fragmentation. Studies support the hypothesis that delivering shock waves at a slower rate improves fragmentation [16].

Fatigue is a bulk action process and may occur anywhere in the stone. Its hallmark is the progressive development of cracks. The cracks are nucleated at sites of small imperfections that occur in almost all materials. The stresses near the imperfections result in a local amplification of the stress which makes the imperfections grow into microcracks. With an increasing number of shock waves the microcracks grow into macrocracks and eventually produce cracks large enough to induce failure. Fatigue cracks often grow by tensile mode or in shear modes, and therefore regions of high tensile stress or shear stress may be more likely to initiate fatigue. The fact that thousands of shock waves are required for stone comminution is indicative of a fatigue process [17].

Damage to tissue is generally accepted to be dominated by a cavitation process. The violent growth and collapse of bubbles has been shown to in a variety of biological systems. Lithotripsy waveforms that mitigate cavitation also show a reduction in tissue injury [16]. However, it is also plausible that direct stress could effect damage and the most likely scenario is through some sort of shear mechanism [18].

CONCLUSIONS

Shock wave lithotripters generate shock waves with peak pressures on the order of 40 to 100 MPa. The region of high pressure is 5 to 15 mm wide and 40 to 80 mm long.

Lithotripters with high pressure and narrow focal spots do not appear to result in improved clinical performance. The mechanisms of stone comminution and tissue damage are still not fully understood. Further understanding may lead to an improvement in lithotripter design. Knowledge of the physics of shock wave lithotripsy also provides insight to improving current practice, for example, ensuring good coupling and firing shock waves at lower rates.

ACKNOWLEDGMENTS

The author thanks fellow members of the Consortium for Shock Waves in Medicine. The work was supported by a grant from the NIH DK43881 and a grant from the Whitaker Foundation RG01-0084.

REFERENCES

1. Cleveland, R.O. and J.A. McAteer, The Physics of Shock Wave Lithotripsy, in *Smith's Textbook on Endourology*, G.H.B. A. D. Smith, D. H. Bagley, R. V. Clayman, S. G. Docimo, G. H. Jordan, L. R. Kavoussi, B. R. Lee, J. E. Lingeman, G. M. Preminger, J. W. Segura, Editor. 2007, BC Decker: Hamilton, ON, Canada. p. 317-332.
2. IEC-TC-87, IEC 61846 Ultrasonics - Pressure pulse lithotripters - Characteristics of fields. 1998, International Electrotechnical Commission: Geneva, Swizterland.
3. Cleveland, R.O., D.A. Lifshitz, B.A. Connors, A.P. Evan, L.R. Willis, and L.A. Crum, In vivo pressure measurements of lithotripsy shock waves in pigs. *Ultrasound Med.Biol.*, 1998. 24: p. 293-306.
4. Coleman, A.J. and J.E. Saunders, A survey of the acoustic output of commercial extracorporeal shock wave lithotripters. *Ultrasound Med.Biol.*, 1989. 15: p. 213-227.
5. Buizza, A., T. Dell'Aquila, P. Giribona, and C. Spagno, The performance of different pressure pulse generators for extracorporeal lithotripsy: a comparison based on commercial lithotripters for kidney stones. *Ultrasound in Medicine & Biology*, 1995. 21(2): p. 259-72.
6. Kerbl, K., J. Rehman, J. Landman, D. Lee, C. Sundaram, and R.V. Clayman, Current management of urolithisasis: Progress or regress? *Journal of Endourology*, 2002. 16(5): p. 281-288.
7. Cleveland, R.O., A. R, and R.K. Babayan, Effect of stone motion on in vitro comminution efficiency of a Storx Modulith SLX. *J. Endourology*, 2004. 18: p. 629-633.
8. Pishchal'nikov, Y.A., J.S. Neucks, R.J. Von der Haar, I.V. Pishchalnikova, J.C. Williams Jr., and J.A. McAteer, Air Pockets Trapped During Routine Coupling in Dry Head Lithotripsy Can Significantly Decrease the Delivery of Shock Wave Energy. *J. Urol.*, 2006. 176: p. 2706-2710.
9. Cleveland, R.O. and O.A. Sapozhnikov, Modeling elastic wave propagation in kidney stones with application to shock wave lithotripsy. *J. Acoust. Soc. Am.*, 2005. 118: p. 2667-2676.
10. Eisenmenger, W., The mechanisms of stone fragmentation in ESWL. *Ultrasound In Medicine And Biology*, 2001. 27(5): p. 683-693.
11. Dahake, G. and S.M. Gracewski, Finite difference predictions of P-SV wave propagation inside submerged solids. II. Effect of geometry. *J Acoust Soc Amer*, 1997. 102(4): p. 2138-45.
12. Xi, X. and P. Zhong. Transient stress in solids during shock wave lithotripsy. in *Proceedings of the First Joint BMES/EMBS Conference*. 1999. Piscataway, NJ, USA: IEEE.
13. Crum, L.A., Cavitation microjets as a contributory mechanism for renal calculi disintegration in ESWL. *J.Urol.*, 1988. 140: p. 1587-1590.
14. Delius, M., W. Brendel, and G. Heine, A mechanism of gallstone destruction by extracorporeal shock waves. *Naturwissenschaften*, 1988. 75: p. 200-201.

15. Sass, W., M. Braunlich, H.-P. Dreyer, E. Matura, W. Folberth, H.-G. Priesmeyer, and J. Seifert, The mechanisms of stone disintegration by shock waves. *Ultrasound in Medicine & Biology*, 1991. 17(3): p. 239-43.
16. Evan, A.P., L.R. Willis, J.A. McAteer, M.R. Bailey, B.A. Connors, Y. Shao, J.E. Lingeman, J.C. Williams, Jr., N.S. Fineberg, and L.A. Crum, Kidney damage and renal functional changes are minimized by waveform control that suppresses cavitation in shock wave lithotripsy. *J.Urol.*, 2002. 168(Oct): p. 1556-1562.
17. Lokhandwalla, M. and B. Sturtevant, Fracture mechanics model of stone comminution in ESWL and implications for tissue damage. *Physics In Medicine And Biology*, 2000. 45(7): p. 1923-1940.
18. Freund, J., in this volume.

Innovations in Lithotripsy Technology

Pei Zhong

Department of Mechanical Engineering and Materials Science, Duke University, Box 90300 Durham, North Carolina 27708

Abstract. The introduction of shock wave lithotripsy (SWL) in the early 1980's revolutionized the surgical management for kidney stone disease. Since then, although numerous 2nd- and 3rd-generation lithotripters have been developed using various means for shock wave generation, focusing, patient coupling and stone localization, the technical improvements in these devices were largely made based on practical concerns for user convenience and multifunctionality of the system rather than a clear understanding of the working principles of SWL. In this paper, the fundamental mechanisms of stone comminution and tissue injury in SWL revealed by basic studies in the past two decades are first reviewed. This is followed by a summary of the innovations in SWL technology developed in recent years that have been demonstrated to provide improved stone comminution with concomitantly reduced tissue injury both *in vitro* using phantom systems and *in vivo* in animal models. Furthermore, the role of treatment strategy in determining the overall outcome of clinical lithotripsy is emphasized, and future prospects for lithotripsy research and technological innovations are discussed.

Keywords: shock wave lithotripsy, acoustic bioeffects, medical applications
PACS: 43.25.Cb, 87.54.Hk.

HISTORY AND EVOLUTION OF SWL TECHNOLOGY

Dornier Medical Systems in Germany invented shock wave lithotripsy in the early 1980's. The first lithotripter, the Dornier HM-3, was built based on electrohydraulic (EH) principles using an underwater spark discharge for shockwave generation and a truncated ellipsoidal reflector for wave focusing. The patient was immersed in a large water tub filled with degassed and deinoized water for acoustic coupling, and stone location was realized with bi-planar fluoroscopy. The FDA approved the clinical use of the HM-3 in the United States in 1984, and since then SWL has become the treatment of choice for upper urinary stone disease with widespread clinical applications [1].

The initial success of SWL prompted several manufacturers to introduce in the late 1980's the 2nd-generation lithotripters, using different techniques for shock wave generation, wave focusing and patient coupling. Representative 2nd-generation lithotripters include the Siemens Lithostar, which uses an electromagnetic (EM) generator with an acoustic lens, both enclosed in a water cushion ("dry" lithotripter), and the Richard Wolf Piezolith-2300 that utilizes a self-focusing piezoelectric (PE) generator placed at the bottom of a small water basin. The primary changes in the design of the 2nd-generation lithotripters were the increased aperture angle of the shock

CP900, *Renal Stone Disease, 1st Annual International Urolithiasis Research Symposium,* edited by A. P. Evan, J. E. Lingeman, and J. C. Williams, Jr.

wave source and reduced acoustic output energy [2] so that SWL could be performed under intravenous sedation rather than regional or general anesthesia as for the HM-3 [3]. Continued evolution in lithotripter design in the 1990's led to the introduction of the 3rd-generation lithotripters, which are characterized by their multifunctional use for SWL, ureteroscopic and percutanous procedures [4]. Up to now, more than 30 different models of commercial lithotripters have been designed and marketed. However, it should be noted that the technical improvements in the 2nd- and 3rd-generation lithotripters were largely made based on practical concerns for user convenience and multifunctionality of the system rather than a rigorous understanding of the underlying mechanisms in SWL [3,5].

Limitations of Current SWL Technology

Although the means for shock wave generation, focusing, patient coupling, and stone localization in lithotripter design have evolved significantly in the past two decades, the fundamental principle of SWL remains unchanged. Independent of the technologies used, almost all commercial lithotripters produce a similar pressure waveform at the focus, which can be characterized by a leading shock front with a compressive wave followed by a trailing tensile wave. The acoustic fields produced by different lithotripters differ from each other in peak amplitude and pulse profile of the pressure waveform, beam size, pulse energy, and therefore, their overall performance [2]. Moreover, the evolution of lithotripter design thus far has overwhelmingly, and perhaps mistakenly, relied on the importance of the compressive component of the lithotripter shock wave (LSW) with almost total neglect of the contribution of the tensile component of the waveform [5]. Further, a growing number of clinical studies have demonstrated that the 2nd- and 3rd-generation lithotripters are often less effective in stone comminution yet with increased propensity for tissue injury and higher stone recurrence rate, compared to the original Dornier HM-3 lithotripter [3,6,7]. Although multiple factors (e.g., beam size, total acoustic energy, and coupling condition, etc.) may contribute to the reduced effectiveness of the newer generation lithotripters, it is critical to gain a fundamental understanding of the mechanisms of stone comminution and tissue injury before better and improved SWL technologies can be developed.

MECHANISMS OF STONE COMMINUTION IN SWL

In the past two decades, significant progress has been made in understanding how SWL works. At the fundamental level, several mechanisms have been proposed as contributory factors for stone comminution in SWL. These include stress gradients built up in the target stone near wave entry and exit sites [8], spalling at the posterior surface due to acoustic impedance mismatch and geometric focusing [8-10], cavitation [11-13], shear stress [10,14], squeezing [15], and dynamic fatigue [16]. In general, these multiple mechanisms can be divided into two categories: stress waves that act inside the stone and cavitation that acts in the surrounding fluid, as revealed by high-speed photoelastic imaging (Fig. 1). Since most kidney stones are brittle materials

[17,18], they fail easily under tension and shear stress or by separation of crystalline-matrix boundaries [19], leading to the formation of relatively large fragments. Cavitation bubbles induced by LSW, in contrast, first expand several hundred times their original size, and then collapse violently, generating strong secondary shock waves and/or high-speed liquid jets impinging toward the stone surface [20-22]. Cavitation damage is characterized by minute pittings as a result of localized stress concentration [12,23].

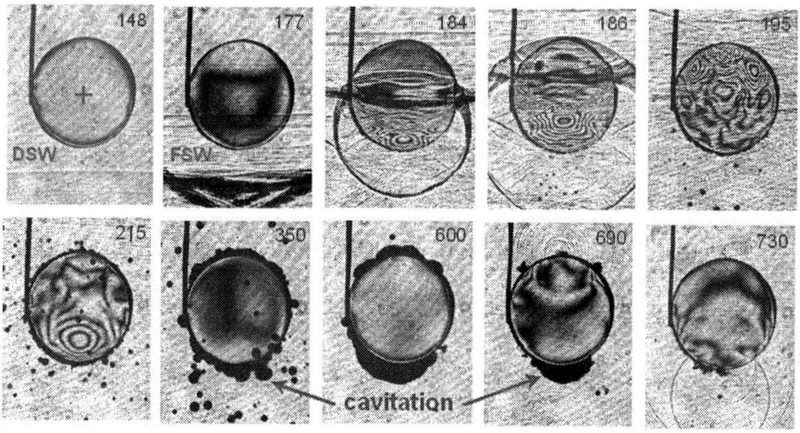

FIGURE 1. High-speed photoelastic imaging sequence demonstrating the transient shock wave-stone interaction with resultant stress wave generation inside an epoxy stone phantom (10 mm in diameter), and the expansion, coalescence, and violent collapse of cavitation bubbles in the fluid surrounding the stone phantom. The incident shock wave propagates from the bottom to the top, and the number in each frame indicates the time delay in microseconds after the spark discharge of the HM-3 lithotripter. DSW: direct shock wave, FSW: focused shock wave.

At the practical level, the contributions of stress waves and cavitation to the overall success of stone comminution in SWL have been investigated [24]. It was found that stress wave-induced fracture dominates the initial disintegration of kidney stones while cavitation is necessary to produce fine, passable fragments that are most critical for the success of clinical SWL. The action of lithotripter-induced stress waves alone was found to be much less effective in comminuting small residual fragments, presumably due to destructive wave superposition. It was suggested that stress waves and cavitation work synergistically, rather than independently, to produce effective stone fragmentation in SWL [24]. Further, cavitation induced pittings could weaken the structure of residual stone fragments, making them much more susceptible under the impact of subsequent lithotripter pulses. This speculation is confirmed by the failure of stone phantoms with geometric configuration that are refractive to spalling and shear-induced damage in castor oil, with damage occurring only when pittings generated by the collapse of laser-induced single bubbles are present on the surface of the phantom before the treatment (Fig. 2).

MECHANISMS OF TISSUE INJURY IN SWL

Tissue injury in SWL is characterized primarily by vascular lesions (damage of endothelial cells and rupture of small blood vessels), which extend along the shock wave propagation path throughout the thickness of the kidney [25,26]. Animal studies have identified several risk factors, including lithotripter parameters (shock number, output energy, pulse repetition rate) and kidney status (solitary or pediatric kidneys, renal infection, elderly patients with pre-existing hypertension) [27,28]. Over the years, two primary mechanisms have been postulated for SWL-induced vascular injury: cavitation [29,30] and shear stress [31,32]. However, other than anecdotal evidence, there is no direct proof to substantiate these theories because of the difficulties in measuring cavitation and LSW-induced shear stresses *in vivo*. Using vessel phantoms made of 200 μm cellulose hollow fibers, we have shown via high-speed imaging *in vitro* that LSW-induced bubble dynamics in small vessels are distinctly different from that induced in free field. Specifically, the initial expansion of the bubble is significantly constrained by the vessel wall. The bubble deforms asymmetrically, leading to substantially weakened collapse. Conversely, the vessel wall could be dilated substantially by the rapid, large intraluminal expansion of the bubble, which could lead to the rupture of small blood vessels [33]. This hypothesis is supported by animal experiments using inverted lithotripter pulses, which significantly suppress intraluminal bubble expansion and lead to minimal tissue damage even after a clinical dose of shock wave exposure [32]. In addition to the direct mechanical damage caused by LSW, there is also evidence of a secondary injury caused by ischemia/reperfusion [34,35].

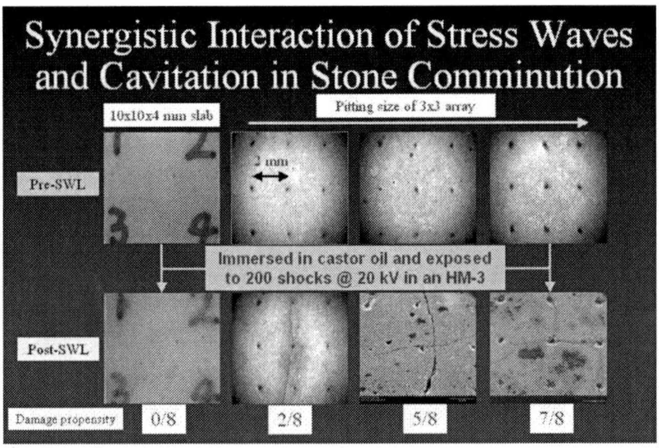

FIGURE 2. Thin slabs of BegoStone phantoms (10x10x3.5 mm, LxWxH), which are refractive to stress wave-induced fracture in castor oil after 200 shocks in an HM-3 at 20 kV, can be damaged (i.e., with new fracture line formation) if cavitation pittings are present on the surface of the phantom before the shock wave treatment. To mimic cavitation damage, the surfaces of the stone samples were treated by laser-induced single bubbles to create 3x3 mm pitting arrays with average pitting size ranging from 100 to 250 μm. The propensity of fracture line formation was found to increase with pitting size.

INNOVATIONS IN SWL TECHNOLOGY

In the past decade, several methods have been proposed to improve the effectiveness and safety of SWL. Most of the improvements have been focused on control of LSW-induced cavitation. Michael Delius first proposed the concept of tandem pulse lithotripsy [36]. Bailey and colleagues have developed a dual head lithotripter design that was intended to concentrate cavitation towards the lithotripter focus while suppressing bubble activities outside the focal volume [37,38]. In Bailey's design, two EH generators, aligned coaxially facing each other, are fired simultaneously and they produce comparable shock waves. We have employed a different approach to achieve cavitation control in SWL. We have designed and fabricated a piezoelectric annular array (PEAA) generator that can be retrofitted around the outer surface of an HM-3 reflector. The PEAA generator is aligned coaxially and confocally with the HM-3, making it convenient for patient coupling. In addition, the PEAA generator is used to produce a time-delayed, much weaker shock wave (~10 MPa) with longer compressive pulse duration (~3 μs). This unique feature of the PEAA generator can be used to selectively intensify the primary collapse of LSW-induced cavitation bubbles near the stone surface for improved stone comminution [5,39]. Microsecond tandem-pulse lithotripsy has also been tested in a piezoelectric shock wave lithotripter with improved stone fragmentation *in vitro* [40]. A second significant development in SWL technology is the *in situ* pulse superposition concept, which can be easily implemented in an EH lithotripter via a reflector insert to reduce large intraluminal bubble expansion and thus the propensity of LSW-induced vascular injury [41,42].

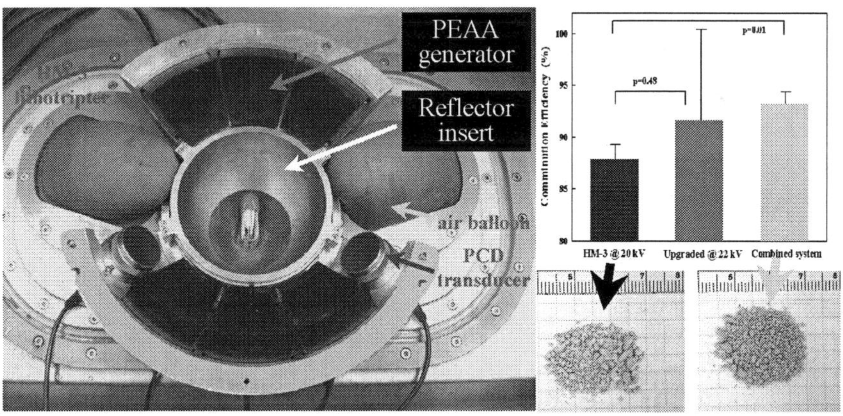

Figure 3. *In vivo* animal experiments comparing stone comminution after 2,000 shocks produced by the original HM-3 at 20 kV, HM-3 with upgraded reflector at 22 kV, and combined system of HM-3 with upgraded reflector at 22 kV and PEAA generator at 4 kV. No stone fragmentation could be produced by using the PEAA generator at 4 kV alone. At least 4 pigs were used in each group.

By upgrading the original HM-3 lithotripter with a reflector insert and a PEAA generator, we have shown in a swine model that *in vivo* stone comminution could be significantly improved (Fig. 3) while collateral tissue injury was substantially reduced following a clinical dose of shock wave treatment. These preliminary results support the hypothesis that optimization of lithotripter pulse profile and sequence may improve the overall stone comminution with reduced tissue injury.

Another interesting development in SWL technology is the introduction of the self-focusing electromagnetic shock wave lithotripter, characterized by wide-focus and low-pressure, which has been shown to be very effective in clinical studies [43].

IMPACT OF TREATMENT STRATEGY ON SWL OUTCOME

An important factor that may influence significantly the outcome of clinical SWL is treatment strategy. For a given total amount of shock waves and acoustic energy, it has been shown that a progressive increase of lithotripter output will produce better stone comminution, compared to other strategies (i.e., progressive decrease or constant output) [44-46]. This result is presumably caused by the impact of treatment strategy on the relative contributions of stress waves and cavitation to the overall stone comminution process in SWL [45]. In addition, it has been shown that a slow pulse repetition rate (i.e., 0.5 Hz) produces better stone fragmentation than a fast rate (i.e., 2.0 Hz). This result has been attributed to the attenuation effect of residual micro-bubbles in the fluid surrounding the stone on the transmission of the tensile component of the ensuing LSW's to the target stone [47,48]. An added benefit of the progressive increase of output energy strategy is that it may also reduce tissue injury. This speculation is supported by recent animal experiments which demonstrate that pre-treatment of the kidney with a few hundreds of low energy shocks can protect the same region of the kidney from a subsequent clinical dose of high-energy shocks, presumably due to SWL-induced vasoconstriction [49].

FUTURE PROSPECTS

The evolution of lithotripsy technology depends critically on our improved understanding of the fundamental mechanisms of stone comminution and tissue injury, as well as on a better appreciation of the critical factors that influence the outcome of clinical lithotripsy procedures. Although much progress has been made in basic research of SWL in the past ten years, new questions have also emerged regarding the interaction of various mechanisms in determining the overall treatment outcome. Specifically, there is a need to better understand the role of various mechanisms in the progressive comminution of residual stones of different size and irregular geometry to fine particles (less than 2 mm) that can be discharged spontaneously following SWL. The interaction between stress waves and cavitation, and how to maximize their synergy to produce more effective stone comminution in SWL needs to be further investigated. Moreover, the influence of the profile of LSW, pressure and energy distribution (i.e., beam size), as well as cavitation activities on lithotripsy outcome should be further examined using more realistic phantoms of the kidney and collecting system, as well as animal models. Furthermore, there is a need for the development of relevant and efficient 3-D numerical models of shock wave generation, propagation, focusing and interaction with kidney stones and renal tissues.

For the practical application of SWL, there are concerns regarding maintaining adequate coupling of the shock wave into the patient, especially for "dry coupling" lithotripters [50]. Therefore, development of techniques to monitor the coupling condition during SWL and/or better coupling methods for shock wave delivery to the patient should directly impact the success of clinical lithotripsy. Further, monitoring of stone comminution progress *in vivo* with concomitant adjustment of lithotripter focusing is another area that needs more thorough investigations. Finally, optimization of treatment strategy to maximize stone comminution and minimize tissue injury should be systematically investigated. Recent studies have already demonstrated the benefit of "priming" with low-energy shock waves on the success of stone comminution and in protecting renal tissues from the treatment of an ensuing clinical dose of high-energy shock waves. Development of better treatment strategies should directly benefit the clinical success of lithotripsy procedures.

Although the feasibility of several novel SWL technologies have already been demonstrated in *in vitro* phantoms and in animal models, these technologies must be further optimized in terms of engineering design (for example, optimization of transducer design, pressure waveform, and reflector insert geometry), system integration, and combination with improved treatment protocols so that their potential can be fully utilized to provide better and safer SWL. As demonstrated clearly by the introduction of SWL technology in the early 1980's, the success of translating novel lithotripsy technologies from academic laboratories to clinical practice in the near future will ultimately depend on multidisciplinary collaborations between academic researchers, urologists, and lithotripter manufacturers.

ACKNOWLEDGMENTS

The author wants to express sincere appreciation to Glenn M. Preminger, Hadley F. Cocks, Xufeng Xi, Songlin Zhu, Yufeng Zhou, Georgy Sankin, Neal Simmons, Jun Qin, Nathan Smith, Mathew Young, Charles G. Marguet, Michaella E. Maloney, and Victor Leitao for their contribution, support, and stimulating discussion about SWL research. This work was supported in part by NIH through grant #: R01-DK25985.

REFERENCES

1. C.G. Chaussy and G.J. Fuchs, Current state and future developments of noninvasive treatment of human urinary stones with extracorporeal shock wave lithotripsy , *J Urol* **141**, 782-792 (1989).
2. A.J. Coleman and J.E. Saunders, A survey of the acoustic output of commercial extracorporeal shock wave lithotripters , *Ultrasound Med. Biol.* **15**, 213-227 (1989).
3. J.E.Lingeman, S.C. Kim, R.L. Kuo, J.A. McAteer and A.P. Evan, Shockwave lithotripsy: Anecdotes and insights , *Journal of Endourology*, **1**, 687-693 (2003).
4. J.E. Lingeman, Extracorporeal shock wave lithotripsy: Development, Instrumentation, and Current status , *Urolithiasis* **24**, 185-211 (1997).

5. Y.F. Zhou, F.H. Cocks, G.M. Preminger, and P. Zhong, Innovations in shock wave lithotripsy technology: Updates in experimental studies , *J Urol*, **172 (5)**, 1892-1898 (2004).
6. S.F. Graber, H. Danuser, W.W. Hochreiter, U.E. Studer, A prospective randomized trial comparing 2 lithotriptors for stone disintegration and induced renal trauma , *J Urol.* **169(1)**, 54-57 (2003).
7. R. Gerber, U.E. Studer, H. Danuser, Is newer always better? A comparative study of 3 lithotriptor generations , *J Urol.* **173(6)**, 2013-2016 (2005).
8. C.G. Chaussy: *Extracorporeal Shock Wave Lithotripsy: New Aspects in the Treatment of Kidney Stone Disease*, Karger, 1982.
9. S.M. Gracewski, G. Dahake, Z. Ding, S.J. Burns, E.C. Everbach, Internal stress wave measurements in solids subjected to lithotripter pulses , *J. Acoust. Soc. Am.* **94**, 652-661 (1993).
10. X.F. Xi and P. Zhong, Dynamic photoelastic study of the transient stress field in solids during SWL , *J. Acoust. Soc. Am.*, **109(3)**, 1226-1239 (2001).
11. A.J. Coleman, J.E. Saunders, L.A. Crum, and M. Dyson, Acoustic cavitation generated by an extracorporeal shockwave lithotripter , *Ultrasound Med. Biol.*; **13**, 69-76 (1987).
12. L.A. Crum, Cavitation microjets as a contributory mechanism for renal calculi disintegration in ESWL, *J. Urol.* **140**,1587-1590 (1988).
13. P. Zhong and C.J. Chuong, Propagation of shock waves in elastic solids caused by the impact of cavitation microjets: Part I. theoretical formulation , *J. Acoust. Soc. Am.*, Vol. 94(1), pp:19-28, 1993.
14. R.O. Cleveland and O.A. Sapozhnikov, Modeling elastic wave propagation in kidney stones with application to shock wave lithotripsy , *J. Acoust. Soc. Am.* **118(4)**, 2667-2676 (2005).
15. W. Eisenmenger, The mechanisms of stone fragmentation in ESWL , *Ultrasound Med. Biol.* **27(5)**, 683-693 (2001).
16. M. Lokhandwalla and B. Sturtevant, Fracture mechanics model of stone comminution in ESWL and implications for tissue damage, *Phys. Med. Biol.* **45(7)**, 1923-1940 (2000).
17. L.G. Jodrde and F.H. Cocks, Fracture strength studies of renal calculi, *J. Mat. Sci. Lett.* **4**, 1264-1265 (1985).
18. P. Zhong, C.J. Chuong and G.M. Preminger, Characterization of fracture toughness of renal calculi using a microindentation technique , *Journal of Materials Science Letters*, **12**, 1460-1462 (1993).
19. S.R. Khan, R.L. Hackett, and B. Finlayson, Morphology of urinary stone particles resulting from ESWL treatment , *J Urol.* **136**, 1367-1372 (1986).
20. C.C. Church, A theoretical study of cavitation generated by an extracorporeal shock wave lithotripter, *J. Acoust. Soc. Am.* **86(1)**, 215-227 (1989).
21. J. R. Blake and D. Gibson, Cavitation bubbles near boundaries, *Ann. Rev. Fluid. Mech.* **19**, 99-123 (1987).
22. G.N. Sankin, W.N. Simmons, S.L. Zhu, and P. Zhong, Shock wave interaction with laser-generated single bubbles , *Physical Review Letters*, **95(3)** Art. No. 034501 JULY 15 2005.
23. P. Zhong, C.J. Chuong and G.M. Preminger, Propagation of shock waves in elastic solids caused by the impact of cavitation microjets: Part II. application to extracorporeal shock wave lithotripsy , *J. Acoust. Soc. Am.*, Vol. 94(1), pp:29-36,1993.
24. S.L. Zhu, F.H. Cocks, G.M. Preminger, and P. Zhong, The role of stress waves and cavitation in stone comminution in shock wave lithotripsy, *Ultrasound Med. Biol.* **28(5)**, 661-671 (2002).
25. M. Delius, Medical applications and bioeffects of extracorporeal shock waves, *Shock Waves* **4**, 55-72 (1994).
26. A. Evan and J.A. McAteer, Q-effects of shock wave lithotripsy , in Kidney Stones: Medical and Surgical Management, Coe FL, Favus MJ, Pak CYC, Parks JH, Preminger GM (eds): Philadelphia, Lippincott-Raven Press 1996, 549-570.
27. A.P. Evan, L.R. Willis, J.E. Lingeman, J.A. McAteer, Renal trauma and the risk of long-term complications in shock wave lithotripsy , *Nephron* **78**, 1–8 (1998).
28. L.R. Willis, A.P. Evan, B.A. Connors, P.M. Blomgren, N.S. Fineberg, J.E. Lingeman, Relationship between kidney size, renal injury, and renal impairment induced by shock wave lithotripsy, *J Am Soc Nephrol* **10**, 1753–1762 (1999).
29. M. Delius, R. Denk, C. Berding, H. Liebich, M. Jordan, and W. Brendel, Biological effects of shock waves: cavitation by shock waves in piglet liver, *Ultrasound Med. Biol.* **16**, 467-472 (1990).

30. D. Dalecki, C.H. Raeman, S.Z. Child, D.P. Penney, R. Mayer, and E.L. Carstensen, The influence of contrast agents on hemorrhage produced by lithotripter fields, *Ultrasound Med. Biol.* **23**, 1435-1439 (1997).
31. D. Howard and B. Sturtevant, In vitro study of the mechanical effects of shock-wave lithotripsy, *Ultrasound Med. Biol.* **23**, 1107-1122 (1997).
32. A.P. Evan, L.R. Willis, J.A. McAteer, M.R. Bailey, B.A. Connors, Y. Shao, *et al.*, Kidney damage and renal functional changes are minimized by waveform control that suppresses cavitation in shock wave lithotripsy, *J Urol.* **168**, 1556–1562 (2002).
33. P. Zhong, Y.F. Zhou, and S.L. Zhu, Dynamics of bubble oscillation in constrained media and mechanisms of vessel rupture in SWL, *Ultrasound Med. Biol.*, **27(1)**, 119-134 (2001).
34. W.L. Strohmaier, K.H. Bichler, J. Koch, N. Balk, D.M. Wilbert, Protective effect of verapamil on shock wave induced renal tubular dysfunction, *J Urol* **150**, 27–29 (1993).
35. R. Munver, C. Delvecchio, R.L. Kuo et al, In vivo assesment of free radical activity during shock wave lithotripsy using a microdialysis system: the renoprotective effect of allopurinol, *J Urol* **167**, 327-334 (2002).
36. M. Delius and W. Brendel, A model of extracorporeal shock wave action: Tandem action of shock waves (Letter to the editor), *Ultrasound Med. Biol.* **14**, 515-518 (1988).
37. M.R. Bailey, Control of acoustic cavitation with application to lithotripsy, Ph.D. Dissertation, University of Texas at Austin, May 1997.
38. D.L. Sokolov, M.R. Bailey and L.A. Crum, Dual-pulse lithotripter accelerates stone fragmentation and reduces cell lysis in vitro, *Ultrasound Med Biol,* **29**, 1045-1052, (2003).
39. X.F. Xi and P. Zhong, Improvement of stone fragmentation during shock wave lithotripsy using a combined EH/PEAA shock wave generator – In vitro experiments, *Ultrasound Med. Biol.* **6**, 457-467 (2000).
40. A.M. Loske, F.E. Prieto, F. Fernandez, J. van Cauwelaert, Tandem shock wave cavitation enhancement for extracorporeal lithotripsy, *Phys. Med. Biol.* **47(22)**, 3945-3957 (2002).
41. P. Zhong and Y.F. Zhou, Suppression of large intraluminal bubble expansion in shock wave lithotripsy without compromising stone comminution: Methodology and in vitro experiments, *J. Acoust. Soc. Am.*, **110(6)**, 3283-3291 (2001).
42. Y.F. Zhou and P. Zhong, Suppression of large intraluminal bubble expansion in shock wave lithotripsy without compromising stone comminution: Refinement of reflector geometry, *J. Acoust. Soc. Am.* **113 (1)**, 586-597 (2003).
43. W. Eisenmenger, X.X. Du, C. Tang, S. Zhao, Y. Wang, F. Rong, *et al.*, The first clinical results of "wide-focus and low-pressure" ESWL, *Ultrasound Med. Biol.*, **28(6)**, 769-774 (2002).
44. J.A. McAteer, T. Baird T, J.C. Williams et al., Voltage-stepping during SWL influences stone breakage independent of total energy delivered: In vitro studies with model stones, *J Urol.* **169 (4)**, 1825 Suppl. S APR 2003.
45. Y.F. Zhou, F.H. Cocks, G.M. Preminger, and P. Zhong, Treatment strategy affects stone comminution efficiency in shock wave lithotripsy, *J Urol*, **172**, 349-354 (2004).
46. M.E. Maloney, C.G. Marguet, Y.F. Zhou, D.E. Kang, J.C. Sung, W.P. Springhart, J. Madden, P. Zhong, and G.M. Preminger, Progressive increase of lithotripter output produces better *in vivo* stone comminution, *Journal of Endourology*, **20**(9), 603-606 (2006).
47. O.A. Sapozhnikov, V.A. Khokhlova, M.R. Bailey, J.C. Williams Jr, J.A. McAteer, R.O. Cleveland, L.A. Crum, Effect of overpressure and pulse repetition frequency on cavitation in shock wave lithotripsy, *J Acoust Soc Am.* **112(3)**, 1183-1195 (2002).
48. Y.A. Pishchalnikov, J.A. McAteer, J.C. Williams, et al., Why stones break better at slow shockwave rates than at fast rates: In vitro study with a research electrohydraulic lithotripter, *Journal of Endourology* **20 (8)**, 537-541 (2006).
49. L.R. Willis, A.P. Evan, B.A. Connors, et al. Prevention of lithotripsy-induced renal injury by pretreating kidneys with low-energy shock waves, *J Amer Soc Nephrol* **17 (3)**, 663-673 (2006).
50. Y.A. Pishchalnikov, J.S. Neucks, R.J. VonDerHaar, et al. Air pockets trapped during routine coupling in dry head lithotripsy can significantly decrease the delivery of shock wave energy, *J Urol.* **176(6)**, 2706-2710 (2006).

Using Helical CT to Predict Stone Fragility in Shock Wave Lithotripsy (SWL)

James C. Williams, Jr.[*], Chad A. Zarse[*], Molly E. Jackson[*], James E. Lingeman[†], and James A. McAteer[*]

[*]*Department of Anatomy and Cell Biology, Indiana University School of Medicine, Indianapolis, IN 46202, USA*
[†]*Methodist Hospital Institute for Kidney Stone Disease, 1801 North Senate Boulevard, Suite 220, Indianapolis, Indiana 46202. USA*

Abstract. Great variability exists in the response of urinary stones to SWL, and this is true even for stones composed of the same mineral. Efforts have been made to predict stone fragility to shock waves using computed tomography (CT) patient images, but most work to date has focused on the use of stone CT number (i.e., Hounsfield units). This is an easy number to measure on a patient stone, but its value depends on a number of factors, including the relationship of the size of the stone to the resolution (i.e., the slicewidth) of the CT scan. Studies that have shown a relationship between stone CT number and failure in SWL are reviewed, and all are shown to suffer from error due to stone size, which was not accounted for in the use of Hounsfield unit values. Preliminary data are then presented for a study of calcium oxalate monohydrate (COM) stones, in which stone structure—rather than simple CT number values—is shown to correlate with fragility to shock waves. COM stones that were observed to have structure by micro CT (e.g., voids, apatite regions, unusual shapes) broke to completion in about half the number of shock waves required for COM stones that were observed to be homogeneous in structure by CT. This result suggests another direction for the use of CT in predicting success of SWL: the use of CT to view stone structure, rather than simply measuring stone CT number. Viewing stone structure by CT requires the use of different viewing windows than those typically used for examining patient scans, but much research to date indicates that stone structure can be observed in the clinical setting. Future clinical studies will need to be done to verify the relationship between stone structure observed by CT and stone fragility in SWL.

Keywords: shock wave lithotripsy; kidney stones; computed tomography; micro CT; Hounsfield unit
PACS: 43.40.Ng, 81.70.Tx, 87.54.Hk

INTRODUCTION

Since the earliest days of shock wave lithotripsy (SWL), it has been known that some stones respond to lithotripsy more readily than do others, and this quality was correlated to the radiological appearance of the stones. For example, Chaussy has been quoted as saying that stones with x-ray density greater than that of spinal bone were generally more difficult to break [1]. As x-ray computed tomography (CT) began to be used for diagnosis and identification of urinary stones, the power of CT seemed to be ideal for identifying the fragility of stones before treatment [2].

CP900, *Renal Stone Disease, 1st Annual International Urolithiasis Research Symposium,* edited by A. P. Evan, J. E. Lingeman, and J. C. Williams, Jr.

Decisions about treatment of stones include more than just whether the stone is amenable to treatment by SWL. There is now ample evidence to show that shock waves can be injurious to renal tissue [3], and that long-term consequences of lithotripsy can be significant, and are related to the number of shock waves received by the patient [4,5]. Thus, there is a need to be able to judge the number of shock waves required to break a given stone, so that the patient will not receive unnecessary shock waves over what is required to comminute the stone. Ideally, this could be done by monitoring the stone during lithotripsy, and stopping lithotripsy when the stone was sufficiently broken. However, present imaging modalities make it difficult to distinguish large stone fragments from small ones, and techniques to more directly monitor stone breakage are still in their infancy [6].

Two directions have been taken for prediction of stone fragility using CT. The first is to use CT to identify the primary composition of the stone. Then, for example, if a stone was identified as uric acid, it would be predicted to break easily with shock waves, while a stone identified as calcium oxalate monohydrate (COM) would be suspected as a difficult-to-break stone. A number of studies have attempted to use CT for compositional determination of stones [7-17]. These attempts are described as more or less successful by most workers, although the most specific determinations take into account the impact of stone size on the Hounsfield unit value [9], or utilize multiple x-ray energies to distinguish some stone types [7].

An overall problem with this approach is that knowing the composition of the stone does not necessarily allow prediction of the fragility of the stone to shock waves. That is, there is a tremendous variability of stone fragility within all types of stone [18]. So, knowing that a stone is composed primarily of COM indicates that it may be difficult to break, but certainly many COM stones respond quite well to SWL [19]. Thus, knowing that a stone is composed primarily of COM really does not help in making decisions about treatment.

The second approach for using CT to help with this problem has been to use the CT number (Hounsfield unit) values directly for predicting stone fragility in SWL. This has been done by a number of groups [20-25], but there are real problems with this sort of approach, as the Hounsfield unit values in clinical CT are profoundly affected by stone size [26,27]. In general, the results show a correlation between high values of Hounsfield unit in stones and failure of lithotripsy, but this correlation is entirely attributable to artifact of stone size on Hounsfield unit values. CT has tremendous potential to help guide treatment planning in SWL, but this can only be realized if the inherent limitations are thoroughly understood.

THE EFFECT OF STONE SIZE ON HOUNSFIELD UNIT VALUES IN HELICAL CT

CT number values in clinical CT are measured in Hounsfield units (HU), on a scale in which air has a value of -1000, water a value of 0, and bone a value of +1000. These values are calculated from the x-ray absorptions measured as the scan is taken, and are used for display of the reconstructed images of the body, with a specific range of Hounsfield unit values being assigned levels of gray according to the 'windows' and 'levels' selected by the viewer.

The computation of these Hounsfield unit values is affected by the resolution of the scanning system and by the x-ray attenuation coefficients of both the material surrounding the objects of interest, and that of the objects themselves. In the case of urinary stones, the x-ray attenuation of the surrounding material (urine and tissue), is much lower than that of the stone, and the CT system 'confuses' the edge of the stone with the surrounding urine and tissue, introducing error in the apparent x-ray attenuation of the stone's edge [26,28]. The distance over which this error extends depends on the spatial resolution of the CT scan. The spatial resolution of scanners continues to improve, but for now, a true 'error zone' of about 2 mm is about the best that can be expected from an abdominal patient scan [29].

This 2 mm error is large in comparison to the size of urinary stones. The error is even more significant when it is realized that the error zone extends over the entire surface of the stone; that is, CT is a three-dimensional imaging method, so that errors must be considered in three dimensions, and not just in two.

The relative volume occupied by such an error zone is surprisingly large. For example, in a sphere of 20 mm diameter, fully half of its volume resides in an outer layer just little more than 2 mm in thickness (Fig. 1). Thus, for a 20 mm stone, scanned with helical CT using a high-resolution protocol, half of the stone volume will be displayed with Hounsfield unit values confused by volume averaging error from the surrounding urine and tissue.

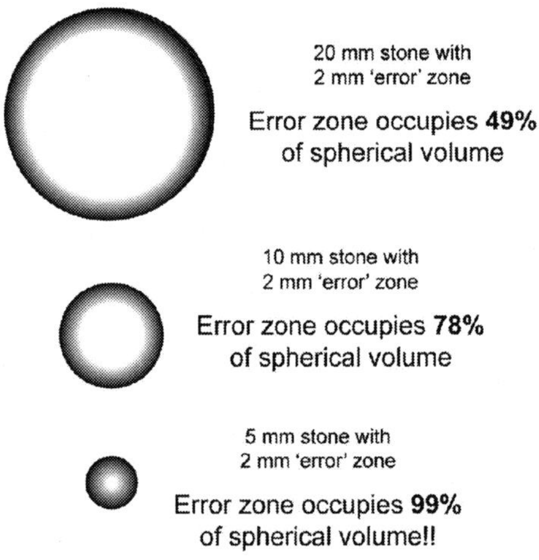

FIGURE 1. The impact of volume averaging error with presently available high-resolution abdominal CT scans. Examples show the portion of a spherical stone affected by CT volume averaging error when spatial uncertainty of x-ray attenuation values extends 2 mm into the stone. Note that the volume of the stone represented in the outermost 2 mm region is substantial, even for larger stones.

The fraction of the stone image affected by this error will, of course, be larger as the stone size decreases. For stones between 5 and 10 mm in diameter, 80-99% of the image volume will be affected by the volume averaging error. If the stone is non-spherical (which is likely), the fraction of the stone image affected by volume averaging with the surround will be even greater.

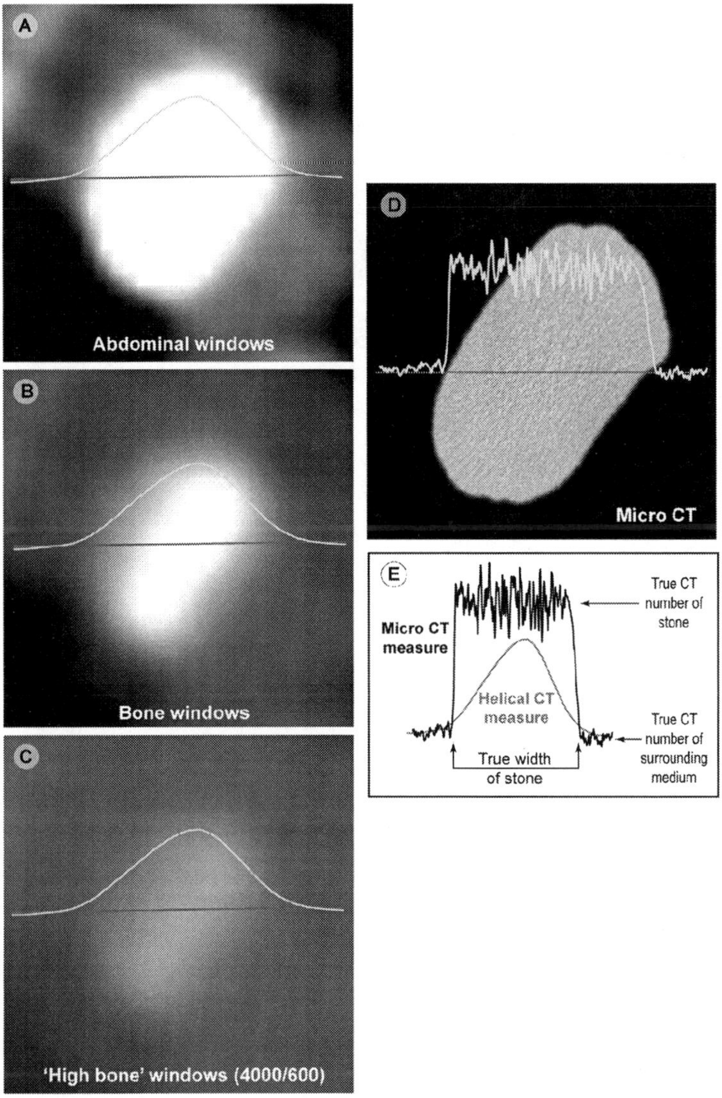

FIGURE 2. Images of a calcium oxalate monohydrate (COM) stone, scanned using 64 detector-row clinical CT with 2.5mm slicewidth (panels A-C) and micro CT (panel D).

Images of a stone are shown in Fig. 2, with the measured Hounsfield unit values shown along a line through the center of the stone. The images on the left are from the same helical CT scan, and demonstrate how different the stone can look using different viewing windows. The curve shown over each image is a graph of the measured Hounsfield unit values, which are, of course, the same for all viewing windows, as these are basic to the scan, and not to the viewing windows. As can be seen by the micro CT image of the same stone (panel D), the mineral in the stone is actually quite uniform, and thus would ideally yield uniform measures of Hounsfield units throughout the stone. Such is not the case, however, and the clinical CT scan of this stone shows the sort of error in CT number illustrated schematically in Fig. 1. The curve for Hounsfield units measured by helical CT in Fig. 2 shows a peak value of about 1400 HU, for a scan using 2.5 mm slicewidth; the same stone scanned at 0.7 mm yielded a consistently higher value through the center of the stone (mean of 1938±43 HU), demonstrating that *all* of the Hounsfield unit values in this 6 mm COM stone were artifactually reduced in the 2.5 mm scan—which is likely the smallest slicewidth that would be used for an abdominal scan in a patient setting. Indeed, most abdominal scans are done at a slicewidth of 3 mm or more, as shown in the cases explored below.

So, we see from Figs. 1 and 2 that error in CT measurement of Hounsfield units in kidney stones can be significant, and that this error will be worse for smaller stones than for larger ones. Putting these two ideas together, one can see that, for stones made of similar material, small stones will yield lower values for Hounsfield units than will large stones, as has been shown previously [26]. How does this affect interpretation of published studies? Six published studies are reviewed here to show the variety of effects.

Specific case studies

Case 1. *Joseph et al., Computerized tomography attenuation value of renal calculus: can it predict successful fragmentation of the calculus by extracorporeal shock wave lithotripsy? A preliminary study.* J Urol *167: 1968, 2002* [20]

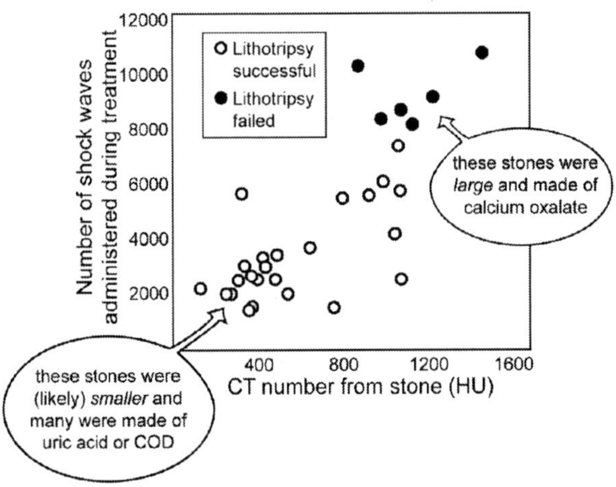

FIGURE 3. Results from Joseph et al. [20] showing a relationship between the CT number for kidney stones (in Hounsfield units, HU) and the resistance of the stones to treatment by SWL. However, this relationship is not fundamental to the Hounsfield unit values of the stones, being a combination of size artifact on CT and the effects of different stone compositions.

This study was performed using 30 patients having solitary renal stones, with a range of stone size of 5-20 mm. The CT scans were reconstructed with 2 mm slices, but the setting for patient scans was not given. Regions of interest were chosen while viewing stones using abdominal windows, and Hounsfield unit values were recorded. Patients were treated with as many as three sessions of SWL, with each session limited to a maximum of 3500 shock waves. In 6 cases lithotripsy failed, as judged by detection of residual fragments larger than 3 mm after 6 weeks. These 6 stones were large (15±5 mm), and the 4 for which analysis was done were composed of calcium oxalate. For stones successfully treated, composition was determined in 16 cases, with 7 of those stones being made of uric acid or calcium oxalate dihydrate, both of which are known to respond well to SWL.

The study showed a significant relationship between the number of shock waves required for treatment (or administered without successful stone comminution) and the Hounsfield unit values of the stones, pre-treatment, as reproduced in Fig. 3. However, this relationship of shock wave dose to Hounsfield units can be accounted for by stone size effects, with a probable additional effect of stone composition, and does not support the principle that x-ray density of stones is in itself a predictor of lithotripsy success.

Case 2. *Pareek et al., Hounsfield units on computerized tomography predict stone-free rates after extracorporeal shock wave lithotripsy.* J Urol *169: 1679, 2003* [21]

50 patients with solitary renal or ureteral stones were studied, first being scanned with CT at 5 mm collimation, and images examined following reconstruction using 2.5 mm slices. All stones were 5-10 mm in size, and Hounsfield unit values were recorded for each. Patients were treated with a single session of lithotripsy, and stone fragments were recovered for analysis. Success was evaluated by plain x-ray at 6 weeks, and fragments of 3 mm were taken as indication of failure of lithotripsy treatment.

Although stone size was measured in this study, no test of size effect was reported. The authors suggest that using patients with stones in between 5 and 10 mm represent a 'homogeneous group,' but this is exactly the range in which one sees a dramatic effect of stone size on Hounsfield unit values [26]. The results showed that stones successfully treated had a lower value for Hounsfield units than those stones that left residual fragments, and this is easily explained by the successfully treated stones being smaller, and—in the case of 7 stones that broke well—being composed of uric acid. Thus, like Case 1, the correlation of lithotripsy success with Hounsfield unit values in this study resulted from a fortuitous combination of compositional and size effects, and does not represent a general principle that can be applied to lithotripsy treatment.

Case 3. *Gupta et al., Role of computed tomography with no contrast medium enhancement in predicting the outcome of extracorporeal shock wave lithotripsy for urinary calculi.* BJU Int *95: 1285, 2005* [22]

108 patients, each having a solitary calculus of 5-20 mm (5-10 mm in the lower pole or ureter), were imaged using helical CT with 3 mm image sections (scan

parameters were not reported). Stones were viewed using abdominal windows, and longest dimension and average Hounsfield units were recorded for each stone. Note that the dimensions of stones were also measured in the longitudinal direction by counting the slices in which the stone was apparent, a measure that is typically less accurate than in lateral directions [30].

Lithotripsy was done in as many as 7 sessions, with 3000 shock waves per session, each 14 days apart. X-rays were taken before and after each lithotripsy session, and also 12 weeks after the last session. Stone fragments were recovered and analyzed from 72 of the patients.

Results showed that lithotripsy success—defined either by complete clearance of fragments or by treatment requiring fewer than 4 lithotripsy sessions—was significantly related both to smaller stone size and lower Hounsfield unit values. However, data were shown only in terms of two size domains (≤1.1 cm or >1.1 cm) and two Hounsfield unit domains (≤750 HU or >750 HU), and complete regression analyses were apparently not done. Despite this, the authors concluded that Hounsfield unit values are the more important predictor of lithotripsy success.

Criticism of this work came in the form of letters to the editor, and a quote from one of these sums up the problems with the study:

> *...the concept of isolating stone density alone as a predictive factor for fragmentation will result in misleading conclusions in the practical setting. Size and density are not mutually exclusive as predictors but linked in the context of CT attenuation values....* [31]

Again, as with the previous two cases, the relationship reported here between Hounsfield unit values of stones and success in lithotripsy was almost certainly due to a combination of stone size and stone compositional variation, and does not represent a principle that can be universally applied to predicting lithotripsy outcomes.

Case 4. *Magnuson et al., Hounsfield unit density accurately predicts ESWL success.* Alaska Med *47: 6, 2005.* [23]

This study included 101 patients with renal or ureteral stones ranging from 5-15 mm in size. Patients were treated with a single lithotripsy session, and stone-free status was determined either by CT or plain x-ray during the period of 6 to 12 weeks following treatment. No details were given on the pre-lithotripsy CT scanning or analysis parameters used, but Hounsfield unit values were normalized to stone diameter.

The results showed a highly significant difference between the stone-free and residual fragment groups, averaging 94 and 123 HU/mm, respectively. No data were given on stone composition (even though all patients were said to have brought in stone fragments for analysis post-lithotripsy).

In one sense, this paper is an improvement over those previously described, as the authors attempted to account for stone size effects by dividing the measured Hounsfield unit values by the stone diameter. However, this measure does not yield a number that is consistent for stones of same composition but of different sizes. As shown in Fig. 4, if the Hounsfield unit value for a stone is accurately measured, then dividing that value by the stone diameter creates a measure that declines with increasing stone size. If one calculates the predicted effect of volume averaging on smaller stones (shown in the gray region in Fig. 4), the measured Hounsfield units divided by the stone diameter still varies with stone size, though in a manner that is somewhat flat for smaller stones, as division by the stone diameter corrects in a rough way for the decrease in apparent Hounsfield units when stone size is less than about twice the slicewidth of the CT scan [26].

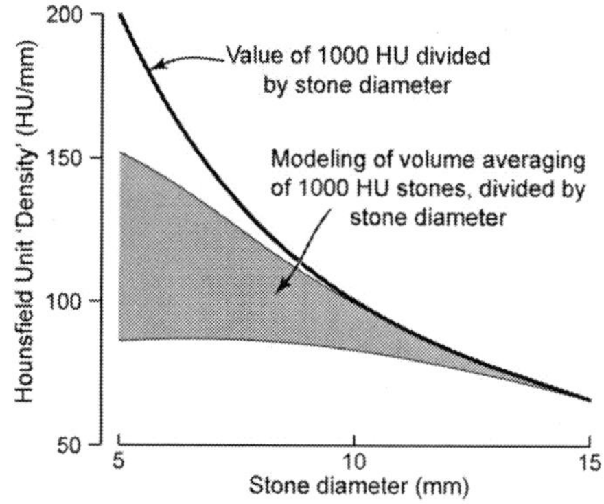

FIGURE 4. Variation of Hounsfield unit 'density' with stone diameter. (Hounsfield unit 'density' is calculated as the measured value of average Hounsfield units for a stone, divided by the stone's diameter.) Note that if the true CT number for the stone is known—shown here for a true value of 1000 Hounsfield units—then division by the diameter yields a hyperbolic relationship. However, at smaller stone sizes, apparent CT number will be reduced by volume averaging. This effect was modeled as per Hu and Fox [28] for maximum and minimum values expected for stones of each size [26], assuming a true CT number of 1000 HU, and the range of results is shown in gray.

Thus, the use of a 'Hounsfield density' value helps in correcting for volume averaging effects in smaller stones, but it artificially depresses this value for larger stones, and this two-fold effect results in data that are difficult to interpret. So, for the results of Magnuson et al., we are left with the possibility that many of the stones that broke more easily were composed of uric acid, and thus yielded a low CT density [9], and there is no indication that the use of this density measure would be valuable for general prediction of success in SWL.

Case 5. *Wang et al., Predictions of outcomes of renal stones after extracorporeal shock wave lithotripsy from stone characteristics determined by unenhanced helical computed tomography: a multivariate analysis.* Eur Radiol *15: 2238, 2005* [24]

This study included 80 patients, many of whom had multiple stones (mean of 2.3 stones per patient). Each patient was scanned by multi-detector helical CT, using 3.75 mm slicewidth, and reconstructions at 2.5 mm. Images were viewed (apparently using only abdominal windows) for measure of stone dimensions, and average Hounsfield unit values for each stone were taken using the largest possible region of interest. Patients were treated using a single session of SWL, and re-scanned by CT for follow-up at 3 months. The presence of any fragments measuring 4 mm or greater was considered a mark of failure of the lithotripsy treatment, with a total failure rate of 48%.

The results showed highly significant correlations between the outcome of lithotripsy and all of the following measures: stone number, stone size, total stone burden, stone shape being non-oval, and Hounsfield unit measure. The authors used multivariate analysis to suggest that stone burden, stone shape, and the Hounsfield unit measure of the brightest stone were all statistically significant predictors of lithotripsy success or failure. The dependence of Hounsfield unit measure on stone size was not acknowledged in this, and the two were treated as independent measures.

Although the authors place a great deal of emphasis on the usefulness of Hounsfield unit values, their results are much more supportive of the relationship between stone size, stone number, and total stone burden as predictors of failure in SWL. The authors may have been unaware of the impact of stone size on apparent values of Hounsfield units. Similarly, their use of regions-of-interest just smaller than the stone image does not acknowledge the probable effects of volume averaging.

The paper also shows no information about the structure of stones, which could have been obtained by using alternative viewing windows [32]. Although the radiologist took time to view the stones in both cross-sectional and coronal views, there was no mention of the use of windows and levels other than those for typical abdominal viewing.

Case 6. *Yoshida et al., Role of volume and attenuation value histogram of urinary stone on noncontrast helical computed tomography as predictor of fragility by extracorporeal shock wave lithotripsy.* Urology *68: 33, 2006* [25]

This study used 56 stones in 49 patients, with all stones evaluated before lithotripsy using an 8-detector row scanner, with 1.25 mm beam collimation, a pitch of 5.0, and 1.25 mm slices on reconstruction. All stones were between 5 and 20 mm in maximum dimension (by plain x-ray). The volume of each stone was selected using a threshold of 100 HU, and histograms created for each stone, as described further below.

Each patient was treated using a Siemens Lithostar, with a maximum of 3500 shock waves per session. Plain x-ray was done within 3 weeks after the session to look for residual fragments, which were the indication for another treatment session. A maximum of 3 sessions were done for each patient, and fragments greater than 3 mm visible after that indicated failure of lithotripsy treatment.

The results showed 17 failures and 39 successes. The stones on which lithotripsy failed were significantly larger (both by maximal dimension and by volume) and higher in measured CT number (in Hounsfield units). The failed stones also showed a higher incidence of a 'hump' in the histogram, as illustrated in Fig. 5.

Although the idea of identifying a hump in the histogram provides a tantalizing quantitative measure in CT analysis of stones, this ends up being just another measure of stone size. Only stones made of materials that absorb x-rays well (calcium minerals) and also are greater than about 10 mm in diameter, would be expected to show a hump in this way. The hump shows the portion of the calcium stone measured without significant volume averaging error, and calcium stones above 10 mm in diameter would be expected to have at least 20% of their volume measured correctly (calculated as per Fig. 1) and thus showing a hump in the histogram of Hounsfield unit values. Smaller stones, regardless of their composition, would have such significant volume averaging error so as to not have many voxels of high value, and thus would be less likely to show a 'hump,' even if they were made of calcium oxalate. Thus, the Yoshida data use Hounsfield units in a new way, but still primarily as an indicator of stone size, which was not acknowledged directly in the paper, and which also can be measured more directly, and more simply, by other methods.

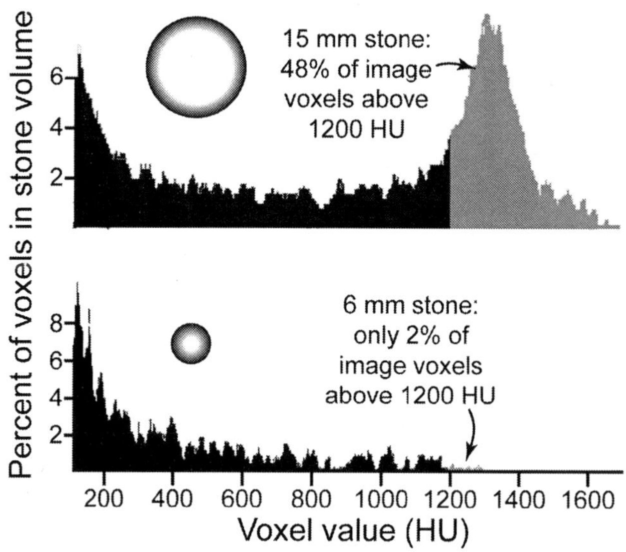

FIGURE 5. Histograms of helical CT Hounsfield unit values for two stones, based upon data from Yoshida et al. [25] (In the paper, histograms were shown, but stone size was mentioned only in the figure legend.) The larger stone apparently had a significant quantity of calcium oxalate (or perhaps calcium phosphate), as shown by the number of voxels above 1200 HU [13]. The scan of the smaller stone shows few voxels above 1200 HU, but this can be explained entirely by volume averaging. That is, the smaller stone could have been pure calcium oxalate, but still show only a few percent of voxels with high HU values, as described above in Fig. 1. The histogram of the larger stone was referred to by Yoshida et al. as having a 'hump' in the region greater than 1200 HU. If all stones were made of calcium oxalate, then the 'hump' would be an indicator of a stone being large enough that a significant portion of its volume was reported with accurately high Hounsfield units.

ANOTHER APPROACH: VIEWING STONE STRUCTURE BY CT TO PREDICT FRAGILITY OF COM CALCULI

We have taken a different approach in recent work, described in preliminary form here. Briefly, the idea was to examine the fragility of COM stones with the hypothesis that stones that looked homogeneous by CT would break differently from those that were not homogeneous. The kind of structure that was observed as indicating inhomogeneity included the presence of significant amounts of calcium phosphate (which shows up brighter than COM on CT), the presence of voids in the stone, and irregular shapes, such as in stones having significant protuberances from their surfaces.

This study was done on COM stones, with the rationale that calcium oxalate stones are the most common stones treated using SWL, and that the monohydrate form of these stones can be especially resistant to shock wave treatment.

Methods

Urinary stones were obtained as discards from a stone lab, with no patient identification, but with the mineral analysis obtained from each stone (either using part of that stone, or another stone from that patient event). Stones were selected that had been determined to be ≥96% COM (whewellite). Stones were scanned by micro CT and the micro CT scans judged by independent observers as indicating a COM stone that was homogeneous in structure, or one that had visible, internal structural features, as indicated in Fig. 6. Only those stones that were consistently judged by four independent observers as being either homogeneous or heterogeneous in structure by micro CT were included in this study.

Stones were hydrated for 4 days, and broken *in vitro* in a Dornier Doli-50 Lithotripter, power level 4, 120 SW/min) over 2 mm mesh, and shock waves to comminution counted for each stone. Order of stone breakage was randomized, and personnel carrying out the lithotripsy had no knowledge of the structural classification of stones by micro CT. Data were analyzed using Student's *t*-test.

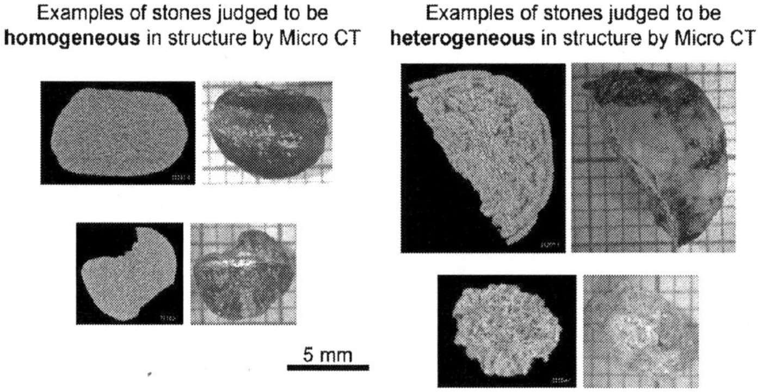

FIGURE 6. Representative examples of COM stones used for *in vitro* lithotripsy experiment. 16 stones were found that were judged by all four observers, independently, as homogeneous in structure by micro CT. 25 stones were consistently judged to be heterogeneous by micro CT.

Results and Discussion

Stones judged to be homogeneous showed micro CT profiles that were characterized by evenness of x-ray attenuation, suggesting a uniform distribution of mineral within each stone. Stones judged to 'show structure' exhibited regions of low x-ray attenuation (voids [33]), regions of high attenuation (indicating the presence of calcium phosphate [34]), and sometimes irregularity of surface contour. Examples of all of these structural forms can be seen in Fig. 6.

Stones that appeared homogeneous in structure by micro CT required, on average, twice as many shock waves for comminution as those showing observable structure, as shown in Table 1.

TABLE 1. Results of in vitro lithotripsy breakage of COM stones.

Structure classification	Shock waves per gram stone (±S.D.)
Homogeneous	1874±821 (n=16)
Heterogeneous	912±678 (n=25)
t-test	p=0.0005

These preliminary results show a significant relationship between structure visible by CT in COM stones and stone susceptibility to shock waves. The difference in fragility of stones in the two groups was quite dramatic, with the homogenous stones requiring an average of nearly 1900 shock waves per gram, while the stones that were identified as having structure by CT required half as many shock waves.

In this study, micro CT was used, which provides better resolution of stone structure than does helical CT [13]. However, stone structure is quite visible by helical CT *in vitro* [32], and stone structure can be seen in patient scans, as well [35,36]. Moreover, the viewing of stone structure, rather than measuring Hounsfield unit value, avoids most of the problems caused by the interaction of stone size with CT resolution. Thus, it is possible that patient scans could be used to view stone structure (using bone windows [27,32]) for identifying COM stones that would be susceptible or resistant to SWL.

CONCLUSIONS

Efforts to predict stone fragility to shock waves using CT number have fallen short because they have not recognized the effect of stone size on CT number in the clinical setting. The preliminary data presented here for COM stones shows that stone structure—rather than simple CT number values—correlates with fragility to shock waves. COM stones that were observed to have structure by micro CT (e.g., voids, apatite regions, unusual shapes) broke to completion in about half the number of shock waves required for COM stones that were observed to be homogeneous in structure by CT. This result suggests another direction for the use of CT in predicting success of SWL: the use of CT to view stone structure, rather than measuring stone CT number alone. Viewing stone structure by CT requires the use of different viewing windows than those typically used for examining patient scans, but studies have clearly demonstrated the ability of CT to show the internal structural features of stones in patient scans. We believe that these data provide a sound rationale for moving ahead with clinical studies to determine the relationship between stone structure observed by CT and stone fragility in shock wave lithotripsy.

ACKNOWLEDGMENTS

This work was funded by NIH R01DK59933.

REFERENCES

1. S.P. Dretler. Stone fragility—a new therapeutic distinction, *J Urol* 139, 1124 (1988).
2. S.P. Dretler and B.A. Spencer. CT and stone fragility, *J Endourol* 15 (1), 31 (2001).
3. A.P. Evan, L.R. Willis, J.E. Lingeman et al. Renal trauma and the risk of long-term complications in shock wave lithotripsy, *Nephron* 78, 1 (1998).
4. G. Janetschek, F. Frauscher, R. Knapp et al. New onset hypertension after extracorporeal shock wave lithotripsy: age related incidence and prediction by intrarenal resistive index, Journal Of *Urology* 158 (2), 346 (1997).
5. A.E. Krambeck, M.T. Gettman, A.L. Rohlinger et al. Diabetes Mellitus and Hypertension Associated with Shock Wave Lithotripsy of Renal and Proximal Ureteral Stones at 19 Years Follow-up *J Urol* 175 (May), 1742 (2006).
6. N.R. Owen, M.R. Bailey, and L.A. Crum. Characterization of a vibro-acoustography system designed to detect kidney stones during lithotripsy, *J Acoust Soc Am* 117, 2588 (2005).
7. M.R. Mostafavi, R.D. Ernst, and B. Saltzman. Accurate determination of chemical composition of urinary calculi by spiral computerized tomography, *J Urol* 159, 673 (1998).
8. K.C. Saw, J.A. McAteer, A.G. Monga et al. Helical CT of urinary calculi: Effect of stone composition, stone size, and scan collimation, *AJR Am J Roentgenol* 175 (August), 329 (2000).
9. S.Y. Nakada, D.G. Hoff, S. Attai et al. Determination of stone composition by noncontrast spiral computed tomography in the clinical setting, *Urology* 55, 816 (2000).
10. G. Motley, N. Dalrymple, C. Keesling et al. Hounsfield unit density in the determination of urinary stone composition, *Urology* 58 (2), 170 (2001).
11. C. Gonzalez Enguita, J.L. Rodriguez Minon-Cifuentes, J. Cabrera Perez et al. La litiasis resistente a LEOC [ESWL-resistant lithiasis], *Actas Urologicas Espanolas*. 23 (3), 247 (1999).
12. A. Demirel and S. Suma. The efficacy of non-contrast helical computed tomography in the prediction of urinary stone composition in vivo, *J Int Med Res* 31, 1 (2003).
13. C.A. Zarse, J.A. McAteer, M. Tann et al. Helical CT accurately reports urinary stone composition using attenuation values: *In vitro* verification using high resolution micro CT calibrated to FT-IR microspectroscopy, *Urology* 63, 828 (2004).
14. M.-F. Bellin, R. Renard-Penna, P. Conort et al. Helical CT evaluation of the chemical composition of urinary tract calculi with a discriminant analysis of CT-attenuation values and density, *European Radiology* 14, 2134 (2004).
15. S. Deveci, M. Coskun, M.I. Tekin et al. Spiral computed tomography: role in determination of chemical compositions of pure and mixed urinary stones—an in vitro study, *Urology* 64, 237 (2004).
16. K.Z. Sheir, O. Mansour, K. Madbouly et al. Determination of the chemical composition of urinary calculi by noncontrast spiral computerized tomography, *Urol Res* 33, 99 (2005).
17. F.J. Burgos, J. Sanchez, S. Avila et al. [The usefulness of computerized axial tomography (CT) in establishing the composition of calculi], *Arch Esp Urol* 46 (5), 383 (1993).

18. J.C. Williams, Jr., K.C. Saw, R.F. Paterson et al. Variability of renal stone fragility in shock wave lithotripsy, *Urology* 61 (6), 1092 (2003).
19. C.G. Chaussy and G.J. Fuchs. Extracorporeal shock wave lithotripsy, *Monographs in Urology* 8, 80 (1987).
20. P. Joseph, A.K. Mandal, S.K. Singh et al. Computerized tomography attenuation value of renal calculus: can it predict successful fragmentation of the calculus by extracorporeal shock wave lithotripsy? A preliminary study, *J Urol* 167 (May), 1968 (2002).
21. G. Pareek, N.A. Armenakas, and J.A. Fracchia. Hounsfield units on computerized tomography predict stone-free rates after extracorporeal shock wave lithotripsy, *J Urol* 169 (May), 1679 (2003).
22. N.P. Gupta, M.S. Ansari, P. Kesarvani et al. Role of computed tomography with no contrast medium enhancement in predicting the outcome of extracorporeal shock wave lithotripsy for urinary calculi, *BJU Int* 95 (9), 1285 (2005).
23. W.J. Magnuson, K.M. Tomera, and R.S. Lance. Hounsfield unit density accurately predicts ESWL success, *Alaska Med* 47 (2), 6 (2005).
24. L.-J. Wang, Y.-C. Wong, C.-K. Chuang et al. Predictions of outcomes of renal stones after extracorporeal shock wave lithotripsy from stone characteristics determined by unenhanced helical computed tomography: a multivariate analysis, *European Radiology* 15 (11), 2238 (2005).
25. S. Yoshida, T. Hayashi, J. Ikeda et al. Role of volume and attenuation value histogram of urinary stone on noncontrast helical computed tomography as predictor of fragility by extracorporeal shock wave lithotripsy, *Urology* 68 (1), 33 (2006).
26. J.C. Williams, Jr., K.C. Saw, A.G. Monga et al. Correction of helical CT attenuation values with wide beam collimation, *Academic Radiology* 8, 478 (2001).
27. J.C. Williams, Jr., S.C. Kim, C.A. Zarse et al. Progress in the use of helical CT for imaging urinary calculi, *J Endourol* 18 (10), 937 (2004).
28. H. Hu and S.H. Fox. The effect of helical pitch and beam collimation on the lesion contrast and slice profile in helical CT imaging, *Med Phys* 23, 1943 (1996).
29. E. Rollano-Hijarrubia, R. Stokking, F. van der Meer et al. Imaging of Small High-Density Structures in CT: A Phantom Study, *Academic Radiology* 13 (7), 893 (2006).
30. N. Narepalem, C.P. Sundaram, I.C. Boridy et al. Comparison of helical computerized tomography and plain radiography for estimating urinary stone size, *J Urol* 167 (March), 1235 (2002).
31. Z.R. Zaman, S.S. Kommu, and N.A. Watkin. Role of computed tomography with no contrast medium enhancement in predicting the outcome of extracorporeal shock wave lithotripsy for urinary calculi, *BJU International* 96 (4), 685 (2005).
32. J.C. Williams, Jr., R.F. Paterson, K.K. Kopecky et al. High resolution detection of internal structure in renal calculi by helical computerized tomography, *J Urol* 167, 322 (2002).
33. S.C. Kim, E.K. Hatt, J.E. Lingeman et al. Cystine: helical computerized tomography characterization of rough and smooth calculi in vitro, *J Urol* 174 (October), 1468 (2005).
34. C.A. Zarse, J.A. McAteer, A.J. Sommer et al. Nondestructive analysis of urinary calculi using micro computed tomography, *BMC Urology* 4, 15 (2004).
35. N. Jacobsen, D. Ng, V. Varma et al. Does internal structure of renal calculi on high resolution CT predict SWL treatment outcome?, *Can J Urol* 11 (3), 2274 (abstract) (2004).
36. S.C. Kim, C.A. Zarse, J.A. McAteer et al. Stone internal structure is visible in patients by helical CT, *J Urol* 171 (4suppl), 509 (2004).

The Future of SWL: A Global Perspective

Kai Uwe Köhrmann

Department. of Urology, Theresienkrankenhaus, Bassermannstr. 1, 68165 Mannheim, Germany

Abstract. The future relevance of shock wave lithotripsy (SWL) to the treatment of urinary stones has been questioned by some. This paper reviews recent developments with an aim to predict the level of usefulness of SWL for the future. The incidence of urolithiasis is increasing throughout the world, and existing metaphylaxis is not widely effective. This results in an increasing need for active stone removal. SWL was and is a well established treatment modality for urolithiasis in the upper urinary tract. For most stone situations there will remain a reasonable choice between SWL versus endoscopic procedures, and it is unlikely that endoscopic procedures will displace SWL completely in general practice. In conclusion, SWL will continue to play an established, if slightly reduced, role in stone treatment in the future.

Keywords: kidney stones, lithotripsy, ureteroscopy, percutaneous nephrolithotomy
PACS: 87.54.Hk

A perspective on the future of SWL can only be developed from the extrapolation of the past and an analysis from the present. This includes not only evidence from the actual literature but also some subjective estimations by the author.

HISTORICAL DEVELOPMENT OF SWL

Within a very short time period after the first clinical treatment of a patient with a kidney stone in February 1980 using the prototype lithotripter Dornier HM1, the first serial-type HM3 was installed in Germany (in 1983) and thereafter distributed all over the world. The revolution of SWL was so successful that this treatment option shortly was accepted as a reasonable alternative to surgical procedures [1,2]. Already five years after its introduction, SWL was the first-choice treatment for nearly all calculi located in the upper urinary tract. Despite the necessity of general anesthesia, the low morbidity for the patient with this non-invasive procedure justified re-treatment when the stone was not completely disintegrated by the first session. Therefore SWL was applied for almost all renal and ureteral stones, excepting staghorn stones, diverticular stones, asymptomatic stones, and nephrocalcinosis. The parallel development of the endoscopic techniques of percutaneous (PCNL) and transureteral (URS) lithotripsy was significantly slower. Only after the availability of highly effective intracorporeal lithotripters and baskets was their range of indications increased. Certainly the short learning curve for SWL compared to endoscopic procedures has been an important reason for the fast spread of shock wave lithotripters. The application of shock waves was possible after a short training period for young urologists and has sometimes been

CP900, *Renal Stone Disease, 1st Annual International Urolithiasis Research Symposium,* edited by A. P. Evan, J. E. Lingeman, and J. C. Williams, Jr.

performed successfully by medical technicians. This is explained by the low risk of severe complications in SWL, even when it is mishandled.

In the first phase of its introduction, SWL seemed to cause no adverse side effects [1] but with time and the arrival of CT and MRI the risk for the kidney became apparent [3,4]. The rate of hematoma has been calculated to be around 0.5%.

The further development of lithotripters was intended to improve stone disintegration and to reduce side effects [5]. Concerning the side effects, on the one hand the trauma to the kidney and adjacent organs should be reduced. On the other hand pain during shock wave application had to be reduced to avoid general anesthesia. Both effects were thought to be reached by concentrating the shock wave energy to a smaller focal area. Under this intention the electrohydraulic shock wave generator has been modified, but also electromagnetic and piezoelectric sources were developed. The development was successful since pain was limited and SWL without anesthesia became possible [6].

Improvement of the disintegrative efficacy was not so prosperous. Some *in vitro* and *ex vivo* studies seemed to prove an advantage in stone comminution by the modern shock wave machines. But no clinical, prospective randomized trial could confirm a benefit compared with the unmodified Dornier HM3.

Nevertheless, some further improvements were gained:

- Stone localization by X-ray and/or sonography enabled the treatment of stones with weak or no radiodensity. Additionally, ultrasound localization reduced X-ray exposure to the patient. But sonographic localization did not became widely accepted since this procedure is more time consuming and ureteral stones usually are not detectable by ultrasound. In the US, urologists usually are not so experienced using sonography. All this has argued against the expensive addition of ultrasound.
- The optimal medium for transmission of acoustic shock waves is degassed water. In the Dornier HM3 the patient was immersed in a large water basin. This was also technically elaborate and costly. Therefore the basin was reduced to a water cushion to be coupled by a membrane and jelly between the water and the skin surface. On the downside, it has been shown that this coupling method reduces shock wave energy and can impair disintegration efficacy significantly.
- The upgrading of lithotripters to a multifunctional workstation or the integration of the shock wave generator into a urological workstation necessitated compromises. But this was driven by economic demands to enable the acquisition of a lithotripter by smaller hospitals. Therefore modular systems were developed with the possibility to use different parts of the workstation (e.g., the C-arm) separately from the lithotripsy system or to upgrade a urologic table by addition of a shock wave generator.

THE ACTUAL SITUATION OF SWL

Today there is a large variety of lithotripter systems, from expensive high-end devices down to low-budget machines. In a lot of cases financial limits influence the choice of the lithotripter significantly. Beyond that, there are no hard criteria for selecting the "best" lithotripter. In the following listing, some essential details of lithotripters are discussed from the present point of view as a basis for developing optimized units for the future:

- The configuration of the optimal pressure and energy distribution in the focus area for the most efficient disintegration and lowest side effects is still not known. The reason for that is that the parameters that control the different effects (disintegration and trauma) specifically are not defined. A larger focal zone with a higher energy density seems to increase stone comminution but also aggravate pain (and thus the need for anesthesia) and tissue damage. A machine with a small focal point, despite having a very high peak pressure, can be applied without narcotics, but the higher re-treatment rate of such systems indicates their lower clinical success.
- Additionally it is not clear what is the ideal system for generating shock waves: electrohydraulic, electromagnetic or piezoelectric. Several lithotripter manufacturers now offer a flexible focal zone (large and small focus), and that is possible now with all three technologies. Moreover, it is beneficial to provide a homogeneous shock wave and low maintenance costs, which is possible especially by electromagnetic and piezoelectric systems.
- Coupling of the shock wave from the generator to the body surface is an essential factor in lithotripsy. The best shock wave is not successful when it doesn't reach the stone undisturbed. Concerning this, the Dornier HM3 provided the optimal way by immersing the patient in a water tub. In this design there is no interface to alter the shock wave. Most present-day lithotripters couple to the patient using water cushions, which is technically and practically easier to handle. But the addition of a silicon layer and the potential of adherent air bubbles (probably a frequent reason for poor SWL results in clinical practice) can decrease the shock wave energy significantly. The way back to the tub could be the future for ensuring optimal coupling, but that is not compatible with integration into a urological workstation.
- To localize the stone, fluoroscopy is the standard. Here the rotatable x-ray tube mounted on a C-arm is less expensive and more practical compared to the two fixed tubes of the HM3. For the option of ultrasound localization we should expect that in-line localization is more precise as compared with off-line.

Since there is no ideal lithotripter we have to choose between the different options, making technical and economic compromises.

THE DEVELOPMENT OF COMPETITIVE PROCEDURES: URS AND PCNL

While SWL showed a continuous increase in usage up to its culmination in the early 1990's, endoscopic procedures have since that time been continuously progressing in technical precision and clinical application [7,8]. By means of miniaturization, more effective devices can be passed through to the stone (e.g., 6-8 French ureteroscopes, holmium laser, etc.) by URS [9] or PCNL [10]. By using flexible endoscopes (together with access sheaths and nitinol baskets) all parts of the upper urinary tract can be accessed. The crucial advantage of endoscopy compared to SWL is the potential for immediate removal of the concretions. Even optimal fragmentation by SWL is followed by a time period for the clearing of the fragments, with the associated risk of colic and obstruction. Particular for kidney stones the time for fragment clearance is unpredictable. But nowadays patients are less willing to accept a course of treatment with unpredictable outcomes. This disadvantage of SWL has to be balanced against the risks of complications of endoscopic methods, which are higher than for SWL.

CHANGES IN INDICATIONS FOR SWL

After the first application of SWL to kidney stones, the indications were expanded rapidly to nearly all stone situations. After the development of lithotripters with the possibility of ventral coupling, stones in the mid ureter could also be treated. "Soft" struvite stones were disintegrated just as were hard cystine or brushite stones. Therefore SWL was the first-choice treatment for all these stones, except for complex staghorn stones, in the early 1990's. At that time some studies appeared which indicated limitations of SWL efficiency [11]. For stones larger than 2 cm and for staghorn calculi the re-treatment rate, auxiliary measures and complications are too frequent (http://www.auanet.org/guidelines/staghorncalculi05.cfm). For stones located in the lower pole the clearance of fragments can be reduced. Therefore for this stone position the indication for SWL is restricted to a stone size of less than 2 cm in case of a narrow, long and steep calyceal neck [12,13]. In the ureter, URS and SWL seem to be equally effective for stones up to 1 cm in size. For larger stones endoscopic procedures are preferred (http://www.auanet.org/guidelines/main_reports/UreStnMain8_16.pdf). For large ureteral or pelvic stones, laparoscopic procedures are increasingly used.

THE FUTURE ROLE OF SWL

Technical development of shock wave lithotripsy

The "mechanisms of shock wave action and strategies for improved SWL" have been presented excellently in this symposium (session 7). Meanwhile there are some important results for the clinical routine to be respected for an more effective and safer

SWL. With respect to this the frequency of shock wave application should be restricted to around 90 SW/min [14,15]. Furthermore, during the SWL session the shock wave energy should be increased progressively [16]. In this manner the initial atraumatic low energy induces vasoconstriction to protect the kidney when the energy is raised. Respecting this, the efficacy of the available lithotripters could be optimized. But the difficult challenge is to surpass that which was already achieved and is still the gold standard since more than 25 years ago.

Because the historical development of a smaller focal zone with high peak pressure was accompanied by loss of disintegrative capacity [17] the tendency is now toward a flexible shock wave generator providing different configurations of the focal zone.

The temporal and spatial pressure distribution of the shock wave determines its disintegrative efficacy on the stone and its traumatizing capacity in the tissue. The induction of cavitation plays a crucial role for both effects [18-21]. But, there may be a conformation of the shock wave that can allow both results; that is, it has been hypothesized that stone disintegration can be improved while tissue trauma is diminished by manipulating the dynamic of cavitation activity [22-24]. Since the possibilities are limited for changing the relevant parameters specifically using a single source, studies have also been performed by combining different generators. One of the first devices used clinically was a "Twin-Head" lithotripter. In this design two identical electrohydraulic sources are integrated to have the same focal point but the shockwave axes are perpendicular to each other [25]. Another option is the double-layer piezoelectric element in which two layers are activated with a short delay and with different energy parameter [26]. Both of these innovative lithotripters have not been shown to be superior to conventional machines with respect to disintegration and trauma. A very new and promising unit is the combination of an electrohydraulic with a piezoelectric generator. With this design a variety of parameters can be controlled specifically to evaluate the ideal pulse profile and shock wave sequence. For *in vitro* application the optimization was successful but this has to be confirmed *in vivo* and in the clinical setting [27].

As already mentioned, coupling and changes of the shock wave parameter during the intracorporeal path is a critical point in SWL [28,29]. These challenges may explain in part why it has been so difficult to improve SWL.

Adverse side effects of SWL

Just recently, reports about long-term side effects of SWL were published and were discussed intensively in this symposium [30] (session 7). Even though the author of this article speculates that the observation that SWL induces significant diabetes won't be confirmed by further studies, we still have to await the definite results. For the moment we draw the conclusion that the side effects of SWL may not be disregarded in the discussion on changing and improving shock wave generators. And we are encouraged to search after the factors and parameters to distinguish between disintegration and side effects [22,31,32].

Stone localization and positioning

Besides shock wave generation and coupling the precise localization of the stone and its positioning in the focal point is essential for SWL success [33]. There are efforts to enable automatic positioning and continuous observation of stone location. The complete protection of the patient from x-rays can only be realized by using ultrasound imaging, and the first study to attempt to use ultrasound to track and target stones is promising [34]. But, automatic adjustment of localization of therapeutic energy in an actual patient is likely to be more difficult than in experimental models.

DEVELOPMENT OF COMPETITIVE ENDOSCOPIC TECHNIQUES

The next stage of progress in endoscopy technology will happen in the field of video imaging. The diameter of the endoscope can be reduced when the light and video-transmission channel requires a smaller part of the instrument cross section. Additional space for improved irrigation flow to improve the view will be achieved by smaller tools (laser fiber, baskets, grasper). The working channel cannot be reduced even more, since otherwise removal of stones and therefore the advantage of the endoscopic technique would be reduced. The reduction of the diameter in ureteroscopy will enable the elimination of postoperative stenting and therefore significantly reduce morbidity and avoid re-intervention for stent removal. PCNL has the advantage that a 26F access can be used without significant trauma to the kidney, when inserted properly. Mini-PCNL will become the alternative for smaller kidney stones and will fill the gap between flexible URS up to 1 cm kidney stones and 2cm stones to be treated by conventional PCNL. Therefore there are reasonable endoscopic options for all urinary stones. If PCNL clears the stone definitively, a postoperative nephrostomy can be avoided in some cases to reduce morbidity even more.

PREDICTION OF SUCCESS

Different stone materials vary in their susceptibility to fragmentation by SWL. Therefore efforts are being made to predict the stone composition *in situ* especially using CT scans. Hounsfield units have been correlated with disintegration by SWL [35], but there are problems with this (see Williams *et al.* in this volume). Additionally, such measurements are not yet standardized and the correlations that have been reported are not specific enough to be used in clinical cases. One reason for this is that other parameters of the stone situation also affect the efficacy of SWL. This multifactorial situation may be able to be analyzed and predicted by "artificial neural networks" [36]. This approach can include not only stone composition but also size, location and other specifications of the stone. These computer programs can be trained and continue to learn with new data. The intention of this is to provide an electronic version of the physician's experience. But in medicine we are far from the situation that human expertise based on knowledge and experience can be exceeded by computers. One critical point is usually not considered: The personal preference of the surgeon founded in operating experience is an essential predictive factor for success. But according to "Evidence Based Medicine" this preference factor has to be discounted. Evidence-based medicine, what it is and what it isn't: It's about integrating individual clinical expertise and the best external evidence [37].

TREATMENT PHILOSOPHY: SWL VS. ENDOUROLOGY

For most of the calculi in the upper urinary tract different options are offered as reasonable and successful treatments. The physician's experience is the next essential factor. But the final decision is set by the patient's preference. In general, patients have to decide among three different strategies (Table 1).

Table 1. The three strategies for treating stones in the upper urinary tract.

Strategy	Advantage	Disadvantage
SWL without anesthesia	o No anesthesia o Low complication rate by procedure o Low treatment costs o No drainage (stent, PCNL)	o Lower stone clearance rate o Longer follow-up to stone clearance o Risk of complication during passage of residual fragments o Higher costs in follow-up
SWL under anesthesia	o Better disintegration rate o Low complication rate by procedure o Moderate treatment costs o No drainage (stent, PCNL)	o Moderate duration up to stone clearance o Risk of complication during passage of residual fragments o Moderate costs in follow-up
Endourology under anesthesia	o Highest immediate stone clearance rate o Shortest treatment time o Shortest and least expensive follow-up	o Risk for severe complications o Anesthesia o Drainage (stent, PCNL) re-intervention for removal of drainage

In Europe the advantage of SWL being able to be used without anesthesia is highly appreciated [38]. Therefore the second generation lithotripters were favored even if they had limited efficacy compared to the HM3 under analgesia. In contrast, in the USA the application of general or spinal anesthesia for a comfortable shock wave treatment is not assessed as an disadvantage. Under anesthesia maximal energy can be applied with the intention to reach the highest rate of stone disintegration independently of the induced pain. The solitary limit is the tissue trauma.

The difference in using anesthesia has resulted in a bias in the competition for the nomination of the "gold standard" lithotripter. Until now the unmodified Dornier HM3 is seen to provide the highest disintegrative efficacy and is usually run under anesthesia. The high-end second or third generation lithotripters (Storz Modulith, Siemens Lithostar, Wolf Piezolith etc.) did not exceed this, but treatment was usually applied usually under analgesia-sedation. Studies should be conducted to compare all these machines (including the flexible focal zones of the latest machines) under the same conditions (general anesthesia) with respect to disintegration and trauma. The results would then provide a basis for the next comparison against the endoscopic procedures.

ADDITIONAL PARAMETERS INFLUENCING THE FUTURE OF SWL

Epidemiology

Urologists should not fear that the occurrence of urinary stones will decline. In fact, the worldwide prevalence, incidence and number of treatments for urinary stones is growing continuously in industrialized nations. For example the prevalence and incidence rose from 4 to 7% and from 0.54 to 1.47 in Germany between 1979 and 2001 [39-44]. A primary reason for this could well be prosperity, which is also evidenced by the spread of the "metabolic syndrome" correlated with body mass index [45,46], diabetes mellitus [47,48] and gout [49-51] as independent risk factors (see also Session 1 from this Symposium).

Metabolic evaluation and metaphylaxis

The highest risk for the future of SWL would be the successful medical treatment of calcium oxalate stones. There are many new insights into the pathogenesis of urinary stones (sessions 1, 3, 5, 6 of this Symposium). We are waiting for a "Viagra-solution" for urinary stones. But the stone surgeons can be confident of keeping their employment, since only a few patients will pay so much money and side effects to avoid the occasional case of renal colic. Because of that, the pharmaceutical industry has limited interest in this field.

Economic factors

There is no doubt that economic factors play a distinct role in deciding between different treatment options [52]. Multiple trials have tried to calculate costs and remuneration for SWL and endourologic procedures, but have not been able to present consistent results. In some studies SWL was more cost effective [53] and in others URS [54-56]. Remuneration is determined by the health system and therefore differs significantly with the country [57]. The consequence is that cost-effectiveness cannot be calculated generally. Therefore a major factor in decision making is locally specific, but there is a general tendency toward endoscopy.

SUMMARY OF THE GLOBAL PERSPECTIVE

- The incidence of urolithiasis is continuously increasing along with the metabolic syndrome, which is correlated with prosperity.

- Efficient metaphylaxis is missing due to low effectiveness, low acceptance and compliance by the patient or due to costs.
- Knowledge about pathogenesis of urolithiasis is growing dramatically. Therefore the possibility to develop a sufficient medical treatment is imminent. But that would primarily reduce the prevalence, since treatment is not likely to be started until the first stone episode happens.
- All this results in a increasing need for active stone removal.
- SWL was and already is a well-established treatment modality for urolithiasis in the upper urinary tract.
- For most stone situations there will remain a reasonable choice between SWL versus endoscopic procedures.
- Concerning their efficiency, lithotripter development seems to have reached a peak level in recent years. A further increase is not to be expected. But attention should be paid to the clinical results of the "tailored shock wave configuration" using new generator concepts.
- The evolution of tools for endoscopic stone removal is proceeding. The major point is to keep the advantage of immediate clearance of all concretions by maximal disintegration and removal via a sufficient working channel in the endoscope
- Adverse side effects of both treatment concepts are minimized. Reactivated discussions will show the harmlessness even in long term follow up.
- Patients can expect a nearly 100% success rate. But additionally they expect more and more a very comfortable treatment. Therefore the tendency is to be treated under general anesthesia even for SWL to ensure pain-free and rapid (by using highly effective shock waves) therapy. Also for general anesthesia the morbidity could be reduced significantly as compared to the past
- Facing the choice between medically reasonable options, two other points will crucially influence the decision: expertise of the surgeon and costs. Parameters with respect to this in the calculation of efficiency have to be established.
- In conclusion SWL will continue to play an established, if slightly reduced, role in stone treatment in the future.

REFERENCES

1. Chaussy C. & Schmiedt E. (1984) *Urol.Radiol.* 6, 80-87
2. Chaussy C.G. & Fuchs G.J. (1989) *J.Urol.* 141, 782-789
3. Rubin J.I., Arger P.H., Pollack H.M., Banner M.P., Coleman B.G., Mintz M.C. & VanArsdalen K.N. (1987) *Radiology* 162, 21-24
4. Kaude J.V., Williams C.M., Millner M.R., Scott K.N. & Finlayson B. (1985) *AJR Am.J.Roentgenol.* 145, 305-313
5. Chow G.K. & Streem S.B. (2000) *Urol.Clin.North Am.* 27, 315-322
6. Rassweiler J., Schmidt A., Gumpinger R., Mayer R. & Eisenberger F. (1990) *J.Urol.(Paris)* 96, 149-153
7. Basillote J.B., Lee D.I., Eichel L. & Clayman R.V. (2004) *Urol.Clin.North Am.* 31, 21-32
8. Auge B.K. & Preminger G.M. (2002) *Endocrinol.Metab Clin.North Am.* 31, 1065-1082

9. Krambeck A.E., Murat F.J., Gettman M.T., Chow G.K., Patterson D.E. & Segura J.W. (2006) *Mayo Clin.Proc.* 81, 468-473
10. Kim S.C., Kuo R.L. & Lingeman J.E. (2003) *Curr.Opin.Urol.* 13, 235-241
11. Rassweiler J. & Alken P. (1990) *Urol.Res.* 18 Suppl 1, S13-S23
12. Clayman R.V. (1998) *J.Urol.* 160, 629
13. Preminger G.M. (2006) *Urol.Res.* 34, 108-111
14. Pace K.T., Ghiculete D., Harju M. & Honey R.J. (2005) *J.Urol.* 174, 595-599
15. McAteer J.A., Williams J.C., Jr., Cleveland R.O., van Cauwelaert J., Bailey M.R., Lifshitz D.A. & Evan A.P. (2005) *Urol.Res.* 33, 429-434
16. Zhou Y., Cocks F.H., Preminger G.M. & Zhong P. (2004) *J.Urol.* 172, 349-354
17. Graber S.F., Danuser H., Hochreiter W.W. & Studer U.E. (2003) *J.Urol.* 169, 54-57
18. Bailey M.R., Pishchalnikov Y.A., Sapozhnikov O.A., Cleveland R.O., McAteer J.A., Miller N.A., Pishchalnikova I.V., Connors B.A., Crum L.A. & Evan A.P. (2005) *UltrasoundMedBiol.* 31, 1245-1256
19. McAteer J.A., Bailey M.R., Williams Jr J.C., Cleveland R.O. & Evan A.P. (2005) *Minerva Urol.Nefrol.* 57, 271-287
20. Chitnis P.V. & Cleveland R.O. (2006) *J.Acoust.Soc.Am.* 119, 1929-1932
21. Lokhandwalla M. & Sturtevant B. (2000) *Phys.Med.Biol.* 45, 1923-1940
22. Zhou Y., Cocks F.H., Preminger G.M. & Zhong P. (2004) *J.Urol.* 172, 1892-1898
23. Eisenmenger W. (2001) *UltrasoundMed.Biol.* 27, 683-693
24. Evan A.P., Willis L.R., McAteer J.A., Bailey M.R., Connors B.A., Shao Y., Lingeman J.E., Williams J.C., Jr., Fineberg N.S. & Crum L.A. (2002) *J.Urol.* 168, 1556-1562
25. Sheir K.Z., El Diasty T.A. & Ismail A.M. (2005) *BJU.Int.* 95, 389-393
26. Loske A.M., Fernandez F., Zendejas H., Paredes M. & Castano-Tostado E. (2005) *J.Urol.* 174, 2388-2392
27. Talic R.F. & Rabah D.M. (2006) *Curr.Opin.Urol.* 16, 83-87
28. Cleveland R.O., Lifshitz D.A., Connors B.A., Evan A.P., Willis L.R. & Crum L.A. (1998) *UltrasoundMed.Biol.* 24, 293-306
29. Averkiou M.A. & Cleveland R.O. (1999) *J.Acoust.Soc.Am.* 106, 102-112
30. Krambeck A.E., Gettman M.T., Rohlinger A.L., Lohse C.M., Patterson D.E. & Segura J.W. (2006) *J.Urol.* 175, 1742-1747
31. Zhu S., Dreyer T., Liebler M., Riedlinger R., Preminger G.M. & Zhong P. (2004) *Ultrasound Med.Biol.* 30, 675-682
32. Heimbach D., Munver R., Zhong P., Jacobs J., Hesse A., Muller S.C. & Preminger G.M. (2000) *J.Urol.* 164, 537-544
33. Cartledge J.J., Cross W.R., Lloyd S.N. & Joyce A.D. (2001) *BJU.Int.* 88, 321-324
34. Chang C.C., Manousakas I., Pu Y.R., Liang S.M., Chen C.H., Chen T.S., Yu F.M., Yang W.H., Tong Y.C. & Kuo C.L. (2002) *J.Urol.* 167, 2594-2597
35. Joseph P., Mandal A.K., Singh S.K., Mandal P., Sankhwar S.N. & Sharma S.K. (2002) *J.Urol.* 167, 1968-1971
36. Hamid A., Dwivedi U.S., Singh T.N., Gopi K.M., Mahmood M., Singh H., Tandon V. & Singh P.B. (2003) *BJU.Int.* 91, 821-824
37. Sackett D.L., Rosenberg W.M., Gray J.A., Haynes R.B. & Richardson W.S. (1996) *BMJ* 312, 71-72
38. Tiselius H.G. (2005) *Urol.Res.* 33, 185-190
39. Pearle M.S., Calhoun E.A. & Curhan G.C. (2005) *J.Urol.* 173, 848-857
40. Sheir K.Z., Zabihi N., Lee D., Teichman J.M., Rehman J., Sundaram C.P., Heimbach D., Hesse A., Delvecchio F., Zhong P., Preminger G.M. & Clayman R.V. (2003) *J.Urol.* 170, 2190-2194
41. Stamatelou K.K., Francis M.E., Jones C.A., Nyberg L.M. & Curhan G.C. (2003) *Kidney Int.* 63, 1817-1823
42. Yoshimura K. & Okuyama A. (2004) *Hinyokika Kiyo* 50, 583-586
43. Hesse A. (2005) *World J.Urol.* 23, 302-303
44. Hesse A., Brandle E., Wilbert D., Kohrmann K.U. & Alken P. (2003) *Eur.Urol.* 44, 709-713
45. Gillen D.L., Coe F.L. & Worcester E.M. (2005) *Am.J.Kidney Dis.* 46, 263-269

46. Taylor E.N., Stampfer M.J. & Curhan G.C. (2005) *JAMA* 293, 455-462
47. Sakhaee K., Adams-Huet B., Moe O.W. & Pak C.Y. (2002) *Kidney Int.* 62, 971-979
48. Taylor E.N., Stampfer M.J. & Curhan G.C. (2005) *Kidney Int.* 68, 1230-1235
49. Abate N., Chandalia M., Cabo-Chan A.V., Jr., Moe O.W. & Sakhaee K. (2004) *Kidney Int.* 65, 386-392
50. Kramer H.M. & Curhan G. (2002) *Am.J.Kidney Dis.* 40, 37-42
51. Pak C.Y., Moe O.W., Sakhaee K., Peterson R.D. & Poindexter J.R. (2005) *J.Urol.* 173, 1606-1609
52. Chandhoke P.S. (2002) *J.Urol.* 168, 937-940
53. Carlsson P. & Tiselius H.G. (1989) *Scand.J.Urol.Nephrol.Suppl* 122, 34-43
54. Lee Y.H., Tsai J.Y., Jiaan B.P., Wu T. & Yu C.C. (2006) *Urology* 67, 480-484
55. Lotan Y., Cadeddu J.A., Roehrborn C.G. & Stage K.H. (2004) *J.Urol.* 172, 1958-1962
56. Lotan Y., Gettman M.T., Roehrborn C.G., Cadeddu J.A. & Pearle M.S. (2002) *J.Urol.* 167, 1621-1629
57. Lotan Y., Cadeddu J.A. & Pearle M.S. (2005) *Urol.Res.* 33, 223-230

Advantage of a Broad Focal Zone in SWL: Synergism Between Squeezing and Shear

Oleg A. Sapozhnikov[*†], Michael R. Bailey[*], Adam D. Maxwell[*], Brian MacConaghy[*], Robin O. Cleveland[‡], James A. McAteer[¶], and Lawrence A. Crum[*]

[*]*Center for Industrial and Medical Ultrasound, Applied Physics Laboratory, University of Washington, Seattle, WA, USA*
[†]*Dept. of Acoustics, Faculty of Physics, Moscow State University, Moscow, Russia*
[‡]*Dept. of Aerospace and Mechanical Engineering, Boston University, Boston, USA*
[¶]*Dept. of Anatomy and Cell Biology, Indiana University School of Medicine, Indianapolis, IN, USA*

Abstract. Objective: The focal zone width appears to be a critical factor in lithotripsy. Narrow focus machines have a higher occurrence of adverse effects, and arguably no greater comminution efficiency. Manufacturers have introduced new machines and upgrades to broaden the focus. Still, little data exists on how focal width plays a role in stone fracture. Thus, our aim was to determine if focal width interacts with established mechanisms known to contribute to stone fracture. Method: A series of experiments were undertaken with changes made to the stone in an effort to determine which is most important, the shock wave (SW) reflected from the back end of the stone (spallation), the SW ringing the stone (squeezing), the shear wave generated at surface of the stone and concentrated in the bulk of it (shear), or SWs generated from bubble collapse (cavitation). Shock waves were generated by a Dornier HM3-style lithotripter, and stones were made from U30 cement. Baffles were used to block specific waves that contribute to spallation, shear, or squeezing, and glycerol was used to suppress cavitation. Numerical simulation and high-speed imaging allowed for visualization of specific waves as they traveled within the stone. Results: For brevity, one result is explained. A reflective baffle was placed around the front edge of a cylindrical stone. The proximal baffle prevented squeezing by preventing the SW from traveling over the stone, but permitted the SW entering the stone through the proximal face and did not affect the other mechanisms. The distal baffle behaved the same as no baffle. The proximal baffle dramatically reduced the stress, and the stone did not break (stone broke after 45±10 SWs without the baffle and did not break after 400 SWs when the experiment stopped). The result implies that since removing squeezing halted comminution, squeezing is dominant. However, there is much more to the story. For example, if the cylindrical stone was pointed, it broke with the point on the distal end but not with the point on the proximal end. In both cases, squeezing was the same, so if squeezing were dominant, both stones should have broken. But the pointed front edge prevents the shear wave. The squeezing wave and its product – the shear wave - are both needed and work synergistically in a way explained by the model. Conclusions: A broad focus enhances the synergism of squeezing and shear waves without altering cavitation's effects, and thus accelerates stone fracture in SWL.

Keywords: lithotripsy, comminution, fracture, stress
PACS: 43.80.Gx, 43.25.Yw, 43.25.Cb

CP900, *Renal Stone Disease, 1st Annual International Urolithiasis Research Symposium,* edited by A. P. Evan, J. E. Lingeman, and J. C. Williams, Jr.

INTRODUCTION

Despite over 20 years of clinical practice and fundamental research, a complete physical explanation of stone comminution by lithotripsy is lacking. Incomplete understanding is evidenced by rising re-treatment rates despite the release of over 40 lithotripter designs over the history of shock wave lithotripsy (SWL) [1-3]. The goal of this paper is to explain how a specific stone fractures by using a theoretical model to simulate the combined effect of many mechanisms and by using the model and experiment to test the role of individual already-described mechanisms of inducing the stress that leads to stone fracture.

Stone fracture is similar to fracture of any brittle object and can be considered as a process whereby cracks form, grow, and coalesce as a result of internal stresses, in this case, generated by the externally applied lithotripter shock wave. Cracks are presumed to initiate at locations where the stress exceeds a critical value. Cracks grow and coalesce under the repetitive loading and unloading in a process called dynamic fatigue, and common practice indicates several lithotripter shock waves are required to fracture stones [4]. Although the described scenario of fracture is agreed upon, this knowledge in itself does not help in predicting stone fragmentation without knowing the mechanisms of how appropriate stresses are generated inside the stone.

Spallation, squeezing, and cavitation are mechanisms by which the lithotripter SW induces stress in the stone. In spallation, the lithotripter SW (a positive pressure spike followed by a negative pressure trough) travels through the stone, reflects at the distal surface, and inverts. On a planar surface, a maximum tension appears where the inverted spike adds to the incident negative tail. In squeezing, the SW enters the stone and moves faster than in water, which leaves the SW in water encircling the stone and creating a hoop stress on the stone. In cavitation, tiny bubbles create points of stress on the stone surface leading to surface cracks and diverging internal stresses. Cavitation is not addressed in this paper but is included in a more complete report [5].

Visualization of the internal stresses in a stone calculated with a numerical model reveals a fracture mechanism called dynamic squeezing [6]. We propose that the visualization is more useful than either of the simple terms “spallation” or “squeezing” and better explains how the stresses are produced that lead to the first fracture of a cylindrical U30 model stone.

THEORY AND METHODS

The numerical images of the stresses were calculated using the linear elastic equations [5]. A planar lithotripter SW enters a cylindrical U30 model stone from the left (see Fig. 1). The stress seen in a central slice through the stone at various time points is shown. Red is high tension (70 MPa) and blue is high compression (-70 MPa). Fracture is most likely to extend from the maximum tensile stress radially along the shortest path to the stress release of the surface.

A minimally obtrusive fixture held a cylindrical U30 model stone [7] fixed axially at the focus of a research lithotripter modeled after the Dornier HM3. The number of

SWs necessary to cause the distal end to separate was recorded and compared to the maximum stress calculated in the stone. The location of fracture was compared to the location of calculated maximum tension. Baffles were placed on the stones to remove the waves responsible for either spallation or squeezing to test the role of each mechanism.

RESULTS

Figure 1 shows a summary of dynamic squeezing. The spallation wave creates little stress. Squeezing statically has little contribution. But the shear wave initiated at the proximal corner focuses because of the squeezing wave traveling along the stone surface and creates the maximum stress at the location where the U30 stones fracture. Calculated maximum stress was 100 MPa, 3.5 mm from the distal end. Measured fracture occurred at 3.6±0.2 mm after 45±10 SWs (N=10).

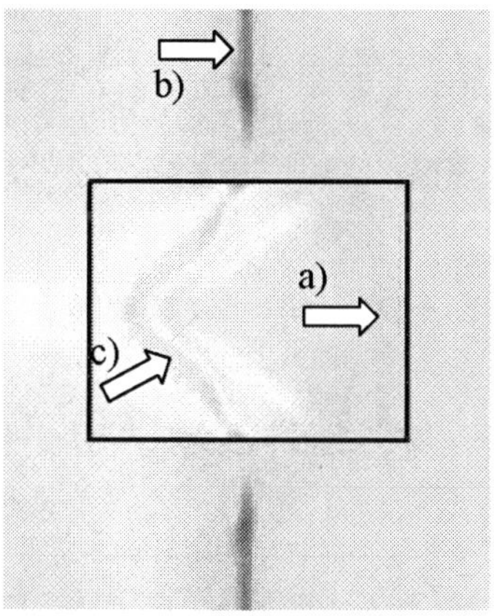

FIGURE 1. Arrow a) indicates the longitudinal wave responsible for spallation. Even when it reflects the tension is low (light yellow). Arrow b) indicates the squeezing wave (the SW outside the stone encircling the stone. Arrow c) indicates the shear wave responsible for "dynamic squeezing" generated at the proximal corner and reinforced as the squeezing wave travels along the stone surface. It focuses in the distal end along the path of the arrow and creates the highest tension (red). Other waves are waves from the longitudinal wave which is supersonic compared to the water sound speed.

Stones were modified as in Fig. 2. The proximal baffle prevented the longitudinal wave, responsible for spallation, from entering the stone, yet calculated pressures (100 MPa) and number of SWs to fracture (50 ± 20) were unchanged. Hence we conclude spallation was not a major contributor to this fracture. Stones did not break with the squeezing wave blocked by baffle (c). The squeezing wave due to the SW beam being broader than the stone is necessary for fracture. Thus, the maximum stress calculated within the stone decreases when the beam width decreases (Fig. 3). However, the quasi-static squeezing stress is present in the pointed stone (d); although these stones did not break. The reason is the squeezing wave must travel some distance from the proximal corner along the stone surface to strengthen the focusing shear wave responsible for dynamic squeezing.

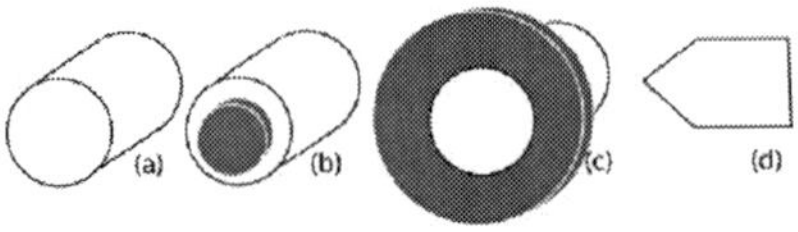

FIGURE 2. U30 stone (a), baffled to prevent spallation (b), baffled to prevent squeezing (c) and front end pointed to prevent dynamic squeezing (d).

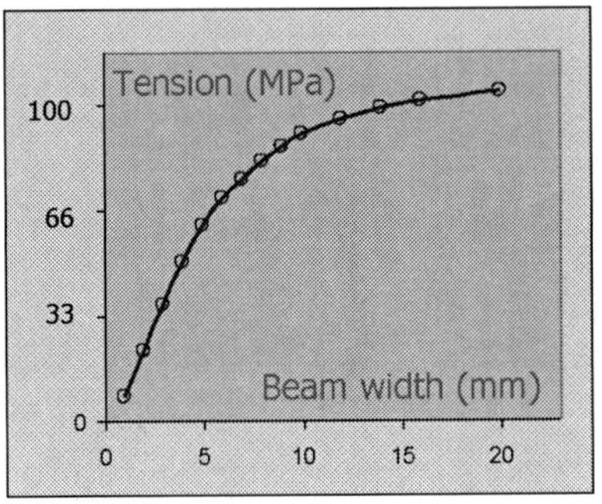

FIGURE 3. The maximum calculated stress in the U30 stone decreases with beam width of the lithotripter (the SW peak pressure, 50 MPa, is fixed).

CONCLUSIONS

A new mechanistic description of stress and fracture in cylindrical U30 stones in lithotripsy was reported. The description is that shear waves generated at corners in the boundary of the stone are reinforced by the SW in water traveling along the surface of the stone and focus to generate the highest stress in the distal end of the stone. It was argued that a fracture plane results between the maximum stress and the stone surface. The description is the result of calculations based on linear elasticity theory. Although some in the lithotripsy community have been content that Energy Density (temporal and spatial integral of the pressure squared divided by the focal beam width [8]) of the conventional lithotripsy shock wave correlates with stone comminution, [9] this model shows that it is not the energy itself but how the energy is applied that is important and that leads to different mechanisms of action. The important energy is that associated with the tension in the stone and not the initial energy in the shock wave applied to the stone. The tension in the stone was adequately described by the model but is not simply related to the SW energy or energy density: it depends on the shock waveform as shown by Cleveland and Sapozhnikov [6] and on beam width as shown here as well. If the beam width of the lithotripter is narrower than the stone then dynamic squeezing—the dominant mechanism in this study—cannot contribute.

ACKNOWLEDGMENTS

The authors thank our fellow members of the Consortium for Shock Waves in Medicine and the Center for Industrial and Medical Ultrasound for discussions, research help, and guidance on this paper. In particular, we would like to thank Dr. Yuriy A. Pishchalnikov and Prof. James C. Williams, Jr. (Indiana University School of Medicine) for guidance in preparing U30 stones, and Mr. Fran Olson (Applied Physics Laboratory) for design and fabrication of much of the experimental apparatus. The work was supported by NIH grants DK43881 and DK55674, NSBRI grant SMS00402, an NIH Fogarty International Research Collaboration Award, an ONR International Field Office Visiting Scientist grant, a CRDF grant, and RFBR grants.

REFERENCES

1. K. Kerbl, J. Rehman, J. Landman, D. Lee, C. Sundaram, and R.V. Clayman, Journal of Endourology 16(5), 281-288 (2002.).
2. A.P. Evan, J.A. McAteer, J.C. Williams, L.R. Willis, M.R. Bailey, L.A. Crum, J.E. Lingeman, and R.O Cleveland, "Shock wave physics of lithotripsy: Mechanisms of shock wave action and progress toward improved SWL," In: Textbook of Minimally Invasive Urology, R. Moore, J.T. Bishoff, S. Loening and S.G. Docimo Eds, Martin Dunitz Limited, London, chapter 28, 425-438 (2004).
3. J.A. McAteer, J.C. Williams, Jr., M.R. Bailey, R.O. Cleveland, and A.P. Evan, Minerva Urologica E Neffrologica 57, 271-279 (2005).
4. B. Sturtevant, "Shock wave physics of lithotripters." In Smith's Textbook of Endourology. Edit. A.D. Smith (Quality Medical Publishing, Inc. St. Louis 1996) 529-52.
5. O.A. Sapozhnikov, A.D. Maxwell, B. MacConaghy, M.R. Bailey, J. Acoust. Soc. Am.112(2) (2007 in press).
7. J.A. McAteer, J.C. Williams, Jr., R.O. Cleveland, J. Van Cauwelaert, M.R. Bailey, D.A. Lifshitz, A.P. Evan, Urol Res 33, 429–434 (2005).
8. International Electrotechnical Committee, IEC Standard 61846 1998 .
9. J.J. Rassweiler, G.G. Tailly, and C. Chaussy, EAU Update Series 3, 17-36 (2005).
6. R.O. Cleveland, O.A. Sapozhnikov, J Acoust Soc Am 118(4), 2667-76 (2005).

A Possible Cumulative Shear Mechanism For Tissue Damage Initiation In SWL

Jonathan B. Freund

University of Illinois at Urbana-Champaign, Urbana, IL 61801

Abstract. In shock-wave lithotripsy, inertial cavitation is observed in kidney tissue after hundreds of shocks are delivered, which seems to correspond with the onset of wide-spread injury. However, it is unclear what initiates the process. It is possible, and has been suggested before, that hemorrhage is a prelude to cavitation damage. We investigate the possibility that the net shear of multiple shocks can accumulate to cause this initial hemorrhage. A mathematical model is used to show that the larger interstitial volume fraction in the medulla toward the papilla tip would make it particularly sensitive there to this mechanism. This is consistent with observations.

Keywords: Shock-wave lithotripsy, tissue damage
PACS: 43.80.Sh, 87.19.Tt

BACKGROUND

There is evidence [1] that inertial cavitation is responsible for the greatest part of the observed damage in SWL [2, 3]. Inverted shock waves generated via a pressure release reflector significantly reduce injury [4], presumably because the trailing part of the wave is compressive and therefore suppresses cavitation. The acoustic signature of inertial cavitation has been observed in pig kidney tissue after about 1000 shocks [5], which is comparable to the number necessary for significant tissue injury [3], though specific thresholds have not yet been determined, nor have detector sensitivities been studied for tissue cavitation.

It remains unclear, however, why so many shock waves are necessary before cavitation signatures are observed in tissue [5]. It has been suggested that bleeding is a necessary prelude to extensive cavitation [6]. In this view, the pooled blood in the lesion would provide favorable conditions for extensive and spreading cavitation damage. It has been proposed that the initial rupture might be caused by expanding cavitation bubbles [7], though this has not been observed *in vivo* and inverted waves still caused small hemorrhages near the papilla tip [4]. Shock-wave induced shearing is another proposed mechanism [8], but the shear of a single shock in that study is anticipated to be insufficient to tear basement membranes.

In this paper we propose a cumulative-shear mechanism, whereby the accumulated shear of hundreds of shocks would produce damaging strains. The key to this mechanism is how much the elasticity of the tissue can return it toward its relaxed, un-sheared state before the next shock. If this relaxation is insufficient, then shear can accumulate with each shock delivered. An assessment of this is made with a simple mathematical model of the tissue of the inner medulla.

CP900, *Renal Stone Disease, 1st Annual International Urolithiasis Research Symposium,* edited by A. P. Evan, J. E. Lingeman, and J. C. Williams, Jr.

TISSUE MODEL

From a mechanical perspective, the most important part of the inner medulla appears to be the basement membranes of the ducts, limbs, and vessels, which we refer to collectively simply as tubes. The pressure-diameter relation of rabbit renal tubule basement membranes has been measured by Welling et al. [9]. These membranes are relatively stiff, with elasticity comparable to that of tendons. Their data allow us to estimate the tension ($T = 0.16$N/m) and bending ($M = 5.2 \times 10^{-16}$Nm) moduli that parametrize the dynamics response of the material to deformation for our model.

The cells and extracellular matrix in the interstitial region between the tubes will also play a structural role. However, it is well known that cells and extracellular matrix material have slow relaxation properties. That is, if deformed, they return slowly to their undeformed state. Extensive measurements on a variety of cells all show about 1 second or larger relaxation times [10, 11]. Cyclically applied forces at 1 Hz, which is close to typical treatment rates, have been observed to cause a significant shear accumulation in fibroblasts [11]. The measured viscoelastic properties of extracellular interstitial gels also indicate a greater than 1 second relaxation time [12]. In this study, we neglect the elastic character of the interstitial material and model it simply as a viscous fluid, assuming that any elastic recovery would be incomplete before the next shock is delivered. For simplicity, the same viscosity (that of blood) was assumed inside and out. These estimates are all sufficient for qualitative assessment of mechanisms; more shock-specific experiments would be needed to quantify the precise tissue response. The governing equations for this membrane-fluid model system are solved numerically with a boundary integral algorithm similar to that used in a previous study of microcirculatory mechanics [13].

We model the structure of the medulla tissue as parallel tubular membranes. As shown in figure 1 (a), we focus on a small periodic sub-region of the medulla. This sub-region is significantly smaller than the region over which the shear would occur in a kidney, but it satisfies the two conditions needed for the results to be applicable: its tube diameters are significantly smaller than the shear's length scale and its shear recovery rate can be related to the shear relaxation of larger regions. It was confirmed with tests of the model that relaxation is independent of transverse length scale, as expected for a linear material.

It is observed in rabbit kidneys [14] that the interstitial volume fraction Γ_i changes from about 0.4 toward the papilla tip to 0.2 midway up the medulla. These changes are also clear in images of the inner medulla, such as shown by Jamison and Kriz [15]. These extrema set the three cases we consider: $\Gamma_i = 0.2$, 0.3 and 0.4. The model's average tube diameters were about 14μm with uniform distribution of $\pm 20\%$.

NET SHEAR DUE TO A FOCUSED SHOCK

In the past, shock induced shear has been estimated for the compressive portion of the wave [8], but it is unlikely that a single shock will produce the high strains needed to rupture basement membranes [9]. This compressive-wave shear is mostly, but not entirely, canceled by the trailing expansive portion of the wave. The residual net shear is

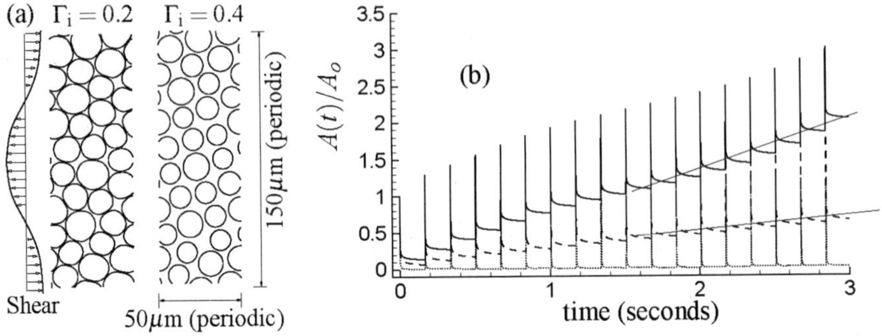

FIGURE 1. (a) Schematic of simulation model configuration. (b) Displacement shear amplitude versus time for shocks applied at 6 Hz: ——— $\Gamma_i = 0.4$; - - - - $\Gamma_i = 0.3$; and ········ $\Gamma_i = 0.2$.

what can accumulate with subsequent shocks if it is not removed by the tissue's elasticity. We estimate the net displacements of the entire focused shock by time integrating the velocity fields computed by Tanguay and Colonius [16] with their virtual lithotriptor. These predict that about a 0.1 percent strain remains after the wave has completely passed, which therefore has the potential to accumulate over the hundreds of shocks of a typical treatment. We apply such a strain to our model as an instantaneous deformation and study the subsequent evolution of the material.

RESULTS AND CONCLUSIONS

The effect of repeated shocks is shown in figure 1 (b). Since nearly all the observed relaxation is in the first 0.15s after the deformation, the delivery rate was set to be 6 Hz in order to reduce the computation time. It is clear that the $\Gamma_i = 0.4$ case shows significantly more accumulated deformation than the $\Gamma_i = 0.3$ case, and that the $\Gamma_i = 0.2$ case shows none.

These results suggest that the approximately 0.1 percent net shear deformation per shock would be completely relaxed when the basement membranes of the renal structures are nearly in contact, as when $\Gamma_i = 0.2$. However, for larger interstitial volume the relaxation is both slower and, in absence of interstitial elasticity, incomplete. For zero interstitial elasticity, 1000 shocks would yield a strain of approximately 15 percent, assuming a homogeneous material. Such strains could cause damage even in absence of cavitation.

We can anticipate that the actual viscoelasticity of the interstitial material, with a relaxation time $\sim$ 1s, would introduce a sensitivity to the shock delivery rate: the greater the time between shocks, the more the deformation could slowly recover via the interstitial material's small elasticity. The cumulative shear mechanism clearly predicts that hemorrhage should first appear in the inner medulla where Γ_i is larger, and sectioning does indeed suggest that this might be the case [17]. Another prediction of the model is that broader focal zones, even at the same peak pressure, should be less damaging. Preliminary results with broader focal zones at lower peak shock pressures and slower rate (27/min) show a marked decreased in injury [18] but focal zone width, shock strength and delivery rate have not been studied independently in animal models. Reducing shock strength of a standard narrower focus lithotriptor also reduces injury [19] and would also reduce shear accumulation. More tests are needed to clarify the mechanisms, but all current results appear consistent with a cumulative shear hypothesis. If this mechanism is confirmed in animal models, slower rates and wave tailoring to reduce net shear might offer means of mitigating injury.

ACKNOWLEDGMENTS

The author is grateful for fruitful discussions about kidneys and shock waves with A. Evan, T. Colonius and J. McAteer.

REFERENCES

1. M. R. Bailey, L. A. Crum, A. P. Evan, J. A. McAteer, J. C. Williams Jr., O. A. Sapozhnikov, R. O. Cleveland, and T. Colonius, "Cavitation in shock wave lithotripsy," in *The Fifth International Symposium on Cavitation,* Cav03-OS-2-1-006, Osaka, Japan, 2003.
2. A. P. Evan, and J. A. McAteer, "Q-effects of shock-wave lithotripsy," in *Kidney stones: medical and surgical management,* edited by F. L. Coe, M. J. Favus, C. Y. C. Pak, J. H. Parks, and G. M. Preminger, Lippincott-Raven, Philadelphia, 1996, pp. 549–570.
3. A. P. Evan, L. R. Willis, J. E. Lingeman, and J. A. McAteer, *Nephron* **78**, 1–8 (1998).
4. A. P. Evan, L. R. Willis, J. A. McAteer, M. R. Bailey, B. A. Connors, Y. Shao, J. E. Lingeman, J. C. Williams, Jr., N. S. Fineberg, and L. A. Crum, *The Journal of Urology* **168**, 1556–1562 (2002).
5. M. R. Bailey, Y. A. Pishchalnikov, O. A. Sapozhnikov, R. O. Cleveland, J. A. McAteer, N. A. Miller, I. V. Pishchalnikova, B. A. Connors, L. A. Crum, and A. P. Evan, *Ultrasound in Med. & Biol.* **31**, 1245–1256 (2005).
6. Y. Shao, B. A. Connors, A. P. Evan, L. R. Willis, D. A. Lifshitz, and J. E. Lingeman, *The Anatomical Record Part A* **275A**, 979–989 (2003).
7. P. Zhong, Y. Zhou, and S. Zhu, *Ultrasound in Med. & Biol.* **27**, 119–134 (2001).
8. M. Lokhandwalla, and B. Sturtevant, *Physics in Med. and Bio.* **46**, 413–437 (2001).
9. L. W. Welling, M. T. Zupka, and D. J. Welling, *News In Physiological Sciences* **10**, 30–35 (1995).
10. T. D. Brown, *J. Biomech.* **33**, 3–14 (2000).
11. H. Karcher, J. Lammerding, H. Huang, R. T. Lee, R. D. Kamm, and M. Kaazempur-Mofrad, *Biophysical J.* **85**, 3336–3349 (2003).
12. D. Zeng, A. Ferrari, J. Ulmer, A. Veligodskiy, P. Fischer, J. Spatz, Y. Ventikos, D. Poulikakos, and R. Kroschewski, *Biophysical J.* **90**, 4380–4391 (2006).
13. J. B. Freund, Leukocyte margination in a model microvessel, in press Physics of Fluids (2007).
14. M. A. Knepper, R. A. Danielson, G. M. Saidel, and R. S. Post, *Kidney International* **12**, 313–323 (1977).
15. R. L. Jamison, and W. Kriz, *Urinary concentrating mechanism: structure and function,* Oxford University Press, New York, 1982.
16. M. Tanguay, and T. Colonius, "Progress in modeling and simulation of shock wave lithotripsy (SWL)," in *Fifth International Symposium on Cavitation (CAV2003),* Osaka, Japan, 2003, pp. 1–11.
17. P. M. Blomgren, B. A. Connors, J. E. Lingeman, L. R. Willis, and A. P. Evan, *Anatomical Record* **249**, 341–348 (1997).
18. A. P. Evan, Y. A. Pishchalnikov, J. C. Williams Jr., J. A. McAteer, B. A. Connors, R. Handa, L. R. Willis, S. Kim, and J. E. Lingeman, *Journal of Urology* **175**, 1668 Suppl. 538–538 (2006).
19. B. A. Connors, A. P. Evan, L. R. Willis, P. M. Blomgren, J. E. Lingeman, and N. S. Fineberg, *J. Am. Soc. Nephrol* **11**, 310–318 (2000).

Numerical study of the collapse of a bubble subjected to a lithotripter pulse

Eric Johnsen and Tim Colonius

Division of Engineering and Applied Science, California Institute of Technology, Pasadena, CA 91125

Abstract.
The collapse of a bubble subjected to a lithotripter pulse is studied numerically. The goal is to record the pressure exerted along the stone, as a measure of potential stone damage. It is found that the pressure due to buble collapse is much larger than that of the lithotripter pulse. Furthermore, the pressure greatly depends on the geometry of the problem (initial stand-off distance and bubble size) and on the properties of the pulse (amplitude and width).

Keywords: Bubble collapse, shockwave lithotripsy
PACS: 47.55.dd, 87.54.Hk

INTRODUCTION

In shockwave lithotripsy (SWL), shockwaves followed by a long expansion tail are focused near kidney stones in order to break them. The tensile part of the pulse causes pre-existing bubble nuclei to grow and subsequently collapse near a stone [1]. When a bubble collapses near a solid surface, a high-speed re-entrant jet directed towards the surface forms and penetrates the bubble. The jet eventually hits the distal side, thereby generating a large water-hammer pressure; for bubbles close enough to the stone, the direct impact of the jet onto the stone can cause significant damage [2]. The goal of the present study is to provide a quantitative understanding of the effect of bubble collapse in the stone comminution mechanism. To do so, the collapse of an air bubble subjected to a lithotripter pulse near a wall was studied numerically in [3].

NUMERICAL MODEL

Numerical simulations of compressible multiphase flows are particularly challenging. Interfaces separating fluids of very different densities can undergo large non-spherical deformations and interact with shockwaves; other complex physical phenomena such as diffusion, surface tension or phase change are important. Since the main features of the flow are interactions between various types of waves with interfaces, compressible multicomponent flows are considered. The fluid components are assumed immiscible, and phase change, surface tension and diffusive effects are neglected. The Euler equations, closed by a stiffened equation of state with appropriate advection equations, govern these flows. Because of shortcomings of current shock-capturing schemes, a new numerical method was developed in [4].

CP900, *Renal Stone Disease, 1st Annual International Urolithiasis Research Symposium*, edited by A. P. Evan, J. E. Lingeman, and J. C. Williams, Jr.

PROBLEM SET-UP

A typical set-up for SWL is taken as the initial conditions: the initial bubble radius is $R_o = 50\mu$m, the pulse width is $\sigma = 6.6$mm, and the pressure amplitude is $P = 357$atm. The bubble is initially located at some distance, H, from a wall. Because the model equations do not include phase change, an exponentially decaying waveform is used, where the initial expansion matches the decay of a lithotripter pulse.

RESULTS AND DISCUSSION

Overall bubble behavior

Figure 1 shows Schlieren contours (norm of the density gradient), in order to visualize both interfaces and shockwaves. When the left-moving lithotripter pulse hits the bubble, an expansion wave is reflected, while a weak shockwave is transmitted into the bubble (frame 1). The pulse is then reflected off the wall on the left, as the bubble starts its aspherical collapse (frames 2-3). When the jet hits the distal side (frame 4), a large water-hammer pressure is generated, propagating radially outwards (frame 5). It is then reflected off the wall back onto the bubble (frame 6). After the water-hammer, the bubble becomes a vortex ring, which rebounds as it convects towards the wall (frames 7-8). The entire process occurs as the compressive part of the pulse is still entering the domain.

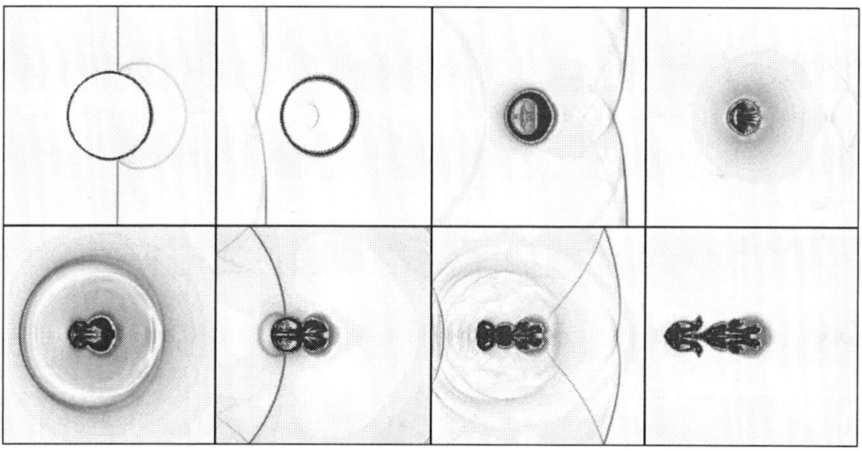

FIGURE 1. Idealized Schlieren contours of the collapse of an air bubble near a solid surface.

Geometrical effects

The effect of the initial stand-off distance from the wall is considered in the left frame of Figure 2. At the center of the domain, the wall pressure is much larger when the bubble is initially located close to the wall. At the top of the domain, the pressure is almost constant, since the distance from the location of the water-hammer does not vary significantly, yet still much larger than the pressure due to the pulse. The wall pressure for small H/R_o is much larger than analytical results for underwater explosions; in this specific case, the bubble collides with the wall at a high speed.

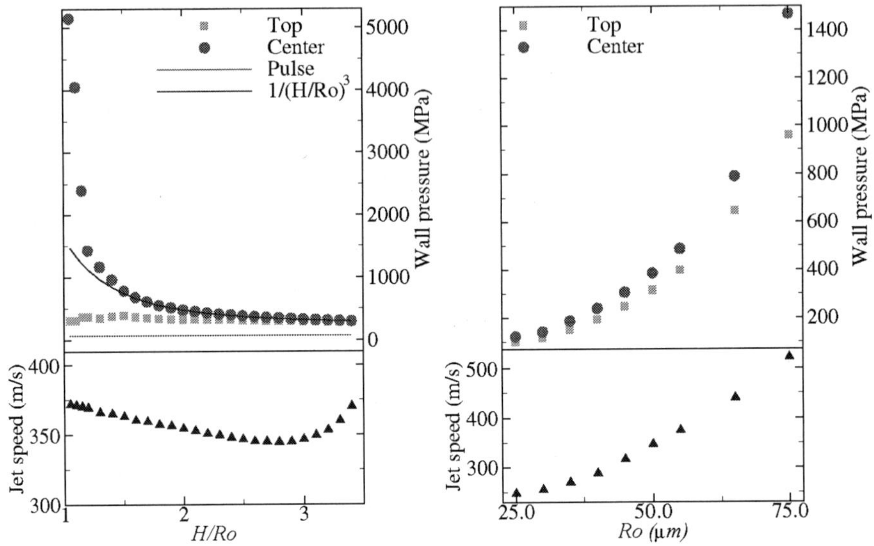

FIGURE 2. Maximum wall pressure and jet speed as a function of H/R_o and R_o.

The effect of the initial bubble radius is considered in the right frame of Figure 2. The jet speed increases with the bubble radius, so that the measured pressure increases accordingly. For a given pressure difference, a larger bubble will collapse to a smaller size (relative to its initial radius) than a smaller bubble.

Effects of the pulse properties

The effect of the pulse amplitude is considered in the left frame of Figure 3. The wall pressure increases linearly with the Mach number [1]. At the top of the domain, the full effect of the incoming lithotripter pulse is felt; the computed data matches the linearized theory well. The wall pressure due to the lithotripter pulse is smaller at the center than at the top of the domain, because the bubble "shields" the wall from the pulse. On the other hand, the wall pressure due to the bubble collapse is greater at the center than at the top of the domain.

Finally, the effect of the pulse width is considered in the right frame of Figure 3. The wall pressure increases with pulse width, since the bubble is subjected to a higher pressure for a longer time. As the width is increased, the pulse looks more and more

[1] The Mach number is related to the pressure ratio across the shock via normal shock relations.

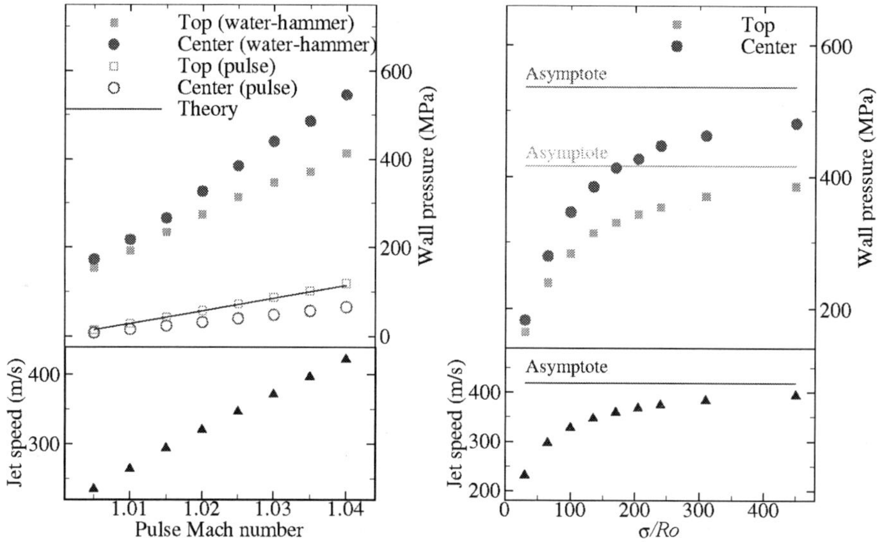

FIGURE 3. Maximum wall pressure and jet speed as a function of M and σ/R_o.

like a shockwave (with no expansion tail) to the bubble. This asymptotic value is shown using the straight lines, which are in reality a point located at $\sigma/R_o \to \infty$.

CONCLUSIONS

The presence of bubbles greatly amplifies the pressure measured at the surface of the stone in SWL. The pressure due to the bubble collapse (impact of the re-entrant jet onto the distal side) is much larger than that due to the initial pulse, even when the jet does not hit the stone. The geometry and properties of the pulse have important effects on the bubble dynamics. In future work, we will explore how the lithotripter design could be modified for optimal performance.

ACKNOWLEDGMENTS

This work was supported by NIH grant PO1 DK043881.

REFERENCES

1. Y. A. Pishchalnikov, O. A. Sapozhnikov, M. R. Bailey, J. C. Williams, R. O. Cleveland, T. Colonius, L. A. Crum, A. P. Evan, and J. A. McAteer, *J. Endourol.* **17** 435-446 (2003).
2. L. A. Crum, *J. Urol.* **140**, 1587-1590 (1988).
3. E. Johnsen and T. Colonius, *J. Acoust. Soc. Am.* in preparation (2007).
4. E. Johnsen and T. Colonius, *J. Comput. Phys.* **219**, 715-732 (2006).

A Passive Technique to Identify Stone Comminution During Shock Wave Lithotripsy

Neil R. Owen[*†], Oleg A. Sapozhnikov[*‡], Michael R. Bailey[*], Leonid Trusov[‡], and Lawrence A. Crum[*†]

**Applied Physics Laboratory, University of Washington, Seattle, WA, USA*
†Department of Electrical Engineering, University of Washington, Seattle, WA, USA
‡Department of Acoustics, Faculty of Physics, Moscow State University, Moscow 119992, Russia

Abstract. The identification of comminution during shock wave lithotripsy can be difficult using fluoroscopy or other imaging modalities. However, correct interpretation is necessary to determine if a stone is breaking and to evaluate the endpoint of therapy. Reported here is a passive method to detect acoustic signals generated by shock wave (SW) impact on a model stone and to correlate the spectrum of the detected signals to stone size. Acoustic scatter from model stones in an electrohydraulic lithotripter was measured in water with a passive, focused receiver before and after the application of either 20 SWs or 50 SWs. The five stones used for each case were dehydrated after the experiment, separated with 3 mm, 2 mm, and 1 mm sequential sieves, and weighed to quantify comminution. The detection method was first successfully used to differentiate broken and unbroken stones. Then the system tracked the decreasing size of particles and clearly showed the presence of particles smaller than 2 mm, which was considered passable size. Thus, the detection system gives feedback on whether stones are breaking and when they may be considered fully comminuted.

Keywords: lithotripsy, comminution, passive detection
PACS: 43.25.Vt, 43.20.Gp, 43.25.Jh, 43.80.Vj

INTRODUCTION AND OBJECTIVES

The identification of comminution during shock wave lithotripsy (SWL) is currently performed using fluoroscopy images taken every 300 to 500 shock waves (SWs). The extent of comminution can be estimated by comparing the most recent images to a baseline taken before any SWs were applied, where a comminuted stone generally appears granular [1]. This analysis can be difficult and depends largely on image quality and a physician's experience. Further, identifying comminution early in a procedure can be more challenging. If it were known that a stone was not breaking, stopping the procedure could spare a patient excessive SW dose and potentially reduce tissue injury and the risk of other side effects [2-4]. It could also save time.

Several ultrasound-based methods have been reported to target stones during lithotripsy. Generally, these account for stone motion and intend to increase comminution efficiency by increasing the number of SWs that hit the stone. These methods are described in more detail in [5] and the references therein. To target the stone and monitor comminution, Fedele *et al.* [6] report a passive method, under patent

CP900, *Renal Stone Disease, 1st Annual International Urolithiasis Research Symposium*, edited by A. P. Evan, J. E. Lingeman, and J. C. Williams, Jr.

review, that employs the acoustic signals generated by cavitation, where emissions related to bubble collapse are dependent upon stone size.

Our method also uses a passive receiver but we avoid cavitation and isolate a segment of resonant acoustic scatter that occurs directly after the SW reflects off the stone's surface and before cavitation bubbles collapse. Energy in the SW is transferred to the stone, which causes reverberations within the stone, where the period of reverberation depends on the stone's size and elastic properties [7]. As SWs break stones into smaller pieces, the period of resonant acoustic scatter becomes shorter. Therefore, comminution can be identified by measuring signals while a stone is still intact and comparing them to signals measured during SWL.

METHODS

Spherical model stones made with cement were held in a low-density polyethylene pipette and placed at the focus of a research lithotripter patterned after the Dornier HM3 [8]. SWs were generated with 18 kV charging potential and fired in water degassed to less than 10% of saturation. The model stones had 10 mm diameter, 2.7 mm/μs sound speed, and 1.15 g/cm^3 density. Prior to the experiment, each stone was weighed and then soaked in de-ionized water for 48 hours. The model stones were subjected to SWs according to two protocols, summarized in Table 1, to measure scatter at different stages of comminution. In Phase 1, scatter from 5 SW was measured, processed, and then averaged to establish baseline data for the intact model stone. During Phase 2, either 20 SW or 50 SW were applied at a clinical rate of 30 SW/min (0.5 Hz). Phase 4 was a post-comminution measurement conducted identically to Phase 1. Slow rates during measurement and 5 min of inactivity between Phases 3 and 4 were used to avoid cavitation.

TABLE 1. Experimental Protocol

Phase	Group 1 (n = 5 stones)	Group 2 (n = 5 stones)
1	5 SW at 1/min	5 SW at 1/min
2	20 SW at 30/min (0.5 Hz)	50 SW at 30/min (0.5 Hz)
3	5 min of inactivity	5 min of inactivity
4	5 SW at 1/min	5 SW at 1/min

Acoustic scatter from the model stones was measured with a broadband, spherical receiver placed outside the aperture of the lithotripter, as shown in Fig. 1. The receiver had 150 mm curvature, 50 mm diameter, and was made with a 25 μm-thickness PVDF membrane. With a differential preamplifier, the full-width half-maximum bandwidth was 100 kHz to 10 MHz. Signals measured with the receiver were high-pass filtered at 100 kHz, digitized at 50 MHz, and saved in a computer.

After the experiment, stones were dehydrated at room temperature for 5 days, then sieved and weighed. The mass of the sieved particles was divided by the mass of the intact stone, measured before the experiment, to calculate a histogram based on particle size. Detected acoustic signals were processed offline with MATLAB, where frequency analysis was used to compare energy in specific frequency bands before and after comminution. A ratio of energies, intended to show the shift of energy to higher frequencies after comminution, was calculated by dividing energy calculated from the

Phase 4 measurements by energy calculated from the Phase 1 measurements. The signal processing method is described with more detail in [5].

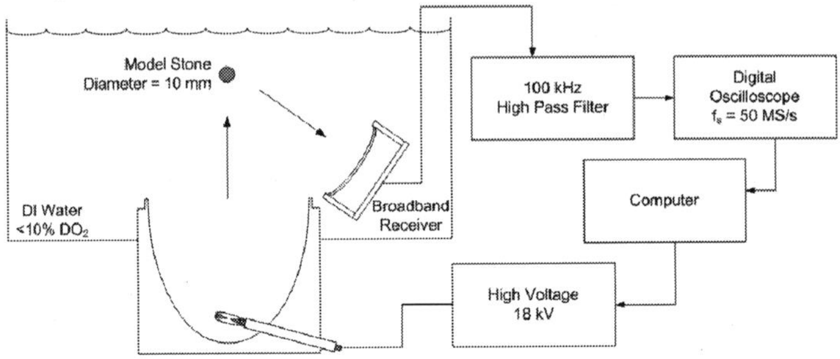

FIGURE 1. The experimental arrangement.

RESULTS

Figures 2A and 2B show histograms of particle size for the 20-SW and 50-SW groups. The percentage of particles smaller than 2 mm, the size considered passable, was 23% and 57% after the application of 20 SW and 50 SW, respectively. Figures 3A and 3B show output of our detection device, a comparison of frequency content of acoustic resonant scattering before and after lithotripsy treatment. Specifically, the ratio of energy in frequency bands corresponding to stone size is shown for the 20-SW and 50-SW groups. Ratio values [5] above 1 in both 3A and 3B indicate a shift of energy to higher frequencies and therefore can be used to identify comminution. Higher ratio values above 675 kHz in Fig. 3B, consistent with an increase in percent comminution for the 50-SW group, suggest the possibility of assessing the extent of comminution. The frequency value of 675 kHz corresponds to particles that are 2 mm in diameter based on the equation, $f=c\cdot(2d)^{-1}$, where d is diameter, c is the speed of sound of the model stone (2.7 mm/μs), and f is the frequency. Similarly, 450 kHz corresponds to particles that are 3 mm in diameter. The difference in ratio values between the 20-SW and 50-SW groups is generally associated with the percent comminution measurements. As the particles become smaller, energy in the measured acoustic scatter signals shifts to higher frequencies.

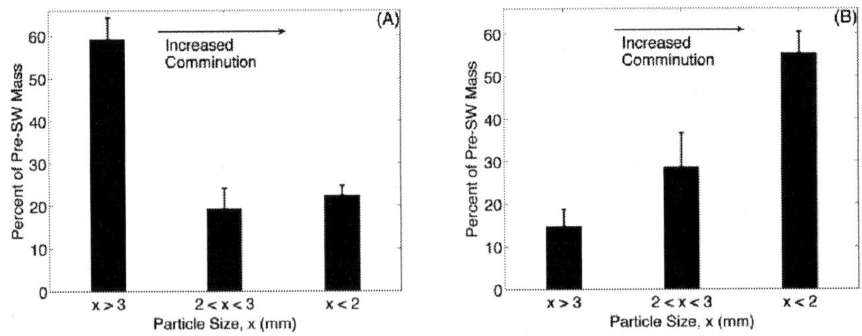

FIGURE 2. Distribution of mass by particle size for (A), the 20-SW group, and (B), the 50-SW group. Each bar shown is an average of data from five stones; lines above the bars indicate standard deviation.

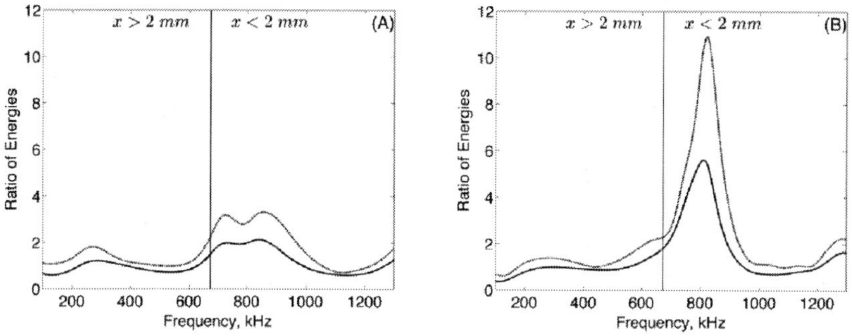

FIGURE 3. The ratio of energies calculated for (A), the 20-SW group, and (B), the 50-SW group. The vertical line at 675 kHz separates particle size, x, that is bigger, to the left, or smaller, to the right, than 2 mm. Solid lines are mean spectra for the five stones, and dotted lines are one standard deviation above the mean.

CONCLUSIONS

Model stones in water were subjected to SWs to test a new method and device to track shifts in resonant scattering and correlate the shift with stone fracture and stone fragment size. Through the frequency analysis method, using a ratio of energies, it was possible to identify comminution for both exposure levels. Data suggest the possibility of assessing the extent of comminution. Future work includes the use of real kidney stones and *ex vivo* tissue to learn the capabilities of this passive method in more realistic conditions.

ACKNOWLEDGMENTS

The authors thank the Consortium for Shock Waves in Medicine. This work was supported by: NIH DK43881, DK55674, NSBRI SMS00402, and RFBR 05-02-16987.

REFERENCES

1. P. N. Rao, *World J. Urol.* 22, 323-327 (2004)
2. J. E. Lingeman and J. R. Newmark, *Kidney Stones: Medical and Surgical Management*, edited by F. L. Coe et al. (Lippencott-Raven, Philidelphia, 1996), pp. 605–614.
3. L. R. Willis, A. P. Evan, B. A. Connors, Y. Z. Shao, P. M. Blomgren, J. H. Pratt, N. S. Fineberg, and J. E. Lingeman, *J. Endourol.* 19, 90-101 (2005)
4. A. P. Evan, L. R. Willis, J. E. Lingeman, and J. A. McAteer, *Nephron* 78, 1-8 (1998)
5. N. R. Owen, O. A. Sapozhnikov, M. R. Bailey, L. Trusov, and L. A. Crum, *J. Acoust. Soc. Am.* 120, in press (2006)
6. F. Fedele, A. J. Coleman, T. G. Leighton, P. R. White, and A. M. Hurrell, *Proceedings of the First Mediterranean Conference on Medical and Biological Engineering, "Health in the Information Society,"* Naples, Italy, 134–139 (2004)
7. R. O. Cleveland and O. A. Sapozhnikov, *J.Acoust. Soc. Am.* 118, 2667–2676 (2005)
8. R. O. Cleveland, M. R. Bailey, N. S. Fineberg, B. Hartenbaum, M. Lokhandwalla, J. A. McAteer, and B. Sturtevant, *Rev. Sci. Instr.* 71, 2514-2525 (2000)

The problem of coupling in dry-head lithotripsy

Yuri A. Pishchalnikov, James A. McAteer, Joshua S. Neucks, Irina V. Pishchalnikova, and James C. Williams, Jr.

Department of Anatomy and Cell Biology, Indiana University School of Medicine, 635 Barnhill Drive, Indianapolis, IN 46202, USA

Abstract. Recent in vitro studies have shown that air pockets can get trapped at the coupling interface of the treatment head in dry-head lithotripsy, and this can pose a significant barrier to transmission of shock wave energy to the focal zone. Breakage of model stones is very sensitive to the presence of air pockets at the coupling interface. The quality of routine coupling is highly variable, and it seems quite feasible that the way in which the coupling gel is applied may have a significant effect on the quality of coupling. Therefore, attempts to find the best coupling regime may be valuable to perform, and preliminary results of *in vitro* tests are presented in this report. Experiments were conducted using gel or castor oil as coupling agents. The test tank was coupled through a transparent Mylar membrane to the water-filled cushion of the treatment head, so that pockets of air trapped between the two coupling surfaces could be observed and photographed. It is shown that the quality of coupling can be improved by applying an excessive amount of gel to just the water cushion of the lithotripter, while applying gel to both the water cushion and the Mylar membrane typically gives poor coupling. Repeat decoupling and re-coupling substantially degraded the quality of coupling, reducing shock wave energy density at the target by ~80%. It was also observed that using castor oil as a coupling medium does not guarantee air-free coupling.

Keywords: shock wave lithotripsy, coupling, bubbles, air pockets, coupling gel, castor oil.
PACS: 43.80.Vj, 43.25.Zx, 43.35.Yb, 43.20.El.

INTRODUCTION

In the first clinical lithotripters the patient was submerged in a water bath. This provided excellent acoustic coupling for transmission of shock waves to the patient, but these water-tub style lithotripters were short lived. To make lithotripters transportable and more convenient to use, the water bath has been replaced by a water-filled cushion that must be coupled to the patient's skin using gel or oil. As convenient as the dry treatment head may be, it is not very efficient. Air pockets get trapped in the coupling medium when the cushion (boot or bellows) is brought into contact with the skin. Because the intensity transmission coefficient for an acoustic wave moving from water to air is only 0.1%, air pockets at the coupling interface pose a substantial barrier. In a recent in vitro study we determined that breakage of model stones is very sensitive to the presence of defects in coupling, and coverage of only 15% of the coupling interface by air pockets reduced the efficiency of stone comminution by 80% compared to air-free coupling [1].

CP900, *Renal Stone Disease, 1st Annual International Urolithiasis Research Symposium*, edited by A. P. Evan, J. E. Lingeman, and J. C. Williams, Jr.

The quality of routine coupling is highly variable [1], and it seems quite feasible that the way in which the coupling gel is applied may have a significant effect on the quality of coupling. Therefore, attempts to find the best coupling regime may be valuable to perform, and preliminary results of in vitro tests are presented in this report. It is shown that coupling can be improved by applying an excessive amount of gel to just the water cushion of the lithotripter, while applying gel to both the water cushion and the test membrane typically gives poor coupling.

Both gel and oil have been used as coupling agents, but gels tend to be more popular because they are easier to handle. One might expect that oil would provide a more consistent interface, however, this study shows that using oil does not guarantee air-free coupling.

MATERIALS AND METHODS

Studies were performed with an electromagnetic clinical lithotripter Dornier DoLi-50 (Dornier MedTech, Kennesaw, GA, USA). The water-filled cushion of the lithotripter treatment head was coupled to a Mylar membrane of the test tank (Fig. 2, left panel) using LithoClear gel (Sonotech Inc., Bellingham, WA). The coupling interface (Fig. 1) was photographed through the test tank. This setup has been used previously to quantify stone breakage efficiency as a function of surface area occupied by air pockets trapped at the coupling interface [1]. Shock waves were measured using a fiber-optic probe hydrophone (FOPH-500, RP Acoustics, Leutenbach, Germany) as previously described [2].

To assess whether the occurrence of air pockets at the coupling interface is related exclusively to use of gel as a coupling agent, some experiments were performed with castor oil. The test system consisted of a spare rubber boot for the DoLi treatment head, clamped to the closed end of a Lexan cylinder (Fig. 3a). The cylinder was mounted at 45°, and the boot was inflated with water. A volunteer (one of the investigators) on a motorized treatment table was moved into contact with the rubber boot, and the coupling interface was photographed through the open end of the cylinder (Fig. 3b).

RESULTS AND DISCUSSION

The coupling interface was susceptible to formation of air pockets, and when coupling was established as might be done prior to treating a patient—smoothing gel over both the treatment head and the Mylar window (surrogate body surface)—the interface always contained defects (Fig. 1a). If, once coupling was established, the treatment head was pulled back and then re-coupled—as would occur in repositioning a patient—air pockets increased. It took special handling to improve the quality of coupling. One procedure that worked well was to apply gel only to the treatment head and, at that, it was necessary to use what seemed to be an excessive amount of gel (~250 ml) deposited as a mound. When the water cushion was inflated and brought into contact with the Mylar window, the gel spread from the center, and air pockets tended to be pushed to the periphery. This method of coupling, and the consequences of decoupling and re-coupling are demonstrated in Fig. 1.

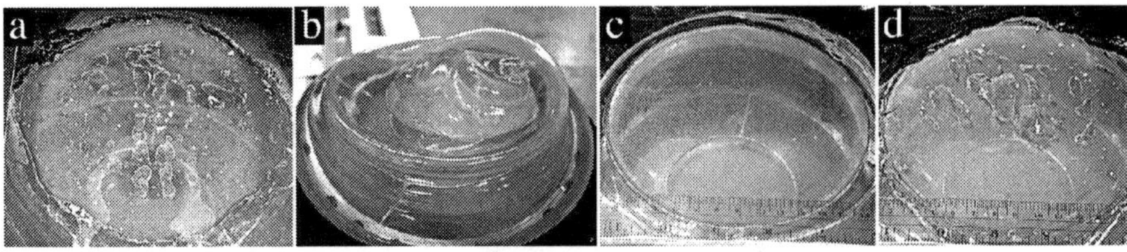

FIGURE 1. A method for improved coupling, and the effect of decoupling and re-coupling. When gel was applied to both the treatment head and the Mylar membrane, coupling was generally quite poor, and the interface contained numerous air pockets **(a)**. Gel applied as a mound, and only to the treatment cushion **(b)** resulted in fewer defects **(c)**. Decoupling and re-coupling, as might be done in repositioning a patient, created more defects **(d)**. The area occupied by air pockets for coupling conditions **(c)** and **(d)** was 0.1% and 17.5%, respectively.

Poor coupling had a measurable effect on waveform and the amplitude of shock waves. Peak positive pressure when coupling was pristine (Fig. 1c) was 51 MPa. Uncoupling and re-coupling created air pockets, and this reduced shock wave amplitude (24 MPa for Fig. 1d). This had a dramatic effect on shock wave energy density (integral of pressure squared over time), and for the examples shown in Fig. 1 (frames c and d), values were 703 and 172 $(\mathrm{MPa})^2 \times \mu s$, respectively. Thus, repeated decoupling and re-coupling (example 1d) substantially degraded the quality of coupling, reducing shock wave energy at the target by 76%.

Air pockets at the coupling interface also affected shock wave focusing. This is illustrated in Fig. 2, where a waveform for the example of poor coupling shows that not only was amplitude reduced, but the arrival of the pulse maximum was also delayed. Thus, air pockets at the coupling interface may be altering the distribution of shock wave energy within the acoustic field of the lithotripter.

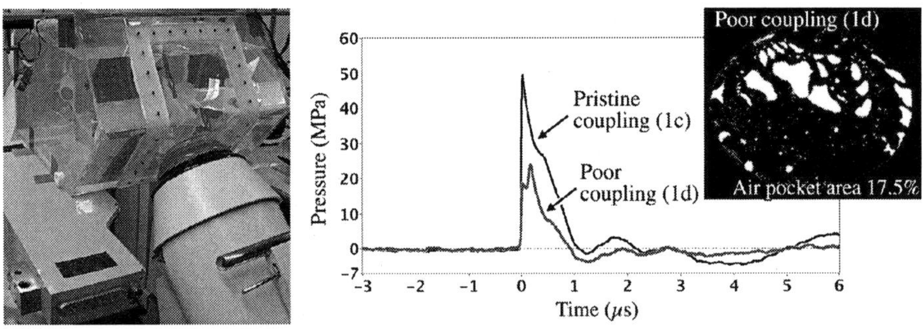

FIGURE 2. Left panel—in vitro test system to assess coupling regimes using the fiber-optic probe hydrophone. Right panel—average of 50 shock waves recorded at coupling conditions **1c** and **1d** from Fig. 1, with the digitized image of the coupling interface **(1d)** shown in the inset. Data in [1] shows that when air pockets occupied 17.5% surface area, as in condition **(1d)**, the efficiency of stone comminution was reduced by 80% compared to breakage when coupling was pristine (as in **1c**).

Castor oil is also prone to coupling artifact. Figure 3 shows the experimental apparatus and representative images of the coupling interface with castor oil at initial contact (Fig. 3c), and when the cushion was decoupled and re-coupled (Fig. 3d).

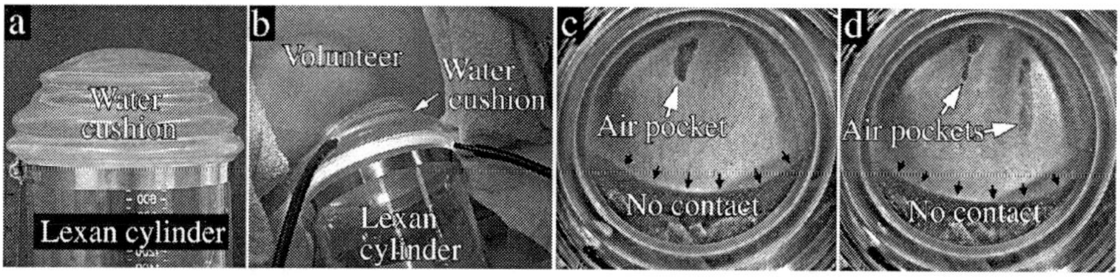

FIGURE 3. Use of castor oil as a coupling agent does not guarantee air-free coupling. **a)** and **b)**—Experimental setup: a spare water cushion was clamped to the closed end of a cylindrical container, allowing visual access of the coupling interface with the skin of one of the investigators lying on the treatment table. **c)**—Air pocket (shown by white arrow) trapped at the coupling interface upon initial contact. **d)**—The cushion was decoupled and re-coupled, introducing additional defects (white arrows). Black arrows in Figures **c** and **d** mark a large defect (no contact zone) in the coupling interface.

It has been shown that the nature of the coupling agent used in dry-head lithotripsy can affect the efficiency of stone fragmentation *in vitro* [3]. This was not investigated in the present study. However even with the same coupling agent, transmitted acoustic energy can vary significantly depending on the number and size of trapped bubbles [1,4]. This underscores the value of controlling coupling quality in dry-head lithotripters. The current study shows that applying gel to both the water cushion and the test membrane gives poor coupling, but that coupling is improved by applying an excessive amount of gel to just the water cushion. This suggests that how a coupling agent is applied makes a difference. Re-coupling was particularly disruptive, suggesting that repositioning the patient could degrade the quality of coupling. This demonstrates that attention needs to be paid to how coupling is accomplished in order to avoid or minimize acoustic shielding by air bubbles trapped at the coupling interface.

ACKNOWLEDGMENTS

Supported by a grant from the National Institutes of Health (DK-43881).

REFERENCES

1. Y.A. Pishchalnikov, J.S. Neucks, R.J. VonDerHaar, et al., *J. Urology* **176**, 2706-2710 (2006).
2. Y.A. Pishchalnikov, J.A. McAteer, R.J. VonDerHaar, et al., *J. Urology* **176**, 2294-2298 (2006).
3. J.J. Cartledge, W.R. Cross, S.N. Lloyd, A.D. Joyce, *BJU International* **88(4),** 321-324 (2001).
4. Y.A. Pishchalnikov, S. Beard, J.C. Williams, Jr., et al., "Bubbles trapped at coupling surface of wave generator significantly reduce acoustic energy delivered in shock wave lithotripsy" in *Therapeutic Ultrasound: 5th International Symposium on Therapeutic Ultrasound,* edited by G.T. Clement et al., AIP Conference Proceedings 829, American Institute of Physics, Melville, NY, 2005, pp. 643-647.

In Vitro Comparison between HM-3 and MODULARIS Lithotripters

Victor A. Leitao[†], W. Neal Simmons[*], Yufeng Zhou[*], Jun Qin[*], Franklin H. Cocks[*], and Jens Fehre[‡], Bernd Granz[‡], Ralf Nanke[‡], Glenn M. Preminger[†], and Pei Zhong[*]

[*]*Duke University Pratt School of Engineering; Durham, NC*
[†]*Duke University Medical Center; Durham, NC*
[‡]*Siemens Medical Solutions; Erlangen, Germany*

Abstract. Shockwave lithotripsy (SWL) is currently the preferred method of treatment for renal calculi < 10 mm in size. Dornier introduced the electrohydraulic HM-3 in 1983, which has become the "gold standard" for SWL. Since then other types of lithotripters (electromagnetic and piezoelectric) have been developed. We compared the third-generation electromagnetic shockwave lithotripter Siemens MODULARIS to the HM-3 *in vitro* assessing acoustic measurement and stone comminution in a holder. Similar results were encountered.

Keywords: Lithotripsy, shock-wave.
PACS: 43.25.Cb, 43.40.Jc; 87.54.Hk

INTRODUCTION

The Dornier HM-3 was the first lithotripter developed [1] and is considered the gold standard for comparison between lithotripters.[2,3] It uses a electrohydraulic shockwave generator and its wet coupling is one of the main reasons why its results are superior to most new generation lithotripters. The main drawbacks of this equipment are its large size, the need in most cases for anesthesia and/or sedation and its inability to allow for multifunctional use. Newer lithotripters have been developed in order to overcome the disadvantages of this first generation device, using different shock generators and coupling systems.[4] The Siemens MODULARIS is a third generation electromagnetic lithotripter which features a compact system design. Its dry coupling using only a water cushion-coupled shockwave generator reduces space requirements to a minimum, whereas patient comfort is increased; for example, treatments are mainly performed under low analgesia. Furthermore, MODULARIS offers multifunctional usage for urodiagnostics and urologic interventions and is a mobile system. However, the stone comminution efficiency at different energy settings has not been evaluated in comparison to the HM-3 standard. By evaluating the acoustic pressure characteristics and in vitro stone comminution, we have determined the MODULARIS' energy setting that closely matches the in vitro performance of the HM-3.

CP900, *Renal Stone Disease, 1st Annual International Urolithiasis Research Symposium,*
edited by A. P. Evan, J. E. Lingeman, and J. C. Williams, Jr.

MATERIALS AND METHODS

The acoustic fields of the MODULARIS and HM-3 lithotripters were characterized by pressure measurement using a Light Spot Hydrophone (LSHD) [5]. Pressure waveforms in the focal plane (X-Y) were captured in degassed water using a digital storage oscilloscope, and transferred to a computer. Pressure analysis determined peak positive and negative pressures and the resulting energy density. Pressure data for the HM-3 was collected using a 20 kilovolt (kV) output setting and pressure data for the MODULARIS was collected at energy settings of E3.0, E4.0, and E5.0, respectively. A minimum of six measurements was collected at each position for the HM-3 because of the large shot-to-shot variation, while only three measurements were done at each point for the MODULARIS due to its stable output. Stone comminution was assessed at 250, 500, 1,000, 1,500 shocks at 20 kV for the HM-3 and at energy settings of E3.0, E4.0 and E5.0 for the MODULARIS. Spherical BegoStone phantoms [6] with one centimeter in diameter and an average dry weight of 1.12 gram (g) ± 0.02 g were held in medium-size finger cots filled with degassed water. Six stones were treated at each shock number and an output energy combination using a pulse repetition rate of one hertz. The stone fragments were allowed to dry at room temperature and then sieved through three meshes (4mm, 2.8mm and 2mm), resulting in four groups of fragment sizes: > 4.0, 4.0 to 2.8, 2.8 to 2.0, and < 2.0 millimeter (mm). Fragmentation efficiency is reported as the mass fraction that passes through the 2.0 mm sieve.

RESULTS

Several differences in the energy fields of the HM-3 (electrohydraulic) and the MODULARIS (electromagnetic) lithotripters have been observed (Figs. 1 and 2). As shown in Fig. 3, the profiles of the pressure waveforms are different. Furthermore, it can be noticed that the variation in the acoustic field of the HM-3 is large because of the instability of the shock discharge from electrohydraulic lithotripters. Because there is inherent randomness in the path the plasma discharge takes between electrodes, the energy discharge does not always occur exactly at the same location. The discharge path and distance also play an important role in the intensity of the energy discharge. These two factors create changing pressure fields for the focus of the HM-3. The 'jumping focus' results in an average -6 decibel (dB) focal size of approximately 12 mm, which is apparently larger than the real beam size of the HM-3 from each shock. Electromagnetic machines such as the MODULARIS are not susceptible to these factors and therefore provide a more stable pressure field. The -6 dB focal size of the MODULARIS at E4.0 referring to the energy density is approximately 10 mm.

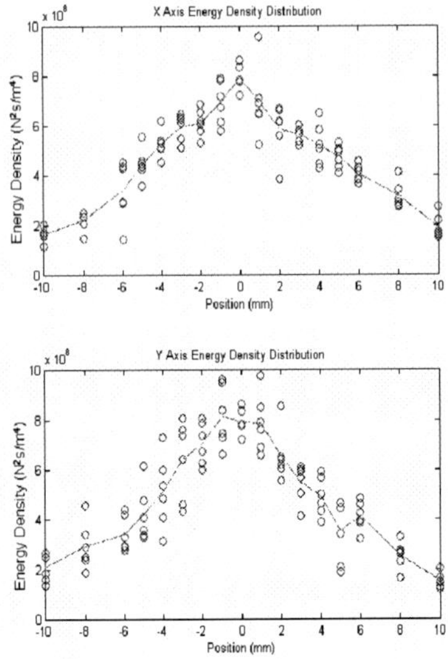

FIGURE 1. Energy distribution at Dornier HM-3 at 20kV.

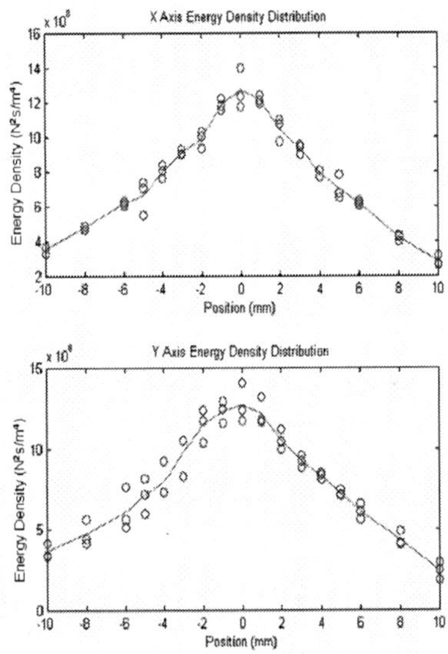

FIGURE 2. Energy distribution at Siemens MODULARIS at E4.0.

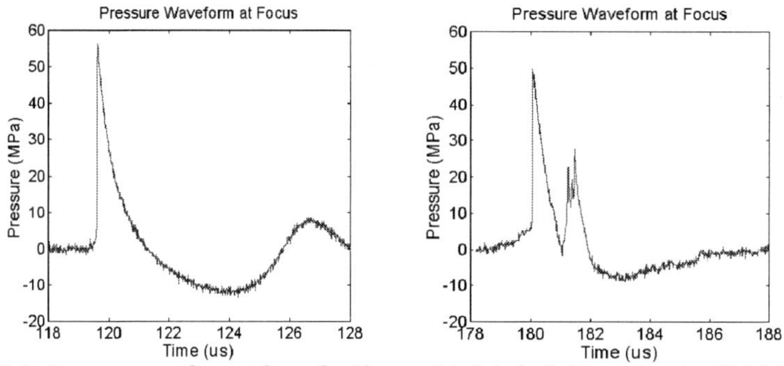

FIGURE 3. Pressure waveform at focus for Siemens Modularis (left) and Dornier HM-3 (right).

The peak positive (P+) and peak negative (P-) pressures are shown in Table 1. The MODULARIS was found to have slightly greater peak positive and peak negative pressures than the HM-3 at all energies examined (E3.0, E4.0, and E5.0).

TABLE 1. Pressure data for HM-3 and MODULARIS lithotripters.

	P+ (MPa)	P- (MPa)
HM-3 at 20kV	48.9±6.4	10.7±0.5
MODULARIS at E3.0	51.3±0.6	12.9±0.5
MODULARIS at E4.0	56.2±1.5	13.6±0.5
MODULARIS at E5.0	59.6±1.3	14.6±0.4

Overall, there is a progressive increase in stone comminution for both lithotripters as the shock number increases. For the MODULARIS, stone fragmentation also increases significantly with the output energy setting between 250 and 500 shocks. The difference in stone comminution produced by different energy levels becomes less significant as the shock number exceeds 1,000. In comparison, it was found that the stone comminution produced by MODULARIS at an energy setting of E4.0 is comparable and E5.0 is better than the HM-3 at 20 kV after 500 shocks (Table 2).

TABLE 2. Stone comminution (% fragments <2mm).

	250 Shocks	500 Shocks	1000 Shocks	1500 Shocks
HM-3 at 20kV	56.23	75.86	91.32	100
MODULARIS at E3.0	44.15	63.47	90.38	98.20
MODULARIS at E4.0	48.44	72.34	91.35	100
MODULARIS at E5.0	58.02	90.42	100	100

CONCLUSION

Regarding acoustic properties, the MODULARIS was found to have slightly higher peak positive and negative pressure values at all energies measured (E3.0-E5.0). In vitro stone comminution in the finger cot was found to be similar between the HM-3 at 20 kV and the MODULARIS at an energy setting of E4.0, and better at E5.0 for greater than 500 shocks. Future work is needed to compare the MODULARIS and the HM-3 in vivo.

REFERENCES

1. C. Chaussy, E. Schmiedt, D. Jocham, W. Brendel, B. Forssmann, V. Walther, "First clinical experience with extracorporeally induced destruction of kidney stones by shock waves", *J Urol* **127**, 471-20 (1982).
2. C. Renner and J. Rassweiler, Treatment of renal stones by extracorporeal shock wave lithotripsy. *Nephron* **81**, 71-81 (1999).
3. J. E. Lingeman, S. C. Kim, R. L. Kuo, J. A. McAteer, A. P. Evan. Shockwave lithotripsy: Anecdotes and insights. *J Endourol* **17**, 687-693 (2003).
4. B. Granz, R. Nanke, J. Fehre, T. Pfister, R. Engelbrecht. Light Spot Hydrophone, Innovation in Lithotripsy. Medical Solutions, **June**, 86-88 (2004).
5. Y. F. Zhou, F. H. Cocks, G. M. Preminger, P. Zhong, Innovations in shock wave lithotripsy technology: Updates in experimental results. *J Urol* **172**, 1892-1898 (2004).
6. Y. Liu and P. Zhong. BegoStone - a new stone phantom for shock wave lithotripsy research. *Journal of the Acoustical Society of America* **112**, 1265-1268 (2002).

Comparison of Light Spot Hydrophone (LSHD) and Fiber Optic Probe Hydrophone (FOPH) for Lithotripter Field Characterization

Victor A. Leitao[*], W. Neal Simmons[†], Yufeng Zhou[†], Jun Qin[†], Georgii Sankin[†], Franklin H. Cocks[†], and Jens Fehre[‡], Bernd Granz[‡], Ralf Nanke[3], Glenn M. Preminger[*], Pei Zhong[†]

[*] *Duke University Medical Center; Durham, NC*
[†] *Duke University Pratt School of Engineering; Durham, NC*
[‡] *Siemens Medical Solutions; Erlangen, Germany*

Abstract. Characterization of the acoustic field of a shock wave lithotripter is important for determining the performance of the device. In this study, we compare the performance of a newly developed Light Spot Hydrophone (LSHD) with the current standard, i.e., the Fiber Optic Probe Hydrophone (FOPH). An electromagnetic (EM) shock wave lithotripter was selected and each hydrophone was used to map the acoustic field of the lithotripter. The peak positive pressure P+, peak negative pressure P-, pulse duration, and effective acoustic energy were calculated using the collected data. Both the LSHD and the FOPH have similar measurement characteristics. They both provide excellent P+ measurement accuracy and response. Although the LSHD was found to provide more repeatable P- pressure measurements, both devices provide excellent pressure measurement of lithotripter shock fields.

Keywords: Lithotripsy, hydrophone, acoustic field.
PACS: 43.38.Pf; 87.54.Hk

INTRODUCTION

Characterization of the acoustic field of a shock wave lithotripter is important for determining the performance of the device. The measurements of lithotripsy shock waves require specialized hydrophones to meet the following demanding characteristics: pressure amplitudes in the range of 2-150MPa, bandwidths in excess of 10MHz, and spatial resolution preferably less than 200μm. In addition, the hydrophone must be durable enough to withstand multiple shocks without significant damage, and if damage occurs, the sensor of the hydrophone can be easily replaced.

Such a hydrophone was first developed by Staudenraus and Eisenmenger [1] who used a fiber optic light source to measure pressure fluctuations. This device was termed Fiber Optic Hydrophone (FOPH). Recently Granz *et. al.* developed a similar device, the Light Spot Hydrophone (LSHD) which uses a focused laser spot on a massive glass block rather than a glass fiber.[2]

CP900, *Renal Stone Disease, 1st Annual International Urolithiasis Research Symposium,* edited by A. P. Evan, J. E. Lingeman, and J. C. Williams, Jr.

Both the FOPH and the LSHD operate on the same principle. Laser light is transmitted to a glass-fluid interface and the intensity of the reflected light is measured. Pressure changes in the fluid create a change of its refraction index and concomitantly the amount of light reflected.

In this study, we compare the performance of a newly developed LSHD with the current standard, i.e., the FOPH.

APPARATUS AND METHODS

An electromagnetic (EM) shock wave lithotripter (Siemens Modularis) was used as an acoustic source for the comparison. The electromagnetic source was chosen because of its output stability from shot to shot.

We used the LSHD (University of Erlangen, Nuremberg, Germany) and a fiber-optic hydrophone FOPH-500 (RP Acoustics, Leutenbach, Germany) to perform the study (Fig. 1).

Each hydrophone was used to map the acoustic field of the lithotripter at several energy output settings. The hydrophones were positioned using a motorized 3-D translation stage. The pressure signals were collected using a digital storage oscilloscope. The focal point was first determined by an iterative method of scanning the X axis until a maximum was found, re-zeroing, and then scanning the Y axis. This process was repeated until the focus was found. Positioning in the Z axis was accomplished after finding the focal point in the X and Y planes. The time from the electromagnetic discharge to the pressure wave was measured. The hydrophone was moved in the Z axis until this time delay matched the manufacturer's specified delay time.

The peak positive pressure P^+, peak negative pressure P^-, pulse duration, and effective acoustic energy were calculated offline using a Matlab program (The MathWorks, Inc, Natick, MA). Acoustic energy was defined by integrating the pressure waveforms over an area defined by a 12mm circle around the focal point (International Standard IEC 61846).

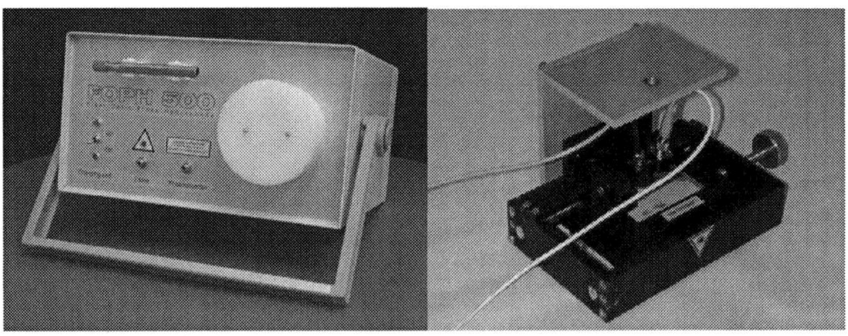

FIGURE 1. Left: Fiber Optic Probe Hydrophone (Controller). Right: Light Spot Hydrophone (Sensor Only).

RESULTS

Using a medium energy setting on the Modularis the maximum pressures recorded were 56 MPa and 57 MPa for the LSHD and FOPH respectively. The peak negative pressures were 14 MPa and 9.3 MPa for the LSHD and FOPH respectively. For reliable P^- measurements several samples were required when using the FOPH because of the formation of cavitation bubbles on the tip of optical fiber (Fig. 2). When using the LSHD bubble formation was not a problem and the measured P^- pulse was stable from shot to shot. The pulse duration (8.7 μs) was similar for both devices. The effective acoustic energy was integrated from the pressure pulses and was found to be 80mJ for the LSHD and 58mJ for the FOPH.

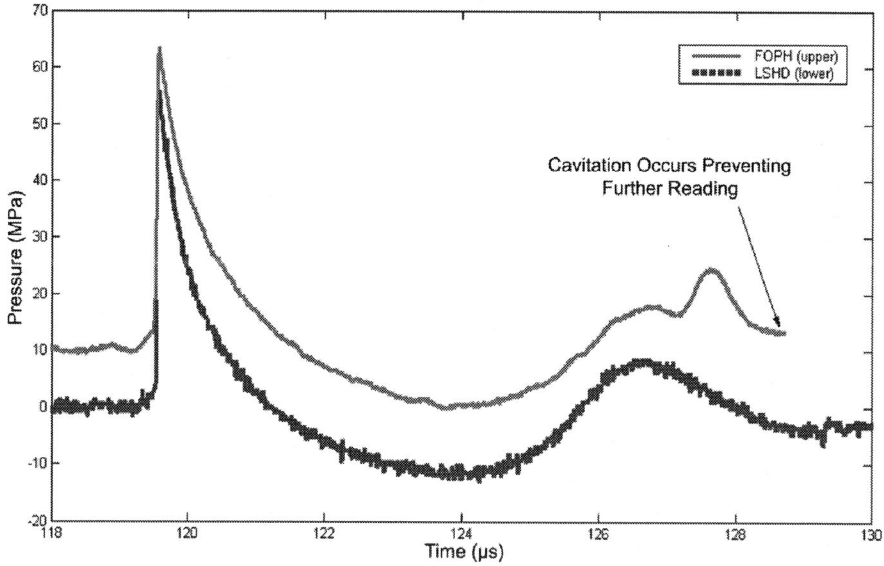

FIGURE 2. Pressure wave from the Siemens Modularis at focus measured with the LSHD (Blue) and the FOPH (Red).

DISCUSSION

Accurate localization and targeting of shock waves are necessary for successful stone comminution. In order to map the acoustic field characteristics, a reliable hydrophone is needed. Both the FOPH and the LSHD provide accurate measurement for characterizing lithotripter acoustic fields.

FOPH has been used broadly for pressure measurement in lithotripters, proving to be accurate and reliable.[3] LSHD has been recently described [2], providing similar indications.

It has been reported that the LSHD provides high-accuracy measurements of both single and broadband pressure pulses. It was used to compare different lithotripters, yielding results with great precision.[4]

The geometric and mechanical differences provide each with specific advantages:

LSHD

Due to its design, it uses a glass bulk as an interface, which is much less susceptible cavitation formation and damage than the FOPH. Whenever there is a crack in the glass surface secondary to cavitation damage and it interferes with the readings, the glass can be moved, without changing the focal point. It allows repetitive measurements devoid of the trouble of finding focus or having to change the fiber. It also has a higher sensitivity and slightly higher spatial resolution.

FOPH

Size and geometry allow for easy measurement setup in any orientation, while the LSHD cannot be positioned for readings from a lateral or inverted shock head. Measured focal point can be easily and precisely marked by the tip of the fiber, allowing placement of focal point markers for later positioning of stone phantoms.

CONCLUSION

Both the LSHD and the FOPH have similar measurement characteristics. They both provide excellent P+ measurement accuracy and response. However, the LSHD provides more repeatable and accurate P- pressure measurements because it is not as susceptible to cavitation bubble error. This is especially important in SWL when trying to measure the total energy of both the P+ and P- regions.

REFERENCES

1. J. Staudenraus and W. Eisenmeger, "Fibre-optic probe hydrophone for ultrasonic and shock-wave measurement in water", *Ultrasonics* **31**, 267-272 (1993).
2. B. Granz, R. Nanke, J. Fehre,T. Pfister, R. Engelbrecht, "Light Spot Hydrophone, innovation in lithotripsy", Medical Solutions June, 86-87 (2004).
3. J. E. Parsons, C. A. Cain, J,. B. Fowlkes, "Cost-effective assembly of a basic fiber-optic hydrophone for measurement of high-amplitude therapeutic ultrasound fields", *J Acoust Soc Am* **119** 1432-1440 (2006).
4. M. B. Gubenko, M. V. Nagulina, N. E. Stankevich. " Targeting and adjustment systems in lithotripsy". *Biomed Eng 39, 256-241 (2005).*

VIII. OTHER TOPICS IN UROLITHIASIS RESEARCH

The Urologist's Guide to the Galaxy

Michael E. Moran

Capital Region Urologic Surgeons, Albany, NY USA

Abstract. "Far out in the uncharted backwaters of the unfashionable end of the Western Spiral arm of the Galaxy…." Stone disease has affected mankind since earliest recorded history and will trouble us as we strive for the stars. Zero and microgravity are risk factors for urolithiasis, but the incidence is not yet known. Yet, the possible "century of space exploration" lies before us if payloads can be inexpensively offloaded from Earth's surface to orbit. The scientific publications about medical conditions of astronauts, deep water environments (submarine) and extreme conditions (Arctic and Antarctic) were reviewed to better understand the urologic risks. Actual events were next sought and any scientific data regarding therapeutic intent was carefully scrutinized. Incidence and risk potential could then be calculated and potential for intervention would then be known. The National Space Biomedical Research Institute has classified space health hazards and stone disease as "Risk 12." Combined statistics from NASA's Gemini, Apollo, and Space Shuttle flights and long-term missions such as Shuttle-Mir or Skylab fail to reveal any "disclosed" emergency stone events. One published article suggests that some cosmonauts have in fact formed stones during space missions. Detailed data from 79 U.S. space missions, involving 219 person-flights, and 175 astronauts show 23 genitourinary problems (1.2 % or 0.07 incidence for 7 days). Submarine encounters are different, however, with 1.8 to 2.6 actual emergency evacuations per 1,000 person months and 23 kidney stone events (data from all subs in U.S. Atlantic Fleet 1993-1996). Extreme environment data appears more similar to that of spaceflight (despite full Earth's gravity) with 1,967 person-years distribution showing no definite stone formation/evacuation (but 335 or 3.6% were not-specified). Pak and co-workers at the University of Texas, Southwestern have extensively evaluated the metabolic consequences of bone-mineral loss and urinary parameters associated with the increased risk of stone formation in space. Astronauts are at significantly greater risk of forming calcium oxalate, calcium phosphate and uric acid stones, and this persists for a period of time following return to normal gravity. Conflicting data exists regarding submarine and extreme environmental databases as to the "actual" space mission risks but the hazard is real. Attempts to evaluate both diagnostic and therapeutic interventions are being pursued. As the number of space visitors increases, so should the incidence of urolithiasis. Both diagnostic and therapeutic methods need to be developed coincident to our further efforts in space.

Keywords: space exploration, zero gravity, urolithiasis.
PACS: 01.30.Cc

INTRODUCTION

The title of this paper comes, of course, from the late Douglas Adams' famous work of science fiction entitled *The Hitchhiker's Guide to the Galaxy* and this is appropriate because our actual knowledge of stone formation in space is shrouded in secrecy and speculation [1]. But the science of urinary supersaturation, physiology of bone resorption, and many of the deleterious effects of prolonged zero-gravity

CP900, *Renal Stone Disease, 1st Annual International Urolithiasis Research Symposium,* edited by A. P. Evan, J. E. Lingeman, and J. C. Williams, Jr.

exposure are well described. We are now entering what many perceive as the "The Century of Space Exploration" and it behooves those of us interested in urinary calculus disease to review our current understanding of what lies ahead, and to review related hazardous environmental experiences in order to form some realistic expectations as mankind approaches Kardashev's level I civilization [2]. Another possible reason for this exercise for many (like the author's) is an absolute fascination about the potential for continued space exploration, sparked by Neil Armstrong's memorable descent upon our moon [3].

SCIENCE FICTION

"*There is no way back into the past. The choice is the Universe—or nothing.*" stated H.G. Wells. Space rock 84001 is a piece of Mars ejected an estimated 3.6 billion years ago and which landed upon this third planet from the sun at the South Pole approximately 13,000 years ago. It appears to have organic tubes that indicate the strong possibility that there was life on that planet some time ago. Our interest in space is as old as the genre of science fiction itself, and quite probably older. We are currently in the midst of intense interest in Mars and some of Jupiter's moons as they might hold basic knowledge on the origins of life. In addition, it has been postulated that our home world is prone to periodic, and perhaps sudden catastrophic impacts, from space debris that would behoove a knowledgeable species to figure out methods of space exploration, colonization and/or expeditious transportation.

Our current problem with these science fiction-like endeavors is the costs of placing payloads into outer space. It has been estimated that 800 million dollars per space shuttle launch, which can carry about 27 tons, costs us about $15,000 per pound (or roughly twice the cost of gold). There are promising technologies that quite likely will solve these huge financial hurdles and allow us to rapidly and far less expensively have access to near Earth orbit. These include the Lockheed Martin X-33 VentureStar, NASA's collaborative hypersonic scramjet, the X-43A (which recently hit Mach 10) and my personal favorite, the "space elevator." Using nanotechnology, carbon nanotubes might be created that would allow a fixed terrestrial point on the equator to be attached to an orbiting platform that would literally run payloads into outer space at a fraction of current costs. If any of these technologies (and assuredly others not listed) manages to prove feasible, the doorway to space will become wide open and our exploration of space will shift into high gear. In fact, the probability that this might be so has prompted many scientists to prematurely call our current century "The Century of Space Exploration."

There are many hazards to space existence for terrestrial humans. The focus of this discussion will be upon the known risks of urolithiasis formation in outer space. The published literature will be reviewed, the physiology summarized and unpublished, but widespread, speculations shall be aired. In the end, our knowledge is not exact and the methods of dealing with colic in space are unknown and as speculative as science fiction itself.

SCIENCE FACT

Early in the clinical literature of urolithiasis it was documented that humans who are incapacitated and bed ridden are prone to kidney stones. In 1922, Paul from Toronto reported on 20 cases of nephrolithiasis occurring in men aged 22 to 37 (average 28.5) who developed renal calculi following war wounds. The average time from the wound to the first symptoms of stones was 17.7 months. All patients had extensive injuries, including osteomyelitis. Most of these patients were bedridden for prolonged times [4]. Fowweather, followed by Pulvertaft, both indicated that recumbency appeared to be the critical problem associated with calcium stone formation, not the degree of trauma [5-6]. The primary event increasing the risk of nephrolithiasis appears to be an acute mobilization of calcium from the skeletal reserves [7]. In some patients, hypercalciuria may be pronounced [8]. In these patients, indwelling Foley catheterization is also common and subsequent bladder infection makes upper tract seeding commonplace. Recurrent urinary tract infection therefore changes the primary stone risk in these patients with high urinary pH with the potential for ammonium production to form struvite stones (magnesium ammonium phosphate hexahydrate) [9]. In current practice with the emphasis on early mobilization and vigorous rehabilitation, no patients except perhaps those with global trauma (i.e. multiple organ injured individuals) run this risk. One current investigation on immobilization-related hypercalemia in a mere 5 patients tried to ameliorate bone mineral loss [10]. In all of this immobilized group, the hypercalcemia during three months of observation could be reversed by administration of low dose pamidronate (10 mg). In a review by Gordon and Reinstein, a discussion of common secondary problems associated with the management of complex trauma victims revealed that urolithiasis was a significant problem. In addition, the costs in managing this secondary problem was significant [11]. It would seem reasonable, despite a paucity of published data, that immobilized patients are at higher risk and maintenance of adequate hydration would be a minimal recommendation. The use of bisphosphonates is more uncertain but indicated if hypercalcemia or urolithiasis develops. A final area of consideration is the effect of physical activity on calcium balance, calcium requirements, and upon bone mineral mass. Because of the aging population and the increasing risk of osteoporosis-induced fractures, a significant volume of research is becoming focused upon these issues. In some studies, physical activity has been noted to have a more profound role in affecting enhanced bone mineral density prior to puberty [12]. The need for greater research and the potential for physical activity itself to have an effect upon calcium balance is critical and the application of these findings to zero-gravity environments is just beginning [13].

A corollary to the immobilization-related hypercalemia and stone formation scenario is the possibility of placing humans in microgravity activity in outer space. With the advent of cooperative international endeavors such as the Space Station, plans for a manned mission to Mars, and the real probability that China might attempt a mission to the moon, these considerations have assumed a more vigorous scientific scrutiny. The physiologic changes that occur to astronauts exposed to microgravity during space flight have been increasingly investigated. Body fluid volumes, electrolyte levels, and bone and muscle undergo significant changes as the body adapts to the weightless environment. There are both short-term space missions similar to those of Gemini, Apollo, and Space Shuttle flights and long-term missions such as Shuttle-Mir or Skylab [14]. In the former short-term space missions, negative calcium balance with bone mineral loss and associated hypercalciuria was noted during Gemini, Apollo, and Space Shuttle missions [14]. Additional alterations include elevated urinary phosphate, decreased fluid intake secondary to early flight space sickness (associated nausea and vomiting) with resulting decreased urinary volume and rising formation product [15]. Citrate has been shown to fall during space flight [16]. Whitson and coworkers have demonstrated that astronauts are at greater risk of forming calcium oxalate, calcium phosphate, and uric acid stones. In follow-up investigations, this same group studied more carefully 6 male astronauts with a mean age of 42.5 (range 36- 49 years old) flying Space Shuttle missions of 11 to 16 days [16]. Urine specimens were collected before, early in the mission (2-4 days), late in the mission (10-13 days), landing day, and 7 to 10 days after landing. Nutrition recommendations were rigorously controlled. Urine volume declined during the early flight but tended to equilibrate by post flight measurements. Urine output declined by 22-52% during spaceflight. Urine pH had a tendency toward increased acidity (lower pH) which also normalized by 7-10 days post flight. Urinary calcium levels increased for all members with individual variation being large (38 to 253 mg/d). Calcium excretion continued to increase during the flight. Urinary potassium was less during the early flight and urinary citrate was lower during the flight but neither were statistically different. The relative supersaturation of calcium oxalate, brushite, sodium urate, and uric acid all rose during early space flight. The calcium oxalate and brushite supersaturations remained statistically elevated throughout the entire space flight [16].

Whitson and colleagues further speculate that dietary factors of the astronauts also play a role in risk for urolithiasis formation. Fluid restriction, protein and calorie ingestion all increase urinary calcium and uric acid concentrations while decreasing urinary citrate. Dietary sodium can also promote renal calculus disease. Diets high in potassium and magnesium may have beneficial effects [16]. Zerwekh reviewed this metabolic data and generated specific nutritional recommendations for crew members on longer space missions. Pharmacologic intervention can raise urinary volumes, diminish bone losses and prevent reductions in urine pH and citrate levels [17].

There exists one published article suggesting that some cosmonauts have in fact formed stones during space missions [18-19]. Another report from NASA's Life Sciences Division suggests this to be a real probability [20]. In Pak's earlier investigations in stone formation by astronauts, he suggested that stone risk factors among applicants for spaceflight programs were environmental in origin [21].

STONES IN SPACE

Space flight is a hazardous activity. There are published well documented investigations into the pathophysiologic problems encountered [22]. In flight medical events for U.S. astronauts during the space shuttle program from April 1981 to January 1998 show a 42% incidence of space sickness but no definite reports of urinary colic and/or urolithiasis. Medical events reported from Russia's Mir from March 1995 to June 1998 likewise fail to reveal any stone events. But space exploration and manned flights are still infrequent compared to terrestrial explorations in other hazardous environments, such as deep sea and polar. Antarctic databases on health hazards also disclose no episodes of evacuation for urinary colic. The incidence of evacuation from U.S. submarines from 1993 to 1996 reveal 23 episodes of acute colic and stone passage out of 332 total emergency evacuations.

Stone disease represents a real risk to our human habitation in micro- or zero-gravity environments. The physiology behind this increased risk is well known and preventative strategies have been developed. The fact that stones in space have not been reported does not mean that they have not occurred. Astronauts as well as pilots in general have an obvious bias against coming forward in reporting these episodes, due to the fear of being grounded. In addition, the system would find that the cost of training specific individuals might outweigh the risk of stone formation in the "highly selected" individuals and efforts to keep them flying might outweigh and justify avoiding reporting. But stone disease in space is potentially serious, especially if exploration expands and extraterrestrial work environments are created that would prolong microgravity exposure times. NASA's "Bioastronautics Roadmap" calls renal stone formation "Risk 4." [23] The National Space Biomedical Research Institute calls stone disease "Risk 12." One published article only suggests that some cosmonauts have, in fact, formed stones during space missions. Detailed data from 79 U.S. space missions, involving 219 person-flights, and 175 astronauts do demonstrate 23 genitourinary problems (1.2% or 0.07 incidence per 7 days) but no further details are available. Conflicting data exists regarding actual space mission risk and stone incidence during submarine duty, but all would agree that the risk of stone disease in space is real. Attempts to evaluate both diagnostic and therapeutic interventions are being pursued actively and the funding for such endeavors is ongoing. As mankind strives to gain access to the final frontier of outer space, hazards must be assumed and methods for adapting to these risks must be found. Arthur C. Clarke stated, "*Two possibilities exist: either we are alone in the Universe—or we are not. Both are equally terrifying.*"

REFERENCES

1. Adams,D: *Hitchhikers Guide To The Galaxy*. Ballantine Books, NY, NY, 1979.
2. Kaku,M: *Visions. How Science Will Revolutionize the 21st Century*. Anchor Books. NY, NY, 1997.
3. Cadbury,D: *Space Race. The Epic Battle Between America and the Soviet Union For Dominion of Space*. Harper Collins Publishers, NY, NY, 2006.
4. Paul,HE. Bone suppuration the basic cause of renal calculus in twenty cases following war wounds. *J Urol* 9:345-362,1922.
5. Pyrah,LN, Fowweather,FS. Urinary calculi developing in recumbent patients. *Brit J Surg* 26:98-112,1938.
6. Pulvertaft,RG. Nephrolithiasis occurring in recumbency. *J Bone Joint Surg* 21:559-75,1939.
7. Deitrick,JE, Wheden,GD, Shorr,E. Effect of immobilization upon various metabolic and physiologic functions in normal men. *Am J Med* 4:3-36,1948.
8. Smith,PH, Cook,JB, Roberston,WG. Stone formation in paraplegia. *Paraplegia* 7:77-85,1969.

9. Elliot,JS, Todd,HE. Calculus disease in patients with poliomyelitis. *J Urol* 86:484-8,1961.
10. Gallacher,SJ, Ralston,SH, Dryburgh,FJ, Logue,FL, Allam,BF, Boyce,BF, Boyle,IT. Immobilization-related hypercalceemia- a possible novel mechanism and response to pamidronate. *Postgrad Med J* 66:918-22,1990.
11. Gordon,DL, Reinstein,L. Rehabilitation of the trauma patient. *Am Surg* 45:223-7,1979.
12. Slemenda,CW, Reister,TK, Hui,SL, Miller,JZ, Christian,JC, Johnston,CC Jr. Influences on skeletal mineralization in children and adolescents: evidence for varying effects of sexual maturation and physical activity. *J Pediatr* 125:201-7,1994.
13. Weaver,CM. Calcium requirements of physically active people. *Am J Clin Nutr* 72:579S-84S,2000.
14. Whitson,PA, Pietrzyk,RA, Pak,CYC, Cintron,NM. Alterations in renal stone risk factors after space flight. *J Urol* 150:803,1993.
15. Pietrzyk,RA, Feiveson,AH, Whitson,PA. Mathematical model to estimate risk of calcium-containing renal stones. *Mineral Electrol Metab* 25:199-203,1999.
16. Whitson,PA, Pietrzyk,RA, Pak,CYC. Renal stone risk assessment during Space Shuttle flights. *J Urol* 158:2305-10,1997.
17. Zerwekh,JE. Nutrition and renal stone disease in space. *Nutrition* 18:857-63,2002.
18. Garilevich,BA, Olefir,IuV. Urolithiasis in flight personnel. *Aviak Ekolog Medit* 36:49-53,2002.
19. Arzamazov,GS, Witson,PA, Lavina,ON, Pastushkova,LKh, Pak,CT. Assessment of the risk factors for urolithiasis in cosmonauts during long space flights. *Aviak Ekolog Medit* 30:24-32,1996.
20. Niccogossian,AE, Rummel,JD, Leveton,L Teeter,R. Development of countereasures for medical problems encountered in space flight. *Adv Space Res* 12:329-37,1992.
21. Pak,CY, Hill,K, Cintron,NM, Huntoon,C. Assessing applicants to the NASA flight program for their renal stone-forming potential. *Aviat Space Environ Med* 60:157-61,1989.
22. Bell,JR, Evens,Jr.,CH: *Safe Passage: Astronaut Care for Exploration Missions*. IOM, The National Academies Press, 2001.
23. NASA's *Bioastranautics Roadmap*: http//bioastroroadmap.nasa.gov

Aromatase Deficient Female Mice Demonstrate Altered Expression of Molecules Critical for Renal Calcium Reabsorption

Orhan K. Öz[*†], Asghar Hajibeigi[*†], Carolyn Cummins[‡], Monique van Abel[#], René J. Bindels[#], Makoto Kuro-o[¶], Charles Y.C. Pak[†§] and Joseph E. Zerwekh[†§]

[*]Radiology, [†]Center for Mineral Metabolism and Clinical Research, [‡]Howard Hughes Medical Institute, Pharmacology,, [¶]Pathology, [§]Internal Medicine, University of Texas Southwestern Medical Center, Dallas, TX, USA, [#]Physiology, University Medical Center Nijmegen, Nijmegen, Netherlands

Abstract. The incidence of kidney stones increases in women after the menopause, suggesting a role for estrogen deficiency. In order to determine if estrogen may be exerting an effect on renal calcium reabsorption, we measured urinary calcium excretion in the aromatase-deficient female mouse (ArKO) before and following estrogen therapy. ArKO mice had hypercalciuria that corrected during estrogen administration. To evaluate the mechanism by which estrogen deficiency leads to hypercalciuria, we examined the expression of several proteins involved in distal tubule renal calcium reabsorption, both at the message and protein levels. Messenger RNA levels of TRPV5, TRPV6, calbindin-D_{28K}, the Na^+/Ca^{++} exchanger (NCX1), and the plasma membrane calcium ATPase (PMCA1b) were significantly decreased in kidneys of ArKO mice. On the other hand, klotho mRNA levels were elevated in kidneys of ArKO mice. ArKO renal protein extracts had lower levels of calbindin-D_{28K} but higher levels of the klotho protein. Immunochemistry demonstrated increased klotho expression in ArKO kidneys. Estradiol therapy normalized the expression of TRPV5, calbindin-D_{28K}, PMCA1b and klotho. Taken together, these results demonstrate that estrogen deficiency produced by aromatase inactivation is sufficient to produce a renal leak of calcium and consequent hypercalciuria. This may represent one mechanism leading to the increased incidence of kidney stones following the menopause in women.

Keywords: aromatase, estrogen, kidney, calcium transport proteins, klotho
PACS: 87.19.Xx

INTRODUCTION

Premenopausal women have about one-half the prevalence of calcium stone disease than men of comparable age. However, this gender difference disappears rapidly after the onset of menopause. By age 55-60 the prevalence of calcium stone disease is equal in men and women and remains equal henceforth [1]. Several studies have provided evidence that urinary calcium excretion increases at menopause and could represent a major risk factor for calcium stone disease [2-4]. The rise in urinary calcium excretion appears to be the result of a renal leak of calcium and suggests that estrogen deficiency

CP900, *Renal Stone Disease, 1st Annual International Urolithiasis Research Symposium,* edited by A. P. Evan, J. E. Lingeman, and J. C. Williams, Jr.

may impair the tubular reabsorption of calcium. The mechanism by which estrogen might regulate calcium reabsorption is incompletely understood. Although our understanding of the normal mechanism by which the renal distal tubule cell reabsorbs calcium has been greatly enhanced in recent years [5], it is not known if estrogen can affect the expression or activity of any of these calcium transporting proteins. To address this issue we utilized the ArKO mouse model of estrogen deficiency to determine whether estrogen deficiency, as opposed to complete gonadal failure of ovariectomized models, is sufficient to alter renal calcium reabsorption and to investigate potential underlying mechanisms.

MATERIALS AND METHODS

Animals: The inactivated aromatase gene was maintained on the hybrid 129SvEV/C57Bl6. Animals used in all studies were 10-13 weeks of age. In some studies, 10 week old animals were treated 3 times/week with 20μg estradiol/mouse, or with sesame oil only (placebo) for 3 weeks. All procedures were approved by the UT Southwestern IACUC.

Analytical studies: Urine was collected from wild-type (WT) and ArKO age-matched mice in metabolic cages during an 18 hour fast or as 2 hour spontaneous voids. Kidneys were powdered under liquid nitrogen and the powder homogenized in TriReagent to obtain protein, DNA, and RNA in 3 different phases. After reverse transcription of the RNA fraction, quantitative real-time PCR was performed using appropriate primers. Messenger RNAs quantitated included TRPV5, TRPV6, calbindin-D_{28K}, PMCA1b and NCX1. Renal proteins were obtained from the organic phase of the TriReagent extract and subjected to SDS-PAGE on 12.5% polyacrylamide gels or Tris-Tricine gels (for calbindin-D_{28K} only). After transfer onto PVDF membranes, the proteins were visualized via incubation with specific antibodies and horse radish peroxidase (HRP) conjugated secondary antibody. Immunohistochemistry for some of the renal proteins was performed on bisected kidneys following dehydration and embedding in paraffin. Proteins of interest were detected after incubation with primary antibodies and the antibody detected using HRP conjugated secondary. Data are expressed as mean ± SEM. Comparison of mean values for statistical significance was accomplished by one-way ANOVA and post hoc analysis via the two-tailed Dunnett's test.

RESULTS AND CONCLUSIONS

Urinary calcium, expressed relative to creatinine, was significantly higher in ArKO mice as compared to WT (Table 1). This was true for spot urines as well as a longer fasting collection. Estradiol treatment reduced urinary calcium excretion to a value not significantly different from WT.

Real-time PCR analysis of mRNA levels for the proteins involved in transepithelial calcium reabsorption, disclosed significantly reduced expression for TRPV5, TRPV6, calbindin-D_{28K}, NCX1, and PMCA1b. Estradiol therapy raised TRPV5, calbindin-

D_{28K}, and PMCA1b mRNA to values not significantly different from WT (Fig. 1). NCX1 mRNA levels in ArKO kidneys remained significantly lower than WT after estradiol therapy. At the protein level calbindin-D_{28K} was significantly decreased in ArKO mice.

TABLE 1. Urinary calcium/creatinine ratios in ArKO and WT mice

Group	Ca/Cr		
	Spontaneous (mg/mg)	**Fasting (mg/mg)**	**GF corrected**
WT	0.123 ± 0.020 (n=10)	0.108 ± 0.022 (n=5)	0.011 ± 0.002 (n=5)
ArKO	0.181 ± 0.020[a] (n=10)	0.277 ± 0.050[a] (n=5)	0.034 ± 0.008[b] (n=5)
ArKO + E_2	—	0.078 ± 0.011 (n=5)	0.012 ± 0.003 (n=5)

[a]Significantly different from WT at $p<0.001$; [b]significantly different from WT at $p=0.03$.

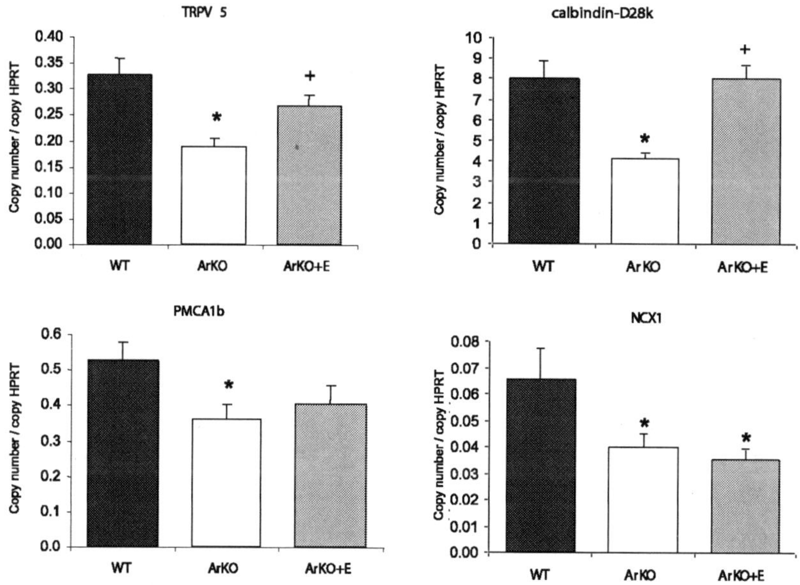

Figure 1. Effect of aromatase deficiency on mRNA levels of genes encoding proteins that regulate calcium transport in the kidney. *$p<0.05$ vs WT; + Not significantly different compared to WT.

Estradiol therapy raised the levels to those of WT (Fig. 2). Immunohistochemistry was performed to examine renal klotho expression. There was intense staining in the distal convoluted tubule but ArKO animals demonstrated much greater area of staining and with greater intensity. This was confirmed by real-time PCR and western blot analysis (Fig. 3). Estradiol treatment of ArKO mice decreased klotho expression in the kidney at both the mRNA and protein level.

Estrogen deficiency, produced by aromatase inactivation, is sufficient to cause renal calcium loss. The decreased reabsorption is associated with decreased expression of the proteins involved in the renal transcellular Ca reabsorption pathway including TRPV5 and 6, calbindin D_{28K}, and PMCA. These findings may provide a mechanism for the increased risk of nephrolithiasis and the observed increased incidence in females at the menopause.

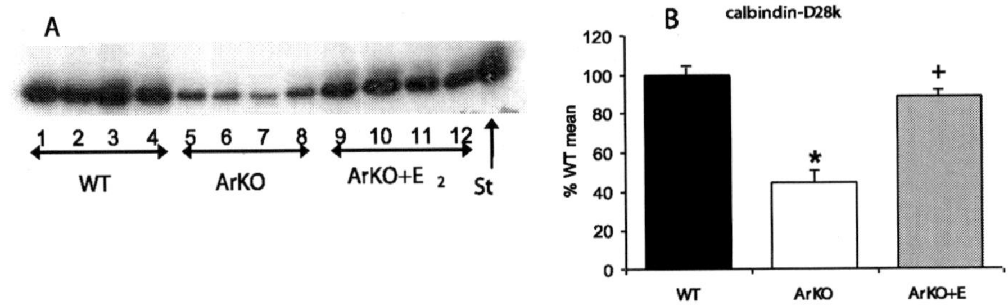

Figure 2. Effect of aromatase deficiency and estradiol supplementation on protein expression of calbindin-D_{28K}. (A) Membranes were probed with antibody to calbindin-D_{28K}. (B) Quantitative analysis of protein expression expressed as the ratio of band intensity for experimental groups to that for WT. *$p<0.05$ vs WT; + Not significantly different compared to WT

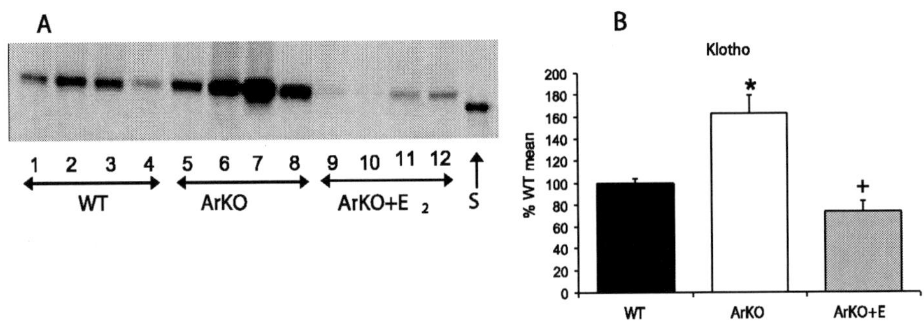

Figure 3. Effect of aromatase deficiency and estradiol supplementation on protein expression of klotho. (A) Membranes were probed with antibody to klotho. (B) Quantitative analysis of protein expression expressed as the ratio of band intensity for experimental groups to that for WT. *$p<0.05$ vs WT; + Not significantly different compared to WT.

ACKNOWLEDGMENTS

This work was supported in part by a grant from the seed account of the Center for Mineral Metabolism and Clinical Research at UT Southwestern Medical Center, in part by NIH HD01463, P01DK20543 and unrestricted funds from the endowment of the Effie and Wofford Cain Distinguished Chair in Diagnostic Imaging.

REFERENCES

1. Robertson WG, S.E. l, H.N. W 1999 The changing pattern of the age of onset of urinary stone disease in the UK. *Eighth European Symposium Urolithiasis*:165-168.
2. Heller HJ, Sakhaee K, Moe OW, Pak CY *J Urol* **168**(5):1923-1927 (2002).
3. Sakhaee K, Nicar MJ, Glass K, Pak CY *J Clin Endocrinol Metab* **61**(2):368-73 (1985).
4. Nordin BE, Polley KJ *Calcif Tissue Int* **41 Suppl 1**:S1-S9 (1987).
5. Hoenderop JG, Nilius B, Bindels RJ Annu Rev Physiol **64:**529-49 (2002).

Subcutaneous Marcaine Infiltration and Post-Operative Pain Perception after Percutaneous Nephrolithotomy

George E Haleblian, Victor A Leitao, Marnie R Robinson, Sean A Pierre, Roger L Sur and Glenn M Preminger

Duke University Medical Center – Division of Urology
Box 3167 Med Ctr, Durham, NC 27710

Abstract. Recent studies have shown a significant decrease in patient reported pain scores when operative incisions are infiltrated with subcutaneous local anesthetic. We hypothesize that patient reported pain and narcotic use could be further decreased for patients with post-percutaneous nephrolithotomy nephrostomy tubes if the nephrostomy tract and incision are infiltrated with local anesthetic.

Keywords: Percutaneous nephrolithotomy, pain
PACS: 87.19.Xx

INTRODUCTION

Since the first report from Fernström and Johansson on percutaneous stone removal in 1976 [1], percutaneous nephrolithotomy (PNL) has become the preferred approach for renal calculi greater than 2 cm [2]. PNL usually requires the placement of a percutaneous nephrostomy for renal drainage post-operatively, which is usually removed within 24-48 hours. Post-operative discomfort secondary to the nephrostomy tube remains a major concern.

Recently, it has been demonstrated that smaller nephrostomy tubes (10F *versus* 22F) decrease pain and analgesic requirements [3]. Decreasing the size of the nephrostomy tube also reduces urinary leak and length of hospital stay [4].

Infiltration of the surgical wound with marcaine following operative procedures has become a more common practice to improve post-operative analgesia and reduce narcotic use [5-7]. To our knowledge, no prospective, placebo-controlled study has been performed to assess the effect of subcutaneous infiltration of marcaine in the nephrostomy tract on post-operative pain perception and narcotic use.

MATERIALS AND METHODS

Twenty-five patients with renal stones greater than 2cm undergoing single access PNL were prospectively enrolled in the study. Informed consent was obtained prior to

CP900, *Renal Stone Disease, 1st Annual International Urolithiasis Research Symposium,* edited by A. P. Evan, J. E. Lingeman, and J. C. Williams, Jr.

enrollment. Patients were randomized in a single blinded manner to one of two groups (group 1: marcaine treatment and group 2: saline).

After completion of stone removal, a percutaneous nephrostomy tube (10F Cope loop pigtail catheter) was placed in all patients. Patients in group 1 received 1.5 mg/kg of 0.25% marcaine infiltrated subcutaneously into the nephrostomy tract using a 23G needle. Patients in group 2 received 60 ml of sterile saline infiltrated subcutaneously into the nephrostomy tract.

Pain scores were assessed using a validated linear visual analogue scale (VAS) at 2 hours, 6 hours, 24 hours, and 48 hours post-operatively. Post-operative narcotic analgesic consumption was recorded and converted into morphine equivalents. The nephrostomy tube was removed on the second day prior to discharge.

RESULTS

Twenty two patients were analyzed, with 10 patients in group 1 (marcaine) and 12 patients in group 2 (saline). Two patients were excluded due to insufficient data and one because of hydrothorax. Patients in group 1 had a mean age of 45.7 years and patients on group 2 a mean age of 45 years. There was no significant difference in mean operative times or blood loss between the two groups.

Scores from subjective pain assessment with VAS did not achieve statistical significance between the two groups at any time interval (2h, 6h, 24h and 48h). Although narcotic consumption tended to be lower in the marcaine group (24.7 mg *versus* 32.1 mg), it also did not reach statistical significance ($p=0.46$).

DISCUSSION

PNL has undergone many technological advances in access material and technique, as well as in lithotripters and in related equipment. It has improved the efficacy and safety of the procedure such that it is the standard of care for treatment of complex staghorn calculi or renal stones >2 cm in size [2]. Traditionally, after completion of PNL, a nephrostomy tube is placed for 48 hours and removed prior to patient discharge.

Studies have been performed demonstrating that decreased nephrostomy tube size has a significant impact on pain and analgesic consumption. Pietrow and associates have shown that the use of a 10 F Cope loop catheter has decreased patient reported pain scores post operatively, and a trend toward lower narcotic consumption post operatively when compared to the 22 F nephrostomy tube [3]. Maheshwire *et al.* also demonstrated that a 9F pigtail nephrostomy catheter decreases pain and medication demand [4]. Belmann reported that in selected cases the nephrostomy tube could be avoided [9], and recently this approach has been used more frequently [10, 11], although avoiding the use of a nephrostomy tube is not routine in treatment of complex calculi [12,13].

Studies in anesthesia, surgery and gynecology literature have described the efficacy of local anesthetic infiltration in surgical incisions. These include efficacy in cesarean sections, thyroid surgery, and mastectomy [14-16]. In the urologic literature, further evidence of efficacy of local anesthesia has been shown in cases involving varicocele ligation under local anesthesia [17].

To our knowledge, this study is the first to compare pain score and analgesic consumption between marcaine and saline subcutaneous infiltration of the nephrostomy tract after PNL. Post-operative pain scores did not differ significantly between the two groups. Narcotic use showed a trend towards decreased requirements in the marcaine group, but this difference did not reach statistical significance. One of the potential confounding factors in this study may be the relatively small number of patients in each group.

CONCLUSION

No significant difference in patient reported pain scores was observed in this pilot study. A trend towards reduced narcotic use was seen in the marcaine group, although this did not reach statistical significance. Additional studies are warranted to define additional measures to reduce patient discomfort for those requiring a nephrostomy tube following PNL.

REFERENCES

1. I. Fernstrom and B. Johansson. Percutaneous pyelolithotomy. A new extraction technique. *Scand J Urol Nephrol* **10,** 257-9 (1976).
2. G. M. Preminger, D. G. Assimos, J. E. Lingeman, S. Y. Nakada, M. S. Pearle, J. S. Wolf Jr, AUA Nephrolithiasis Guideline Panel. Chapter 1: AUA guideline on management of staghorn calculi: diagnosis and treatment recommendations. *J Urol* **173**, 1991-2000 (2005).
3. P. K. Pietrow, B. K. Auge, C. D. Lallas, R. W. Santa-Cruz, G. E. Newman, D. M. Albala , G. M. Preminger. Pain after percutaneous nephrolithotomy: impact of nephrostomy tube size. *J Endourol* **17**, 411-414 (2003).
4. P. N. Maheshwari, M. G. Andankar, M. Bansal. Nephrostomy tube after percutaneous nephrolithotomy: large-bore or pigtail catheter? *J Endourol* **14,** 735-737 (2000).
5. P. Biboulet, D. Morau, P. Aubas, S. Bringuier-Branchereau, X. P. Capdevila. Postoperative analgesia after total-hip arthroplasty: Comparison of intravenous patient-controlled analgesia with morphine and single injection of femoral nerve or psoas compartment block. a prospective, randomized, double-blind study. *Reg Anesth Pain Med* **29,** 102-109 (2004).
6. A. Ng, A. Swami, G. Smith, A. C. Davidson, J. Emembolu. The analgesic effects of intraperitoneal and incisional bupivacaine with epinephrine after total abdominal hysterectomy. *Anesth Analg* **95**, 158-162 (2002).
7. L. H. Pobereskin and J. R. Sneyd. Wound infiltration with bupivacaine after surgery to the cervical spine using a posterior approach. *Br J Anaesth* **84,** 87-88 (2000).
8. E. N. Liatsikos, D. Hom, C. Z. Dinlenc, R. Kapoor, M. Alexianu, P. Yohannes, A. D. Smith. Tail stent versus re-entry tube: a randomized comparison after percutaneous stone extraction. *Urology* **59,** 15-19 (2002).
9. G. C. Bellman, R. Davidoff, J. Candela, J. Gerspach, S. Kurtz, L. Stout. Tubeless percutaneous renal surgery. *J Urol* **157**, 1578-82 (1997).
10. J. Limb and G. C. Bellman GC. Tubeless percutaneous renal surgery: review of first 112 patients. *Urology* **59**, 527-31 (2002)

11. A. Tefekli, F. Altunrende, K. Tepeler, A. Tas, S. Aydin, A. Y. Muslumanoglu. Tubeless percutaneous nephrolithotomy in selected patients: a prospective randomized comparison. *Int Urol Nephrol.* 2006 Dec 14; [Epub ahead of print]
12. S. C. Kim, W. W. Tinmouth, R. L. Kuo, R. F. Paterson, J. E. Lingeman. Using and Choosing a Nephrostomy Tube after Percutaneous Nephrolithotomy for Large or Complex Stone Disease: A Treatment Strategy. *J Endourol* **19,** 348-352 (2005).
13. H. N. Shah, V. B. Kausik, S. S. Hegde, J. N. Shah, M. B. Bansal. Safety and efficacy of bilateral simultaneous tubeless percutaneous nephrolithotomy. *Urology* **66,** 500-504 (2005).
14. A. Bagul, R. Taha, M. S. Metcalfe, N. R. Brook, M. L. Nicholson. Pre-incision infiltration of local anesthetic reduces postoperative pain with no effects on bruising and wound cosmesis after thyroid surgery. *Thyroid* **15:** 1245-1248 (2005).
15. P. O, Ranta, T. I. Ala-Kokko, J. E. Kukkonen, P. P. Ohtonen, T. H. Raudaskoski TH, P. K. Reponen, N. J. Rawal. Incisional and epidural analgesia after caesarean delivery: a prospective, placebo-controlled, randomised clinical study. *Int J Obstet Anesth* **15:** 189-194 (2006).
16. N. Rawal, A. Gupta, M. Helsing, K. Grell, R. Allvin. Pain relief following breast augmentation surgery: a comparison between incisional patient-controlled regional analgesia and traditional oral analgesia. *Eur J Anaesthesiol* **23**, 1010-1017 (2006).
17. P. Gontero, G. Pretti,, F. Fontana, A. Zitella, G. Marchioro, B. Frea. Inguinal versus subinguinal varicocele vein ligation using magnifying loupe under local anesthesia: which technique is preferable in clinical practice? *Urology* **66**, 1075-1079 (2005).

It Pays to Read the Old Dead Guy's Papers: Triggering Doses of Oxalate and Calcium Oxalate Nephrocalcinosis

Susan Ruth Marengo and Ailin Zhang

Department of Urology, Case School of Medicine, Cleveland, OH 44106-4931

Abstract. It has been hypothesized that high triggering doses of hyperoxaluria induce crystal formation, while lower maintenance doses promote crystal growth. We confirmed this using minipumps secreting 30 to 60 µmol potassium oxalate per day to induce modest, continuous hyperoxaluria for 28 days after the triggering dose (288 µmol oxalate) was given as an i.p. injection or infused over 24hr. Calcium oxalate crystal deposition was induced in 6/6 rats. This hypothesis could explain the modest clinical correlation between oxalate excretion and calcium oxalate stone disease.

Keywords: oxalate, nephrocalcinosis, rat, stone disease
PACS: 81.10.Dn

INTRODUCTION

The role of oxalate in calcium oxalate (CaOx) stone disease is somewhat of an enigma. Although oxalate excretion is an important factor in the calculation of CaOx urolithiasis risk indices and in a stone former's medical work up, it is not tightly tied to stone former status. One explanation for this apparent paradox is that many such patients have transient spikes in oxalate excretion—probably induced by dietary indiscretions—which trigger the formation of CaOx crystals. Consuming the amount of oxalate in a standard serving of spinach can increase plasma oxalate concentrations and raise oxalate excretion 3-4 fold over fasting values [1]. A modestly elevated basal oxalate excretion could then foster crystal growth.

Vermeulen's laboratory developed the triggering/maintenance hypothesis of hyperoxaluria in the 1960's [2]. Rats fed a diet of 1.2% oxamide for 3 days (triggering dose) followed by a diet of 0.4% oxamide for 25 days (maintenance dose) developed intratubular CaOx nephrocalcinosis and papillary CaOx surface deposits. The triggering and maintenance doses did not induce CaOx nephrocalcinosis if given alone. We used the minipump model of continuous hyperoxaluria to reappraise this hypothesis. In this model minipumps are implanted subcutaneously and deliver a standard dose of oxalate [3-4]. This direct delivery avoids potential problems due to variation in gut absorption or metabolism of precursor to oxalate.

CP900, *Renal Stone Disease, 1st Annual International Urolithiasis Research Symposium,*
edited by A. P. Evan, J. E. Lingeman, and J. C. Williams, Jr.

METHODS

Male Sprague-Dawley rats (197-312 gm) were treated with PBS vehicle or a maintenance dose of potassium oxalate (KOx) ± a triggering dose of oxalate on day 0. Maintenance doses of KOx were administered by constant infusion from an osmotic minipump implanted subcutaneously on days 0 and 14 [3-4]. Treatments were: Control (PBS for 28 days, n=4); Constant KOx (60 μmol KOx/day for 28 days, no triggering dose, n=3); StepDown KOx + NaOx Injection (60 μmol KOx/day for days 0-14, 30 μmol KOx/day for days 15-28, 288 μmol NaOx i.p. triggering dose on day 0, n=3); StepDown KOx + KOx 1day Pump (60 μmol KOx/day for days 0-14, 30 μmol KOx/day for days 15-28, 288 KOx minipump triggering dose on day 0-1, n=3). 24hr urine samples were collected in the presence of HCl+azide on day 0-1, day 6-7, day 13-14, day 14-15, day 20-21 & day 27-28. Urine oxalate was determined spectrophotometrically by the oxalate-oxidase assay. The presence or absence of crystals was determined on frozen sections stained with Toluidine blue and observed under polarizing optics.

RESULTS & DISCUSSION

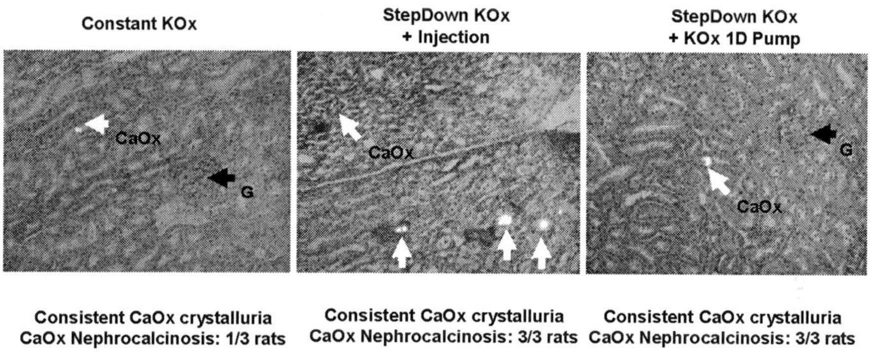

FIGURE 1. Representative CaOx nephrocalcinosis in KOx treated rats. White arrows indicate CaOx nephrocalcinosis, black arrows glomeruli, 20x. CaOx nephrocalcinosis was not observed in controls.

All rats receiving oxalate had frequent-to-persistent CaOx crystalluria. CaOx nephrocalcinosis was present in 0/4 Control rats, 1/3 Constant KOx, 3/3 StepDown KOx + NaOx Injection, and 3/3 StepDown KOx + KOx 1day Pump. Most of the crystals were in the cortex, although a few were in the medulla or, rarely, the papilla (Fig. 1).

Individual profiles for oxalate excretion are shown in Fig. 2. On day 0 or 1, Constant KOx rats averaged 2.5-fold oxalate excretion as compared to Control rats, while StepDown KOx + NaOx Injection rats averaged 4.8-fold and StepDown KOx + KOx 1day Pump averaged 8.3-fold. Averaging oxalate excretion over the rest of the treatment period, the mean daily excretion was less than twice that of Control rats.

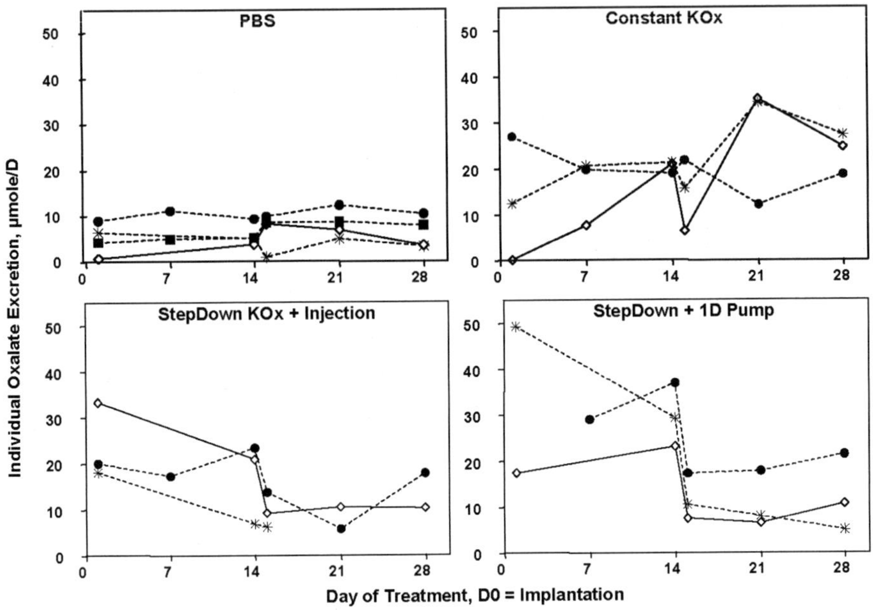

FIGURE 2. Oxalate excretion patterns for individual rats.

The sum of the triggering dose (288 µmol) plus the maintenance dose (60 µmol/day) of oxalate on day0-1 was 348 µmol of oxalate. In previous studies 100% of the rats receiving 360 µmol KOx/day for 13 days developed CaOx nephrocalcinosis [3-4]. A reduction of even 17% in the dose of oxalate reduced CaOx nephrocalcinosis to 27% in these rats, even though CaOx crystalluria remained consistent. This suggests that the initiation of nephrocalcinosis depends on a critical condition other than the mere presence of crystals. Our data suggest that markedly elevated oxalate excretion, even for brief periods, may be of critical importance in this process.

Previous models of oxalate-driven CaOx nephrocalcinosis require either several months of treatment, high levels of continuous hyperoxaluria (> 5 times normal excretion), ancillary metabolites, or the presence of hypercalciuria. Our preliminary data support Vermeulen's "trigger & maintenance" hypothesis of hyperoxaluria, in that a triggering dose of oxalate over 24 hr plus a modest level of hyperoxaluria for 28 days consistently induced CaOx nephrocalcinosis. After further development, this model seems likely to be clinically relevant for patients with CaOx stone disease and persistent, mild hyperoxaluria.

ACKNOWLEDGMENTS

This work was supported by an American Foundation for Urologic Research Bridge Grant and NIH-NIDDK R01 DK073730.

REFERENCES

1. R.P. Holmes, W.T. Ambrosius, and D.G. Assimos, *J Urol* 174, 943 (2005).
2. C.W. Vermeulen, E.S. Lyon, J.E. Ellis et al., *J Urol* 97, 573 (1967).
3. S.R. Marengo, D.H-C. Chen, G.T. MacLennan et al., *J Urol* 171, 1304 (2004)
4. S.R. Marengo, D.H.-C. Chen, A.P. Evan et al., *Urol Res* 34, 200 (2006).

Labouring Under The Stone—A Literary Legacy of Lithiasis

Michael E. Moran

Capital Region Urologic Surgeons, Albany, NY USA

Abstract. The history of mankind's suffering greatly from calculus disease has been one of excruciating longevity. Since the first historical records, humans have formed stones and endured the wrath of these concretions' passage via the delicate mechanisms of the urinary tract. This study involved detailed investigations of historical writings of famous stone sufferers to better appreciate the circumstances of our patients. Collected histories both of textbooks and articles were scrutinized for the accounts of famous stone sufferers. Once identified, primary resources were sought with English translations given preference. Cross-referencing all informational sources was attempted. The accounts were then classified as lower urinary tract (BS), upper urinary tract (KS), by century of the individual, and whether these were ancient (before 100 years ago) or recent (from the 20th Century onwards). Many of these great men and woman suffered in relative silence. Not much is available on descriptions of their colic. However, there are others such as Michel Montaigne, Erasmus of Rotterdam, Benjamin Franklin, Thomas Sydenham, Sir William Osler and Richard Selzer who were able to transform their suffering into ethereal expressions of pure pain and suffering. The ancient descriptions are twofold fascinating, as the victims of stone disease faced quackery and profound ignorance from the medical profession and no effective remedy for the pain. Here again, there are two typical responses: the enlightened cerebral concerns of Montaigne, Sydenham, and Franklin versus the punitive, religious overtones from Erasmus and Pepys. Lower and upper tract stones produced equal horrors to those once thought to incur punishment from the gods, or turning to stone-like "living statues." No amount of literary expression can capture the true essence of renal colic. Medical texts from their earliest times place stone passage near the top of the pantheon of medical suffering. Each of these prolific and erudite stone sufferers provides us, the next generation, a unique window into the perception of colic. "The colic was followed by an ulcer, or more accurately, by a hard swelling which first extended all along the lower right groin. Then it centered on the pit of my stomach, almost like a dragon with its teeth biting my navel while the rest of its body was writhing and its tail stretching towards my loins…it causes constant, sometimes, unbearable pain." [Erasmus]

Keywords: urolithiasis, history
PACS: 01.01.00; 01.65.+g; 87.19.Xx

INTRODUCTION

The history of mankind's suffering from disease has no more eloquent tale, than that of its suffering from urolithiasis. Humans have experienced urinary colic from the beginnings of recorded civilization. In addition, our knowledge that humans have been afflicted with urinary tract stones date from an El Amrah boy, about age 16, dating from 4800 BC from Prof. G. Elliott Smith in the Hunterian Museum [1]. This

CP900, *Renal Stone Disease, 1st Annual International Urolithiasis Research Symposium,* edited by A. P. Evan, J. E. Lingeman, and J. C. Williams, Jr.

represents a scholarly review of early writings, some personal (i.e. journals), some essays, and others direct observations from eye witnesses of people suffering from urinary colic who could not do so in silence. These are explorations of written accounts of suffering from stone disease for those of us who today are still attendant upon those who suffer. This is a story of renal colic, expressed by those who have experience firsthand. Attempts at expressing their suffering in their own words can provide remarkably poignant insights into those who suffer. Some, such as Montaigne, have left such a vast array of literature expressing their pain and suffering that it is difficult to judge which parts to include. Stone sufferers also probably had to deal with the added anxiety that, at least up until the 1920's, the medical profession had almost nothing to offer. (Laudnum was introduced for pain and suffering by Paracelsus in the 16th century [2].) Stone sufferers were thus doubly entrapped: lack of medical knowledge and a surgical armamentarium that was even worse—more torture than therapy.

EARLY MODERN SUFFERING

"I want to be seen here in my simple, natural, ordinary fashion, without straining or artifice, for it is myself that I portray." Thus begins Michel de Montaigne's accounts of his life and studies [3]. From 1577-78 this extraordinary man journeyed throughout Europe to both discover himself and learn to live his life of recurrent suffering from urolithiasis. "I am in the grips with the worst of all maladies, the most sudden, the most painful, the most mortal, and most irremediable." Montaigne traversed on horseback most of Europe and continued eloquently to document his torment, but developed a stoic, almost conversational ability to see himself outside of his body. He is an early enlightened mind that is skeptical of the medical profession of the time. He does not believe anything that has been told to him about his disease and has queried others about their medical therapies. Unfortunately, he will be forced to consult with these "professionals" out of sheer necessity.

Desiderius Erasmus lived between 1466 and 1536 and was widely believed to be the most brilliant mind of the age. He was a "classic scholar" and was recruited by almost every royal court to "lend counsel."

> *This is now the fourth month of my illness. First I suffered from colic, then from vomiting. This poor little body of mine does not get along very well with the doctors. All the medicines they gave me did me harm...The colic...was followed by a hard swelling which first extended all along the lower right groin. Then it centered on the pit of my stomach, almost a dragon with its teeth biting my navel while the rest of its body was writhing and its tail stretching towards my loins; when its head was fastened tight it coiled around to the left side of my navel, with its tail almost encircling it. It caused constant, sometimes unbearable pain. I could not eat or sleep or write or read.*

Erasmus knew almost all of the "best" physicians of his era and sought help from them, including Paracelsus. Though a known humanist, the suffering for Erasmus took on a more dark, sinister punishing sort of experience for him, versus the more stoic descriptions of Montaigne. "What is this [torture by the stone] but tasting of death again and again? Deliver me, if possible from this evil which is in me." [4]

Finally, the great physician William Harvey himself suffered with stones. One eyewitness account records his suffering.

> *...he made himselfe a way to putt himselfe out of his paine, by opium; not but that, had he laboured under great paines, he had been readie enough to have donne it; I doe not deny that it was not according to his principles upon certain occasions to..."*

The profession had nothing much to offer those suffering under the stone, not even to themselves [1].

WRITERS SUFFERING WITH THE STONE

Stone disease has continued to afflict others throughout the world, and writers form an interesting subject of study. Samuel Pepys kept detailed journals of his life in Elizabethan England. He religiously documented each episode of colic he suffered. "

> *...cold weather, which for these two days has been frost, in some pain in my bladder. Dined at home and then with my wife to the Paynter's...which brings great pain in my back...as it used to when I had the stone...*

In March of 1658 Pepys underwent the dangerous operation for the removal of a bladder stone which was about the size of a golf ball. He kept it in a special display case and he celebrated the anniversary of surviving this ordeal with a party where the "trophy" was passed all around [5].

On September 1, 1997, this literary legacy was recapitulated by Tom Chiarella in Esquire Magazine [6].

> *Enter the kidney stone, the wolverine of pain, mythic in its ferocity, intensity, and blind instinct to maim. One stab of pain from a kidney stone and you'll never want to piss again. Passing one is like digesting a razor blade.*

He continued in this literary vein,

> *The stone can strike at any time. One minute, you're on the couch watching SportsCenter™, the next you're corkscrewing headfirst into the Berber, sucking air, waving the white flag on life. You stand up. You sit down. You curl up. You grip your sides. Nothing helps.* [6]

Finally, in the modern era when electronic entertainment has nearly replaced written media, Kramer of *Seinfeld* fame summarizes his suffering from stone passage as follows: "And this jagged shard of calcium pushes its way through the ureter into the bladder. It's forced out through the urine!" [7]

PHYSICIANS AND SUFFERING

The final contribution in this literary overview comes from our colleagues in medicine who have suffered amongst the lot of the stone afflicted. Benjamin Franklin received an honorary medical degree as well as being a founding father of this country. His father and oldest brother both suffered from stones. Franklin's curiosity about this disease would portend ominously for his own future suffering.

> *Because now disabled by the Stone, which the Easiest Carriage gives me Pain, wounds my bladder, and occasions me to make bloody Urine...I am more afraid of the Medicines than of the Malady.* [8]

Other great medical minds also suffered such as Antonio Scarpa, Johan van Beverwijck, Boerhaave, Thomas Linarce, John Joans, and Philip Syng Physick but they did so silently [9]. Thomas Syndenham though did not:

> *Gout produces calculus in the kidney...the patient has frequently to entertain the painful speculation as to whether gout or stone be the worst disease. Sometimes the stone, on passing...kills the patient, without waiting for the gout...* [10]

Sir William Osler likewise followed in his idol's footsteps, suffering in like fashion. His textbook of medicine, referred by many to be the bible of disease at the turn of the 20th century has a particular feel of empathy, since pen and patient were known sufferers.

> *And then abruptly, or working out of the steady pain, came the paroxysm, like a twisting, tearing hurricane, with its well-known radiation, followed by the vasovagal features, the pallor, cold extremities, feeble pulse, sweating, nausea, vomiting, and in two attacks, a final, not altogether unpleasant period, when unconsciousness and pain seemed wrestling for a victory reached with the help of God's own medicine—morphia.* [11]

One final physician/author is worth presenting here, a surgeon by trade who would know best what types of descriptive metaphors might best sum up his personal agony. Richard Selzer penned this:

> *Delicate durability describes the human body, and nowhere is this more apparent that in the urinary tract. If the liver is all bulk and thunder, the heart fist and thrust and piston, and the brain a foamy paste of insubstantial electricity, the parts of the urinary tract-namely the kidneys, ureters, and bladder- are a tracery of tubules and ducts of such fineness as would lay mad a master plumber, more, a Venetian glassblower.*

He warms to his topic, by introducing the reader to the pathophysiology of supersaturation:

> *What is man, the son of man, asks the biochemist, but a container of salt solution in a state of more or less saturation?*

Finally he winds his way into personal torment:

> *Thus is agony born. The speck hardens, concretes, is overlaid with more salt dust, becomes compressed. Spikes extend from it, pits are excavated, until it has a shape as distinctive as a face...There in the dank and humid corners of the kidney, the dragony thing lurks until weaned from its cache by the horrid principles of physics and chemistry.*

And the pain is experienced:

> *Then there is Pain. But such a pain as defies words of mouth or pen to set it down, pain that, by its intensity, elects the sufferer to an aristocracy of endurance, from which all mere mortals are excluded. He who has not felt the boiling grip of colic in back or side or belly has not the language of this elite, is illiterate of their tongue.* [12]

CONCLUSIONS

Colic has been described as the most intense and severe pain that a human can appreciate. That said, it is commonly quoted that no one has ever died of pain. Stones have afflicted mankind since the alluvial beginnings. Though those of us who treat, study, investigate, and research the spectrum of urolithiasis genuinely know that these patients do indeed suffer, it is not widely appreciated to what extent. We have a priceless legacy of stone formers who have heroically suffered and written of their misery. Their legacy is a window into the patients who still suffer mostly silently, awaiting our medical wisdom; whether palliation of pain and suffering while attempting to pass these concretions, or bravely harrowing the modern surgical environment of mid-infrared lasers and high energy shock waves or ultrasonic disruption.

REFERENCES

1. Ellis,H: *A History of Bladder Stone*. Blackwell Scientific Publ., Oxford, 1969.
2. Ball,P: *The Devil's Doctor. Paracelsus and the World of Renaissance Magic and Science*. Farrar, Straus and Giroux, New York, 2006.
3. Montaigne, M: *The Complete Works: Essays, Travel Journal, Letters*. Transl. Donald M. Fram, Hamish Hamilton, London, 1957.
4. Healy,M: Journeying with the "Stone": Montaigne's healing travel journal. *Lit and Med* 24(2):231-249,2006.
5. Samuel Pepys *Biography*. http://www.pepys/info
6. Chiarella, T, Leclerc, A: Stranded in midstream. *Esquire* 128 (3):134, 1997.
7. *Seinfeld.* The Gymnast. Sony Pictures, Season 6, Episode 6, November 3, 1994.
8. Comer,GW, Goodwin,WE: Benjamin Franklin's bladder stone. *J Hist Med All Scie* Oct:361-377,1953.
9. *A Bicentennial History of the Practice of Urology in the United States*. Medical Communications Inc, Northfield, IL, 1976.
10. Sydenham,T: *A treatise on gout and dropsy*. Transl by R.G. Latham, 1688.
11. Bliss,M: *William Osler. A life in medicine*. Oxford Univ Press, Oxford, 1999.
12. Slezer,R: *Mortal Lessons: Notes on the art of surgery*. Simon and Schuster, NY, 1974.

Calcium Oxalate Accumulation in Malpighian Tubules of Silkworm (*Bombyx mori*)

Aaron J. Wyman and Mary Alice Webb

Department of Botany and Plant Pathology, Purdue University, West Lafayette, IN 47907

Abstract. Silkworm provides an ideal model system for study of calcium oxalate crystallization in kidney-like organs, called Malpighian tubules. During their growth and development, silkworm larvae accumulate massive amounts of calcium oxalate crystals in their Malpighian tubules with no apparent harm to the organism. This manuscript reports studies of crystal structure in the tubules along with analyses identifying molecular constituents of tubule exudate.

Keywords: Calcium oxalate (CaOx), silkworm, *Bombyx mori*, Malpighian tubules
PACS: 87.68.+z

INTRODUCTION

Research into kidney stone diseases would greatly benefit by having a simple, easily manipulated genetic model system allowing for direct analyses of factors affecting calcium oxalate crystallization. Silkworms (*Bombyx mori*) provide an ideal candidate, as they accumulate large amounts of calcium oxalate crystals in their Malpighian tubules [1,2], organs that function like mammalian kidneys and are considered analogous to kidney epithelium [3]. Previous studies of silkworm tubules established that the calcium oxalate crystals developed in association with an organic matrix of unknown composition [1,2]. A myriad of cytological, molecular, and genetic tools, including a complete genome sequence, are now available for studying silkworm [4,5]. We are currently developing silkworm as a model experimental organism to examine factors, including genetic mutations and diet, which can influence calcium oxalate crystallization in mammalian kidney stone disease.

RESULTS AND DISCUSSION

Crystallization of calcium oxalate is a normal feature of tubule development in silkworms feeding on their native diet of mulberry leaves (Fig. 1). Shortly after larvae hatch and begin feeding, calcium oxalate crystals develop inside the Malpighian tubules, which form closed loops (Fig. 1). As crystals accumulate, the tubules begin to appear birefringent in the light microscope under crossed polarizers, and by 24 hours after hatching crystals fill the lumen of the tubules, which become highly birefringent (data not shown). Silkworm larvae go through five developmental stages, or instars,

CP900, *Renal Stone Disease, 1st Annual International Urolithiasis Research Symposium,* edited by A. P. Evan, J. E. Lingeman, and J. C. Williams, Jr.

which are separated by a molting cycle in which the larval "skin" is shed. Initial studies have indicated that crystals persist in the Malpighian tubules through all five instars (data not shown). In related species, fluxes in calcium oxalate within the Malpighian tubules occur in relation to molting [6]. However, similar fluxes have not been reported in silkworm, and it is not known whether they occur.

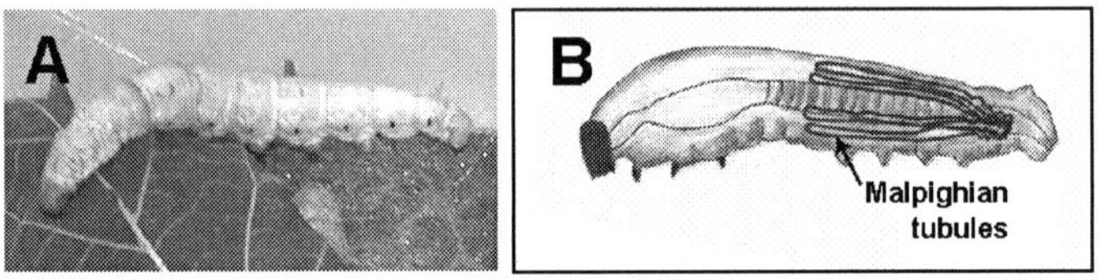

FIGURE 1. **A:** Mature silkworm larva on a mulberry leaf just before pupation (0.5X). **B:** Tracing of Malpighian tubules in 72 hr larva viewed under crossed polarizers (7X).

Structural Studies

To observe calcium oxalate crystals in the lumen of the Malpighian tubules, second instar larvae were prepared for cryo-SEM by rapid freezing followed by fracturing of the frozen sample and sublimation of the fractured surface. Phenomenal accumulations of tablet-shaped crystals of calcium oxalate were observed in the tubule lumen (Fig. 2). Crystals are not randomly arranged, but rather occur in oriented stacks, indicating that they do not float free within the lumen. Strands of matrix of unknown composition were observed on and between individual crystals. Crystals isolated from second instar larvae were also observed in the SEM. Isolated crystals had a regular characteristic structure, consisting of thin rectangular tablets with rounded corners and variable length to width ratios (Fig. 3). A small proportion of the crystals form spherical aggregates (arrow) apparently resulting from interpenetrant twinning. Crystals isolated from fifth instar larvae were similar but had a more elongate shape with pointed ends (not shown). At both stages observed, parallel faces of the tablets appeared smooth relative to the edges, which had a coarse appearance.

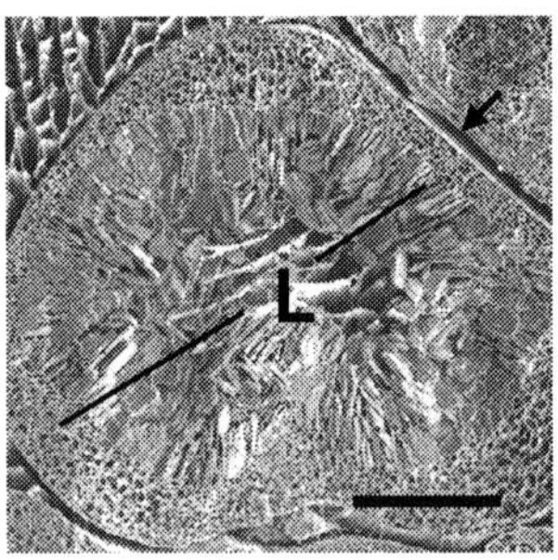

FIGURE 2. Transverse fracture of a second instar silkworm, showing a Malpighian tubule with its lumen filled with calcium oxalate crystals. In insects a single cell layer forms the tubules with a

basement membrane on the outside (arrow) and microvilli (obscured by crystals) on the inside bordering the lumen (–L–). Bar = 30 μm.

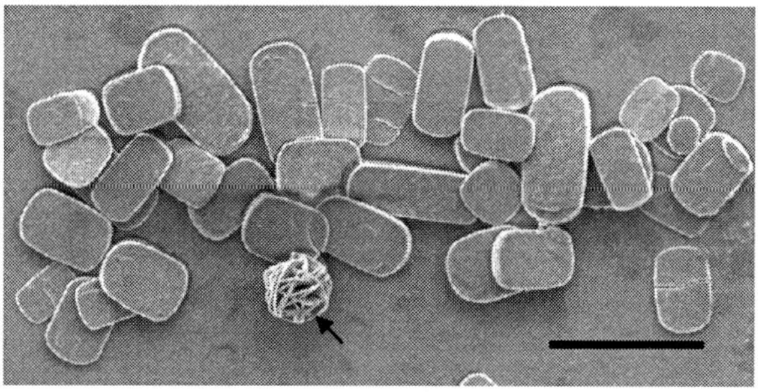

FIGURE 3. Calcium oxalate crystals isolated from Malpighian tubules of silkworm. Bar = 10 μm.

Analysis of Tubule Exudate

When Malpighian tubules dissected from silkworms were cut, a yellowish fluid was released along with calcium oxalate crystals. Samples of fluid exudate were analyzed for proteins and small molecules. Exudate proteins separated by SDS-PAGE (sodium dodecyl sulfate-polyacrylamide gel electrophoresis) consisted of a complex mixture of polypeptides. Selected polypeptide bands were excised from gels and were prepared by standard methods [7] for analysis by MALDI-TOF MS (matrix-assisted laser desorption/ionization-time of flight mass spectrometry). Homologous sequences were identified with the MASCOT search engine, a probability-based scoring system [8], using the NCBI (National Center for Biotechnology Information) non-redundant protein database. Sequences identified with significant MASCOT scores (Table 1) included membrane transport proteins, chaperones, enzymes, regulatory or signaling proteins, and cytoskeletal elements. With the exception of the signaling proteins, all proteins listed in Table 1 have also been found in the proteome of human urine [9]. Their common presence in both urine and Malpighian tubule exudate further supports the utility of silkworm as a model system for kidney stone disease.

TABLE 1. Selected Proteins Identified in Silkworm Tubule Exudate

Function/Identity (organism)	Accession #	MASCOT Score
Chaperones		
DnaJ (*Theileria annuata*)	gi|65302773	55
Hsc70 (*Bombyx mori*)	gi| 112982828	74
Hsp90 (*B. mori*)	gi|112983556	404
Transporters		
H^+-ATPase (*Manduca sexta*)	gi|9714	85
V-ATPase (*B. mori*)	gi|114052088	52
Enzymes		
Hydroxypyruvate isomerase (*B. mori*)	gi|114052328	80
Glutathione-S-transferase (*B. mori*)	gi|61287207	55
Signaling/Regulatory Proteins		

cAMP-regulated phosphoprotein 19 (*Danio rerio*)	gi|34783815	59
Ankyrin repeat protein 26 (*Mus musculus*)	gi|109940218	52
Calcium-regulated protein (*Strongylocentrotus purpuratus*)	gi|72085956	73
Numerous cytoskeletal elements	--	>55

To identify other constituents of the tubule exudate, samples of exudate were collected in absolute ethanol and derivatized for analysis by GC-MS (gas chromatography-mass spectrometry). Among the most abundant small molecules in the exudate (Table 2) were the five amino acids listed, but other amino acids were present at lower concentrations, including phenylalanine, lysine, glutamine, glycine, methionine, asparagine, and proline. Citrate and other organic acids were also prominent. Many of these molecules are also characteristically abundant in normal human urine and may influence calcium oxalate crystallization [10,11]. Oxalate and mineral ions were not detectable with this methodology but will be targeted in future analyses using ion chromatography.

Preliminary studies not included in this manuscript have examined the effects of diet on calcium oxalate accumulation in silkworm larvae. Distinct differences in tubule size and birefringence were observed between larvae fed their natural diet of mulberry leaves, which contain substantial amounts of oxalate, and larvae fed an alternative diet of low-oxalate lettuce (Wyman and Webb, unpublished data). Studies similar to those reported here will be used to compare the effects of diet on calcium oxalate crystallization and constituents of the Malpighian tubules in silkworms.

TABLE 2. Constituents of Silkworm Exudate Identified by GC-MS Analysis

Abundant Amino Acids	Organic Acids	Other
leucine	citric acid	putreanine
isoleucine	malonic acid	insect hormones
tyrosine	succinic acid	fatty acids
serine		wax components
threonine		

SUMMARY AND CONCLUSIONS

Silkworm larvae raised on their natural diet of mulberry leaves accumulate massive amounts of tablet-shaped calcium oxalate crystals in their Malpighian tubules. Constituents of exudate collected from Malpighian tubules include proteins, amino acids, organic acids, and other small molecules. Many of the molecules identified in this study are also present in human urine. Use of silkworm to study factors affecting calcium oxalate crystallization provides a simple model system for kidney stone disease in humans.

ACKNOWLEDGMENTS

We thank Ed Simpson for his help with maintaining silkworm stocks. We also thank Amber Hopf, Kevin Kowalski, and Dorota Inerowicz (Bindley Biosciences) for their aid with the GC-MS and MALDI-TOF-MS analyses, respectively. We acknowledge use of the Life Sciences Electron Microscopy Center and thank Debby Sherman for her assistance. Thanks also to Jo Anne Fisher for help with Figure 1. We are grateful for the support provided by the College of Agriculture and the Department of Botany and Plant Pathology at Purdue University.

REFERENCES

1. D. J. Teigler, H. J. Arnott, *Nature* **235**, 166-167 (1972a)
2. D. J. Teigler, H. J. Arnott, *Tissue Cell* **4**, 173-185 (1972b)
3. R. Cagan, *Curr Opin Nephrol Hypertens* **12**, 11-17 (2003)
4. M. R. Goldsmith, T. Shimada, H. Abe, *Annu Rev Entomol* **50**, 71-100 (2005)
5. J. Wang, Q. Xia, X. He et al., *Nucleic Acids Res* **33**, D399-D402 (2005)
6. R. Barbier, B. Le Garff, *Int J Insect Morphol & Embryol* **14**, 3-20 (1985)
7. M.C. Hall, M. P. Torres, G. K. Schroeder, C. H. Borchers, *J Biol Chem* **278**, 16698-16705 (2003)
8. D. N. Perkins, D. J. C. Pappin, D. M. Creasy, J. S. Cottrell, *Electrophoresis* **20**, 3551-3567 (1999)
9. J. Adachi, C. Kumar, Y. Zhang, J. V. Olsen, M. Mann, *Genome Biol* **7**, R80 (2006)
10. I. K. Tan, B. Gajra, *Ann Acad Med Singapore* **35**, 468-475 (2006)
11. A. Guerra, T. Meschi, F. Allegri et al., *Urol Res* **34**, 359-364 (2006)

Famous Stone Patients and Their Disease

Michael E. Moran

Capital Region Urologic Surgeons, Albany, NY USA

Abstract: The fact that stone patients have endured much throughout the ages and that prior to our current era, when the ultimate horror, "being cut for the stone" was the only alternative to the repeated episodes of colic, should be recalled from time to time. Urolithiasis has affected humanity throughout the ages and has been indiscriminate to those lives it touched. A full accounting of those who have suffered and recorded their agonies is beyond the scope of this investigation; however, even a partial accounting is valuable for present day physicians who care for those with stone disease. For the present work, the historical accounts of stone disease literature were scrutinized for individual sufferers who could be cross-referenced from other sources as legitimately afflicted by stones. Only those patients that could be documented and were (or are) well known were included, because the internet is now a verdant repository of thousands of "not so well knowns." Reliable historical data was found for a variety of persons from the pre-Christian era to the present, including those remembered as philosophers and scientists, physicians, clergy, leaders and rulers, entertainers, athletes and fictitious/Hollywood-type individuals. Verified accounts of famous stone formers were chosen for this paper, and are presented in chronological order. The list of urolithiasis sufferers presented here is undoubtedly incomplete, but it is not through lack of trying that they are missing. Most often, the suffering do so silently, and that is always allowed.

Keywords: urolithiasis, history
PACS: 01.01.00; 01.65.+g; 87.19.Xx

INTRODUCTION

The literature is strewn with the flotsam and jetsam of diatribes regarding the cause and effects of urolithiasis. But in the final accounting of disease, human beings contract each episode and suffer individually. An investigator deals with statistics, and patient lists generate clinical series. Often overlooked is the individual. It is almost impossible to write a scientific paper any longer about an individual without crossing the threshold of impropriety or now federal legislation concerning HIPAA violation (Health Insurance Portability and Accountability Act of 1996, public law 104-191). Yet the individual is the unique endpoint of all discussions of disease, the final common denominator between treatment and outcome. So it behooves those whose mission it remains to become knowledgeable about stone disease to have at least passing knowledge of a catalog of the only patients one can discuss outside of these realms of impropriety and Federal jurisdiction: those who suffered in the historic past. Our society has already bypassed the acceptable boundaries of this indiscretion for a more tabloid notoriety. This represents an attempt at scholarly, chronologic listing of famous urolithiasis sufferers.

CP900, *Renal Stone Disease, 1st Annual International Urolithiasis Research Symposium*,
edited by A. P. Evan, J. E. Lingeman, and J. C. Williams, Jr.

METHODS

The Internet and historical literature regarding urolithiasis provides the student of history a list of famous stone sufferers. Any cross-referenced confirmation of these patients' stone sufferings were then traced. If there is identified confirmatory information from secondary sources, they were included in this list. Recognizing that the list, no matter what details could be found, is likely to be incomplete, this author leaves additions to the list to fall upon the shoulders of others in the future. The particular emphasis of the present search was upon science writing and articles from the past, as the modern current literature suffers from the society-imposed necessity to make anonymous the identity of present-day stone sufferers. In this article, there will be no emphasis on the suffering or treatment of these people. The purpose is to just generate a single list, as comprehensive as possible, of famous stone patients.

RESULTS

The following table represents a verified list of famous stone patients. They are classified by the category or profession that each individual would be most identified. Some well-known stone patients, such as Ben Franklin, could be listed in several categories, but only one was chosen here. (For example, Franklin is listed as a physician, because of his particular medical interests in stone disease.) In addition, within each classification, persons are listed in chronological order.

CONCLUSIONS

From the very earliest records, humans have been plagued by urolithiasis. There are no known ancient manuscripts that document individuals who have suffered, but the first known instance comes to us from Diogenes Laertius regarding the philosopher, Epicurus [2]. His stone disease would result in loss of life. Some histories describe that the stone disease itself had affected the outcomes of wars, as in the case of Napoleon III [3]. Others have had their suffering transformed into miraculous cures requiring sainthood (Saint Henry of Bavaria, Fig. 1). Some have taken the desperate route of surgical lithotomy and lived to tell about it (Pepys and Marshall). Some suffered enough to brave the knife, but were not so lucky, like Leopold of Belgium. Stones have afflicted the poor, the evil, the wealthy and the most devout without discrimination (Fig. 2, Pope Innocent XI's stone, 1689). Stone sufferers have publicly aired their sufferings, which represent a literary legacy that has seldom been mentioned at stone meetings (see my paper on this elsewhere in this Proceedings, pp. 402-405). Some writers have brazenly described their suffering from colic in magazines such as *Esquire* or in reference to their works (Alan Ginsberg and Richard Selzer). The notion of the stone patient's suffering has most recently become a somewhat *cause célèbre* might be illustrated by the fictional characters that have been cropping up on sitcoms and TV shows, including Kramer from *Seinfeld* and Joey from *Friends*.

TABLE 1. Famous stone formers.

Pre-Christian era	
El Amrah boy age 16 dated about 4800 B.C. (Prof. G. Elliott Smith in Hunterian Museum)[1]	
Epicurus (270 B.C.)[2]	
Philosophers/Scientists	
Erasmus of Rotterdam[3]	Michel de Montaigne [4]
Francis Bacon (and his brother) [5]	Galileo
Johan van Beverwijck [3]	Isaac Newton [6]
George-Louis Leclerc (Count of Buffon)	Horace Walpole
Isaac Asimov [7]	
Physicians	
Boerhaave	Thomas Syndenham [8]
Antonio Scarpa	Benjamin Franklin [9]
Thomas Linacre	William Harvey
John Jones	Philip Syng Physick [1]
Sir William Osler [10]	Richard Selzer [11]
Clergy	
Pope Innocent XI	John Wilkins
Pope Clement XI	
Leaders	
Henry II of Bavaria	Frederick III (King of Saxony)
Peter the Great	Louis XIV
Oliver Cromwell	Sir Kenelm Digby
John Marshall [1]	King George IV
John Hart (signer of the Declaration of Independence)	Napoleon Bonaparte
King Leopold I of Belgium	Napoleon III
Lyndon Johnson	Dennis Hastert (House Speaker)
John Prescott	
Artists/Entertainers	
Alan Ginsberg (poet)	Ava Gardner
Gay Talese	John Derek (husband of Bo)
Suzanne Strempek Shea	William Shatner
Bruce Springsteen	Tito El Bambino
Karl Pilkington	John Wilkins
Athletes	
Joe Mauer (baseball)	
Fictitious TV/Movie Characters	
Kramer (6th episode of *Seinfeld*)	Joey of *Friends*
Al Swearengen in TV series *Deadwood*	Muddy Waters in *Family Guy*
Duckman (from the cartoon *Duckman*)	Brock (TV series *Reva*)

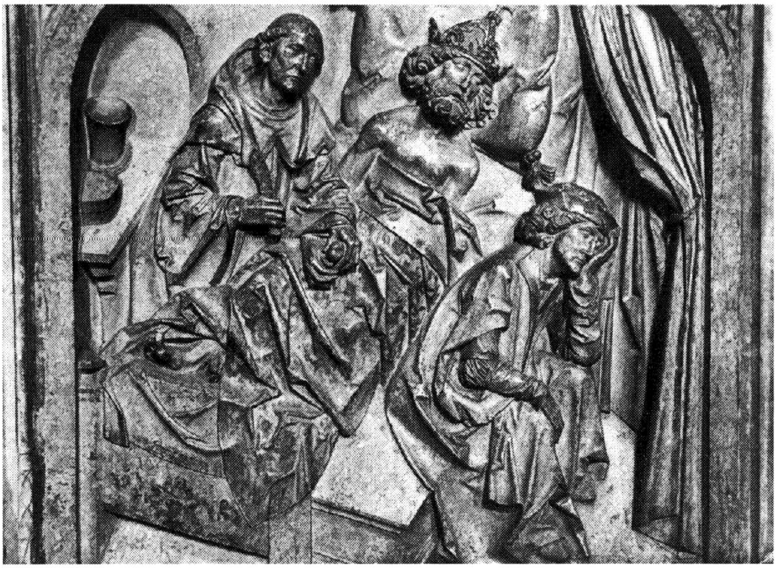

FIGURE 1. Sculpture of Henry II of Bavaria (by Riemenscheider, circa 1499-1513). Later canonized as St. Henry, he suffered from bladder stones and is said to have been cured in his sleep by St. Benedict, the figure at left, who is placing the stone in Henry's hand. The figure at the right is that of a doctor, sleeping. Wellcome Library, London; used by permission.

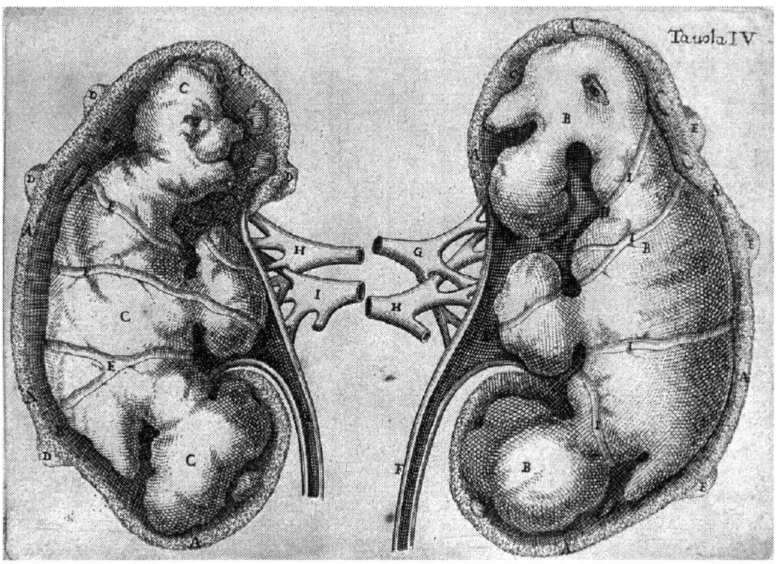

Figure 2. Drawing of the kidneys of Pope Innocent XI, who died of urolithiasis. The illustration was published in 1707 by Tommaso Alghisi. On the left is the right kidney, with the large stone marked as **C**; the letter **E** marks channels through the stone, which evidently carried what little urine was produced by the remaining renal tissue (**A**). The left kidney (on the right) shows similar structure, with the stone marked by **B**, and the channels through the stone by **I**. Wellcome Library, London; used by permission.

Whatever the interest in urolithiasis at scientific meetings, the focus is rightly on pathophysiology, preventative strategies, incidence, therapeutics and surgery. But the lessons of the past should not be forgotten, and the legacy of the individual might yet be introduced by knowledge of those who have suffered. Famous stone sufferers do not lead us to knowledge that will change the disease, but their legacy should not be lost.

REFERENCES

1. Ellis,H: A History of Bladder Stone. Blackwell Scientific Publ., Oxford, 1969.
2. Bitsori,M, Galanakis,E: Epicurus' death. *World J Urol* 22(6):466-469,2004.
3. Engel,RM: *De Historia Lithomiae*. http://www.urolog.nl/urolog/php/content.php?doc=lithotomia &profmenu=yes
4. Healy,M: Journeying with the "stone": Montaigne's healing travel journal. *Literature and Med* 24(2):231-249,2006.
5. Winer,R: Comments on Francis Bacon's 1625 essay on a "...Regimen of Health." http://www.gesher.org/Articles/Health/Comments%20on%Bacon's%20Regimen%of
6. Ostad,E, Wise,GJ: Celestial bodies and urinary stones: Isaac Newton (1641-1727)- health and urological problems. *BJU Internat* 95:24-26,2005.
7. Asimov, I.: *It's Been a Good Life*, Prometheus Books, Amherst, NY, 2002.
8. Dehurst,K: *Dr. Thomas Sydenham, his life and original writings*. Wellcome Institute, London, 1966.
9. Bliss,M: *Sir William Osler. A Life in Medicine*. Oxford University Press, Oxford,1999.
10. Corner,GW, Goodwin,WE: Benjamin Franklin's bladder stone. *J Hist Med All Sci* Oct:361-377, 1953.
11. Selzer,R: *Mortal Lessons: notes on the art of surgery*. Simon and Shuster, NY, 1974.

Evaluation of Medical Cystine Stone Prevention in an Animal Model

Sreedhar Sagi, Gunnar Wendt-Nordahl, Peter Alken, and Thomas Knoll

Department of Urology, University Hospital Mannheim, Theodor-Kutzer-Ufer 1-3 68135 Mannheim, Germany

Abstract. Medical treatment for cystinuria aims to decrease the concentration of cystine in the urine, increase its solubility and therefore prevent stone formation. Ascorbic acid and captopril have been recommended as alternatives to thiol drugs, though conflicting data undermining their efficacy has been widely reported, too. The aim of this study was to verify the effects of ascorbic acid and captopril on cystine stone formation in the cystinuria mouse model. A total of 28 male homozygous *pebbles* mice were used for characterizing the mice on normal diet, ascorbic acid and captopril supplemented diets. The *baseline* physiological parameters of the mice were determined initially. The normal diet was then replaced with the supplemented diet (ascorbic acid/captopril) for the next 48 weeks and various biochemical parameters in urine and plasma were analyzed. All homozygous mice developed urinary cystine stones during the first year of life. No reduction in the urinary cystine concentration was seen with either of the supplemented diets. The stone mass varied widely in the study and a beneficial effect of ascorbic acid in some of the animals was possible though an overall statistical significance was not seen. Conclusions: The cystinuria mouse model provides an ideal tool for evaluation of stone preventive measures in a standardized environment. This study confirms that ascorbic acid and captopril are not effective in cystinuria.

Key words: animal models; ascorbic acid; captopril; cystinuria; inborn genetic diseases; urinary calculi
PACS: 87.19.Xx

INTRODUCTION

Cystinuria, a genetic disorder, is the cause of 1-2% stones observed in adults and up to 10% of those occurring in children [1]. Cystinuria is characterized by an increased urinary excretion of cystine and other dibasic amino acids (lysine, arginine and ornithine). Due to the low solubility of cystine in urine, the increased excretion results in the formation of cystine stones. Patients with cystinuria frequently form urinary cystine calculi and may subsequently require multiple stone removing procedures during their lifetime, which could have an impact on their renal function [2]. The uptake of cystine is mediated by the $b^{o,+}$ heterodimeric amino acid transporter system which is defective in cystinuria. The $b^{o,+}$ system consists of two sub units, the heavy chain rBAT which associates with the light chain $b^{o,+}$ AT. Mutations in the two genes, SLC3A1 (rBAT) and SLC7A9 ($b^{o,+}$ AT) have been shown to lead to the cystinuria phenotype [3-5]. Cystinuria type I, the most common variant of the disease, results

CP900, *Renal Stone Disease, 1st Annual International Urolithiasis Research Symposium,* edited by A. P. Evan, J. E. Lingeman, and J. C. Williams, Jr.

from a defect in the rBAT subunit of the cystinuria transporter [6]. An important target for the prevention of cystine stones is cleavage of the disulfide bond of cystine. The resulting cysteine molecule is significantly more soluble in physiological urine and does not form stones. D-penicillamine and alphamercaptopropionylglycine (α-mpg) are the most widely used drugs for this. D-penicillamine is a thiol drug which creates complexes that are 50 times more soluble than cystine [7]. α-mpg is a mercaptan agent with similar chemical structure and mechanism of action as D-penicillamine, but has been shown to be 50% more effective [8]. However, side-effects of these drugs are common and long-term patient compliance is low. Ascorbic acid (vitamin C) is described as having redox capabilities leading to a reduction of cystine to the more soluble cysteine. Asper and Schmucki first proposed an ascorbic acid therapy for cystinuria in the early 80's [9]. These reports led to the recommendation of mega-doses ascorbic acid by the European Association of Urology (EAU) for patients with mild cystinuria (<3 mmol/d). Captopril, a first-generation angiotensin converting enzyme (ACE) inhibitor has been to shown to reduce urinary cystine concentration in patients with cystinuria [10]. Captopril also contains a free sulfydryl group that can cleave the disulfide bond of cystine. Streem and Hall [11] have concluded captopril can significantly, and at times profoundly, decrease urinary cystine excretion in patients with homozygous cystinuria. However, conflicting data concerning the efficacy of ascorbic acid and captopril has been widely reported too.

The efficacy of these therapies is hard to evaluate as the number of available patients at any one center is low. An established animal model could overcome this problem as it provides adequate numbers for testing in a standardized environment, unlike the testing in human volunteers where cystine concentration can be affected by dietary preferences, sodium and fluid intake. The first mouse model, *pebbles,* which mimics human cystinuria type I, provides an ideal tool for evaluation of stone preventive measures [12]. The aim of this study was to test the effects of ascorbic acid and captopril on cystine stone formation in the *pebbles* cystinuria mouse model.

METHODS

Animals

Pebbles is a murine model for type I cystinuria, created by an N-ethyl-N-nitrosourea-induced mutation in SLC3A1 resulting in a single amino acid substitution in the extracellular domain of rBAT (Ingenium Pharmaceuticals, Munich, Germany). Newborn mice were genotyped for the SLC3A1 mutation and identified as wild type (Wt), heterozygous (Ht) or homozygous (Ho) for the mutation by restriction fragment length polymorphism assay. All the mice were maintained in 12 h light–dark cycles with free access to tap water and standard chow *ad libitum*. Housing facilities and all experimental procedures were conducted in compliance with the EEC Directive 86/609 and with the animal welfare regulations (Tierschutzgesetz, TSG, and The Society of Laboratory Animal Science, GV-SOLAS).

Ascorbic acid and captopril supplemented diets

Homozygous male *pebbles* mice were used to determine the efficacy of ascorbic acid and captopril in the prevention of cystine stones. The mice (n=28) were fed with normal diet (ND) for the first 12 weeks to obtain the *baseline* levels of various biochemical parameters in plasma and urine The normal diet was modified to include 65 mg of ascorbic acid (AA) and 2 mg captopril per kg body weight (ssniff Spezialdiäten, Soest, Germany). The normal diet was replaced with the AA (n=8) and captopril (CP, n=8) supplemented diets and maintained for the next 42 weeks. Homozygous mice (n=12) receiving the ND served as controls. After 42 weeks, the animals were sacrificed. Cystine stones in the urinary tract were identified initially by x-ray and later, after extraction of the stones, by x-ray diffraction analysis.

Biochemical parameters in plasma and urine

Blood was drawn from the orbital sinus of the eyes of the mice and plasma was collected by centrifugation. The mice were housed in metabolic cages to collect the 24-hour urine samples. The levels of creatinine, urea, protein, sodium, potassium in plasma and urine were measured using a Hitachi Auto analyzer 911E. The urinary oxalate levels were determined by ion chromatography. Urinary cystine and cysteine levels were determined by mass spectrometry.

Statistical analyses

All numerical results are expressed as means ± standard deviation (SD) for 'n' animals in each protocol. Differences between means were evaluated by the Scheffé test. A value of $p \leq 0.05$ was considered statistically significant. All calculations were performed with the SAS statistical software package.

RESULTS

Effects of ascorbic acid supplemented diet (AA) on homozygous *pebbles* mice

Renal function was only dependent on the genotype and was not altered with the change in diet (Table 1). AA did not bring about any significant changes in the metabolic or physiological parameters of the homozygous mice. There were no significant differences among the creatinine, urea, protein, potassium and sodium levels in the plasma of the homozygous mice irrespective of the diet. The urinary cystine levels remained unaffected with the change in diet. There was no significant difference in the cystine excretion among mice fed with ND or AA. The cystine levels were consistent in all the mice for the entire duration. All the mice had similar cystine excretion as the *baseline* when normalized at various time intervals (Fig.1). AA did not cause any significant change in the urinary levels of creatinine, urea, sodium, protein and albumin. The oxalate levels in urine tended to be lower in AA mice (29±22 mg/l) compared to ND mice (75±93 mg/l) though this difference was not significant. A significant reduction of the pH was observed in AA mice: The urinary pH in ND mice averaged 7.4±0.6 while it averaged 6.2±0.8 (p=0.047) in AA mice. There was no significant difference in the creatinine clearance (CrCl) among the mice on ND or AA (ND: 0.27±0.22 ml/min; AA: 0.13±0.06 ml/min). Significant progression of renal impairment was observed in all the mice irrespective of the diet. This was evident by observing the high urinary indices of the fractional excretion of sodium (FENa) and renal failure index (RFI).

Table 1. Evaluation of urinary functional parameters in mice fed on normal (ND) and ascorbic acid supplemented diet (AA), showing means ± SD. $^*p=0.047$; $^\dagger p\leq 0.05$

	ND	AA
Cystine (mg/l)	164±19	185±51
Cysteine (mg/l)	99±61	825±2156
Creatinine (mg/dl)	11.39±9.44	5.82±2.24
Urea (mg/dl)	4994±3260	2041±825
Oxalate (mg/l)	75±93	29±22
Sodium (mmol/l)	95.09±54.02	48.55±7.49
Protein (mg/ml)	0.45±0.15	0.43±0.47
Albumin (mg/ml)	11.65±7.0	19.21±25.53
pH	7.4±0.6	6.2±0.8*
Creatinine clearance (ml/min)	0.27±0.22	0.13±0.06
Fractional excretion of sodium	1.03±0.48	2.09±0.74†
Renal fractional (failure) index	1.52±0.71	3.20±1.16

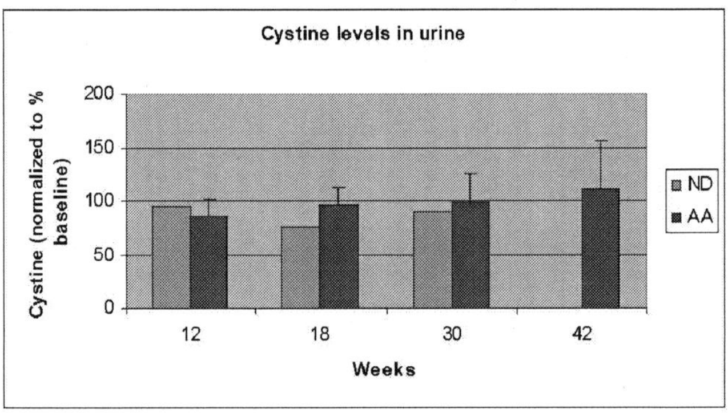

Figure 1. Cystine levels in urine. ND: Normal diet, AA: Ascorbic acid supplemented diet. Cystine values have been normalized to the baseline(100%). The time interval at 42 weeks could not be taken into consideration due to the death of control mice.

X-ray analysis after 42 weeks of therapy revealed the presence of cystine calculi in the urinary bladder of all the homozygous mice irrespective of the diet (Fig.2). No calculi were observed in the kidneys. X-ray diffraction analysis of calculi identified all stones as purely composed of cystine. The weight of the cystine calculi differed significantly between the individuals. Although urinary cystine excretion was comparable, there was a tendency for reduction of stone mass in homozygous males on AA diet (94±68), though the difference was not statistically significant. The stone mass in Ho males on ND (389±292 mg) was highly variable among the individuals (Fig.3). The ascorbic acid supplemented diet did not cause any major impact on the physical characteristics of the mice. No significant increase or decrease in food/diet consumption or in the weight of the mice over the *baseline* was seen in any of the mice irrespective of the diet. The water consumption and urine excretion were not significantly different among the mice.

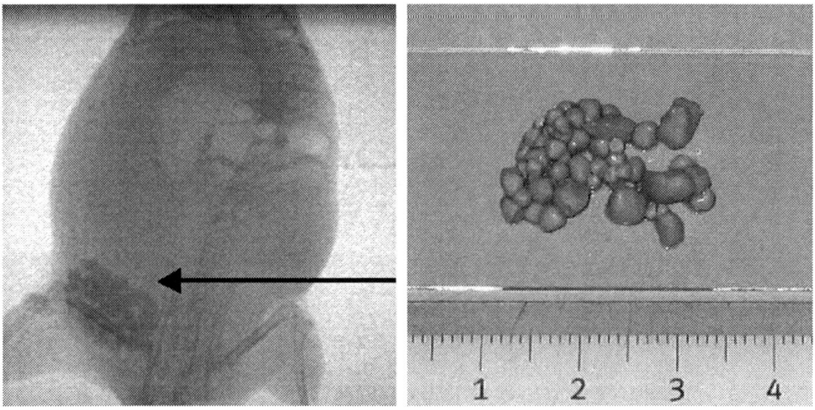

Figure 2. *Left*: X-ray image of the homozygous *pebbles* mouse (60 weeks of age), showing cystine stones in bladder. *Right*: Cystine calculi (stones) extracted from the bladder of the same mouse.

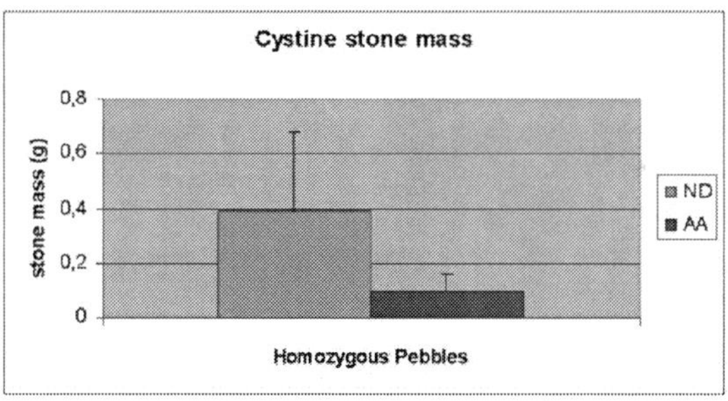

Figure 3. Mean cystine stone mass in ascorbic acid therapy. ND: Normal diet, AA: Ascorbic acid supplemented diet.

Effects of captopril supplemented diet (CP) on homozygous *Pebbles*

The physiological and biochemical parameters were similar in all the mice irrespective of the diet (Table 2). No significant changes were observed in the creatinine, urea and protein levels in the plasma. A significant increase was found in the potassium levels in the plasma of CP mice (4.84±0.25, $p \leq 0.0082$) compared to mice on ND (4.62±0.39). A significant difference was also found in the sodium levels in plasma (ND: 155.28±4.15; SD: 151.09±3.72, $p \leq 0.0004$). There was no significant difference in the urinary cystine excretion among mice fed with ND or CP (Fig.4). Cysteine, the reduced product from cystine was also not significantly different in either of the diet groups. The cysteine values were very variable irrespective of the diet. No significant differences were observed in urea or creatinine in relation to diet. Unlike urea and creatinine, the albumin values were dependent on the individual mice significantly ($p<0.0182$), though they had similar values in the diet groups (ND: 18.08±17.67 mg/ml; CP: 18.30±21.40 mg/ml). There was no significant change in the urinary pH in mice on CP. The CrCl, FENa values were similar both the diet groups. All the mice had high RFI (>1) irrespective of the diet, indicating a post renal failure. X-ray analysis after 48 weeks of treatment revealed the presence of cystine calculi in the urinary bladders of all mice irrespective of the diet. The weight of the cystine calculi did not differ significantly between the groups (ND: 0.1±0.07 g; CP: 0.15±0.1 g; Fig.5). No significant differences were seen in the food and water consumption in the mice. All the mice weighed similar irrespective of the diet. The urine excretion was also similar in all the mice irrespective of the diet.

Table 2. Evaluation of urinary functional parameters in mice fed on normal (ND) and captopril supplemented diet (CP).

	ND	CP
Cystine (mg/l)	211±74	214±53
Cysteine (mg/l)	354±223	463±367
Creatinine (mg/dl)	6.51±3.18	6.30±2.31
Urea (mg/dl)	2264±1618	2152±626
Sodium (mmol/l)	41.80±7.45	46.10±7.93
Potassium (mmol/l)	100.40±22.05	100.47±17.39
Protein (mg/ml)	0.45±0.57	0.40±0.38
Albumin (mg/ml)	18.08±17.67	18.30±21.40
pH	6.12±0.46	6.52±1.06
Creatinine clearance (ml/min)	0.14±0.08	0.15±0.06
Fractional excretion of sodium	0.76±0.42	0.76±0.29
Renal fractional (failure) index	1.18±0.65	1.15±0.44

DISCUSSION

Effects of ascorbic acid supplemented diet on homozygous *pebbles*

Vitamin C (Ascorbic acid) is recommended for stone prevention in patients with moderate cystine excretion. This study was done to ascertain the efficacy of ascorbic acid as a therapeutic agent for cystinuria. Asper and Schmucki first publicized the use of ascorbic acid therapy in cystinuria patients [9]. They used 5 g of ascorbic acid per day and observed 40% decrease in cystine concentration. Lux and May [13] also proposed that ascorbic acid therapy is a practical, inexpensive prophylaxis for cystine stone patients. Birwe et al. [14] have also investigated the efficacy of ascorbic acid therapy. They report only a mild decrease in cystine values in both cystinurics and control patients (11% & 23% respectively). They indicate that AA therapy seems to be of use only in patients excreting 3,000 µmol cystine/ day. In this study in *pebbles* mice with a similar concentration of ascorbic acid in the diet, there was no reduction in the urinary cystine concentration compared to the mice on ND. Reducing the urinary concentration of cystine is considered the primary goal for treatment of cystinuria, thereby reducing the super saturation and crystallization of cystine in urine [15]. It was evident that AA could not reduce the urinary cystine concentration in *pebbles* mice. Ragone [16] strongly contradicts the notion of ascorbic acid in reducing the urinary cystine levels. He points out through the redox equations that ascorbic acid is not capable of transforming cystine into cysteine, which requires a stronger reducing agent.

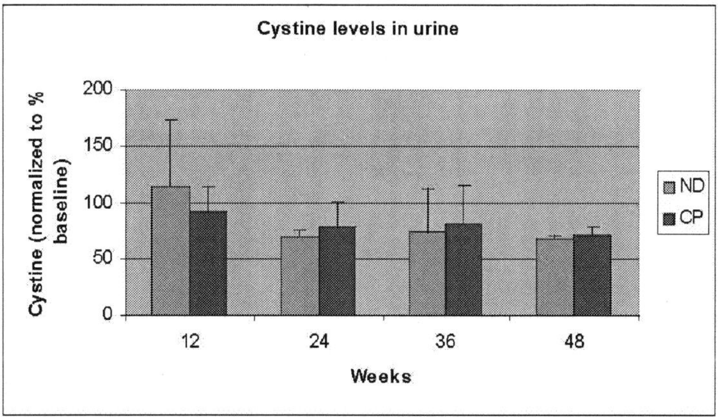

Figure 4. Cystine levels in urine. ND: Normal diet, CP: Captopril supplemented diet. Cystine values have been normalized to the baseline (100%).

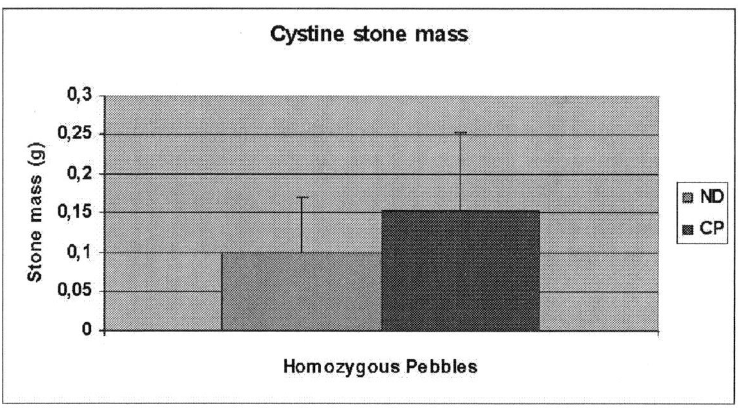

Figure 5. Mean cystine stone mass in captopril therapy. ND: Normal diet, CP: Captopril supplemented diet.

At the end of 42 weeks, when the animals were sacrificed, the stone mass seen in mice with AA was only insignificantly lower than the stone mass found in mice on ND. However, several authors reported stone formation in patients with relatively low cystine excretion and, in contrast, infrequent stone formation in patients with high urinary cystine excretion [17,18]. This may confirm the findings of comparable cystine excretion in treated and non-treated animals but slightly lower stone mass in the AA group. Stone mass did vary largely in the study and a beneficial effect of ascorbic acid in some of the animals is possible but did not lead to an overall statistical relevance.

Urinary pH plays a very important role in cystine stone prevention. Cystine is reported to dissolve more easily in alkaline urine than acidic urine. In medical practice, ascorbic acid may be given in the form of an effervescent tablet. The sodium bicarbonate present in these tablets causes urinary alkalization. It was observed that the pH of the homozygous *pebbles* mice under AA decreased to the acidic range. It is known that AA changes the pH of the urine to acidic in nature [19]. No alkalizing agent was used to increase the pH in contrast to the studies in human subjects by other groups in order to separate the effects of the sodium bicarbonate from ascorbic acid. Lux and May [13] conclude that the beneficial effects of ascorbic acid in reducing cystine which they observed are due to the reducing capabilities of ascorbic acid, alkalizing the urinary pH and super hydration of the patient. In all the human trials, in addition to alkalization, urine was diluted by the increased intake of fluids. Hence, it is hard to distinguish the beneficial effects of ascorbic acid alone in treating cystinuria while super hydration and urinary alkalization have synergistic effects on cystine reduction. Apart from a significant increase in the urine volume with the AA, no other changes were observed in other physical characteristics. The plasma creatinine and urea values remained unaffected by the change in diet. Of particular interest in ascorbic acid therapy is the oxalate elimination in urine. Vitamin C was believed to increase oxalate excretion and may be a risk factor for calcium oxalate nephrolithiasis in individuals consuming "megadoses" of vitamin C. Oxalic acid is one of the chief metabolites of ascorbic acid (50% of total excretion of oxalate). Birwe et al. [14] report an increase in oxalic acid excretion with high intake of ascorbic acid. There have also been reports that excessive amounts of AA in the form of therapy can itself lead to the formation of oxalate stones. However, we did not observe this effect in our study. No oxalate stones were observed in the heterozygous or wild type males, which were fed with AA for the same duration as the homozygous males.

Recent findings by Evan *et al.* [20] show that cystine can crystallize in the lumens of ducts of Bellini, plug them and cause cell injury. This might lead to glomerular injury. However, in our study we could not find any significant albuminuria or proteinuria in homozygous mice compared to the heterozygous or wildtype mice (data not shown). Morphological histological studies of the mice are currently ongoing.

Effects of captopril supplemented diet on homozygous *pebbles*

Captopril, an angiotensin-converting enzyme inhibitor containing a sulfhydryl group was considered an alternative to penicillamine in view of the high side effects of the latter. In 1987, Sloand and Izzo [10] first reported a big reduction in the urinary cystine levels in two siblings treated with captopril for hypertension. Similar to D-penicillamine and α-mpg, captopril is a thiol compound containing a free sulfydryl group that can form a complex with cystine. The resultant captopril-cystine disulfide compound they believed to be 200 times more soluble than cystine alone. As per Sloand and Izzo, renal function remained stable during the duration of the therapy. Discontinuation of the drug led to the return of cystine excretion to the *baseline*, loss of renal function and proteinuria. The subjects were also encouraged to undertake vigorous hydration. The findings from Streem and Hall [11] also coincide with Sloand and Izzo in showing that captopril can at times reduce urinary cystine excretion along with the use of standard regimen of super-hydration and alkalization. In spite of a significant decrease in urinary cystine excretion, stone formation was noted in 4 out of 7 patients on captopril regimen. Since the study of Sloand and Izzo, there have been conflicting reports regarding the efficacy of captopril in decreasing urinary cystine. Dahlberg et al. [21] could not confirm the results of Sloand and Izzo, though they also used 150 mg of Captopril per day apart from alkalization and high fluid intake. Coulthard et al. [22] confirm the fact that when sufficient captopril is added *in vitro* to the urine of cystine patients a tendency toward reduction in the cystine levels was seen but it was not statistically significant. However this phenomenon was not observed in captopril treated patients. They also surmise that the amount of captopril administered would be insufficient to bind cystine in large amounts as cystinuric patients exhibit very large amounts of cystine.

Though Perazella and Buller [23] recommend captopril treatment for cystinuria, they also agree that the dramatic reduction in the amount of urinary cystine excretion cannot occur simply as the result of the formation of captopril-cysteine disulfide compound. Chow and Streem [24] used captopril when the patients reported intolerance to the thiol derivatives They conclude that D-penicillamine and α-mpg are effective in decreasing the stone formation rate on people in whom hydration and alkalization alone fails. While captopril may be beneficial in this setting it does not appear to be as effective as the above two thiols.

Captopril supplemented diet did not cause any significant changes in the metabolic pattern of the homozygous *pebbles* mice. Urinary cystine excretion was not reduced among homozygous *pebbles* mice fed with the CP, showing the inefficiency of captopril to reduce cystine when there is a high amount of cystine excretion. Captopril did not seem to be helpful in reducing the stone mass.

The urinary pH was not affected by the diet. Similarly water/food consumption and urine excretion remain unchanged with the diet. This study was aimed to establish the efficacy of captopril in cystinuria patients as a stand alone therapy. This is due to fact that a few reports indicate captopril as a stand alone therapy was effective in reducing the urinary cystine concentration. From this study it is evident that captopril is ineffective in reducing urinary cystine and it conforms to the view that captopril does not have enough cystine binding capacity to lower urinary cystine values.

CONCLUSION

In cystinuria high levels of motivation and compliance are necessary to drink large volumes of fluid spread throughout the day, every day for life. Effective cystine binding thiol drugs like D-penicillamine and α-mpg have high side effects. While medical management can effectively reduce the rate of stone formation, there is a lack of clear data as to which medical regimen is the most effective. Ascorbic acid treated animals showed a tendency to a lower stone mass though there was no reduction in the urinary cystine values. Further studies have to evaluate the effect of combination therapies. Captopril as an adjuvant therapy might not be helpful in palliating cystinuria.

REFERENCES

1. Knoll T, Zollner A, Wendt-Nordahl G, Michel MS, Alken P. Cystinuria in childhood and adolescence: recommendations for diagnosis, treatment, and follow-up. *Pediatr Nephrol* 2005; 20(1):19-24.
2. Assimos DG, Leslie SW, Ng C, Streem SB, Hart LJ. The impact of cystinuria on renal function. *J Urol* 2002; 168(1):27-30.
3. Mora C, Chillaron J, Calonge MJ, Forgo J, Testar X, Nunes V, Murer H, Zorzano A, Palacin M. The rBAT gene is responsible for L-cystine uptake via the b0,(+)-like amino acid transport system in a "renal proximal tubular" cell line (OK cells). *J Biol Chem* 1996; 271(18):10569-10576.
4. Dello SL, Pras E, Pontesilli C, Beccia E, Ricci-Barbini V, de Sanctis L, Ponzone A, Gallucci M, Bisceglia L, Zelante L, Jimenez-Vidal M, Font M, Zorzano A, Rousaud F, Nunes V, Gasparini P, Palacin M, Rizzoni G. Comparison between SLC3A1 and SLC7A9 cystinuria patients and carriers: a need for a new classification. *J Am Soc Nephrol* 2002; 13(10):2547-2553.
5. Palacin M, Fernandez E, Chillaron J, Zorzano A. The amino acid transport system b(o,+) and cystinuria. *Mol Membr Biol* 2001; 18(1):21-26.
6. Schmidt C, Vester U, Hesse A, Lahme S, Lang F, Zerres K, Eggermann T. The population-specific distribution and frequencies of genomic variants in the SLC3A1 and SLC7A9 genes and their application in molecular genetic testing of cystinuria. *Urol Res* 2004; 32(2):75-78.
7. Lotz M, Potts JT, Jr., Holland JM, Kiser WS, Bartter FC. D-penicillamine therapy in cystinuria. *J Urol* 1966; 95(2):257-263.
8. Harbar JA, Cusworth DC, Lawes LC, Wrong OM. Comparison of 2mercaptopropionylglycine and D-penicillamine in the treatment of cystinuria. *J Urol* 1986; 136(1):146-149.
9. Asper R, Schmucki O. [Cystinuria therapy by ascorbic acid (author's transl)]. *Urol Int* 1982; 37(2):91-109.
10. Sloand JA, Izzo JL, Jr. Captopril reduces urinary cystine excretion in cystinuria. *Arch Intern Med* 1987; 147(8):1409-1412.
11. Streem SB, Hall P. Effect of captopril on urinary cystine excretion in homozygous cystinuria. *J Urol* 1989; 142(6):1522-1524.
12. Peters T, Thaete C, Wolf S, Popp A, Sedlmeier R, Grosse J, Nehls MC, Russ A, Schlueter V. A mouse model for cystinuria type I. *Hum Mol Genet* 2003; 12(17):2109-2120.
13. Lux B, May P. Long-term observation of young cystinuric patients under ascorbic acid therapy. *Urol Int* 1983; 38(2):91-94.
14. Birwe H, Schneeberger W, Hesse A. Investigations of the efficacy of ascorbic acid therapy in cystinuria. *Urol Res* 1991; 19(3):199-201.
15. Soble JJ, Streem SB. Contemporary management of cystinuric patients. *Tech Urol* 1998; 4(2):58-64.
16. Ragone R. Medical treatment of cystinuria with vitamin C. *Am J Kidney Dis* 2000; 35(5):1020.
17. Stoller ML, McDonald MW, Gentle DL, Bruce J, Low RK. Acalculous cystinuria. *J Endourol* 1997; 11(4):233-238.
18. Ng CS, Streem SB. Contemporary management of cystinuria. *J Endourol* 1999; 13(9):647-651.
19. Hess B. Nutritional aspects of stone disease. *Endocrinol Metab Clin North Am* 2002; 31(4):1017-101x.

20. Evan AP, Coe FL, Lingeman JE et al. Renal crystal deposits and histopathology in patients with cystine stones. *Kidney International* (2006) 69, 2227-2235.
21. Dahlberg PJ, Jones JD. Cystinuria: failure of captopril to reduce cystine excretion. *Arch Intern Med* 1989; 149(3):713, 717.
22. Coulthard MG, Richardson J, Fleetwood A. The treatment of cystinuria with captopril. *Am J Kidney Dis* 1995; 25(4):661-662.
23. Perazella MA, Buller GK. Successful treatment of cystinuria with captopril. *Am J Kidney Dis* 1993; 21(5):504-507.
24. Chow GK, Streem SB. Medical treatment of cystinuria: results of contemporary clinical practice. *J Urol* 1996; 156(5):1576-1578.

Does Potassium Citrate Medical Therapy Increase the Risk of Calcium Phosphate Stone Formation?

Victor Leitao, George E Haleblian, Marnie R Robinson, Sean A Pierre, Roger L Sur and Glenn M Preminger

Duke University Medical Center – Division of Urology
Box 3167 Med Ctr, Durham, NC 27710

Abstract. Potassium citrate has been extensively used in the treatment of recurrent nephrolithiasis. Recent evidence suggests that it may contribute to increasing urinary pH and, as such, increase the risk of calcium phosphate stone formation. We performed a retrospective review of our patients to further investigate this phenomenon.

Keywords: Renal calculi, potassium citrate.
PACS: 87.19.Xx

INTRODUCTION

Potassium citrate therapy is a cornerstone in the medical management of urinary lithiasis. It has been demonstrated to increase urinary citrate concentration, as well as decrease ionic calcium concentration in the urine by complexing calcium and by direct inhibition of calcium oxalate stone formation. Citrate, being an alkali, also changes the biochemical characteristics of urine by increasing urinary pH. Some have suggested that this increase in urinary pH may lead to decreased calcium oxalate and uric acid stone formation but may in fact decrease the solubility product of calcium phosphate and consequently an iatrogenic increase in calcium phosphate (Ca Phos) nephrolithiasis may occur.

Our objective is to ascertain the incidence of calcium phosphate stones in our patient population and determine if a phase change in stone type has occurred after institution of potassium citrate therapy.

MATERIALS AND METHODS

A retrospective study of all patients undergoing stone analysis between 1/1/2004 and 1/1/2006 was performed. Institutional Review Board Committee approval was obtained.

One hundred and ten patients were identified, having 120 stones analyzed by spectroscopy at Mission Pharmacal (San Antonio, TX). Patients with a minimum of 2

CP900, *Renal Stone Disease, 1st Annual International Urolithiasis Research Symposium*, edited by A. P. Evan, J. E. Lingeman, and J. C. Williams, Jr.

stone analyses, two 24 hour urine evaluations, and who were on potassium citrate therapy were identified. Within this cohort a subset who demonstrated a change in percentage of calcium phosphate in their stones were identified and analyzed.

All 24 hour urinary metabolic profiles were also performed at Mission Pharmacal (San Antonio, TX).

RESULTS

Forty three stones containing a reportable percentage of calcium phosphate (Ca Phos) were identified in 33 patients. Of these, 7 patients had multiple stone analyses. All had 24 hour urinary metabolic profiles performed. Medical therapy for stone disease was instituted in 6 of the 7 patients. The remaining patient was diagnosed with hyperparathyroidism, treated surgically, and excluded from the review.

Review of patient demographics revealed five males and 1 female, with mean age of 49.8 years (range 37 to 56 years). Five patients had 2 stones analyzed and one had 5 stones submitted for analysis. All exhibited a phase change in stone composition after institution of medical therapy as outlined in table 1. All patients were taking potassium citrate (20-60 mEq daily), four were also taking chlorthalidone, and one was on allopurinol.

Three patients had a decrease in percentage of Ca Phos in the stone analyses (mean 53.3%) while other 3 had an increase in percentage of Ca Phos (mean 86.1%). Urinary pH values increased significantly in only 2 of the 4 patients that exhibited an increase in Ca Phos stone composition. In the 2 patients with decreased Ca Phos composition, urinary pH increased in one patient and decreased in the other.

Table 1: Stone composition and phase changes identified

Pt	Analysis Date	Ca Ox Mono	Ca Ox Di	Ca Phos	Other	pH
1	2/24/2004	40	30	30		6.2
1	11/4/2004	10	20	70		6.58
2	10/10/2004	70	10	20		6.05
2	5/30/2005	50	50	0		6.23
3	4/2/1996	20		80		N/A
3	6/22/1998	15		85		N/A
3	9/17/1999			100		7.14
3	5/19/2003			100		6.88
3	5/16/2005			100		6.96
4	7/1/2002		80	20		5.8
4	10/20/2004	50	10	40		6.1
5	2/7/2005			100		6.7
5	4/3/2005			80	20 (Struvite)	7.0
6	1/12/2004	30	20	50		7.4
6	7/6/2005	40	30	30		6.4

DISCUSSION

Approximately 15% of all kidney stone formers produce calculi that are composed predominantly of calcium phosphate.[1] A report of 1392 stone formers that had their stone compositions analyzed indicated that 38% of stones contained some phosphate [2]. Mandel and associates reported that recurrent stone formers tend to convert calcium oxalate (CaOx) stones to Ca Phos. This was more evident in patients with a higher frequency of stone recurrence, and associated with an increase in Ca Phos stone content as well as a decrease in the interval between episodes [3]. High urinary pH has been linked to an increased risk of Ca Phos stones [4]. $CaHPO_4$ precipitates are formed when the ion product for ionized calcium and divalent phosphate exceeds its solubility product and its ability to remain dissolved in a supersaturated solution; hence, a urine pH of 6.8 increases the potential risk for precipitation of $CaHPO_4$ by 3-fold when compared to a pH of 6.1 [4]. At a pH lower than 6.2 the solubility of calcium phosphate is greatly improved [5].

Citrate therapy has been known to decrease the risk of stone recurrence, by complexing calcium, as well as directly inhibiting crystallization [6-8]. It also causes a rise in urinary pH, with a daily dose of 60 mEq increasing urinary pH by 0.5 units [9]. Thus, initiation of medical therapy with potassium citrate could impart an increased risk of Ca Phos stone formation.

Our study demonstrates that after citrate therapy, the percentage of calcium phosphate in subsequent stones did not increase in all patients. Although there was an increase in pH in 5 patients, only 3 had an increase in their percentage of Ca Phos while the remaining two had a decrease in the percentage of Ca Phos in their stones. Only one patient showed a decrease in pH after potassium citrate, also decreasing the percentage of Ca Phos in their stones.

A recent paper regarding citrate administration and its therapeutic effects was evaluated in a computational program known as Joint Expert Speciation System (JESS). The findings suggested a decrease in the percentages of CaOx and brushite in the urine of patients on citrate therapy [10]. Conversely, an increase in urine pH is associated with an increased risk of formation of hydroxyapatite, octacalcium phosphate and tribasic calcium phosphate stones when studied with JESS. It has been reported that increases in pH are associated with potassium citrate therapy and therefore, the clinical correlation with these theoretical results should be revealing.

CONCLUSION

Our review has suggested that a phase change in urinary stone composition is a complex process. We have seen both increases and decreases in percentage of calcium phosphate in urinary stones and urinary pH in patients treated with potassium citrate therapy that are not necessarily concordant. Further investigations in the form of a collaborative, multi-center trial may help better understand this phenomenon.

REFERENCES

1. F. Coe and J. Parks. "Pathogenesis and treatment of nephrolithiasis." in The Kidney: Physiology & Pathophysiology: edited by D. W. Seldin,, Lippincott Williams & Wilkins, Philadelphia, 2000. pp. 1841-67.

2. C. Y. Pak, J. R. Poindexter, B. Adams-Huet, M. S. Pearle. Predictive value of kidney stone composition in the detection of metabolic abnormalities. Am J Med 115, 26-32 (2003).
3. N. Mandel, I. Mandel, K. Fryjoff, T. Rejniak, G. Mandel. Conversion of calcium oxalate to calcium phosphate with recurrent stone episodes. J Urol, 169, 2026-2029 (2003).
4. K. S. Kamel, M. A. Shafiee,S. Cheema-Dhadli, M. L. Halperin. Studies to identify the basis for an alkaline urine pH in patients with calcium hydrogen phosphate kidney stones. Nephrol Dial Transplant (2006) DOI 10.1093/ndt/gfl588
5. Hesse, A, Heimbach, D. Causes of phosphate stone formation and the importance of metaphylaxis by urinary acidification: A review. World J Urol 17, 308-315 (1999).
6. G. M. Preminger, K. Sakhaee, C. Y. Pak. Alkali action on the urinary crystallization of calcium salts: contrasting responses to sodium citrate and potassium citrate. J Urol 139, 240-242 (1988).
7. G. M. Preminger, K. Sakhaee, C. Skurla, C. Y. Pak. Prevention of recurrent calcium stone formation with potassium citrate therapy in patients with distal renal tubular acidosis. J Urol 134, 20-23 (1985).
8. C. Y. Pak. Citrate and renal calculi. Min Electr Metab 13, 257- 266 (1987).
9. C. Y. Pak. "Physicochemical action and extrarenal manifestations of alkali therapy" in. Proceedings of the Sixth International Symposium on Urolithiasis, edited by V. R. Walker, R. A. L. Sutton, E. C. Bert Cameron, C. Y. Pak, W. G. Robertson, Plenum Press, New York, 1989. pp. 511-516.
10. A. Rodgers, S. Allie-Hamdulay, G. Jackson. Therapeutic action of citrate in urolithiasis explained by chemical speciation: increase in pH is the determinant factor. Nephrol Dial Transplant 21, 361-369 (2006).

Author Index

A

B

C

D

E

F

G

H

J

K

V

W

Y

Z